WP 141 BRO

This book is due for return on or before the last date shown below.

5 JAN 2000

6 FEB 2000

Diagnostic Imaging
and Endoscopy
in Gynecology

Diagnostic Imaging and Endoscopy in Gynecology

A PRACTICAL GUIDE

Edited by

IVO BROSENS MD, PhD, FRCOG
Catholic University of Leuven
Leuven
Belgium

and

KEES WAMSTEKER MD, PhD
Spaarne Hospital
Haarlem
The Netherlands

WB SAUNDERS COMPANY LTD
London Philadelphia Toronto Sydney Tokyo

WB Saunders Company Ltd

24–28 Oval Road
London NW1 7DX, UK

The Curtis Center
Independence Square West
Philadelphia, PA 19106-3399, USA

Harcourt Brace & Company
55 Horner Avenue
Toronto, Ontario M8Z 4X6, Canada

Harcourt Brace & Company, Australia
30-52 Smidmore Street
Marrickville, NSW 2204, Australia

Harcourt Brace & Company, Japan
Ichibancho Central Building, 22-1 Ichibancho
Chiyoda-ku, Tokyo 102, Japan

A catalogue record for this book is available from the British Library

ISBN 0-7020-2105-9

Typeset by J&L Composition Ltd, Filey, North Yorkshire
Printed in Hong Kong by Dah Hua Printing Press Co. Ltd

Contents

PART 2 CLASSIFICATION OF PATHOLOGY

Contributors

MA Allon MD
Hutzel Hospital/Wayne State University
Department of Obstetrics and Gynecology
4707 St Antoine Boulevard
Detroit
Michigan
USA

AL Baert MD
Professor and Chairman
Department of Radiology
Universitaire Ziekenhuizen Leuven
Gasthuisberg
Herestraat 49
Leuven
Belgium

S de Blok MD PhD
Consultant Obstetrician/Gynecologist
Onze Lieve Vrouwe Gasthuis
Department of Obstetrics and Gynecology
PO Box 95500
Amsterdam
The Netherlands

I Brosens MD, PhD, FRCOG
Professor
Faculty of Medicine
Catholic University of Leuven
Leuven
Belgium

JJ Brosens MD, MRCOG
Research Fellow and Honorary Senior Registrar
Institute of Obstetrics and Gynaecology
Royal Postgraduate Medical School
Hammersmith Hospital
Du Cane Road
London
UK

S Campbell MBChB, FRCOG
Professor and Head
Department of Obstetrics and Gynaecology
St George's Hospital Medical School
Cranmer Terrace
London
UK

DM Chernoff MD, PhD
Clinical Instructor
Department of Radiology
University of California San Francisco
Box 0628
505 Parnassus Avenue
San Francisco
California
USA

L Cohen MD
Assistant Professor
Department of Obstetrics and Gynecology
Prentice Women's Hospital and Maternity
Center
Northwestern University Medical School
333 East Superior Street, #490
Chicago
Illinois
USA

ID Cooke FRCOG
Professor and Academic Head
Department of Obstetrics and Gynaecology
The University of Sheffield
Jessop Hospital for Women
Leavygreave Road
Sheffield
UK

M Cosson MD
Gynecologist
Centre Hospitalier de Roubaix
Pavillon Paul Gellé
91 avenue Julien Lagache
Roubaix
France

J Decocq MD
Gynecologist
Centre Hospitalier de Roubaix
Pavillon Paul Gellé
91 avenue Julien Lagache
Roubaix
France

J Deprest MD
Department of Obstetrics and Gynecology
University Hospital Gasthuisberg
Herestraat 49
Leuven
Belgium

MP Diamond MD
Professor of Obstetrics and Gynecology
Director, Division of Reproductive
Endocrinology and Infertility
Hutzel Hospital/Wayne State University
Detroit Medical Center
4707 St Antoine Boulevard
Detroit
Michigan
USA

L Dukel MD
Consultant
Department of Obstetrics and Gynecology
University Hospital Rotterdam `Dijkzigt'
Dr Molewaterplein 40
Rotterdam
The Netherlands

MH Emanuel MD
Consultant
Department of Obstetrics and Gynaecology
Spaarne Ziekenhuis Haarlem
van Heythuizenweg 1
Haarlem
The Netherlands

LTGM Geerts MD
Consultant/Head of Ultrasound Unit
Department of Obstetrics and Gynecology
Faculty of Medicine
University of Stellenbosch
PO Box 19063
Tygerberg
South Africa

N Gleicher MD
Professor of Obstetrics and Gynecology
Professor of Immunology/Microbiology
The Center for Human Reproduction
750 New Orleans Street
Chicago
Illinois
USA

S Gryspeerdt MD
Department of Radiology
Universitaire Ziekenhuizen Leuven
Gasthuisberg
Herestraat 49
Leuven
Belgium

H Hricak MD, PhD
Professor of Radiology, Urology and
Radiation Oncology, Obstetrics, Gynecology
and Reproductive Sciences
Chief, Abdominal Imaging Section
Department of Radiology
University of California San Francisco
Box 0628
505 Parnassus Avenue
San Francisco
California
USA

DA Johns MD
Director of GYN Laparoscopy Center
Harris Methodist Hospital
Fort Worth
Texas
USA

VC Karande MD
Director, Division of GynecoRadiology
The Center for Human Reproduction
750 New Orleans Street
Chicago
Illinois
USA

L Keith MD
Professor
Department of Obstetrics and Gynecology
Prentice Women's Hospital and Maternity
Center
Northwestern University Medical School
333 East Superior Street, #464
Chicago
Illinois
USA

A Kolbenstvedt MD, PhD
Professor
Department of Radiology
Rikshospitalet
University of Oslo
Pilestredet 32
Oslo
Norway

CL Kowalczyk MD
Assistant Professor
Department of Obstetrics and Gynecology
Division of Reproductive Endocrinology and
Infertility
Wayne State University
4707 St Antoine
Detroit
Michigan
USA

S Kupešić MD, PhD
Head, Ultrasonic Institute
Department of Obstetrics and Gynecology
Medical School University of Zagreb
Sveti Duh Hospital
Zagreb
Croatia

A Kurjak MD, PhD
Professor, Head of Department of Obstetrics
and Gynecology
Medical School University of Zagreb
Zagreb
Croatia

B Lunenfeld MD, FRCOG, FACOG (Hon)
Professor
Department of Life Sciences
Bar-Ilan University
Ramat Gan
Israel

E Lunenfeld MD
Senior Lecturer
Fertility and IVF Unit
Department of Obstetrics and Gynecology
Soroka Medical Center
Beer-Sheba
Israel

HJ Odendaal MBChB, MD, FRCOG
Professor and Head, Department of Obstetrics
and Gynaecology
Faculty of Medicine
University of Stellenbosch
PO Box 19063
Tygerberg
South Africa

D Querleu MD
Professor
Chirurgie Gynecologique
Hôpital Jeanne de Flandre
CHRU
59037 Lille
France

S Reddy MD
Department of Obstetrics and Gynecology
Emory University
The School of Medicine
69 Butler Street, SE
Atlanta
Georgia
USA

K Reese MD
Women's Health Center
121 Wakelee Avenue
Ansonia
Connecticut
USA

J Rock MD
Professor and Chairman
Department of Obstetrics and Gynecology
Emory University
The School of Medicine
69 Butler Street, SE
Atlanta
Georgia
USA

JJ Sciarra MD, PhD
Thomas J Watkins Professor and Chairman
Department of Obstetrics and Gynecology
Prentice Women's Hospital and Maternity
Center
Northwestern University Medical School
333 East Superior Street, #490
Chicago
Illinois
USA

IW Scudamore MRACOG, MRCOG
Clinical Lecturer
Department of Obstetrics and Gynaecology
The University of Sheffield
Jessop Hospital for Women
Leavygreave Road
Sheffield
UK

AM Siegler MD DSc
Professor of Obstetrics and Gynecology
Department of Obstetrics and Gynecology
State University of New York
Health Science Center at Brooklyn
450 Clarkson Avenue
Brooklyn
New York
USA

N de Souza BSc, MBBS, FRCR
Senior Lecturer
The Robert Steiner Magnetic Resonance
Unit
Royal Postgraduate Medical School
Hammersmith Hospital
Du Cane Road
London
UK

SL Stanton FRCS, FRCOG
Consultant Urogynaecologist
St George's Hospital Medical School
Urogynaecology Unit, Department of
Obstetrics and Gynaecology
Lanesborough Wing
Cranmer Terrace
London
UK

**SL Tan MBBS, MD, FRCOG, FRCS(C),
MMed(O&G)**
James Edmund Dodds Professor and
Chairman, Department of Obstetrics and
Gynecology
McGill University
Obstetrician and Gynecologist-in-Chief
Royal Victoria Hospital
687 Pine Avenue West
Montreal
Quebec
Canada

D Timmerman MD
Consultant
Department of Obstetrics and Gynecology
Universitaire Ziekenhuizen Leuven
Gasthuisberg
Herestraat 49
Leuven
Belgium

MC Treadwell MD
Assistant Professor
Division of Maternal–Fetal Medicine
Department of Obstetrics and Gynecology
Hutzel Hospital/Wayne State University
4707 St Antoine Boulevard
Detroit
Michigan
USA

L Van Hoe MD
Department of Radiology
Universitaire Ziekenhuizen Leuven
Gasthuisberg
Herestraat 49
Leuven
Belgium

I Vergote MD, PhD
Professor
Gynaecologische Oncologie
Universitaire Ziekenhuizen Leuven
Gasthuisberg
Herestraat 49
Leuven
Belgium

K Wamsteker MD, PhD
Director
Hysteroscopy Training Centre
Department of Obstetrics and Gynecology
Spaarne Hospital
Haarlem
The Netherlands

JW Wladimiroff MD, PhD
Professor
Department of Obstetrics and Gynecology
University Hospital Rotterdam 'Dijkzigt'
Dr Molewaterplein 40
Rotterdam
The Netherlands

J Zaidi MBBS, MRCOG
Senior Registrar
Department of Obstetrics and Gynaecology
The John Radcliffe Hospital
Headley Way
Headington
Oxford
UK

D Zudenigo MD, MSc
Resident
Department of Obstetrics and Gynecology
Medical School University of Zagreb
Sveti Duh Hospital
Zagreb
Croatia

Foreword

The development of imaging and endoscopic techniques over the past few decades has presented gynecologists with a vast array of new tools in diagnostics and therapeutics. Most texts on the subject deal with one technique or another and its applications. There is a need in the field for a textbook that puts all these techniques, imaging and endoscopic, together and discusses their potential application and relative merits in the context of clinical situations faced by the practicing gynecologist. This is what this book, edited by Dr Brosens and Dr Wamsteker, has achieved.

Diagnostic imaging and endoscopy are rapidly advancing fields. The editors should be complimented for assembling 45 knowledgeable experts from 10 countries to cover the various topics.

For gynecologists and their patients, new technology can be a friend, but it can also be a foe. It is a friend when it improves diagnostic ability and allows the use of non-invasive or minimally invasive procedures instead of less convenient and less safe invasive procedures. The new technology can be a foe when it is abused, when its introduction is not evidence-based, when it adds to the cost of medical management without demonstrable additional therapeutic benefits, and, last but not least, when it is put in inexperienced hands.

People have a right to the fruits of science, and practicing physicians are keen that their patients should get the best of what science can offer. We need, however, to keep in mind that there is always an *opportunity cost*. If resources are used in one way, an opportunity to provide some other benefit has to be renounced. Possible alternative uses of resources should always be considered. The individualistic ethic of medicine should take into consideration the social ethic of economics.

This book provides a well-balanced overview of the various imaging and endoscopic procedures. It deals in separate sections with techniques that are established and techniques that are still in the development stage. It provides separate sections on normal appearances, essential to avoid false positive diagnoses and unnecessary treatments. It also emphasizes limitations, potential complications and side effects of the various procedures.

Current and emerging imaging and endoscopic techniques will need continued evaluation to assess their appropriate place and usefulness in various clinical situations. For this international effort to be productive, gynecologists need to adopt standardized classifications to describe their findings and to present their results. The International Federation of Gynecology and Obstetrics (FIGO) encourages the development of these definitions and classifications through its Study Group on Definitions and the work of its various committees, including Gynecological Oncology. However, it is not enough to develop classifications. They have to be accepted and used. It was appropriate that the editors devoted the last chapter in their book to highlight this need.

I hope that this practical guide will help gynecologists in selecting and using the appropriate technologies for their practices, for the clinical conditions they face and for the patients they treat.

Professor Mahmoud F. Fathalla
President, FIGO
Professor of Obstetrics and Gynecology, Assiut
University, Egypt

Acknowledgements

Among the many people we wish to thank for their valuable contribution to this book, we especially would like to extend our gratitude towards, first of all, our families for the time we have invested in the project rather than spent with them, Marie-Rose Puttemans, secretary, Corry Stappers-de Kuijer, HTC staff, Dr Noël Eastham, pathologist, the publisher Margaret Macdonald for bringing us together and designing the project, and the production staff of WB Saunders. Last, but not least, we wish to thank all the authors for their excellent contributions.

IB and KW

Notice

Diagnostic Imaging and Endoscopy in Gynecology is an ever-changing field. Standard safety precautions must be followed, but as new research and clinical experience broaden our knowledge, changes in treatment and drug therapy become necessary or appropriate. Readers are advised to check the product information currently provided by the manufacturer of each drug to be administered to verify the recommended dose, the method and duration of administration, and contraindications. Some of the procedures described in this Work may require specialized training and experience.

It is the responsibility of the treating physician relying on experience, appropriate clinical training and knowledge of the patient to perform these procedures in the intended manner, and to determine drug dosages and the best treatment for the patient. Neither the Publisher nor the editors assume any responsibility for any injury and/or damage to persons or property.

The Publisher

1 *Introduction*
I Brosens and K Wamsteker

Among the many books on gynecological imaging and endoscopic techniques, *Diagnostic Imaging and Endoscopy in Gynecology: A Practical Guide* aims to provide the gynecologist with a comprehensive, practical guide that helps with choosing and applying the most appropriate diagnostic techniques in clinical practice. Since this practice has changed so much over the last few decades through the introduction and evolution of new imaging and endoscopic techniques, the established gynecologist and the resident/trainee are faced with the problem of rational use of these techniques. Although the scope of the instrumentation is impressive, it does have limitations. Therefore its rational and efficient use is of paramount importance. Furthermore, since the new techniques can be expensive and may carry a risk to the patient, they should be used only to benefit the patient and on economically justified grounds.

With the increasing use of combined diagnostic and operative procedures in endoscopy, the risk exists of under-treatment as well as over-treatment. The decision to operate or not should be based on the accurate diagnosis and proper assessment of the extent of the pathology. As editors, we invited leading gynecologists to describe the pathology of major disease entities in relation to their associated symptoms and signs, and to discuss the investigational methods which are most appropriate for visualization and diagnosis of the related pathology. This can be cross-referred to the first section of the book where special attention has been given to a description of the standard techniques and to illustration of normal appearances and their variances.

Although the diagnosis of pathology of the lower genital tract, including cervical dysplasia and malignancy, has for obvious reasons not been included, the official International Federation of Gynecology and Obstetrics (FIGO) staging for cervical cancer has been added to the chapter on classifications as the imaging techniques in some chapters refer to this staging.

For quick reference, the correlation between disease entity and diagnostic techniques is summarized in the penultimate chapter.

Throughout, the authors have followed a template to make the book easy to consult. However, the editors retained diversity of presentation and opinion where this seemed justifiable. The editors have also tried to ensure that the quality of illustrations and the readability of the text are uniformly of the highest possible standard.

Section One: Explorative Techniques

PART 1
STANDARD TECHNIQUES
AND NORMAL APPEARANCES

2 *Ultrasonography*
L Dukel and JW Wladimiroff

■ INTRODUCTION

Ultrasonography of the female genital organs and related structures within the pelvis has become an important diagnostic procedure in gynecological practice, especially since the development of the technique of transvaginal sonography (TVS). The traditional technique of transabdominal sonography (TAS) cannot, however, be abandoned because it can provide vital extra information that would be missed when TVS alone is performed under conditions described later in this chapter. The easy interpretation of the clear images produced by TVS has led to widespread use of this technique in gynecological practice and TVS is even advocated as a routine office procedure complementary to each bimanual pelvic examination in order to improve diagnostic accuracy (Timor-Tritsch, 1990; Carter et al, 1994). In TVS, with its excellent resolution despite high degrees of magnification, we must not overreact to normal physiological conditions that escaped detection in the past because they were not previously imaged (Goldstein, 1990). In this chapter we will describe the necessary instrumentation, the different scanning techniques with their specific advantages and limitations and the sonographic appearances of uterus, ovary and other adnexal and pelvic structures, with emphasis on real time TVS examination.

■ EQUIPMENT

When ultrasound travels through the tissue its intensity and amplitude become reduced (attenuated), resulting in much weaker echoes from deeper structures. This attenuation is caused by reflection, absorption, scattering and refraction. With increased frequency there is more absorption (conversion of sound into heat), resulting in more attenuation. The practical penetration of ultrasound into the tissue is therefore less at higher frequencies. In considering the imaging quality of ultrasound equipment, this is important because another characteristic, the resolution, is also related to the frequency of the ultrasound. Resolution, in particular, affects the detail of the display. Axial resolution is the ability to identify and separate reflecting structures that are positioned in the direction of the sound beam. The smaller the distance between reflecting structures that can be visualized, the higher the resolution. The shorter the spatial pulse length, the less overlap will occur between the reflected pulses. This results in better axial resolution. As spatial pulse length decreases with increased frequency, axial resolution will increase with increased frequency, this at the cost of reduced sound penetration. Lateral resolution is the ability of the system to display separately reflectors in a plane perpendicular to the direction of the transmitted sound beam. Lateral resolution is less affected by frequency, it is merely dependent on the diameter of the sound beam. The smaller the beam, the better the lateral resolution. Beam diameter is to some extent determined by the frequency (higher frequency reduces beam diameter), but is mainly reduced by focusing.

These frequency-related characteristics are important factors to consider when choosing the kind of transducer suited to the distance of the objects to be visualized. The pelvis is filled with many structures of almost similar acoustic impedance and therefore detailed ultrasound imaging is difficult to achieve. In TAS the distance to the organs is relatively large: deeper penetration requires low attenuation and therefore the use of lower frequencies, giving rise to lower resolution. The frequencies used for TAS vary between 3.5 and 5.0 MHz. In TVS the transducer can be placed much closer to the organs to be visualized and, as most of the relevant anatomical structures are within 9 cm of the vaginal fornices, it is possible to increase the frequency up to 7.5 MHz, while

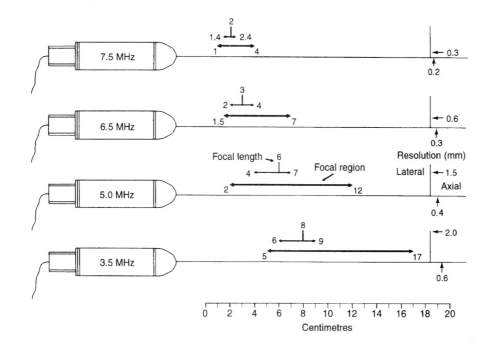

Figure 2.1: Physical properties (axial and lateral resolution, focal length and focal region) of transducers with different emission frequencies. From Schats (1991) with permission of the author.

attenuation is still acceptable. This improves resolution, as illustrated in *Figure 2.1*. Another important advantage is the ability to magnify the image, only at the cost of somewhat decreased resolution.

For TVS, in particular, the field of view or sector angle is very important for interpretation of the image. Wider fields of view provide a better panorama of the pelvis, and sector angles less than 90° must be avoided. End-firing vaginal probes with the beam projected from the center of the transducer tip make proper orientation to pelvic anatomy much easier than angulated firing probes with asymmetrical beams. Some manufacturers provide probes that can steer the field of view as well as the scanning plane. When considering the shape of the transducer probe, it is important that the design allows transvaginal ultrasound guided aspiration and biopsy.

■ TECHNIQUE

A prerequisite for reliable transabdominal pelvic ultrasound is a filled urinary bladder. It provides an acoustic window that actually enhances transmission of the sound beam. As the bladder fills it also pushes loops of bowel cephalad, making interpretation of images much easier because of the absence of the bizarre reflections of fecal matter and gas. Another method of helping to displace

loops of bowel is to place the patient in a slight Trendelenburg position. The distended bladder may cause the patient discomfort, which makes meticulous timing of the examination essential. In transducer selection, the distance to the structures being imaged will determine the frequency, and as TAS requires deeper penetration, generally 3.5 to 5.0 MHz transducers are used, limiting resolution.

Anatomical planes employed to identify images in TAS include the traditional coronal, sagittal (or longitudinal) and transverse planes (Dodson and Deter, 1990). Conventionally, longitudinal images are displayed with the patient's head to the left side of the screen, and transverse images are shown as if the examiner is conducting a pelvic examination, the right side of the screen corresponding with the patient's left side. This orientation corresponds with radiological imaging. In performing ultrasound imaging, sonologists often angle the transducer obliquely, thus aiming to create images containing the most information regardless of orientation. This 'anatomy-derived' orientation is developed in greater detail for TVS as described later in this chapter (Zimmer et al, 1991).

Since TVS is characterized by the very close proximity of the transducer tip to the structures to be imaged, the urinary bladder has to be empty to prevent compression or displacement of these structures and to keep the

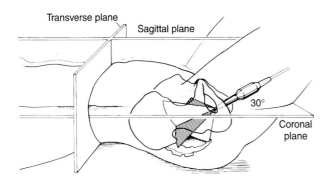

*Figure 2.2: Conventional anatomical planes used to identify images in transabdominal sonography. From Dodson MG & Deter RL (1990). Definition of anatomical planes for use in transvaginal sonography. J Clin Ultrasound **18**: 239–242. Copyright © 1990 John Wiley & Sons Inc. Reprinted with permission of John Wiley & Sons, Inc.*

organs within the focal zone of the transducer. For the examination the lithotomy position enables sufficient manipulation of the probe and a slight reversed Trendelenburg tilt allows any free peritoneal fluid to collect in the pelvic cavity, which aids in imaging fine structures. Because less penetration of the ultrasound is required, high frequency probes up to 7.5 MHz can be used, resulting in high resolution imaging.

In order to bring the transducer as close as possible to the organs under study and to bring them within the focal zone, different manipulations can be performed – for example, pushing and pulling, rotating and tilting the probe at various angles. As in a bimanual examination, the examiner's free hand can be placed on the lower abdomen to shift the pelvic organs toward the tip of the probe. In cases of pelvic pain this 'dynamic use of the probe' also includes the localization of the point of maximal intensity of the pain by gentle touching under direct vision with the tip of the probe. To diagnose pelvic adhesions the different organs can be displaced by pushing and pulling the transducer, while at the same time examining their sliding movements in relation to each other and the pelvic wall ('sliding organ sign') (Timor-Tritsch, 1992). Palpable findings can be made instantly visible by introducing the probe along one finger in the vagina, directing it to the finding in question (Zimmer et al, 1991). If a discrepancy exists between the ultrasound image and the expected diagnosis, or when there is doubt about the scanning results, a pelvic examination

must be performed.

Since the effective focal zone of a 7.5 MHz transducer ends at 4 cm, structures deeper than 4 cm may be missed. Even a fairly large mass may be undiagnosed by TVS if, because of its size, it does not extend far enough into the pelvis. The conclusion is that, whenever a pelvic mass has to be ruled out or is suspected, a 5.0 MHz transvaginal probe could be used and a transabdominal scan must also be performed.

TVS is an endocavitary dynamic scanning technique and therefore the planes of the images obtained by TVS do not generally correspond to the conventional anatomical and radiological planes described for TAS (*Figure 2.2*). The transducer is inserted into the vagina, which runs superiorly and posteriorly, and the pelvis itself is tilted at an angle of 30° to the long axis of the body. In addition, the vagina itself limits the freedom of movement of the transducer, and thus most images are in a plane oblique to the anatomical planes. Dodson and Deter (1990) suggested the terminology of transpelvic plane and AP-pelvic plane. Transpelvic plane images are obtained in planes at different angles above and below the coronal plane when the sound beam is directed across or from side to side in the pelvis (*Figure 2.3a*). AP-pelvic plane images are obtained when the sound beam is directed in an anteroposterior direction in the pelvis (*Figure 2.3b*). Targeted organ scanning without resorting to planes is a different approach to orientation (Rottem et al, 1990a). The main reason for using this 'organ-oriented' scanning is the very short distance to the organs, resulting in close-up images encompassing only a single organ, or even a part of it. Another important reason for this successful concept is the dynamic use of the probe, which includes its rotation and the continual changing of angles between probe and organs. Using this technique the examiner searches for each specific organ as the main target, and it can be considered as a modified bimanual examination providing detailed visual rather than tactile information.

Most sonographers, especially in the United States, display the apex of the sector wedge at the top of the screen. In Europe several centers prefer to display the image turned round, with the apex at the bottom of the screen. A 90° shift of the apex to the right side of the

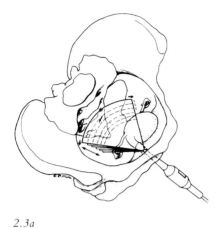

2.3a

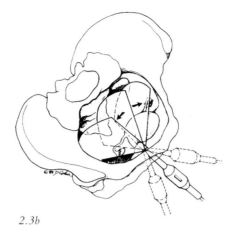

2.3b

Figure 2.3: (a) Transpelvic plane images are obtained when the sound beam is directed from side to side across the pelvis. (b) AP-pelvic plane images are obtained when the sound beam is directed anteroposteriorly in the pelvis. From Dodson MG & Deter RL (1990) Definition of anatomical planes for use in transvaginal sonography. J Clin Ultrasound **18**: 239–242. *Copyright ©1990 John Wiley & Sons Inc. Reprinted by permission of John Wiley & Sons, Inc.*

screen would correlate best with the anatomical situation when the patient is in the supine position, but this display format is not an option on currently available ultrasound machines. Awareness of the differences prevents confusion, but as long as standardization of image display does not exist, it is of utmost importance to label each image taken.

In addition to scanning procedures alone, TVS can be used for interventional purposes like aspiration of ova for in vitro fertilization, aspiration of ovarian cysts and aspiration and drainage of pelvic fluid collections.

Distension of the uterine cavity by instilling a solution imposes sonographic contrast and provides sonographic delineation of uterine contents (*Figure 2.4*). This so-called sonohysterography of the uterine cavity is a method of assisting in the diagnosis of abnormal endometrial echoes that cannot be adequately evaluated by conventional TVS. Excellent discrimination between intracavitary, intramural and diffuse processes can be obtained (Parson and Lense, 1993). A flexible catheter is used – one that is sufficiently long to enter the uterine cavity and of sufficiently small diameter to pass through the cervix without dilatation. Only when a patulous cervix or an enlarged uterus is present is the use of a catheter with a 2 ml cervical balloon advised to maintain adequate pressure to expand the uterine cavity. Isotonic media like normal saline solution or lactated Ringer's solution are instilled at a slow rate to prevent patient discomfort (5–10 ml/min as a function of uterine size and amount of backflow). Gaucherand et al (1995) described a total volume of 5–30 ml of normal saline to provide high quality imaging without provoking pain.

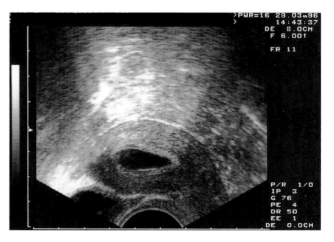

2.4a

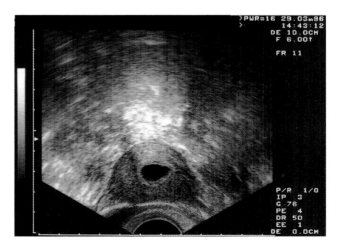

2.4b

Figure 2.4: (a) AP-pelvic plane sonohysterography of an expanded normal uterine cavity with very sharp delineation of the endometrial surface. (b) Transpelvic plane of the same cavity.

▪ LIMITATIONS

TVS characterizes a lesion better than its transabdominal counterpart but penetration is limited because of higher frequency, and the field of view is generally smaller. Lesions outside the relatively short range of the intravaginal probe may be missed if the transabdominal scan is omitted. Transducers with a lower frequency can be used but at the cost of lower resolution. In elderly patients the vagina has less elasticity, limiting maneuverability of the probe; in these patients it is also difficult to localize the ovaries because they are small, without follicles, and there is less pelvic fluid to provide an acoustic interface. An enlarged uterus caused by fibroids sometimes pushes other structures outside the focal range of the transducer, and rigid bulky fibroids limit the maneuverability of the probe. Prepubertal patients and those who are virgins are not suitable candidates for TVS, and patients with acute pelvic pain may not tolerate this examination.

▪ ANATOMY AND NORMAL APPEARANCES

CERVIX

The uterine cervix is best visualized with the endovaginal probe at a distance of 2–3 cm from it in the longitudinal plane. The cervical size varies considerably, and in relation to overall uterine dimensions. In the prepubertal situation the cervix is proportionally large, occupying up to one half of the uterus. As the uterine corpus enlarges more than the cervix at puberty, the cervix occupies about one third of the uterus in the adult woman. The endocervical canal is easy to locate as a continuation of the endometrium. Its appearance depends on the amount and quality of the cervical mucus and may vary between a thin echogenic interface, when the mucus has a low fluid content (*Figure 2.5*), and a very prominent hypoechoic stripe, especially in the preovulatory period (*Figure 2.6*). Nabothian cysts are frequently visualized adjacent to the external cervical os and appear as thin-walled anechoic round structures. Dilated endocervical cysts may be seen beside the cervical canal (*Figure 2.7*).

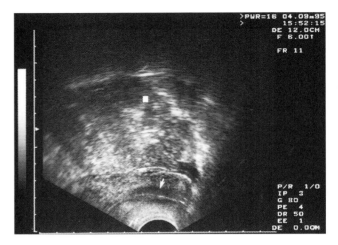

Figure 2.5: Longitudinal view of the normal lower uterus and cervix; the cervical canal shows as a thin echogenic interface (arrow).

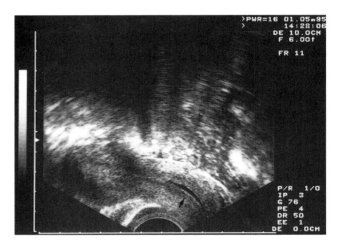

Figure 2.6: Mucus in the cervical canal shows as a prominent hypoechoic stripe (arrow).

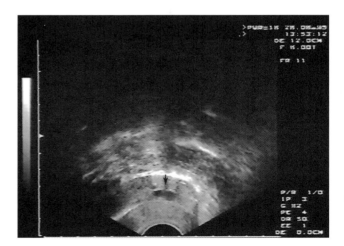

Figure 2.7: Dilated endocervical cysts adjacent to the cervical canal (arrow).

UTERUS

The uterus provides the pear-shaped, central landmark of the female pelvis in TVS pelvic ultrasound examinations (*Figure 2.8*). It is composed mainly of muscle and returns low level echoes, somewhat more than those from the pelvic muscles. The body and fundus may lie to one side of the midline, but the cervix is almost always situated in the midline. The normal size of the uterus depends on the parity and the age of the woman. In nulliparous, postpubertal women the size is approximately 7 cm in the longitudinal dimension and 3–4 cm in anteroposterior and transverse dimensions. In the postmenopausal woman the uterus decreases in size to approximately 5 cm longitudinally. After pregnancy there is a permanent increase in length of about 1 cm (*Figure 2.9*). Merz et al (1996) measured a statistically significant difference in overall uterine length between groups of nulliparous (7.3 cm ± 0.8 SD), primiparous (8.3 cm ± 0.8 SD) and multiparous (9.2 cm ± 0.8 SD) women.

Three zones can be detected in the myometrium. The inner layer is more hypoechoic, which has been attributed to the more vascular, deepest layer of the myometrium. It appears as a hypoechoic halo surrounding the more echogenic endometrium. The thicker and more echogenic middle layer of the myometrium is separated from the outer layer by the arcuate plexus of blood vessels (*Figure 2.10*). Subendometrial contractions can be observed with both TAS and TVS. The peak frequency is approximately three contractions per minute at the time of ovulation, at which time contractions propagate toward the fundus; during menses these contractions propagate in the opposite direction, toward the cervix (Lyons et al, 1991).

Ingoing and outgoing blood vessels can be detected lateral to the uterine margin on either side, and are most prominent at the level of the internal cervical os (*Figure 2.11*). When large pelvic varices are present at the uterine margin it is sometimes difficult not to confuse them with pelvic disease processes.

The endometrium appears as an echogenic interface in the central uterus and can be depicted by TVS in great detail. It varies in echogenicity and thickness, depending on menstrual phase, age and hormonal replacement

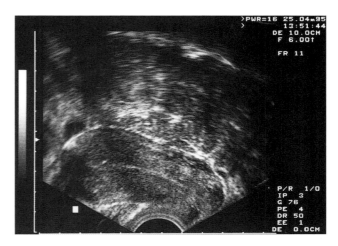

2.8a

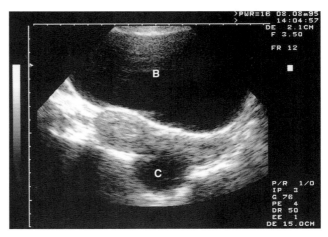

2.8b

Figure 2.8: *Long axis scan of a normal uterus by (a) transvaginal sonography and (b) transabdominal sonography. B, Bladder; C, cyst behind the uterus.*

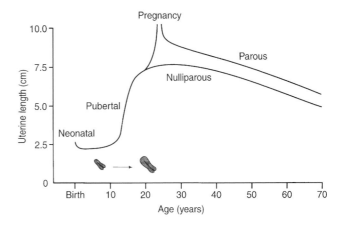

Figure 2.9: *Age changes in the uterus. The length of the uterus is plotted in relation to the changes with age and functional status. From Cosgrove DO (1993) Pelvic anatomy. In Dewbury K et al (eds) Ultrasound in Obstetrics and Gynecology, 1st edn, p 20. Reproduced with permission of the publisher, Churchill Livingstone, Edinburgh.*

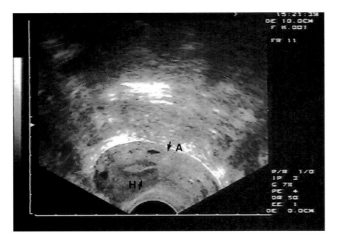

2.10a

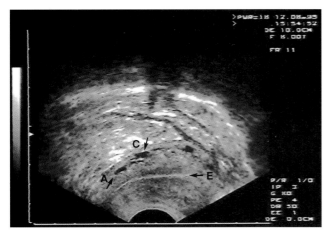

2.10b

Figure 2.10: *(a) The three zones of the myometrium: the halo (H) surrounding the endometrium; the more echogenic middle and outer layers separated by the arcuate plexus (A) of vessels. (b) Postmenopausal uterus with a very thin endometrium (E). Note also the calcifications (C) in the prominent vessels of the arcuate plexus (A).*

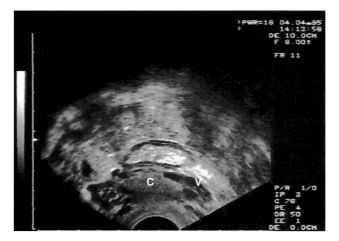

Figure 2.11: *Transpelvic plane image of the region of the internal cervical os (C) with ingoing and outgoing vessels (V).*

therapy. Endometrial thickness measurements should include both layers without the previously described hypoechoic halo that surrounds the endometrium.

As a result of the influence of the amount of circulating estrogen and progesterone during the menstrual cycle, changes in thickness and texture of the endometrium are seen (*Figure 2.12*). During menstruation the endometrium appears as a thin and interrupted echogenic interface; sloughing tissue and hypoechoic structures related to extravasated blood are visualized within the uterine cavity. In the proliferative phase the endometrium thickens (range 4–8 mm) and appears isoechoic to the myometrium. In the periovulatory period the endometrium becomes multilayered: a more echogenic layer surrounds the more hypoechogenic inner endometrium, which represents edema of the compactum layer ('double hairpin sign'). During the secretory phase the endometrium is thickest (range 7–14 mm) and most echogenic because of the mucus and stored glycogen in the tortuous glands. Cyclic changes of the endometrium may aid in the monitoring of infertile patients (Fleischer et al, 1984). In cases of dysfunctional bleeding the appearance of the endometrium may guide the physician to the desired treatment. A thick echogenic endometrium may indicate the use of progesterone; a very thin endometrium may indicate the need for combined estrogen and progesterone treatment (Lewit et al, 1990).

Variations in the anatomy of the endometrial interfaces are present in women who have Müllerian duct fusion abnormalities of the uterus and are best examined in the secretory phase of the menstrual cycle. A bicornuate uterus can easily be diagnosed if two separate echogenic lumina are present. Endometrial contour defects are best examined in the proliferative phase because the hypoechoic endometrium contrasts best against echogenic structures like polyps.

After the menopause the endometrium becomes inactive and thin. In asymptomatic postmenopausal women no consensus exists as to how normal endometria should be differentiated from abnormal: cut off levels for the upper limit of normal vary between 5 and 10 mm (Granberg, 1994; Shipley et al, 1994). In the largest study of endometrial thickness in symptomatic postmenopausal women (the Nordic trial), a cut off level of

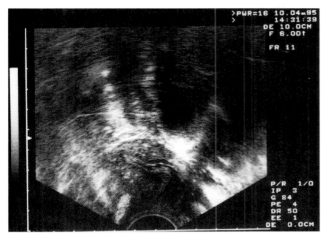

2.12a

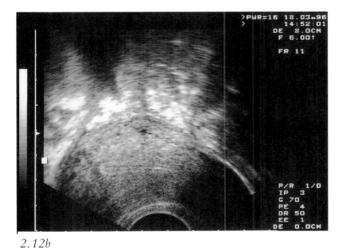

2.12b

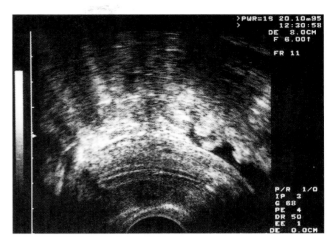

2.12c

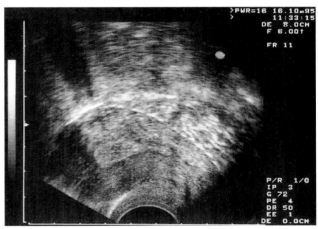

2.12d

Figure 2.12: *Endometrial variation during the menstrual cycle. (a) Sludging of the endometrium during menstruation. (b) Proliferative phase. (c) Multilayered appearance of the preovulatory phase. (d) Secretory phase.*

≤ 4 mm for detecting endometrial abnormality (polyps, hyperplasia or cancer) had a sensitivity of 96.0% and a specificity of 68.0% (Karlsson et al, 1995). The conclusion from this study, using curettage as the gold standard for evaluation of endometrial pathology, is that it would seem justified to refrain from dilatation and curettage in women with postmenopausal bleeding and an endometrial thickness of ≤ 4 mm. Although there is no agreement on this point in the literature (Conoscenti et al, 1995), the false negative rate of the order of 5% for an endometrial scan must be compared with the false negative rates after dilatation and curettage, reported to be 2–6% (Granberg, 1994). It is now clear that hysteroscopy with biopsy is superior to curettage for evaluating endometrial pathology. Emanuel et al (1995) conclude, in a prospective study comparing TVS and diagnostic hysteroscopy, that TVS could be implemented as a routine first-step technique in the evaluation of patients with abnormal uterine bleeding, and that a further diagnostic procedure, preferably hysteroscopy with hystological examination, is indicated in the case of an abnormal or inconclusive sonogram. When complaints persist after a normal sonogram, with or without treatment, a further diagnostic procedure with histological examination should be performed.

A nonmeasurable endometrium can be caused by a very thin endometrium, but also by endometrial cancer with the same echogenicity as the myometrium. To exclude endometrial abnormalities in cases of nonmeasurable endometria (as high as 30%), it is very important to perform further invasive biopsy procedures (Karlsson et al, 1995).

OVARIES

In the premenopausal, nulliparous female the ovaries are usually situated in the ovarian fossa (Waldeyer's fossa), which is on the lateral pelvic wall between the external iliac veins, the internal iliac artery and the obliterated umbilical artery. The ovaries are traced by scanning in the AP plane and transpelvic plane, starting alongside the uterus toward the pelvic side wall; they are often found in close proximity to the pelvic vessels (*Figure 2.13*). In parous women, in particular, ovarian location is more variable and sometimes the ovary can be found behind the uterus or in the pouch of Douglas (*Figure 2.14*). If the ovary is not detected in these places, visualization may be helped by applying gentle pressure with the vaginal probe or with the examiner's free hand on the abdominal wall. This helps to shift the ovary that is located higher than usual toward the focal zone of the transducer and can diminish the effect of intervening bowel gas. Visualization of (follicular) cysts is often the first sign that the ovary has been found, and using these cysts as a guide the entire ovary can be depicted. After the menopause the ovaries may be hard to find because the follicles serving as sonographic markers are absent and the ovaries themselves atrophy.

Ovarian size varies with age, menstrual status, body habitus and phase of menstrual cycle; in general it should not exceed $4 \times 3 \times 2$ cm in the reproductive period. Because of variations in shape the calculation of ovarian volume, using the formula for an ellipsoid ($d_1 \times d_2 \times d_3 \times 0.523$ where d represents diameter), provides a more objective method of assessment of ovarian size. In a representative study (Granberg and Wikland, 1988), mean ovarian volume in the preovulatory phase was 5.8 ± 2.9 cm^3; other investigators reported even larger volumes (Cohen et al, 1990; Merz et al, 1996). *Figure 2.15* shows the variation of ovarian size with age.

Since the ovary changes with the phases of the menstrual cycle, an understanding of this dynamic process is important for the interpretation of ultrasound images. Using the transvaginal route, allowing the use of high frequency probes in close proximity to the ovaries, follicles as small as 2 mm in diameter can be quantified. Follicles appear as echo-free, round or ovoid translucent structures within the uniform texture of the ovarian

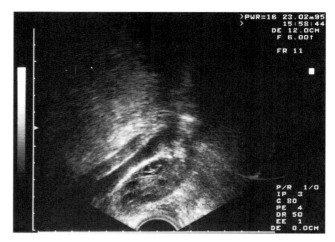

Figure 2.13: Normal ovary showing numerous small follicles and in close proximity to the pelvic vessels.

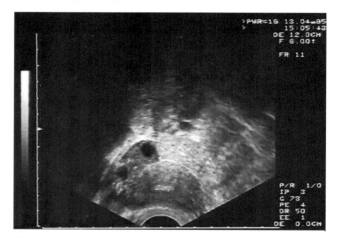

Figure 2.14: Normal ovary situated behind the uterus.

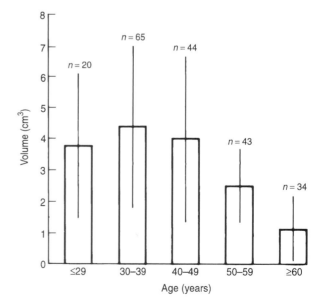

Figure 2.15: Ovarian volume as related to 10-year age cohorts. From Granberg & Wikland (1988) with permission of the publisher, The American Institute for Ultrasound in Medicine.

stroma. Pache et al (1990) carried out a transvaginal ultrasound study to analyze the number of follicles and follicle growth patterns in three successive periods of the menstrual cycle: the early follicular phase (from menses up to and including the day of selection of the dominant follicle), the late follicular phase (between the day of selection and the day of the luteinizing hormone (LH) peak), and the luteal phase (following the LH peak until menses). The mean number of follicles in the different phases varied between 5.9 and 7.4 for the dominant ovary and 5.8 and 7.5 for the nondominant ovary. The presence of a dominant follicle could be ascertained between cycle days 5 and 12 (mean cycle day 8.3) at a follicle diameter between 6.5 and 14.0 mm (mean 9.9 mm). All leading follicles displayed a linear growth rate ranging between 1.4 and 2.2 mm/day (mean 1.7 mm/day); at the time of the LH peak the leading follicle measured between 18.1 and 22.6 mm (mean 20.6 mm). Growth of small follicles was established in both ovaries up to the time of selection; in this study every follicle with a diameter of 11 mm or more was

dominant and the diameter of nondominant follicles always remained less than 11 mm (*Figure 2.16*). van Santbrink et al (1995) showed that the first day of a significant rise in estradiol plasma level correlated strongly with the day on which the dominant follicle appeared sonographically, and a significant correlation existed between the rate of increase in estradiol plasma concentrations and dominant follicle growth (*Figure 2.17*).

After ovulation a small amount of fluid may be visualized in the pouch of Douglas, and shortly after ovulation a characteristic sonographic appearance of the corpus luteum can be recognized. The fresh corpus luteum appears as a hypoechoic, predominantly cystic structure that may assume several shapes. The wall may be thickened and

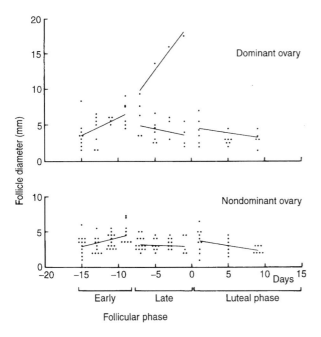

*Figure 2.16: Follicle diameters according to the day of sonographic measurement for both ovaries in a representative normally cycling woman (day 0 = LH surge). From Pache TD, Wladimiroff JW, de Jong FH, Hop WC & Fauser BCJM (1990) Growth patterns of nondominant ovarian follicles during the normal menstrual cycle. Fertil Steril **54**: 638–642. Reproduced with permission of the publisher, the American Society for Reproductive Medicine (The American Fertility Society).*

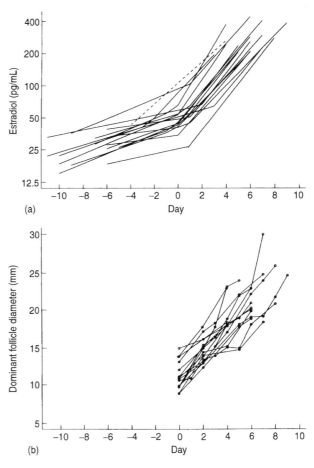

*Figure 2.17: Rise in (a) individual estradiol serum concentrations and (b) diameter of the dominant follicle synchronized around the first day of visualization of the dominant follicle. From van Santbrink EJ, Hop WC, van Dessel TJHM, de Jong FH & Fauser BCJM (1995) Decremental follicle-stimulating hormone and dominant follicle development during the normal menstrual cycle. Fertil Steril **64**: 37–43. Reproduced with permission of the publisher, the American Society for Reproductive Medicine (The American Fertility Society).*

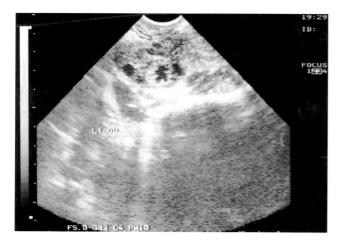

2.18a

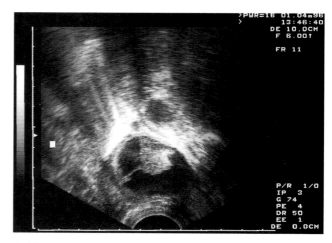

2.18c

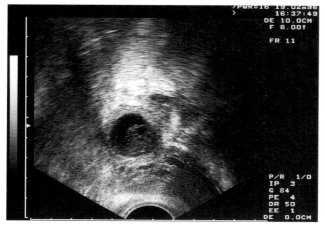

2.18b

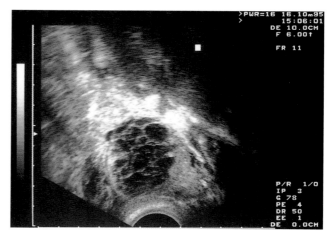

2.18d

Figure 2.18: *Variations in the appearance of the corpus luteum. (a) Small corpus luteum surrounded by normal ovarian tissue. (b) Small corpus luteum cyst. (c) Corpus luteum cyst with bizarrely shaped*

echogenic mass reflecting a retracted blood clot. (d) Corpus luteum cyst with clot formation appearing as a fine mesh-like structure.

irregular and it often contains internal echoes, reflecting hemorrhage. The diameter does not usually exceed 4 cm. Other sonographic appearances include a highly echogenic area (representing a blood clot), in sharp contrast to the remaining liquid-filled echolucent space, or it may appear as a septated cystic mass containing components of different echogenicity. The septa may be solitary or appear as a complex yet delicate network (*Figure 2.18*). These images are a reflection of the process of bleeding, clot formation, retraction and reabsorption (Rottem and Timor-Tritsch, 1991). In cases of a corpus luteum cyst or a hemorrhagic corpus luteum, it may attain 8 cm or more in size (Rottem et al, 1990b). Because of these features the corpus luteum can mimic a number of disease processes.

FALLOPIAN TUBES

The normal Fallopian tube is not usually seen because of its small size and tortuous course. Only when some fluid is present may it be possible to delineate the tube as an undulating structure lateral to the uterus and behind the ovaries or in the pouch of Douglas (*Figure 2.19*). The pathological tube is more easily recognized because it may become dilated and filled with fluid (Timor-Tritsch and Rottem, 1987).

Hysterosalpingo contrast sonography is a new technique for assessing tubal patency. By injecting a highly echogenic suspension of microscopic air bubbles (stabilized by galactose or albumin microparticles) into the uterus it is possible to visualize flow through the tubes

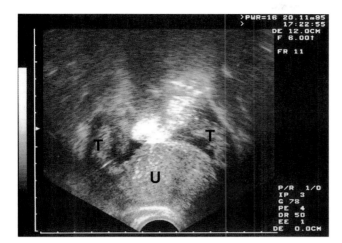

Figure 2.19: Transpelvic view of the uterus(U) and both undulating Fallopian tubes (T) surrounded by some free peritoneal fluid.

and thus indicate tubal patency with an accuracy similar to the standard procedures (Campbell et al, 1994). Uterine malformations can also be detected using the same technique.

LOWER URINARY TRACT

The static and dynamic function of the urethrovesical region can be studied by use of transvaginal ultrasound. Previous methods, including videocystourethrography and lateral bead-chain cystourethrography, require the use of X-rays and carry a significant complication rate (Quinn et al, 1988). Linear array as well as end-firing probes can be used to obtain pictures from several possible sites (rectal, perineal, vulvar and vaginal). The inferior border of the symphysis pubis is the fixed midline landmark and has a hyperechoic appearance; the hypoechoic appearance of the stored urine is immediately apparent when the transducer is placed just within the introitus. The term 'bladder neck' refers to the junction of the bladder and the apposed walls of the proximal urethra. Under normal conditions, specific provocative maneuvers, like coughing, give rise to no, or only minor inferior and posterior, displacement of the bladder neck and are not associated with leakage of hypoechoic urine.

REFERENCES

Campbell S, Bourne TH, Tan SL & Collins WP (1994) Hysterosalpingo contrast sonography (HyCoSy) and its future role within the investigation of infertility in Europe. *Ultrasound Obstet Gynecol* **4**: 245.

Carter J, Fowler J, Carson L, Carlson J & Twiggs LB (1994) How accurate is the pelvic examination as compared to transvaginal sonography? A prospective, comparative study. *J Reprod Med Obstet Gynecol* **39**: 32–34.

Cohen H, Tice H & Mandel F (1990) Ovarian volumes measured by ultrasound: bigger than we think. *Radiology* **177**: 189–192.

Conoscenti G, Meir YJ, Fischer-Tamaro L et al (1995) Endometrial assessment by transvaginal sonography and histological findings after D & C in women with postmenopausal bleeding. *Ultrasound Obstet Gynecol* **6**: 108–115.

Dodson MG & Deter RL (1990) Definition of anatomical planes for use in transvaginal sonography. *J Clin Ultrasound* **18**: 239–242.

Emanuel MH, Verdel Mj, Wamsteker K & Lammes FB (1995) A prospective comparison of transvaginal ultrasonography and diagnostic hysteroscopy in the evaluation of patients with abnormal uterine bleeding: clinical implications. *Am J Obstet Gynecol* **172**: 547–552.

Fleischer AC, Pittaway DE, Beard LA et al (1984) Sonographic depiction of endometrial changes occurring with ovulation induction. *J Ultrasound Med* **3**: 341.

Gaucherand P, Piacenza JM, Salle B & Rudigoz RC (1995) Sonohysterography of the uterine cavity: preliminary investigations. *J Clin Ultrasound* **23**: 339–348.

Goldstein SR (1990) Incorporating ultrasonography into the overall gynecologic examination. *Am J Obstet Gynecol* **162**: 625–632.

Granberg S (1994) Sonography of the endometrium in the postmenopausal women. *Ann Med* **26**: 81–83.

Granberg S & Wikland M (1988) A comparison between ultrasound and gynecologic examination for detection of enlarged ovaries in a group of women at risk for ovarian carcinoma. *J Ultrasound Med* **7**: 59–64.

Karlsson B, Granberg S, Wikland M et al (1995) Transvaginal ultrasonography of the endometrium in women with postmenopausal bleeding: a Nordic multicenter study. *Am J Obstet Gynecol* **172**: 1488–1494.

Lewit N, Thaler I & Rottem S (1990) The uterus: a new look with transvaginal sonography. *J Clin Ultrasound* **18**: 331–336.

Lyons EA, Taylor PJ, Zheng ZH et al (1991) Characterization of subendometrial myometrial contractions throughout the menstrual cycle in normal fertile women. *Fertil Steril* **55**: 771–774.

Merz E, Miric-Tesanic D, Bahlman F, Weber G & Wellek S (1996) Sonographic size of the uterus and ovaries in pre- and postmenopausal women. *Ultrasound Obstet Gynecol* **7**: 38–42.

Pache TD, Wladimiroff YW, de Jong FH, Hop WC & Fauser BCJM (1990) Growth patterns of nondominant ovarian follicles during the normal menstrual cycle. *Fertil Steril* **54**: 638–642.

Parson AK & Lense JJ (1993) Sonohysterography for endometrial abnormalities: preliminary results. *J Clin Ultrasound* **21**: 87–95.

Quinn MJ, Beynon J, Mortensen NM & Smith PBJ (1988) Transvaginal endosonography in the assessment of urinary stress incontinence. *Br J Urol* **62**: 414–418.

Rottem S & Timor-Tritsch IE (1991) Ovarian pathology. In Timor-Tritsch IE & Rottem S (eds) *Transvaginal Sonography*, 2nd edn, pp 145–173. New York: Elsevier.

Rottem S, Thaler I, Goldstein SR, Timor-Tritsch IE & Brandes JM (1990a) Transvaginal sonographic technique: targeted organ scanning without resorting to 'planes'. *J Clin Ultrasound* **18**: 243–247.

Rottem S, Levit N, Thaler I et al (1990b) Classification of ovarian lesions by high-frequency transvaginal sonography. *J Clin Ultrasound* **18**: 359–363.

Schats R (1991) Transvaginal sonography in early pregnancy. MD, PhD Thesis. Erasmus University, Rotterdam.

Shiply CF, Simmons CL & Nelson GH (1994) Comparison of transvaginal sonography with endometrial biopsy in asymptomatic postmenopausal women. *J Ultrasound Med* **13**: 99–104.

Timor-Tritsch IE (1990) Is office use of vaginal sonography feasible? *Am J Obstet Gynecol* **162**: 983–985.

Timor-Tritsch IE (1992) Transvaginal sonography in gynecologic practice. *Curr Opin Obstet Gynecol* **4**: 914–920.

Timor-Tritsch IE & Rottem S (1987) Ultrasonographic study of the fallopian tube. *Obstet Gynecol* **70**: 424–428.

van Santbrink EJP, Hop WC, van Dessel TJHM, de Jong FH & Fauser BCJM (1995) Decremental follicle-stimulating hormone and dominant follicle development during the normal menstrual cycle. *Fertil Steril* **64**: 37–43.

Zimmer EZ, Timor-Tritsch IE & Rottem S (1991) The technique of transvaginal sonography. In Timor-Tritsch IE & Rottem S (eds) *Transvaginal Sonography*, 2nd edn, pp 66–75. New York: Elsevier.

3 *Endoscopy: hysteroscopy*
K Wamsteker

■ INTRODUCTION

Hysteroscopy with directed histological biopsy has appeared to be method of choice for the diagnosis of intrauterine disorders. Direct visualization of the uterine cavity can disclose and identify almost all intracavitary and endometrial abnormalities (Wamsteker, 1977, 1984; Gimpelson and Rappold, 1988; Loffer, 1989; Motashaw and Dave, 1990; Salaz-Lizee et al, 1993; Emanuel et al, 1995a). Although transvaginal ultrasonography (TVS) is an excellent method for screening for intrauterine pathology and for revealing intrauterine abnormalities (Emanuel et al, 1995b), in cases of abnormal findings TVS should be followed by direct hysteroscopic imaging to define the nature, location and extent of the pathology and to assess the most appropriate method of treatment.

In modern gynecological units a curette is no longer used for dilatation and curettage (D & C) procedures alone, but, in conjunction with hysteroscopy, to obtain directed or randomized intrauterine tissue samples for histological examination in specific cases. Learning how to handle the hysteroscope and how to interpret the obtained images are essential parts of hysteroscopic education. Artifacts, generally created by improper instrumental management during the procedure itself, can easily be misinterpreted as abnormalities.

In this chapter the most commonly applied techniques and methods for diagnostic hysteroscopy and normal hysteroscopic appearances, including artifacts, will be described.

■ EQUIPMENT

METHODS

Hysteroscopy can be performed with or without distension of the uterine cavity. Without distension the method is referred to as contact hysteroscopy, a technique originally introduced by Barbot et al (1980). As the uterine cavity is not distended, the hysteroscope is in direct contact with the endocervical or intrauterine mucosa. No general overview image can be obtained, which is a significant disadvantage of the method. Visualization and interpretation are difficult, as is the disclosure of pathology. These are the main reasons why this technique has been almost completely abandoned as a method for routine diagnostic hysteroscopy. Contact hysteroscopy with a microhysteroscope with magnification, however, is still performed occasionally for scientific studies, either in addition to hysteroscopy with uterine distension, or as microcolpohysteroscopy for diagnosis of (endo)cervical dysplasia or malignancy (Hamou, 1981; Gilbert et al, 1990). For clinical practice this method appears to be of limited importance (Tseng et al, 1987; Guerra et al, 1988). As the methods for diagnosis of cervical dysplasia and malignancy are not covered by this book, this technique will not be further discussed.

The most generally applied technique for diagnostic hysteroscopy is panoramic hysteroscopy, with distension of the uterine cavity. For the interpretation of hysteroscopic images it is very important to realize that the different methods and distension media used in panoramic hysteroscopy can produce different images of intrauterine structures.

DISTENSION MEDIA

The media used for distension of the uterine cavity can be divided into three groups, which will be discussed separately: gaseous media, high viscosity fluids (HVF) and low viscosity fluids (LVF).

GASEOUS MEDIA

The gas most generally used for distension of the uterine cavity in hysteroscopy is CO_2 (Lindemann, 1971). CO_2

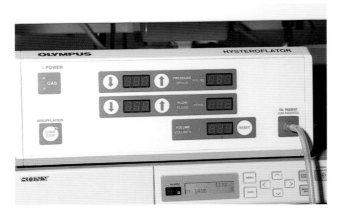

Figure 3.1: CO_2 insufflator for hysteroscopy; insufflation pressure and CO_2 flow can be adjusted separately.

may only be delivered by insufflators specifically developed for hysteroscopy, which operate only within certain safety limits for insufflation pressure and gas flow (*Figure 3.1*). A CO_2 flow rate of up to 100 ml/min and an insufflation pressure of 150 mmHg have appeared to be the maximum levels at which safety can be assured. Although some studies have indicated that minor intravascular CO_2 bubbles can still develop, they do not seem to be harmful (Brundin and Thomasson, 1989; Rythén-Alder et al, 1992). With larger quantities or pressure of CO_2 insufflation, CO_2 emboli can result in serious complications (Lindemann, 1975; Lindemann et al, 1976). The hysteroscopic image with CO_2 distension is very bright and clear, as long as no mucous bubbles develop or blood is present in the uterine cavity. The mucosa is somewhat compressed by the intrauterine pressure. Mucous bubbles can significantly hamper adequate visualization. If blood is present in the uterine cavity, adequate visualization can be even more difficult and some areas of the cavity may not be visualized at all.

CO_2 distension can be used either with flexible or, single flow (SF) and continuous flow (CF), rigid hysteroscopes, and is very useful for office hysteroscopy. Some shoulder pain may develop after the procedure in cases of patent tubes.

HIGH VISCOSITY FLUIDS

The most important high viscosity fluid used in hysteroscopy is 32% dextran 70 in dextrose 5% (Hyskon®) (Edström and Fernström, 1970). This distension

medium is very effective for diagnostic procedures as it can rinse some blood and/or mucus from the uterine cavity and its high viscosity reduces tubal and cervical outflow, which supports a more steady uterine distension. For use with diagnostic hysteroscopes Hyskon should be 10% diluted with saline or dextrose 5% to enhance its flow through the hysteroscope. The dextran concentration is thus reduced to approximately 29%.

Uterine distension with the dextran solution can easily be accomplished through a 20 or 30 ml syringe with Luer-Lok connection, directly attached to the hysteroscope or through a connecting tube.

The use of dextran requires special cleaning procedures for the instruments in order to prevent caramelization of the dextran. They must be rinsed with warm water with a neutral detergent immediately after the procedure and all moving parts must be cleaned very thoroughly both before and after disassembling. Liquid disinfection is to be advised because autoclaving may still allow the moving parts of the instruments to stick. In view of the risk of caramelization and the required special cleaning procedure this distension medium is less suitable for office procedures and diagnostic procedures that require operating instruments. Other disadvantages of working with dextran solutions are that they are rather messy and stick to the video camera, which requires frequent cleaning.

Anaphylactic reactions can occur with dextran. Although the incidence is only approximately 1:10 000 cases (McLucas, 1991), the reaction can be very serious and life threatening.

These disadvantages have reduced the use of Hyskon significantly in favor of LVF with continuous flow hysteroscopes.

LOW VISCOSITY FLUIDS

LVF are the most important distension media in modern hysteroscopy, especially in combination with CF hysteroscopes (Wamsteker and de Blok, 1993).

The most generally used liquids are sorbitol 4 or 5%, glycine 1.5% and dextrose 5%, which are electrolyte-free solutions. Saline can also be used for diagnostic procedures but as it is a conductive fluid it should never be used in combination with electrosurgery. To avoid confusion it is recommended that saline should not be used in hysteroscopy units where electrosurgical procedures may be performed.

LVF should preferably be used with CF hysteroscopes, especially in cases with difficult visualization because of blood and/or mucus in the uterine cavity, and in endo-surgical procedures, as mixing of these fluids with blood or mucus causes blurring of the vision with SF instruments. Some people, however, prefer to use SF hysteroscopes with LVF because of the reduced diameter of the sheath and the possibility of using thin flexible hysteroscopes. If necessary, some overdilatation of the internal cervical os can enable flushing with cervical outflow. We definitely prefer the use of rigid CF hysteroscopes, in spite of their slightly greater diameter, as this method provides for optimal visualization.

LVF must be delivered under pressure, for which different methods can be used, as follows.

- Gravity: a fluid bag suspended at a level of between 1 m (74 mmHg) and 1.5 m (110 mmHg) above the level of the patient; especially useful for diagnostic office procedures.
- Pressure cuffs: manually (*Figure 3.2a*) or automatic (*Figure 3.2b*); the infusion pressure should be 150 mmHg; the standard method for diagnostic procedures and minor interventions; to be used in all cases of impaired visualization due to blood and/or debris.
- Electronic fluid control pumps: generally roller pumps with adjustable pressure and flow and some with liquid loss control (*Figure 3.3*); these pumps are more expensive and are especially designed for endosurgical procedures; they will generally only be used for diagnostic procedures that are performed in the operating room.

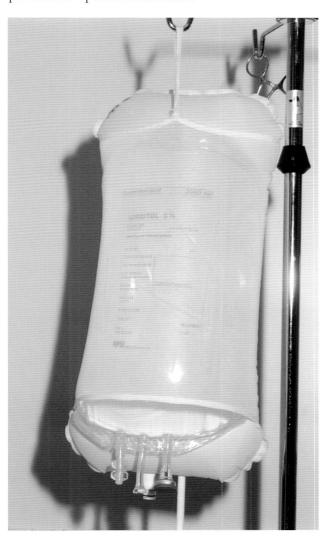

3.2a

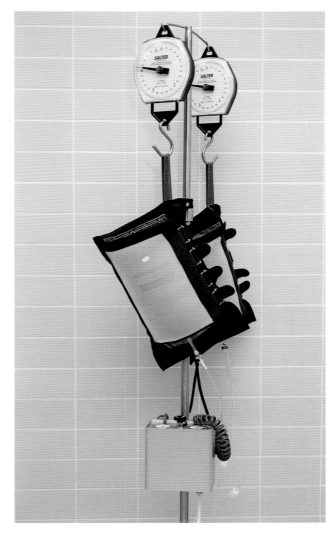

3.2b

Figure 3.2: *(a) Manual pressure cuff for pressurized delivery of low viscosity fluids. (b) Automatic pressure cuff for pressurized delivery of* *low viscosity fluids; double system for rapid change of bags; also available for single fluid bag.*

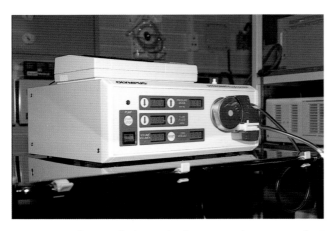

Figure 3.3: *Electronic fluid control roller pump with permanent fluid loss control; the fluid pressure and flow are separately adjustable (Uteromat Fluid Control ™, Olympus). Reproduced with permission of Olympus Winter & Ibe.*

The fluid from the outflow channel and the reflux from the vagina should always be collected and measured continuously and should be subtracted from the infused amount of fluid to determine the fluid loss. This retained fluid loss should be considered to have been intravasated (although some of it may have entered the abdominal cavity through the Fallopian tubes). The total amount of fluid loss should never exceed 1.5 liters. With higher quantities of intravasation, overfilling of the circulation, with pulmonary edema and hyponatremia, may occur (Loffer, 1995). In diagnostic procedures this risk is almost negligible as the amount of fluid loss will seldom be more than 100–150 ml. With minor interventions the fluid loss usually never exceeds 500 ml; however, a false route or a perforation will result in a rapid increase of the fluid loss.

HYSTEROSCOPES

Basically the hysteroscopic equipment for panoramic diagnostic hysteroscopy can be divided into flexible and rigid hysteroscopes. Rigid hysteroscopes are available in two varieties: SF or CF. The outer sheath of SF hysteroscopes has only one channel for the delivery of the distending medium. CF hysteroscopes have an outer sheath with two separated channels, one for the inflow and another for the outflow of the distending medium. Flexible hysteroscopes are only available as single flow instruments.

All these instruments are available for diagnostic hys-

teroscopy. Their specific advantages and disadvantages to this purpose will be discussed.

FLEXIBLE DIAGNOSTIC HYSTEROSCOPES

The principal advantage of flexible diagnostic hysteroscopes, especially for routine office procedures, is the small diameter of 3.6 mm, which eliminates the need for cervical dilatation and/or local anesthesia. The tip of the hysteroscope can be bent manually up to 100° or 120° in either direction (*Figure 3.4*) for visualization of the cornual areas. The honeycomb structure of the image, caused by the fiberoptic image transmission, however, reduces the resolution and the sharpness of the image (*Figure 3.5*). As a result of this limitation minor mucosal abnormalities can be overlooked. For routine diagnostic office screening these hysteroscopes are satisfactory, in

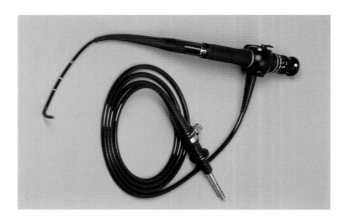

Figure 3.4: *Flexible 3.6 mm diagnostic hysteroscope; the distal tip can be bent manually at the eyepiece.*

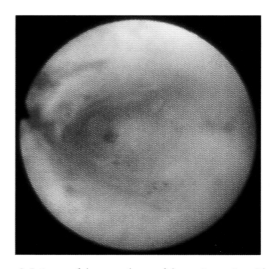

Figure 3.5: *Image of the cornual area of the uterine cavity with a flexible hysteroscope; note the honeycomb structure of the image.*

so far as inadequate visualization will prompt a repeat inspection with rigid and preferably CF instruments.

All flexible hysteroscopes are single flow hysteroscopes, as they only have an inflow channel, and are used with CO_2 gas or low viscosity fluid distension. In the presence of mucus and/or blood, LVF should be used, if necessary with extra cervical dilatation to create some kind of flushing effect with vaginal outflow.

RIGID DIAGNOSTIC HYSTEROSCOPES

Single flow hysteroscopes

SF hysteroscopes must be used with either CO_2 gas or Hyskon distension. The diameter of the diagnostic outer sheaths is 4 mm (3 mm telescope) or 5 mm (4 mm telescope) (*Figure 3.6*). The telescopes have a 30° angle of view for better inspection of the cornual areas. The brightness and angle of view of the new 3 mm Olympus telescopes is significantly increased, eliminating the need for special light sources. The instruments do not have a working channel for biopsies. Biopsies should be taken either with a directed curettage or with the use of an operating sheath; however, SF operating sheaths do not perform very well and are not recommended.

The disadvantages of SF hysteroscopes with CO_2 and Hyskon distension have already been mentioned.

Continuous flow hysteroscopes

CF hysteroscopes are equipped with separated inflow and outflow channels for the distending medium. For optimal fitting in the internal cervical os the sheath should preferably have a round circumference. These instruments can be used both with CO_2 or with liquid distension media, and allow for flushing of the uterine cavity during CO_2 hysteroscopy. Their best performance is with pressurized LVF, producing rapid inflow and outflow and providing excellent visualization in all circumstances, even in the presence of a bleeding endometrium (Wamsteker and de Blok, 1993).

The standard CF hysteroscopes for diagnostic hysteroscopy are equipped with either a 3 mm 30° foreoblique wide angle telescope and a 4.5 mm CF outer sheath, or a 4 mm 30° telescope with a 5.5 mm CF sheath (*Figure 3.7*). The outflow channel also serves as a working channel but the diameter allows only 3 Fr instruments for very small biopsies. For more reliable tissue sampling or interventions the outer sheath should be replaced with a 5.5 or 6.5 mm (3 mm telescope), or 7 or 8 mm (4 mm telescope) CF operating sheath with a working channel for 5 or 7 Fr instruments (*Figures 3.8* and *3.9*) (Wamsteker et al, 1992).

The standard 4.5 and 5.5 mm CF hysteroscopes, either alone or in combination with a 4 or 5 mm single flow sheath, are most likely to become the hysteroscopes of choice for diagnostic procedures. The small diameter of the 4.5 mm instrument make it especially suitable for office and ambulatory procedures without anesthesia, while the 5.5 mm hysteroscope with increased image size is most appropriate for diagnostic procedures in the operating theatre with local or general anesthesia.

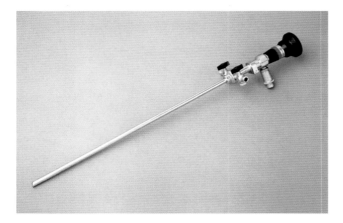

Figure 3.6: Rigid 5 mm single flow diagnostic hysteroscope with 4 mm 30° wide angle telescope: the instrument has two connections that come together in one main channel for the delivery of the distending medium inside the sheath.

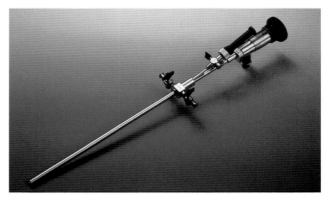

Figure 3.7: Design of rigid 4.5 and 5.5 mm continuous flow diagnostic hysteroscope with 3 or 4 mm 30° foreoblique wide angle telescope (Olympus); the sheath contains two separate channels for the distending medium; one for the inflow and the other for the outflow of the medium; the required flow direction is indicated at the stopcocks; the working channel allows 3 Fr instruments.

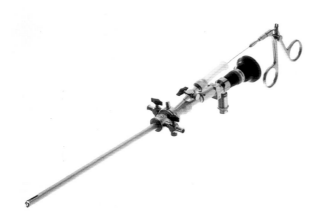

Figure 3.8: *Rigid 7 mm continuous flow operating hysteroscope with 4 mm 30° telescope for minor interventions; the working channel admits 5 Fr instruments.*

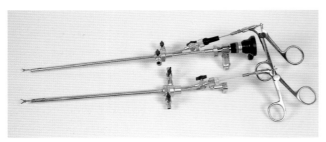

Figure 3.9: *Rigid 5.5 and 6.5 mm continuous flow operating hysteroscopes with 3 mm 30° telescope for minor interventions; the working channels admit 5 and 7 Fr instruments, respectively.*

LIGHT SOURCE

The light source to be used for diagnostic hysteroscopy depends on the requirements and the instruments. A 300 W xenon or 250 W halogen light source should preferably be used (*Figure 3.10*); both of these will suffice in all circumstances in diagnostic procedures, either with or without a video camera. For purely diagnostic office procedures with a 4 mm telescope a 150 W halogen light source can be applied as well. With 3 mm telescopes this light source will not always suffice, especially with video imaging.

VIDEO CAMERA

A highly sensitive CCD (charge-coupled device) or chip camera with high resolution (*Figure 3.11*) must be used with hysteroscopy. Blood in the uterine cavity or congestion of the endometrium will absorb a great deal of light and will lessen the quality of the image significantly

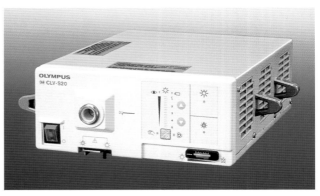

3.10a

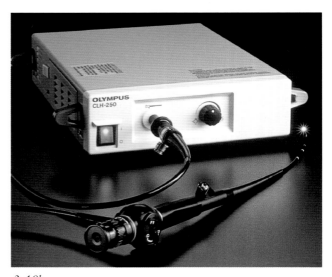

3.10b

Figure 3.10: *(a) 300 W xenon light source. (b) 250 W halogen light source with flexible hysteroscope.*

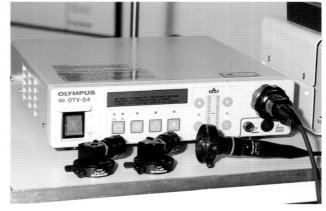

Figure 3.11: *CCD video camera with control unit and three different adapters: (from right to left) straight, hooked and beam splitter.*

if the camera is insufficiently sensitive. Video recordings can be made with S-VHS, VHS or U-matic recorders for documentation and video printers are very useful for instant documentation.

■ TECHNIQUE

GENERAL REMARKS

The hysteroscope should always be introduced into the uterine cavity under visual control from the endocervix on through the internal cervical os. The hysteroscope should never be advanced into the uterine cavity without adequate visibility as this can result in the creation of a false route or even perforation. Touching the mucosa with the hysteroscope sheath should be avoided as much as possible as this readily produces artifacts and/or bleeding. Hysteroscopy is essentially a no-touch technique. For this reason the hysteroscope must also never be advanced inside the uterine cavity without adequate distension of the cavity.

With rigid hysteroscopes it has to be kept in mind that the angle of view is 30°. To visualize the complete endocervix and the internal cervical os (*Figure 3.12*) the hysteroscope has to be moved into a position at an angle of 30° to the endocervical canal.

The hysteroscope should be inserted into the uterine cavity by passing the internal os very carefully under visual control and, if possible, without prior dilatation. It must be remembered that the tip of a rigid hysteroscope has a sharp and a blunt edge because of the 30° viewing angle of the telescope. The sharp edge should not come into contact with the wall of the internal os or the endometrium. With upward viewing the blunt edge must be guided closely underneath the anterior wall, and the posterior wall should not be visible in the lower part of the image (*Figure 3.13*). This will prevent disruption of the endometrium during the passage through the internal os. Once in the uterine cavity the hysteroscope must be lifted upward to re-establish complete panoramic vision.

If the internal os will not open enough for smooth passage of the hysteroscope sheath it must be dilated, preferably using half-size Hegar dilators, or the hysteroscope should be rotated 180° in order to have the blunt angle of the hysteroscope tip sliding smoothly over the posterior ridge. After passing the internal os the hysteroscope must again be rotated backwards. The uterus must never be sounded before the procedure. Rotation of the hysteroscope together with movement of the hysteroscope to the left and the right side enables complete visualization of the whole uterine cavity and both cornual areas (*Figure 3.14*).

Sometimes the tip of a flexible hysteroscope will need guiding with a forceps to overcome the slight resistance of the internal cervical os and to prevent bending of the distal tip. Although rotation of the hysteroscope is necessary for visualization of the uterine cavity and the

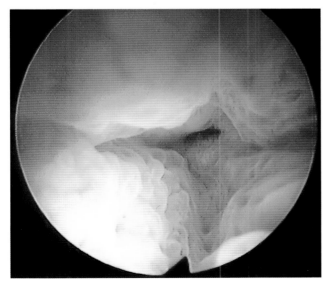

Figure 3.12: Endocervical channel with internal cervical os.

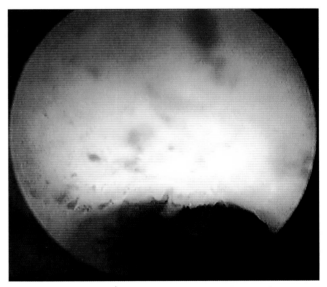

Figure 3.13: Passing the internal cervical os: with upward viewing telescope the hysteroscope is guided closely underneath the anterior wall, avoiding contact of the sharp angle of the tip of the hysteroscope with the posterior wall and the isthmic endometrium; note that the posterior wall is not visible.

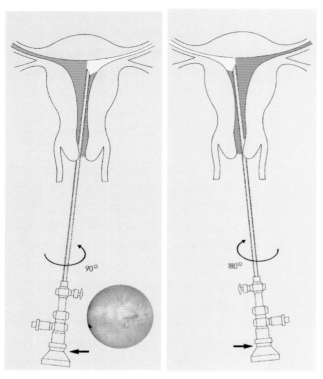

3.14a   3.14b

Figure 3.14: *(a) A 90° rotation of the hysteroscope and a slight lateral movement allow the visualization of the tubal ostium (insert: left tubal ostium). (b) Another rotation of 180° allows the location of the opposite tubal ostium. Reproduced with permission of Olympus Winter & Ibe.*

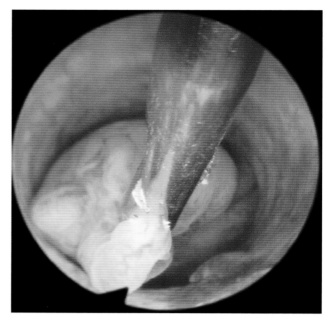

Figure 3.15: *Visually directed biopsy of intracavity polyp.*

cornual areas as well, in contrast to rigid hysteroscopes lateral or downward and upward movements of the instrument are not required as the tip can be bent and directed into the desired position. This method, however, requires experience.

A tissue specimen should always be obtained for histological examination if there is any abnormal finding (*Figure 3.15*).

CO₂ DISTENSION

It is preferable not to dilate the internal cervical os with CO_2 distension as this can cause bleeding, which should be avoided whenever possible. Sometimes very viscous mucus in the endocervix impaires visibility and must be either removed or carefully passed by. Once in the uterine cavity one should pause momentarily until mucous bubbles have dissipated (*Figure 3.16*). In case of persis-

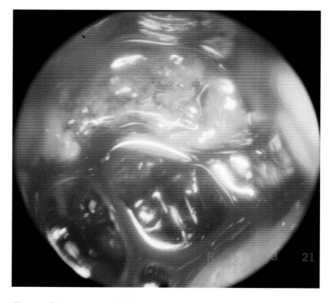

Figure 3.16: *Mucous bubbles in the isthmic area with CO_2 hysteroscopy.*

tent blurring of the vision the telescope tip can be cleared by very gently touching the uterine wall. In case of persistent impaired visibility due to mucus and/or blood a CF hysteroscope must be used, either to flush the uterine cavity or to switch completely to low viscosity fluid distension.

DEXTRAN DISTENSION

The Hyskon solution must be 10% diluted with saline or dextrose 5% to enhance the liquid flow through the hysteroscope channel. The hysteroscope must be prefilled with the dextran solution before introduction into the endocervix. Because of the high viscosity of the solution, advancing the hysteroscope should be delayed a few moments after passing the internal cervical os until full dilatation of the uterine cavity is accomplished.

The uterine cavity can be flushed with the dextran solution from the fundal or cornual areas in order to clear the distending liquid. The instruments must be cleaned carefully after the procedure to prevent caramelization of the dextran.

LOW VISCOSITY FLUID DISTENSION

As the results when using LVF with SF instruments can be disappointing, it is recommended that CF hysteroscopes are used.

After prefilling the hysteroscope with the liquid it is inserted into the endocervical canal with a half opened inflow stopcock and completely opened outflow stopcock. If necessary for adequate distension the inflow stopcock can be opened slightly wider or the outflow stopcock closed partially. Once in the uterine cavity, both inflow and outflow stopcocks are opened completely for rapid flushing of the cavity. If more distension of the uterine cavity is required, the outflow stopcock can be partially closed until adequate distension is achieved. With partial opening and closing of the inflow and outflow stopcocks any desired degree of distension and liquid flow can be attained, according to the circumstances and personal preference (*Figure 3.17*). The outflow stopcock must never be closed completely as this will eliminate the liquid flow which is the most important aspect of the CF principle.

The outflow stopcock must be connected with a tube to a calibrated collection bottle. A collecting basin (beneath the gynecological chair), which is also con-

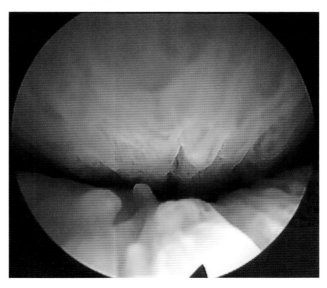

3.17a

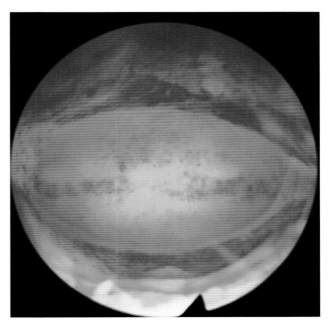

3.17b

Figure 3.17: *(a) Uterine cavity with very low degree of distension: the mucosal membranes are almost in apposition. (b) Uterine cavity with partial distension: the endometrium is flattened; the horizontal red area in the fundus marks the stretched fundal fold of the endometrium.*

nected to the collecting bottle, is recommended in order to collect the vaginal fluid loss (*Figure 3.18*).

LVF can also be used to flush the uterine cavity in cases of inadequate visualization with CO_2 distension. The

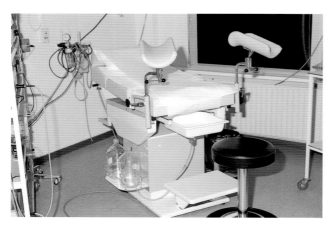

Figure 3.18: Electrically adjustable gynecological chair with basin and calibrated bottles for collection of the return fluid during hysteroscopy with liquid distension.

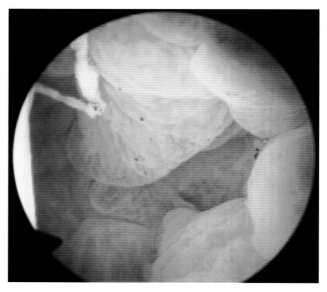

Figure 3.19: Secretory endometrium.

CO_2 must be disconnected or a three-way stopcock must be used. The uterine cavity is flushed with an open outflow stopcock. After reconnection of the CO_2 insufflation tube one must insure that the outflow stopcock remains open to flush out all the liquid, before again closing the outflow stopcock for the CO_2 distension. CO_2 visualization is usually completely restored following this procedure.

■ CONTRAINDICATIONS AND LIMITATIONS

Absolute contraindications for hysteroscopy are acute endometritis or pelvic inflammatory disease (PID). In patients with a history of chronic or recurrent PID, hysteroscopy could provoke an exacerbation. In such patients erythrocyte sedimentation rate (ESR) and C-reactive protein (CRP) values should be obtained before the procedure. If elevated the procedure should be postponed. Antibiotic prophylaxis during the procedure is, however, always recommended in patients with a history of PID. In cases of abnormal vaginal or cervical discharge a vaginal and endocervical culture should be obtained, and in cases of pathology treatment must be completed before the procedure. With a positive endocervical culture, a follow up culture after the antibiotic treatment is recommended.

An intact early pregnancy is a relative contraindication; however, hysteroscopy can be used for the retrieval of 'missing' intrauterine contraceptive devices (IUCDs) in early

pregnancies without obvious negative sequelae.

It is preferable not to perform the hysteroscopic procedure in the second half of the menstrual cycle in cases where the patient does not have adequate contraception because the transportation of a fertilized egg could be disturbed, which could result in an ectopic pregnancy. Performing the procedure in the second half of the cycle is, in any case, discouraged unless the patient is using oral contraceptives. The thick secretory endometrium hampers adequate visualization and can obscure pathology (*Figure 3.19*)(see also *Figure 2.11*).

If there is profuse endometrial bleeding hysteroscopic visualization can be difficult, even with pressurized CF techniques. The uterus can be flushed with a small catheter to evacuate blood clots or these may be removed with a small ovum forceps.

With a very patulous cervix it can be difficult to achieve adequate distension of the uterine cavity. In such cases a cervical vacuum adapter can be applied or the cervix can be narrowed with an extra tenaculum placed in an anteroposterior and slightly lateral position.

HYSTEROSCOPY AND ENDOMETRIAL CANCER

Extensive studies have not indicated any deleterious effect of abdominal escape of the gas or liquid when used for distension of the uterine cavity in panoramic hysteroscopy in cases of endometrial cancer (Wamsteker,

1977; Wamsteker and de Blok, 1993; Neis et al, 1994; Suprun et al, 1994). Although both during D & C and hysteroscopy spill of endometrial cancer cells to the peritoneal cavity may occur (Sagawa et al, 1994; Schmitz and Nahhas, 1984), this does not seem to have an effect on the prognosis. An extensive study by Johnsson (1973) in 606 patients with endometrial cancer stage I and II who underwent hysterography, and 158 patients without hysterography, with a follow-up of between 5 and 14 years, failed to indicate that abdominal spillage of radiographic contrast worsened the prognosis.

Although the intra-abdominal spread of intrauterine particles has been demonstrated during D & C (Barents and vd Kolk, 1975), there does not seem to be an increase in the frequency of recurrences or metastases in cases of endometrial cancer. During curettage and even during bimanual palpation in patients with endometrial cancer, tumor cells have also been identified in the inferior vena cava and the vena cubiti (Roberts et al, 1960), and a review of the literature does not indicate that hysteroscopy with abdominal leakage of the distension medium should be considered to be more hazardous.

Notwithstanding these considerations it is still advisable to try to minimize transabdominal leakage of the distension medium as much as possible in these cases.

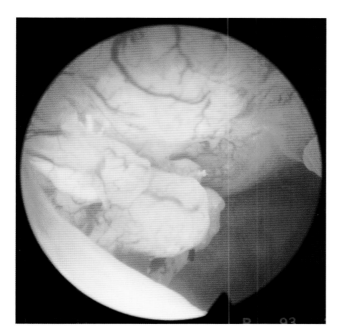

Figure 3.20: Localized early endometrial cancer diagnosed with directed hysteroscopic biopsy.

This could be achieved by reduction of the intrauterine working pressure during the hysteroscopic examination in suspected cases of malignancy.

Although D & C will rarely fail to disclose endometrial cancer and hyperplasia, hysteroscopic investigation increases the chance of early detection of small endometrial cancers (*Figure 3.20*) and facilitates the determination of the location, size and extent of the neoplasia and/or its precursors (Takashima, 1985; Goldberg et al, 1986; Noumoff and Faruqi, 1993; Taddei et al, 1994; Spiewankiewicz et al, 1995).

■ COMPLICATIONS AND SIDE EFFECTS

With proper techniques and adequate experience complications in diagnostic hysteroscopic procedures will be extremely rare (Lindemann, 1975; Raju and Taylor, 1986; de Jong et al, 1990; Hill et al, 1992). It is most important to insure prevention of complications, and their recognition and management if and when they occur. Possible complications can be related to the instrumental procedure itself, the distension medium, inadequate visualization or the anesthetic agent.

Complications from the instrumental procedure itself are the creation of a false route and/or perforation, both of which generally arise from improper instrumental management. Most frequently they will occur during blind sounding and/or dilatation of the internal os before the actual hysteroscopic procedure in a sharply anteverted or retroverted uterus (Valle, 1993). Blind sounding should never be performed before the hysteroscopic procedure and dilatation of the internal os should, when necessary, be done very carefully, paying attention to the uterine position and using half size Hegars. The dilatation of the internal os should produce a springy feeling when the pressure to the Hegar is slowly increased. If there is unexpected resistance, the position of the internal os must first be identified by endocervical hysteroscopic inspection. The hysteroscope must always be guided through the endocervix and the internal os under direct visual control.

During the hysteroscopic examination itself perforation of the uterus is very rare and should not occur. If it does occur, perforation is usually seen in the fundal area and results from improper technique or impaired visibility. This complication can be prevented by never advancing the hysteroscope without adequate distension and panoramic view.

Complications that may arise from the distending media have already been discussed.

To prevent complications due to impaired visibility it is of vital importance to work with only high quality equipment: telescope, light guide cable, light source and video camera. Another prerequisite is to adopt a no-touch technique when and wherever possible.

Complications that could arise from the use of local anesthetics are acute and late toxic reactions and can be prevented by avoiding intravascular injections and by not exceeding the maximum allowed dosage of the anesthetic.

Vasovagal reactions during the procedure, which could occur as a result of manipulations of the internal os in sensitive patients, can be prevented by an intramuscular application of 0.5 mg atropine i.m. 10–15 min before the procedure.

Painful contractions during dilatation of the uterine cavity can be prevented by the oral application of a prostaglandin synthetase inhibitor 2 hours before the procedure.

■ NORMAL APPEARANCES

ENDOCERVIX

The endocervical canal is somewhat spindle shaped and opens into the vagina through the external os. At its upper end the cervical canal communicates with the uterine cavity through a constricted orifice with a well developed muscular coat, the internal os (*Figure 3.21*), which is also the lower margin of the isthmic area of the uterine cavity. The endocervical mucosa consists mainly of columnar epithelium, which penetrates into the stroma, forming deep and branched tubular 'glands'. The surface of the endocervix contains deep infolding clefts within the stroma, known as plicae palmatae (*Figure 3.22*). Anterior and posterior longitudinal ridges can be recognized as the fusion lines of the Müllerian ducts (*Figure 3.12*). The plicae palmatae spread out laterally from these ridges and differ significantly in appearance.

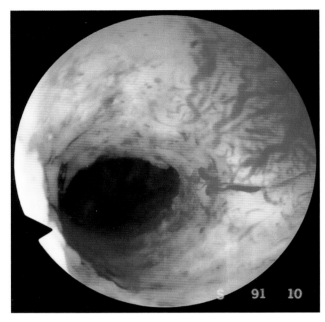

Figure 3.21: *Upper endocervical canal with dilated internal cervical os.*

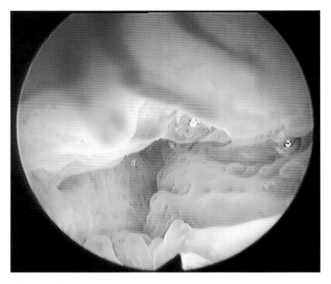

Figure 3.22: *Endocervical mucosa with plicae palmatae.*

The plicae can be rather pronounced and may obstruct a blindly inserted uterine sound or Hegar dilator, leading to the creation of a false route. In fertile women the plicae are rather smooth; after the menopause they can either be flattened or still be clearly seen as more firm, fibrotic structures with interconnecting adhesions (*Figure 3.23*).

To prevent the hysteroscope tip from damaging the endocervical structure and being obstructed by the plicae, the sheath should always be guided through the

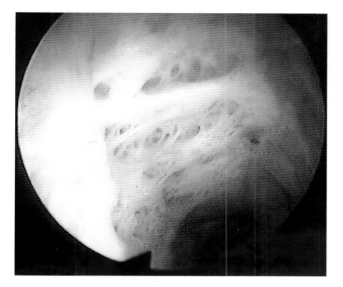

3.23a

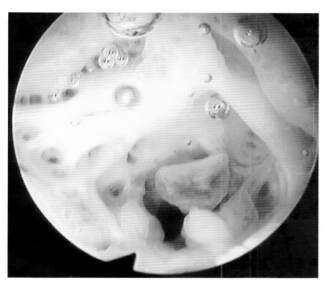

3.23b

Figure 3.23: *(a) Postmenopausal endocervical mucosa with flattened and rigid plicae palmatae. (b) Postmenopausal endocervix with pronounced fibrotic plicae palmatae and adhesions; these plicae could obstruct a blindly inserted sound or Hegar dilator.*

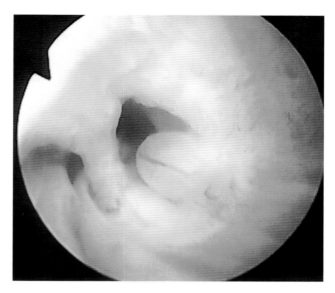

Figure 3.24: *Small endocervical cysts filled with mucus.*

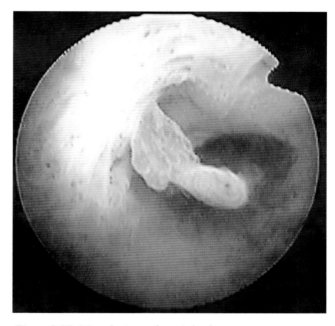

Figure 3.25: *Minor benign endocervical polyp.*

endocervix under visual control. In parous women the internal os will frequently be opened sufficiently by the distension medium alone; in nulliparous and post-menopausal women the internal os sometimes has to be dilated with Hegar probes. Small cysts, similar to those in the ectocervix (Nabothian cysts), and containing mucus, may also be visible in the endocervix (*Figure 3.24*).

Small endocervical polyps may be present but are generally of no clinical significance (*Figure 3.25*). They may be removed for histological examination but must be resected in cases showing an atypical vascular pattern. Larger endocervical polyps causing clinical symptoms will usually have been seen during earlier speculum examination of the ectocervix.

UTERINE CAVITY

The uterine cavity (*Figure 3.26*) is a pear-shaped space within the uterine body (corpus) which has a thick, muscular wall and a very fragile mucosa, the endometrium. The upper dome-like portion of the uterine cavity is the fundal area and the funnel-shaped

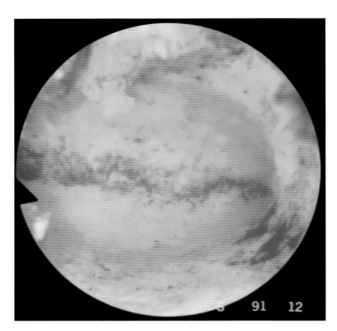

Figure 3.26: Normal fundal region of the uterine cavity with full distension.

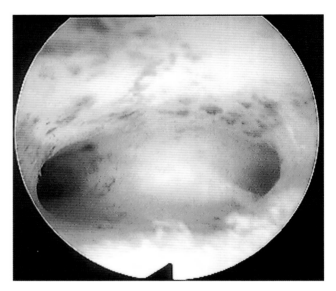

Figure 3.28: Fundal area of the uterine cavity with small central vault and more pronounced cornual areas indicating an arcuate uterus.

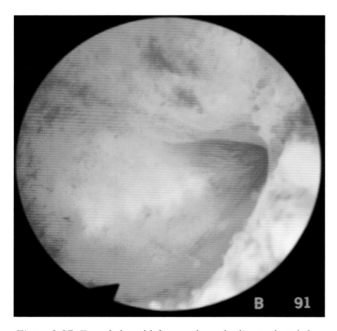

Figure 3.27: Funnel-shaped left cornual area leading to the tubal ostium.

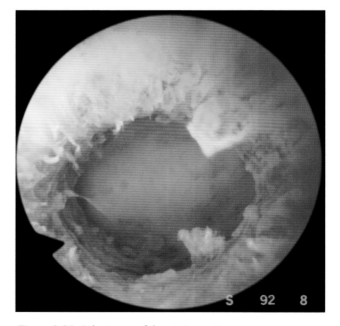

Figure 3.29: Isthmic area of the uterine cavity.

upper lateral parts ending at the tubal orifices are the cornual areas (*Figure 3.27*) leading to the orifices of the Fallopian tubes. Sometimes a small vault may be identified in the fundal area, indicating an arcuate uterus, with somewhat more pronounced cornual areas, which is also considered as being normal (*Figure 3.28*). When in doubt a hysterogram can be considered in order to help distinguish between an arcuate and a subseptate uterus.

The endocervix is separated from the uterine cavity by a slightly constricted area, the isthmus, at the lower margin of which is the internal cervical os. The isthmic portion of the uterine cavity is narrower than the upper uterine cavity (*Figure 3.29*) and its mucosa is less susceptible to hormonal changes than the endometrium of the upper part of the uterine cavity.

Adequate distension is mandatory for reliable hysteroscopic evaluation of the uterine cavity. With CF hys-

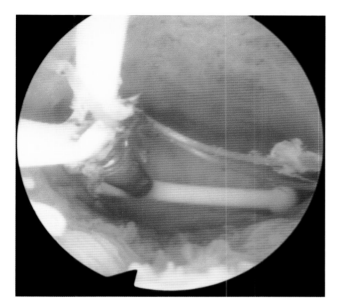

Figure 3.30: 'Lost' IUCD with intracavitary positioned threads.

teroscopy the intrauterine pressure can be changed for better assessment of the endometrial structure and the intramural extent of intrauterine pathology.

Rigid hysteroscopes should be rotated and moved laterally (*Figure 3.14*) for full inspection of the cornual areas and close inspection of the mucosa. With flexible hysteroscopes this can be accomplished by just bending the pliable tip.

IUCDs in the uterine cavity can be located easily (*Figure 3.30*). The hysteroscope should be guided very carefully alongside the stem of the device to prevent pushing the IUCD against the fundus, which could result in perforation.

ENDOMETRIUM

With CO_2 and Hyskon distension the endometrium is usually somewhat compressed as a result of the intrauterine pressure that is required for adequate visualization. CF distension with LVF provides for optimal visualization at any intrauterine pressure and degree of distension. This method enables a much better evaluation of the surface structure of the endometrium, especially with reduced intrauterine pressure (*Figure 3.31*).

The endometrium is very fragile and contact with the hysteroscope during examination should be avoided as much as possible. On contact the endometrium may be partially 'shaved off', producing endometrial fragments that could be interpreted as abnormalities and can obscure the panoramic vision.

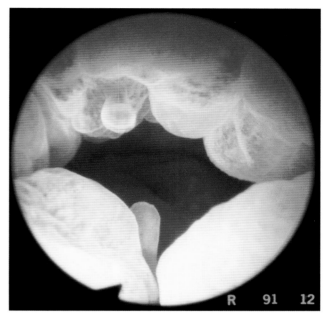

3.31a

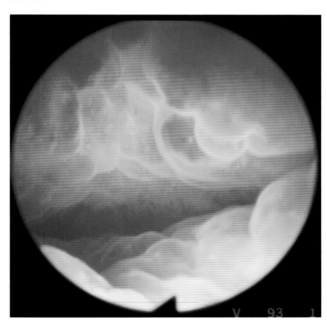

3.31b

Figure 3.31: (a) Mucosa of the isthmic area of the uterine cavity with reduced intrauterine pressure. (b) Uterine cavity and proliferative endometrium with reduced intrauterine pressure.

The thickness of the endometrium can be estimated by compressing it with the hysteroscope sheath, which will leave a ridge in the mucosa, almost equal to the endometrial thickness. With the progression of the menstrual cycle towards the midcycle ovulation, the thickness of the endometrium increases. Endometrial gland openings are clearly visible as small white spots (*Figure 3.32*). After ovulation the well proliferated endometrium will start to secrete and will resemble an undulating landscape (*Figure 3.33*). The endometrium during this period is fragile and very susceptible to contact damage. On the other hand it could be mistaken for hyperplasia and it can obscure intrauterine pathology. For this reason diagnostic hysteroscopy must be performed in the first half of the menstrual cycle. In cases of irregular or continuous bleeding proper scheduling will not be possible. In such cases endometrial hyperplasia due to hormonal dysfunction may be observed. Underlying pathology, such as more permanent hyperplasia, polyps or myomas, can be obscured by the thick,

hyperplastic endometrium. In these cases it is recommended that a repeat hysteroscopic procedure is performed shortly after a withdrawal bleeding, evoked by a 10 day course of a progesterone, to exclude other pathology. When endometrial hyperplasia has existed for some time, blood vessels can readily be seen in the endometrial outgrowths, and either polypoid structures or cysts may have developed. These structures will not be eliminated by a progesterone-induced withdrawal bleeding.

Occasionally, dilated blood vessels can be identified, the clinical significance of which is not yet defined (*Figure*

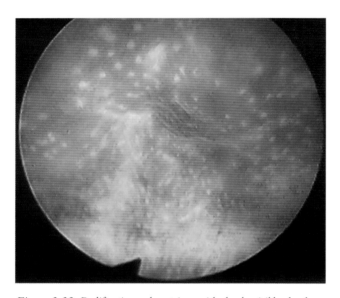

Figure 3.32: Proliferative endometrium with clearly visible gland openings.

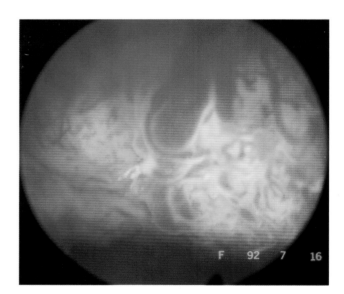

3.34a

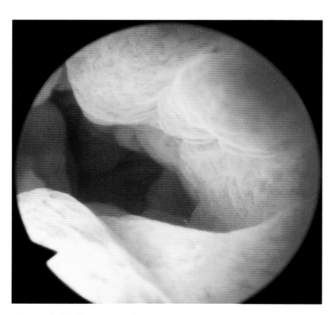

Figure 3.33: Secretory endometrium.

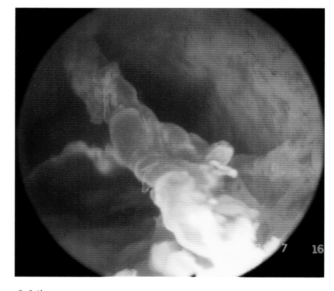

3.34b

Figure 3.34: (a) Dilated endometrial blood vessels.
(b) Endometrial proliferation with dilated blood vessels.

3.34); they may be responsible for intermenstrual bleeding because focal coagulation of these vessels has sometimes appeared to resolve this complaint.

Atrophic endometrium is very thin and flat and is white or yellow, with almost no, or only a very delicate, submucosal vascularization (*Figures 3.35* and *3.36*) (see also *Figure 2.10b*). Sometimes the vascularization can have a somewhat atypical aspect without pathology on histological examination. Even minor abnormalities can be recognized very easily in cases of atrophic endometrium, although 'abnormal' vascularization can lead to macroscopic overdiagnosis, which makes histological examination of biopsies of any abnormal appearance mandatory.

With oral contraception, especially pills with low estrogen content, the endometrium is flat and sometimes even atrophic (*Figure 3.37a*), but can also show different degrees of slight proliferation (*Figure 3.37b,c*). Generally it has a more reddish appearance than real atrophy and sometimes it has a rather pronounced subendometrial vascularization.

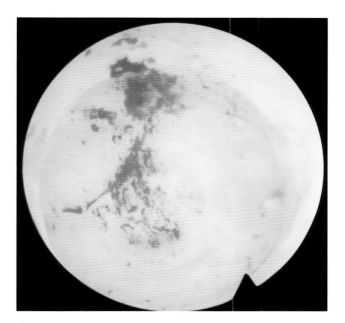

Figure 3.35: *Uterine cavity with atrophic endometrium.*

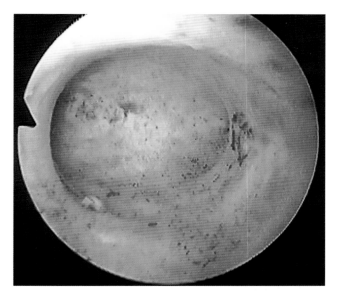

3.37a

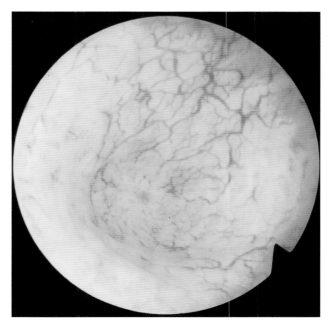

Figure 3.36: *Network of tiny submucosal blood vessels with atrophic endometrium.*

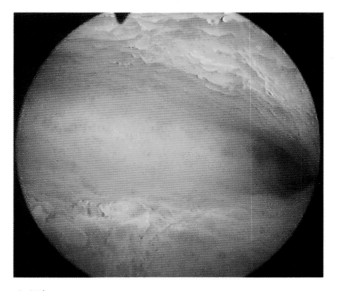

3.37b

Figure 3.37: *(a–c) Different degrees of endometrial proliferation in women with low estrogen-containing oral contraception.*

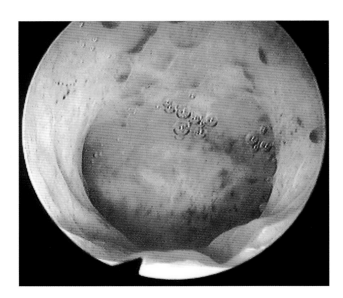

3.37c

Figure 3.37: continued.

TUBAL OSTIA

The tubal orifices differ in appearance from patient to patient and even the tubal ostia on both sides are never the same (*Figure 3.38*). Sometimes a mucosal diaphragm can be seen in front of the actual entrance to the tube, which is familiar from hysterosalpingographic images (*Figure 3.39*) (see also *Figure 5.5*) and the clinical relevance of which, if any, is not yet known (Coeman et al, 1995). Tiny polypoid structures can appear in the ostium and seem to be of no clinical significance. If

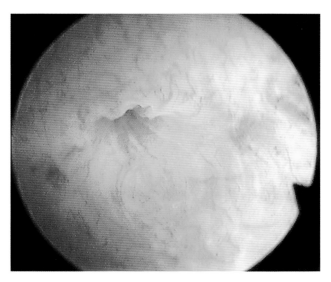

3.38a

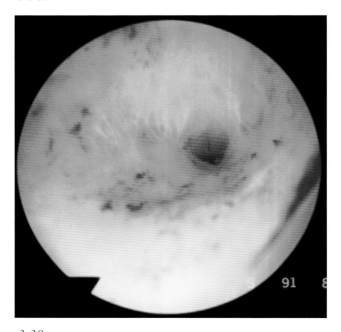

3.38b

3.38c

Figure 3.38: (a) and (b) Normal tubal orifice. (c) Tubal orifice with minor scarring.

larger, they should be considered to be pathological as they can obstruct the ostium mechanically (*Figure 3.40*).

In some cases the very first part of the intramural portion of the tube can be visualized, especially with increased intrauterine pressure and a multiparous uterus. In postmenopausal women the tubal orifices can be rather narrow (*Figure 3.41a,b*) or completely obliterated

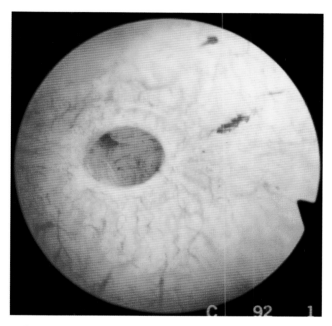

3.39a

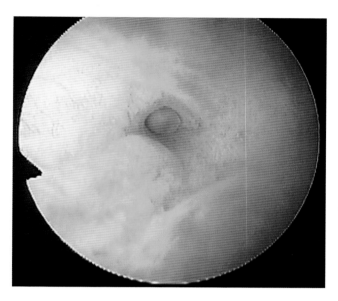

Figure 3.40: *Small polyp located in the entrance of the tube, which could result in functional obstruction.*

salpinx the flow with Hyskon distension will decrease and reflux will be seen when the pressure is discontinued.

With low viscosity fluid distension and CF technique tubal patency cannot be easily recognized because of the low viscosity of the liquid and the rapid circular flow in the uterine cavity.

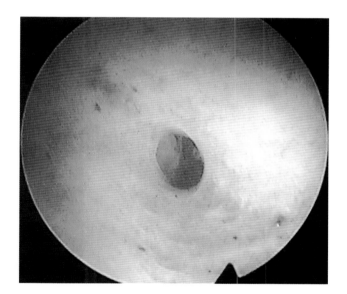

3.39b

Figure 3.39: *(a) and (b) Mucosal diaphragm in front of the actual entrance of the Fallopian tube.*

(*Figure 3.41c*).

With some of the distension media an indication of the tubal patency can be obtained: with CO_2 distension gas bubbles can be seen passing to the tubes and with Hyskon distension a flow with blood fragments or small bubbles through the ostia can be identified. In cases of hydro-

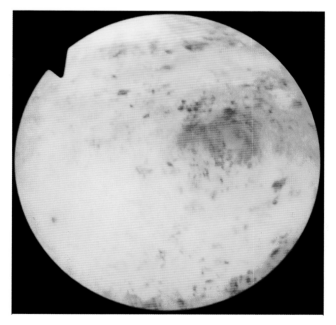

3.41a

Figure 3.41: *(a) Normal tubal ostium in postmenopause.*

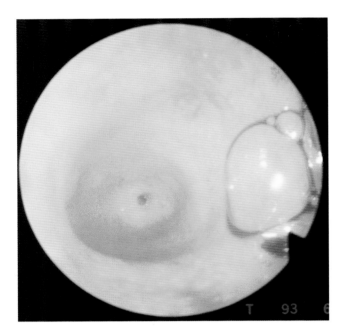

3.41b

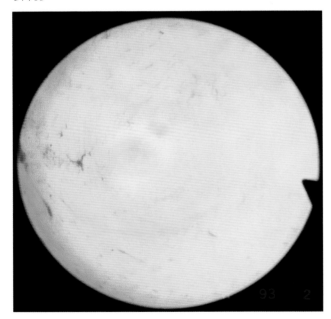

3.41c

Figure 3.41: *(a) and (b) Normal tubal ostium in postmenopause. (c) Obliterated tubal ostium in postmenopause.*

ARTIFACTS

Insertion of the hysteroscope without direct visual control can create a false route, especially if the endocervical wall has very pronounced clefts and ridges, in cases of sharp anteversion or retroversion or if the endocervical canal is abnormal. A false direction may be recognized by observing a 'dimple' in the endocervical wall. After further pro-

gression, where a false route remains unsuspected, penetration into the cervical stroma and the myometrium may eventually occur. The resulting image may be misinterpreted as fibrosis or adhesions. Ultimately, further penetration into the false route will lead to perforation. This is why it is essential to guide the hysteroscope through the

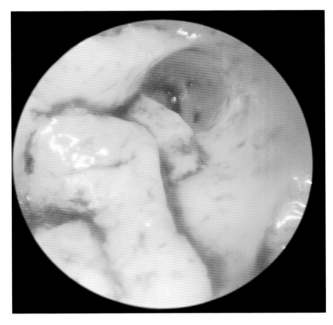

3.42a

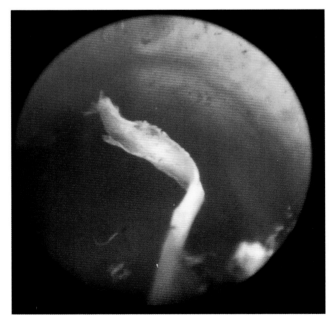

3.42b

Figure 3.42: *(a) Partly detached piece of endometrium with CO_2 distension; the tissue sticks to the wall of the uterine cavity. (b) and (c) Detached strip of endometrium with Hyskon (b) and low viscosity fluid (c) distension; the tissue floats freely in the liquid.*

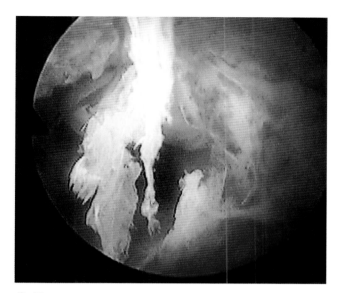

3.42c

Figure 3.42: continued.

endocervix and the internal os under visual control.

In the uterine cavity, contact of the hysteroscope tip with the endometrium can produce partially detached endometrial fragments, which could be misinterpreted as irregular shedding or 'polyps' (*Figure 3.42*).

Finally, in cases of complete perforation, the intestines and yellow mesenteric fat will be seen and the uterine cavity ceases to distend adequately. With CF distension almost no return fluid will be obtained, even with high liquid flow, and the procedure must be discontinued immediately.

REFERENCES

Barbot J, Parent B & Dubuisson JB (1980) Contact hysteroscopy: another method of endoscopic examination of the uterine cavity. *Am J Obstet Gynecol* **136**: 721-726.

Barents JW & vd Kolk G (1975) Iatrogene migratie van cellen en weefselelementen bij curettage. *Ned Tijdschr Geneeskd* **119**: 229–232.

Brundin J & Thomasson K (1989) Cardiac gas embolism during carbon dioxide hysteroscopy: risk and management. *Eur J Obstet Gynecol Reprod Biol* **33**: 241–245.

Coeman D, Van Belle Y & Vanderick G (1995) Tubal ostium membranes and their relation to infertility. *Fertil Steril* **63**: 666–668.

De Jong P, Doel F & Falconer A (1990) Outpatient diagnostic hysteroscopy. *Br J Obstet Gynaecol* **97**: 299.

Edström K & Fernström I (1970) The diagnostic possibilities of a modified hysteroscopic technique. *Acta Obstet Gynecol Scand* **49**: 327–330.

Emanuel MH, Verdel MJC, Stas H, Wamsteker K & Lammes FB (1995a) An audit of true prevalence of intra-uterine pathology: the hysteroscopical findings controlled for patient selection in 1202 patients with abnormal uterine bleeding. *Gynaecol Endosc* **4**: 237–241.

Emanuel MH, Verdel MJ, Wamsteker K & Lammes FB (1995b) A prospective comparison of transvaginal ultrasonography and diagnostic hysteroscopy in the evaluation of patients with abnormal uterine bleeding. *Am J Obstet Gynecol* **172**: 547–552.

Gilbert L, Saunders N & Sharp F (1990) Microcolpohysteroscopic tailoring of cervical conization. *Obstet Gynecol* **76**: 101–105.

Gimpelson RJ & Rappold HO (1988) A comparative study between panoramic hysteroscopy with directed biopsies and dilatation and curettage. *Am J Obstet Gynecol* **158**: 489–492.

Goldberg GL, Altaras MM, Levin W et al (1986) Microhysteroscopy in evaluation of the endocervix in endometrial carcinoma. *Gynecol Oncol* **24**: 189–193.

Guerra B, Mancini L, Linsalata I & Orlandi C (1988) Endocervical extension of cervical intraepithelial neoplasia: the role of microcolpohysteroscopy in clinical practice. *Cervix Lower Female Genital Tract* **6**: 219–224.

Hamou J (1981) Microhysteroscopy: a new procedure and its original applications in gynecology. *J Reprod Med* **26**: 375.

Hill NCW, Broadbent JAM, Magos AL et al (1992) Local anaesthesia and cervical dilatation for outpatient diagnostic hysteroscopy. *J Obstet Gynecol* **12**: 33–37.

Johnsson JE (1973) Hysterography and diagnostic curettage in carcinoma of the uterine body. *Acta Radiol Suppl* **326**: 1.

Lindemann HJ (1971) Eine neue Untersuchungsmethode für die Hysteroskopie. *Endoscopy* **4**: 194.

Lindemann HJ (1975) Komplikationen bei der CO_2 Hysteroskopie. *Arch Gynäkol* **219**: 257.

Lindemann HJ, Mohr J, Gallinat A et al (1976) Der Einfluss von CO_2 Gas während der Hysteroskopie. *Geburtshilfe Frauenheilkd* **36**: 153.

Loffer FD (1989) Hysteroscopy with endometrial sampling compared with D & C for abnormal uterine bleeding. *Obstet Gynecol* **73**: 16–20.

Loffer FD (1995) Complications of hysteroscopy: their cause, prevention and correction. *J Am Assoc Gynecol Laparosc* **3**, 11–26.

McLucas B (1991) Hyskon complications in hysteroscopic surgery. *Obstet Gynecol Surv* **46**: 196.

Motashaw ND & Dave S (1990) Diagnostic and therapeutic hysteroscopy in the management of abnormal uterine bleeding. *J Reprod Med* **35**: 616–620.

Neis KJ, Brandner P & Keppeler U (1994) Tumour cell spread via hysteroscopy? *Geburtshilfe Frauenheilkd* **54**: 651–655.

Noumoff JS & Faruqi S (1993) Endometrial carcinoma. *Microsc Res Tech* **25**: 246–254.

Raju KS & Taylor RW (1986) Routine hysteroscopy for patients with a high risk of uterine malignancy. *Br J Obstet Gynaecol* **93**: 1259.

Roberts S, Long L, Jonasson O et al (1960) The isolation of cancer cells from the bloodstream during uterine curettage. *Surg Gynecol Obstet* **111**: 3.

Rythén-Alder E, Brundin J, Notini-Gudmarsson et al (1992) Detection of carbon dioxide embolism during hysteroscopy. *Gynaecol Endosc* **1**, 207–210.

Sagawa T, Yamada H, Sakuragi N et al (1994) A comparison between the preoperative and operative findings of peritoneal cytology in patients with endometrial cancer. *Asia Oceania J Obstet Gynaecol* **20**: 39–47.

Salaz-Lizee D, Gadonneix P, Van Den Akker M et al (1993) The reliability of various methods for investigating the endometrium. A comparative study in 178 patients. *J Gynecol Obstet Biol Reprod (Paris)* **22**: 593–599.

Schmitz MJ & Nahhas WA (1994) Hysteroscopy may transport malignant cells into the peritoneal cavity. Case report. *Eur J Gynaecol Oncol* **15**: 121–124.

Spiewankiewicz B, Stelmachov J, Sawicki W et al (1995) Hysteroscopy with selective endometrial sampling after unsuccessful dilatation and curettage in diagnosis of symptomatic endometrial cancer and endometrial hyperplasias. *Eur J Gynaecol Oncol* **16**: 26–29.

Suprun HZ, Taendler-Stolero R, Schwartz J et al (1994) Experience with Endopap endometrial sampling in the cytodiagnosis of endometrial carcinoma and its precursor lesions: I. A correlative cytologic–histologic–hysteroscopic diagnostic pilot study. *Acta Cytol* **38**: 319–323.

Taddei GL, Moncini D, Scarselli G et al (1994) Can hysteroscopic evaluation of endometrial carcinoma influence therapeutic treatment? *Ann N Y Acad Sci* **734**: 482–487.

Takashima E (1985) Usefulness of hysteroscopy for detection of cancer in the endocervical canal. *Acta Obstet Gynaecol Jpn* **37**: 2401–2409.

Tseng P, Hunter V, Reed TP III & Wheeles CR Jr (1987) Microcolpohysteroscopy compared with colposcopy in the evaluation of abnormal cervical cytology. *Obstet Gynecol* **69**: 675–678.

Valle RF (1993) Cervical and uterine complications during insertion of the hysteroscope. In Corfman S, Diamond MP & DeCherney A (eds) *Complications of Laparoscopy and Hysteroscopy*, pp 167–176. Oxford: Blackwell Scientific.

Wamsteker K. (1977) *Hysteroscopie*. PhD thesis, University of Leiden.

Wamsteker K (1984) Hysteroscopy in the management of abnormal uterine bleeding in 199 patients. In Siegler AM & Lindemann HJ (eds) *Hysteroscopy, Principles and Practice*, pp 128–131. Philadelphia: JB Lippincott.

Wamsteker K & de Blok S (1993) Diagnostic hysteroscopy: technique and documentation. In Sutton C & Diamond MP (eds) *Endoscopic Surgery for Gynaecologists*, pp 263–276. London: WB Saunders.

Wamsteker K, de Blok S & Emanuel MH (1992) Instrumentation for transcervical hysteroscopic endosurgery. *Gynaecol Endosc* **1**: 59.

4 Endoscopy: laparoscopy
J Deprest and I Brosens

■ INTRODUCTION

Laparoscopy is a well established technique in the routine investigation and treatment of female pelvic pathology and infertility. It allows a complete and detailed examination of the pelvic organs and to a certain extent examination of the bowel, liver and inferior surface of the diaphragm. It is, however, an operative procedure which should be performed by an experienced surgeon who is competent to deal with any complication that may arise. Complications can occur even with experienced operators, although the risk is directly proportional to the skill of the surgeon. It is estimated that it takes 250 laparoscopies to develop the skill to be a safe operator and during the learning period the trainee must be guided by an experienced laparoscopist.

■ EQUIPMENT

The essential equipment for performing diagnostic or operative laparoscopy includes the following items:

- insufflator and insufflating needles
- laparoscope
- light source
- trocars and cannulas
- grasping and dissecting forceps and scissors
- electro- and thermocoagulation
- flushing cannula
- chip camera
- standard laparotomy instrument.

It is not necessary to have a large range of instruments to perform diagnostic laparoscopy; it is, however, necessary to have the correct instruments and to be able to deal properly with complications. The safety of laparoscopy depends on good visibility, gentle instrument and tissue handling, precise tissue dissection and effective control of bleeding. The reader is referred to standard textbooks of gynecological laparoscopy for guidelines about the choice of appropriate instruments: this chapter is restricted to the discussion of the basic principles of diagnostic procedures.

■ TECHNIQUE

Diagnostic laparoscopy must always be performed in a fully equipped operating theatre so that any complication that may arise can be treated without delay. In the case of major vessel laceration, it must be possible to convert immediately to laparotomy without moving the patient to another theatre or hospital. Appropriate instruments for performing laparotomy should be immediately available in the operating room.

As optimal visualization is the key to accurate diagnosis, the following conditions should be fullfilled (*Table 4.1*). A bowel preparation is administered the day before surgery, facilitating the pelvic inspection and reducing the risk and consequences of bowel injury. Minimal bowel preparation includes the prescription of a soft diet, stool softeners and large amounts of fluid 2 days before the procedure to reduce bowel distension. The bladder is emptied and the uterus is cannulated and fixed to allow manipulation.

Table 4.1 *Conditions for optimal visualization at diagnostic laparoscopy*

- Bowel preparation administered the day before surgery
- Empty bladder
- Uterus cannulated and fixed to allow manipulation
- Sufficient pneumoperitoneum
- Access for manipulating instrument
- Safe positioning of the patient, allowing 20–30° Trendelenburg tilt during inspection

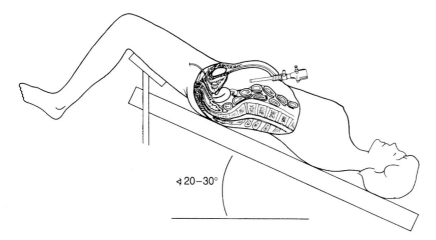

⊲ 20–30°

Figure 4.1: *Positioning of the patient after insertion of first trocar, for inspection and operative endoscopy. The patient is positioned in Trendelenburg, about 25°, with the legs in abduction and flexion at the hips.*

POSITIONING

THE PATIENT

Proper positioning of the patient is essential for:

- increased safety;
- optimal visualization of the pelvic organs;
- comfort of the operator.

Important features of correct positioning of the patient are:

- initial lithotomy position for access to the vagina and rectum;
- knees in flexion, to increase the stability of the patient once she is in the Trendelenburg position;
- Trendelenburg position:
  - ≤ 10° initially for insertion of Veress needle and trocar – more than 10° moves the lower aorta closer to the umbilicus.
  - 20–30° during actual endoscopy in order to prevent the bowel from sliding into the pelvic cavity and provide optimal access to the pouch of Douglas (*Figure 4.1*).

THE OPERATOR, ASSISTANT, NURSE AND INSTRUMENTATION (*Figure 4.2*)

Arrangement of instruments around the operating table depends basically on whether the operator is right or left handed. The description below is valid for a right handed operator. A mirror image would apply for a left handed physician.

- The operator stays at the left side of the patient. If available, the assistant will be on the patient's right side or between her legs. The nurse and instrument table are placed to the left of the operator.

- The instrumentation (i.e. insufflator, light source, etc.) and video monitor are placed to the caudal end of the patient, and thus in front of the operator. This is the most essential point because the operator must be able to monitor, at any given time, such parameters as intra-abdominal pressure and other settings. The operator, the target area (pelvis) and the monitor should be in one line. This line should be aligned as much as possible with the longest axis of the patient to facilitate stereotaxis of the operator and assistant.

LAPAROSCOPIC ENTRY

INSUFFLATION

Insufflation needle

Currently available insufflation needles are based on the Veress needle design. Such needles have a hollow sleeve, with a beveled, sharp needle point and a spring loaded blunt probe within it. When, at introduction, resistance at the tip of the needle is lost, the blunt probe moves

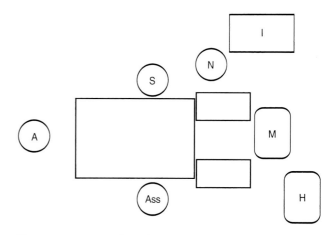

Figure 4.2: *Position of anesthetist (A), surgeon (S), assistant (Ass), nurse (N), monitor (M), hardware (H), and instrumentation (I).*

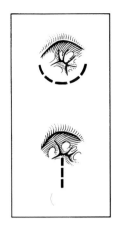

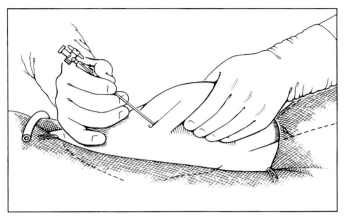

Figure 4.3: (a) Umbilical incisions and (b) correct insertion technique. The left hand elevates the lower abdominal wall; the right hand inserts the needle, holding it in a dart-like fashion. Reproduced with permission from Cusumano PG & Deprest J (1995) Advanced Gynecologic Laparoscopy. *London: The Parthenon Publishing Group. Illustration by Diane Bruyninckx.*

4.3a   4.3b

forward, providing the needle with a less harmful blunt tip, pushing away free-moving hollow viscera. The blunt probe has a distal lateral hole, allowing gas entry. Standard lengths of Veress needle are 100, 120 and 150 mm. When reusable needles are employed, the safety of the needle must be checked at the beginning of each procedure by verification of the spring function. The probe or needle may be bent during maintenance or packing for sterilization, preventing the probe from moving freely in the needle. Furthermore, the needle must be checked for patency by testing the flow of gas or fluid before each use. If it is not patent, there may be false pressure readings, suggesting malposition of the needle. Disposable needles are less likely to malfunction and are always clean, but apart from this they are probably no safer than reusable needles.

Umbilical insertion

Rigorous technique is compulsory: over half of major vessel lacerations are due to the Veress needle. In all patients, whatever their size, the umbilicus remains the thinnest part of the abdominal wall and seems a logical place for entry into the peritoneum. Abdominal palpation excludes large masses to be avoided during access. First an incision is made, large enough to prevent skin resistance during introduction of the Veress needle and subsequently for the trocar (*Figure 4.3*). The incision may be vertical or semilunar. After incision, the abdominal wall should be elevated with the left hand, lifting it in the direction of the pubis and away from the bifurcation. This can only be done in an adequately relaxed patient. Towel clips, Allis clamps, or even Kocher clamps on the anterior rectus sheath, may be used to elevate the abdominal wall. The needle should be held at its base with the right hand between index finger and thumb, in a dart-like fashion. The fifth finger is used as a stop to prevent unintentionally deep insertion of the needle once the fascial resistance is passed. Holding the needle between thumb and index finger allows the surgeon to feel and see the functioning of the spring during insertion. Penetration of the fascia and the peritoneum may be felt and seen separately with the Veress needle resistance and spring movement.

The needle should be inserted while it is open and not connected to the insufflation cable. Perforation of organs may thus be noted, either by sight or by the smell of the back flow of their contents. Further, on entry to the virtual space of the abdominal cavity, an open needle will allow air to enter it, prompting bowels to drop away from the abdominal wall.

The needle is initially directed perpendicular to the fascia, and then pointed towards the uterus. If any organs are to be damaged, the uterus is the most forgiving. By elevation, the axis of the needle pathway is lifted away from the bifurcation. Elevation does not reduce the risk of bowel perforation in cases of adherent bowel as it is lifted together with the abdominal wall.

Tests for peritoneal insertion

When a blind technique with a conventional Veress needle is used, some indirect tests are available to confirm correct positioning. The so-called 'waggling test' is the most frequently used in Western Europe and is based on the principle of tactile confirmation of a freely moving tip. Waggling is, however, potentially dangerous. If the point of the needle is in a major vessel, waggling will worsen a punctiform lesion into a true large laceration of that vessel. Other tests are therefore advocated. The so-called 'drop test' uses a drop of water on the back of the open Veress needle. If the needle is correctly placed, lifting up the abdominal wall will create a decrease in intra-abdominal pressure, and the drop will be suctioned into the cavity. The 'manometer test' is based on the same principle of negative intra-abdominal pressure. The needle is connected to the insufflation cable and, on elevation of the abdominal wall, falling pressure readings are noted when the needle is intraperitoneal. The 'aspiration–instillation–aspiration' test offers a double confirmation. After introduction, the needle is connected to a syringe and the surgeon first aspirates. When any material, such as blood, bile, bladder or bowel contents, is aspirated, the needle should be withdrawn and a clean one inserted. If nothing is aspirated, 10 ml of normal saline is injected and immediately thereafter reaspiration is attempted. When the needle is intraperitoneal and free, the fluid is dispersed in the abdominal cavity and cannot be reaspirated. If, however, the fluid is entrapped preperitoneally, or within abdominal adhesions, it will be possible to reaspirate it almost completely. An advantage of this test is that if a piece of tissue is trapped in the needle during insertion it will be flushed away. When the needle is correctly located, liver dullness will disappear. This sign is useless, however, as it comes fairly late and can even be positive with preperitoneal insufflation. Neither should one rely on the volume insufflated, as it is different for all patients and even large volumes can be insufflated preperitoneally. We tend to keep on insufflating until the preselected intra-abdominal pressure is reached, whatever the volume (or insufflation time) needed. The larger the volume of the pneumoperitoneum, the more comfortable the trocar insertion.

Small optics that allow the surgeon to look through the needle have become available: some diagnostic procedures can be completed through these small access ports (minilaparoscopy). Experience and performance with these operative procedures has not yet been formally evaluated.

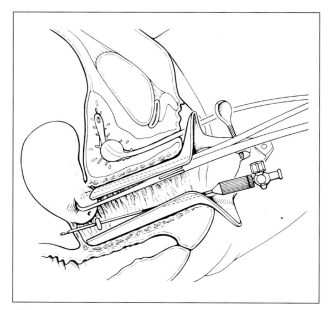

4.4a

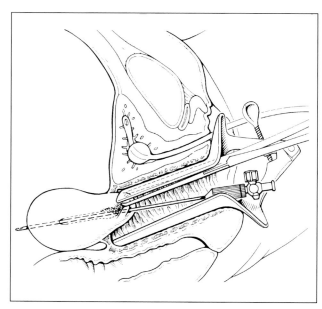

4.4b

Figure 4.4: (a) Posterior fornix insertion. The tenaculum, grasping the posterior part of the cervix, stretches the posterior vaginal fornix. (b) Transuterine insertion. Using a tenaculum, the uterus is pulled along the axis of the pelvis. Reproduced with permission from Cusumano PG & Deprest J (1995) Advanced Gynecologic Laparoscopy. *London: The Parthenon Publishing Group. Illustration by Diane Bruyninckx.*

Alternative needle insertion sites

Other sites of insertion have been described (*Figure 4.4*). Insertion of the needle can be performed through the cul-de-sac (Neely et al, 1975) or the uterus (Morgan, 1979). For both techniques, contraindications are any suspicion of pelvic adhesions, e.g. by previous myomectomy, history of pelvic inflammatory disease, extensive endometriosis, etc. Vaginal needles have a stop about 3 cm proximal to the tip to prevent overintroduction. Suprapubic insertion is also described. The uterus is manipulated against the anterior abdominal wall and the needle is first introduced into the uterine fundus and afterwards disengaged.

Adhesions, particularly to the midline of the anterior abdominal wall or to the umbilicus, may render umbilical access difficult or contraindicated (Childers et al, 1993; Lang et al, 1993). Under these circumstances, a 'left upper quadrant insertion', more accurately intercostal or infracostal, may be preferred. Contraindications are gastric, splenic or transverse colonic surgery. Patients should have a nasogastric tube inserted for aspiration of gastric contents. An incision is made in the ninth intercostal space, in the middle of the midclavicular or the anterior axillary line. Skin and various abdominal wall layers are attached to the ribs and do not move along them when being pierced with the needle. Two distinctive 'pops' can be felt. The adherence of the peritoneum makes preperitoneal insufflation unlikely. Alternatively, the incision and needle insertion can be made at the inferior costal margin. After insufflation, a 5 mm trocar is placed under the last rib, allowing a smaller scope to be used to judge the safety of larger trocar placement elsewhere, or to assist in adhesiolysis at other port sites.

Whenever any problems are met during needle insertion or insufflation, or there is doubt, our policy is to proceed with open laparoscopy (see below).

FIRST TROCAR INSERTION

The pneumoperitoneum provides a buffer space between the abdominal wall and hollow viscera, preventing direct trauma to the abdominal organs. Despite this, the introduction of the trocar remains a blind and dangerous step. The skin incision should be large enough to prevent any resistance at the level of the incision. Indeed, any resistance makes the surgeon lose the feeling of the tip of the instrument and use more force to introduce the trocar, increasing the risk of inadvertent trauma. Trocar blades should always be as sharp as possible. When an adequate pneumoperitoneum is established, lifting up the abdominal wall is not really useful as only the skin, not the entire anterior abdominal wall, is lifted. It is preferable to use both

hands to control the entry of the trocar. One hand is used to force the trocar, the other hand to arrest the forward penetration of the trocar once the fascia is perforated. (If only one hand is used, a stretched middle finger can prevent overinsertion.) When a pyramidal trocar is used, there is no reason to rotate the trocar during introduction. The sharp edges of the trocar will tear the fascia and cause subsequent gas leaks, and more force will be needed to enter the abdomen. The trocar is first moved horizontally under the skin for 1 cm, and then turned back to fix and penetrate the fascia. This is the so-called 'Z technique', which is believed to reduce the number of subsequent umbilical hernias because the skin and fascial defects are not directly aligned (*Figure 4.5*). Once the fascia is penetrated, the trocar should be directed to the uterus and not laterally to the major vessels.

Once the first trocar is inserted, the scope is inserted immediately to confirm appropriate insertion and absence of unintentional trauma. A complete overview of the abdominal cavity should precede any procedure, particularly looking for bleeding or trauma to organs that could have occurred during the first blind steps of the procedure.

OPEN LAPAROSCOPY

Hasson (1974) designed open laparoscopy as an entry method to eliminate the blind steps of insufflation and trocar introduction. This technique can be used primarily, may follow an unsuccessful Veress needle insertion or can be used in selected 'at risk' patients. The original technique consists of making a vertical infraumbilical incision of 2 cm. The fat is dissected away bluntly and specially designed Deaver retractors are used to expose the fascia. The fascia is grasped with a Kocher forceps and incised vertically. The peritoneum is then opened under direct view. Sutures are passed on both sides through the fascia, to secure the Hasson cannula later on. The sleeve, with the blunt obturator, can be introduced through the peritoneal opening, and an acorn-shaped collar is slipped down to seal the opening. Fascial sutures are tied to the special arms on the trocar sleeve. Insufflation can start immediately at a high flow rate. Open laparoscopy in experienced hands should not take much more time than the blind technique.

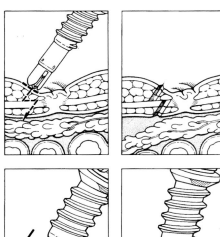
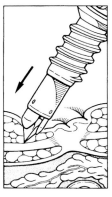
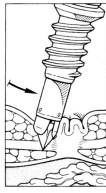
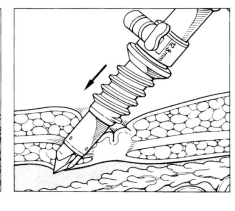

*Figure 4.5: **Z** technique for trocar insertion. Reproduced with permission from Cusumano PG & Deprest J (1995) Advanced Gynecologic Laparoscopy. London: The Parthenon Publishing Group. Illustration by Diane Bruyninckx.*

More recently, disposable modifications of the Hasson cannula have become available (*Figure 4.6*). Sutures are no longer needed; the cannula is anchored to the abdominal wall between expandable arms inside, and a gasket outside, which is screwed downwards to the skin. This gasket prevents gas leakage as long as the angle of the cannula to the skin is not too shallow. Other cannulas have an inflatable balloon at the tip which prevents gas leaks from inside. The abdominal wall is compressed

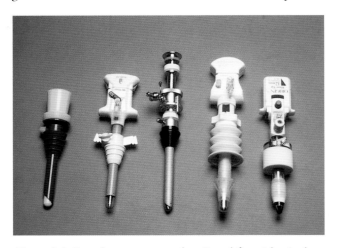

Figure 4.6: Open laparoscopy cannulas. From left to right: Apple and Ethicon modifications of Hasson's cannula (Karl Storz) (centre), Bluntport (Autosuture) and Blunttip (Origin). Reproduced with permission from Cusumano PG & Deprest J (1995) Advanced Gynecologic Laparoscopy. London: The Parthenon Publishing Group.

between the balloon and a rubber ring outside. This system performs well.

SECONDARY TROCAR INSERTIONS

From this point on, further ports are introduced under endoscopic view, minimizing the risk of internal injury. The location of these ports is decided according to the procedure to be performed and takes the anatomy into account (*Figure 4.7*). A general rule, the 'triangle of success' applies. Secondary ports should form a triangle with the target area. The target area is the top of the triangle, the two secondary cannulas form the base. The working ports should never be put closer than one fist from each other because any closer would align introduced instruments, rendering them inefficient. Ports should be inserted about 20 cm from the target area, as most instruments are designed to work at that distance. Because gynecologists usually work in the pelvis, secondary insertions in operative gynecology are into the left and right iliac fossae. A suprapubic insertion is made if a third instrument is used. For most procedures with three secondary ports it is easier to insert iliac ports well laterally. The ports are located to the breadth of two or three fingers above the pubic rim of the symphysis. When voluminous masses reach beyond the pelvis, ports should be inserted higher. During placement of lateral

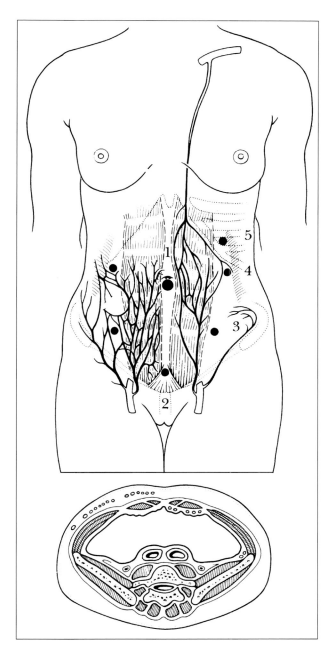

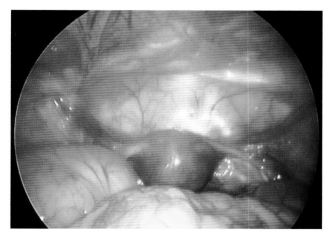

Figure 4.8: Panoramic view of the abdominal cavity.

Figure 4.7: Different insertion sites. Anterior view of the body, showing sites of insertion and anatomical pitfalls: 1, (peri)umbilical; 2, suprapubic; 3, iliac fossa (on the lateral border of the rectus muscle); 4, upper quadrant (3–5 cm under the last rib – called Palmer's point; and 5, inter- or infracostal. Reproduced with permission from Cusumano PG & Deprest J (1995) Advanced Gynecologic Laparoscopy. London: The Parthenon Publishing Group. Drawing by Diane Bruyninckx.

ports, epigastric vessels can easily be lacerated. Precautions, such as transillumination in thin patients, or parietal inspection, may prove to be helpful in identifying these vessels. The deep epigastric vessels arise at the medial borders of the internal inguinal ring, and lateral to the obliterated umbilical ligaments, under the rectus muscle. Superficial epigastric vessels run above the muscle: hitting them will cause percutaneous or subcutaneous bleeding. Trocars are inserted at a 90° angle to the fascia, either lateral or medial to the rectus muscle borders, avoiding these vessels.

INSPECTION

The laparoscopic evaluation includes a systematic inspection of the abdominal cavity and the pelvic organs.

ABDOMINAL CAVITY

With the patient still horizontal, the abdominal cavity is inspected systematically (*Figure 4.8*). The cecum and appendix are identified and their visual normality confirmed. The ascending colon is followed until the hepatic flexure is reached. The paracolic gutters are inspected for evidence of endometriosis or adhesions. The right lobe of the liver and inferior surface of the diaphragm are examined for evidence of adhesions, which may indicate sequelae of pelvic inflammatory disease (*Figure 4.9a*). It may be necessary to place the patient in the reversed Trendelenburg position to allow gas to flow in the upper abdomen for a clearer view of the liver and gallbladder. The telescope is withdrawn to allow it to pass the ligamentum falciparum and reach the left lobe of the liver (*Figure 4.9b*). The anterior aspect of the stomach is inspected. The spleen is

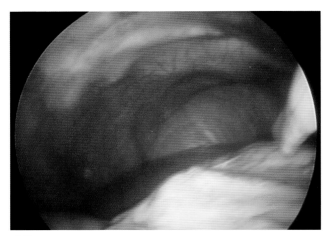

4.9a

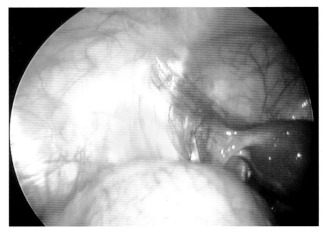

Figure 4.10: *Adhesions between the descending colon and the pelvic side wall are normal and can obscure the access to the left adnexa.*

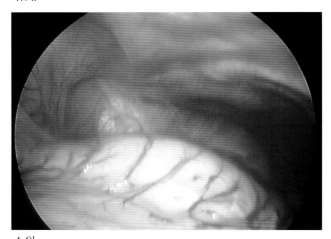

4.9b

Figure 4.9: *Inspection of upper abdomen: (a) right lobe of liver and diaphragm; (b) ligamentum falciparum and stomach.*

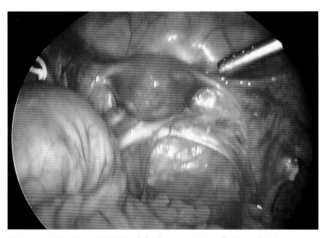

Figure 4.11: *At a 30° Trendelenburg position the bowel is kept above the pelvic brim. The bowel has been moved out of the pelvic cavity and the uterus is manipulated into anteversion, exposing the pouch of Douglas.*

normally not seen without retraction of the stomach, which is rarely indicated. The descending and sigmoid colon are inspected. It should be remembered that there are normally adhesions between the descending colon and the pelvic side wall that may partially obscure the left adnexa (*Figure 4.10*). These adhesions need not be dissected as they are physiological, and an increased Trendelenburg tilt and the use of a probe may be helpful in exposing the left adnexal area. The probe can also be used to palpate the consistency of the bowel.

THE PELVIC ORGANS

After systematic inspection of the abdominal cavity the Trendelenburg position is increased to 30° in order to allow the bowel to slide above the promontorium (*Figure 4.11*). The bowel is moved out of the pelvic cavity and stabilized above the promontorium. Having the

patient's legs in a horizontal or only slightly elevated position preserves the lumbar lordosis, which will prevent the bowel from sliding into the pelvic cavity. It should be stressed that it is impossible to perform a complete examination of the pelvic organs using a simple puncture technique.

Uterus

This is first inspected in its normal position. It is then elevated and anteverted for examination of the size and shape of the corpus and its relationship with the round ligament, Fallopian tube and ovarian ligaments, and to define the presence of the normal anatomy or defects in fusion of the Müllerian ducts, or intramural or subserous fibroids (*Figure 4.11*).

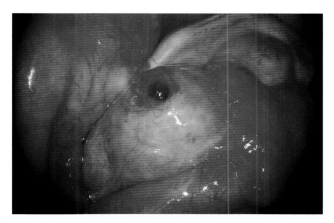

Figure 4.12: A corpus luteum with an ovulation stigma is demonstrated by lifting and rotating the ovary.

Fallopian tubes

After inspection of the uterus, the Fallopian tubes are examined in detail. They must be visualized throughout their length from uterine horn to fimbriae. During the examination the diameter and mobility of the isthmus and ampulla should be noted. The fimbriae are closely inspected for the presence of adhesions. Later on, irrigation and underwater inspection may complete the evaluation.

Ovaries

The ovaries are inspected carefully and their size and any evidence of ovarian activity are noted. Follicular and luteal structures are noted and a recent corpus luteum can be identified by the presence of an ovulation stigma (*Figure 4.12*). The surface of the ovary is fully inspected for the presence of endometriosis or adhesions. Filmy, nonvascularized adhesions can be masked as they collapse against the ovarian surface because of the pneumoperitoneum. The anterior side and the hilus of the ovary are exposed. Grasping the ovary should be avoided as this may cause trauma to the surface epithelium and provoke adhesions. It can be useful to lift the ovary and manipulate the uterus into the fossa ovarica. While it is resting on the anterior surface of the uterus, the ovary can be slowly rotated and fully inspected (*Figure 4.13*).

Pelvic peritoneum

Examination of the pelvic peritoneum should proceed in a schematic direction commencing with the anterior abdominal wall, then moving to the bladder and uterovesical pouch, the anterior side of the right broad ligament,

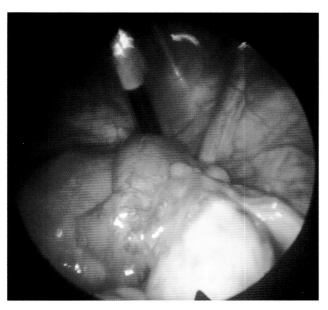

Figure 4.13: The ovary and ampullary segment are lifted and exposed. By moving the uterus into the fossa ovarica the adnexa rests on the anterior surface of the uterus, allowing careful examination of the ovary and fimbriae.

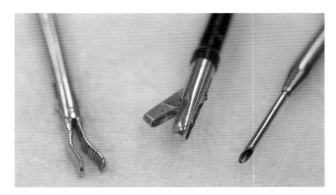

Figure 4.14: Atraumatic and biopsy forceps, and an aspiration needle are essential accessory instruments in diagnostic laparoscopy.

the round ligament, the Fallopian tube, the posterior surface of the broad ligament and the pouch of Douglas and back to the anterior cul-de-sac via the left side.

Additional explorations

- Peritoneal cytology and/or peritoneal washings are sampled whenever indicated in the initial stage of laparoscopy (*Figure 4.14*).
- Tubal patency is controlled by the dye test using a dilated solution of methylene blue or indigo carmine. A 5 mm probe is useful for cannulating the infundibulum whenever a phimosis is suspected.
- Hydroflotation is a very useful technique for controlling the fimbriae and detecting fimbrial adhesions and filmy, avascular ovarian adhesions (*Figure 4.15*).

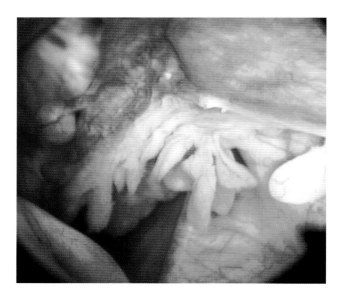

Figure 4.15: *Hydroflotation is a useful technique for exposing the fimbriae and detection of filmy adhesions.*

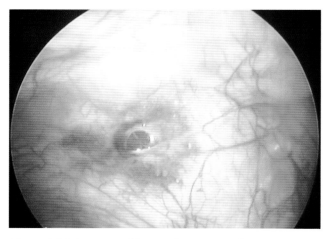

Figure 4.16: *Inspection of the secondary incision after retracting the cannula shows the bruised area.*

■ Punctures to detect hemorrhagic cysts in an enlarged ovary can be useful but if abnormalities are found they should always be confirmed by biopsy. The place of biopsy, puncture and aspiration is discussed in the chapters on adnexal mass (Chapter 21), pelvic inflammatory disease (Chapter 18) and endometriosis (Chapter 19).

■ Biopsies are an integral part of diagnostic laparoscopy (*Figure 4.14*).

■ Diagnostic laparoscopy may necessitate operative procedures such as adhesiolysis to gain access to pelvic organs and to mobilize the ovary or Fallopian tube for full inspection.

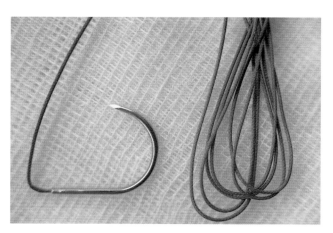

Figure 4.17: *J-shaped needle for closure.*

CLOSING THE ABDOMINAL WALL

At the end of the procedure, and after control of hemostasis, the carbon dioxide should be allowed to escape. Inspection with a partially deflated abdomen may reveal bleeding that was previously invisible because of high intra-abdominal pressure. An underwater examination, as described by Reich, might also be helpful. Secondary incisions might start bleeding when the cannula is withdrawn, so one should look for this before retracting the endoscope (*Figure 4.16*). Some surgeons leave in a drain, and/or local anesthetic, which may be helpful in alleviation of postoperative pain (Narchin et al, 1991; Loughney and Ryall, 1994). When a trocar is pulled out, the obturator is left in the sleeve to prevent the bowel being pushed into the empty cannula by positive intraperitoneal pressure, caused by remnants of pneumoperitoneum, or

coughing if the patient wakes up prematurely.

Small skin incisions, i.e. up to 5 mm, can be approximated superficially with strips or sutures, although very recently a report about omental herniation in a 5 mm port has been published. Even when the fascia and the peritoneum are closed, irrigation fluid may drain through the stab wounds and patients should be informed about this. For incisions larger than 5 mm the fascia is closed separately because both umbilical and lateral incisional hernias have been observed (Kadar et al, 1993). The fascia should be exposed with retractors and closed under view, e.g. with specially designed J-shaped needles (*Figure 4.17*). In obese patients identification of fascia may be difficult, particularly in the lower quadrants. Various instruments for facilitating closure have been described (Phipps and Taranissi, 1995).

■ CONTRAINDICATIONS

The contraindications to laparoscopy have been well established and should be strictly observed.

The *absolute contraindications* include mechanical and paralytic ileus, extremely large abdominal mass, hypovolemic shock, specific medical disorders such as cardiorespiratory failure or myocardial disease, severe obstructive airway disease and irreducible hernia.

The *relative contraindications* include multiple abdominal incisions, abdominal wall sepsis, generalized peritonitis, gross obesity, blood dyscrasia and coagulopathy, and hiatus hernia. The decision to perform or not to perform a laparoscopy will depend on the experience of the surgeon as well as the importance of a laparoscopy to the patient's health.

At risk patients are obese or very thin patients, patients with strong abdominal muscles (sportswomen), patients with a deformed vertebral axis, children and dwarfs. The open laparoscopy technique has been designed as an entry method to eliminate the blind steps of insufflation and trocar introduction and this technique can be used in such patients. Medical conditions should be stabilized before any surgical procedure is performed, and in cases of hiatus hernia the volume of gas can be limited and steep Trendelenburg avoided. Other techniques such as the abdominal wall elevator may also be more suitable in such patients.

■ COMPLICATIONS AND RISKS

Laparoscopy is a potentially dangerous surgical procedure and major complications can only be avoided by meticulous attention to detail, early recognition of problems and correct handling of complications. According to large survey studies, the risk of serious complications of diagnostic laparoscopy decreased in the 1980s as a result of increased experience. With the sudden increase in operative procedures in recent years and inadequate training, the current risk of laparoscopy in general has increased. The risk of complications of diagnostic laparoscopy (Veress needle, trocar) is estimated at 3–4%. Some of the more serious complications are due to anesthesia. Other complications include failed procedures, burns, direct trauma of pelvic organs, bowel and urinary tract, hemorrhage and infection (*Table 4.2*). Death has occurred as a result of damage caused by the laparoscopic entry technique:

- skin knife incision injury to vena cava
- Veress needle in kidney and gas embolism

Table 4.2 *Complications of diagnostic laparoscopy (Chamberlain and Carron Brown, 1978)*

Complications	Rate per 1000 laparoscopies
■ Anesthetic complications	
Anesthetic	0.8
Cardiac arrhythmias	0.4
Cardiac arrest	0.2
■ Failed procedures	
Failed laparoscopy	7.5
Failed abdominal insufflation	3.5
Failed vaginal insufflation	0.0
■ Burns	
Skin	0.3
Other	0.2
■ Direct trauma	
Pelvic organs	3.4
Bowel	1.8
Urinary tract	0.2
■ Hemorrhage	
Pelvic blood vessels and mesosalpinx	2.7
Abdominal wall	2.5
Mesentery of bowel	1.1
Pelvic side wall and ovarian vessels	0.9
■ Infection	
Abdominal wound	0.5
Pelvic	0.5
Urinary tract	0.5
Chest	0.2
■ Other complications	
Chest pain	0.3
Pulmonary embolism	0.2
Deep vein thrombosis	0.2
Late complications	0.1

- Veress needle tear of vena cava
- trocar injury of large vessels
- second-puncture injury to iliac vessels
- abdominal wall bleeding after trocar removal.

A potential danger is that diagnostic laparoscopy is extended to operative laparoscopy with procedures of doubtful or unproven benefit to the patient. The surgeon may be tempted to reason that the diagnostic laparoscopy can be extended with a minor surgical procedure on the basis of potential benefit to the patient. It is evident that any surgical procedure performed at the time of laparoscopy carries an extra risk of complications and that the appropriateness of each procedure must be based on scientific evidence independent of the availability of easy access. All too often, the risks of adhesion formation and its consequences for ovarian and tubal function are underestimated.

REFERENCES

Chamberlain GVP & Carron Brown J (1978) *Gynaecological Laparoscopy*. London: Royal College of Obstetricians and Gynaecologists.

Childers JM, Brzechffa PR & Surwit EA (1993) Laparoscopy using the left upper quadrant as the primary trocar site. *Gynecol Oncol* **50**: 221–225.

Hasson HM (1974) Open laparoscopy: a report of 150 cases. *J Reprod Med* **12**: 234–238.

Kadar N, Reich H, Liu CY, Manko GF & Gimpelson R (1993) Incisional hernias after major laparoscopic gynecologic procedures. *Am J Obstet Gynecol* **168**: 1493–1495.

Lang PFJ, Tamussino K & Hönigl W (1993) Palmer's point: an alternative site for inserting the operative laparoscope in patients with intra-abdominal adhesions. *Gynaecol Endosc* **2**: 35–37.

Loughney AD & Ryall EA (1994) Intraperitoneal bupivacain for the relief of pain following day case laparoscopy. *Br J Obstet Gynaecol* **101**: 449–451.

Morgan HR (1979) Laparoscopy: induction of pneumoperitoneum via transfundal puncture. *Obstet Gynecol* **54**: 260–261.

Narchin P, Benhamou D & Fernandez H (1991) Intraperitoneal local anaesthetic for shoulder pain after day case laparoscopy. *Lancet* **388**: 1569–1570.

Neely MR, McWilliams R & Makhlouf HA (1975) Laparoscopy: routine pneumoperitoneum via the posterior fornix. *Obstet Gynecol* **45**: 459–460.

Phipps JH & Taranissi M (1994) Laparoscopic peritoneal closure needle for prevention of port hernias and management of abdominal wall vessel injury. *Gynaecol Endosc* **3**: 189–191.

5 Hysterosalpingography
AM Siegler

■ INTRODUCTION

The hysterosalpingogram (HSG) is a relatively painless, simple, nonoperative screening procedure. It remains a basic test before undertaking surgical correction of pelvic causes of infertility, despite the arrival of modern diagnostic gynecological techniques, such as laparoscopy, hysteroscopy, ultrasonography (US) and magnetic resonance imaging (MRI).

Although the HSG cannot define the extent of conditions such as endometriosis and periadnexal adhesions, it reveals the shape of the uterine cavity and important characteristics of the tubal lumina besides their patency. Careful performance and interpretation are essential so that the radiological findings can be correlated with endoscopic examinations. When the properly performed hysterogram is interpreted as normal, it is unusual to find significant intrauterine disease at hysteroscopy. With normal fill and spill of the contrast material from both Fallopian tubes, it is uncommon for the laparoscopic examination to detect significant tubal disease.

■ INSTRUMENTS

Various cervical cannulas have been described. The Jarcho has an adjustable steel collar and rubber acorn. The latter are positioned about 0.5 cm from the perforated end of the cannula and the acorn held in place by the metal collar. Alternatively a balloon catheter (Yoder, 1988) can be inserted through the endocervical canal and inflated with about 2 ml of sterile water or air. Its major disadvantage is that it can obscure the lower uterine segment and sometimes makes interpretation of intrauterine lesions difficult (*Figure 5.1*). With a vacuum cannula, a cup adheres to the cervix by suction (Malstrom, 1961). Although this technique enables excellent observation of the endocervical canal and lower uterine segment, there is frequent loss of suction

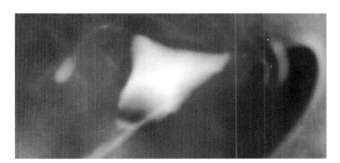

5.1a

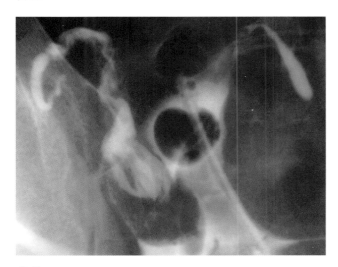

5.1b

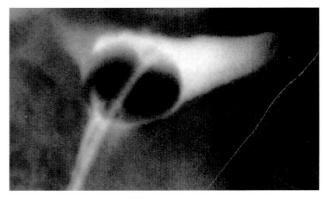

5.1c

Figure 5.1: *(a)–(c) A balloon catheter was used for these hysterosalpingograms: possible intrauterine abnormalities could be obscured.*

during uterine manipulation, and a suction apparatus and cups of different sizes are needed.

■ CONTRAST MEDIA

Many contrast media have been used in HSG since the procedure was first described by Rindfleisch (1910), who injected bismuth solution into the uterine cavity. Subsequently oil-based contrast media (OBCM) like Lipiodol and Ethiodol were developed. Water-based contrast media (WBCM) with various viscous additives are used presently to avoid the risks of oil embolism and granuloma formation. In a comparative study between low-osmolality WBCM and conventional WBCM, no differences were noted concerning the incidence of abdominal pain, allergic reactions, or in the ability to make a radiological diagnosis (Andrew et al, 1981; Rappaport et al, 1982).

All media used for HSG contain iodine, some are soluble in water and others in oil. Both types have certain advantages and disadvantages. The physician should be familiar with their characteristics because the type of medium can influence the technique of the examination and the interpretation of the radiographs. WBCM pass through the uterus and tubes more quickly and greater amounts are needed. With WBCM, normal rugal folds characterized by longitudinal dark lines are seen. In distally obstructed tubes, a dark line is often visible if the endosalpinx is not damaged severely. OBCM will not mix with fluid in a hydrosalpinx so that pear-like formations occur. The proponents of OBCM claim that these media give a clearer, sharper image, cause less abdominal pain after peritoneal spill, and peritubal disease can be detected more accurately in the drainage radiograph.

■ TECHNIQUE

The best radiographs with fewest complications can be obtained by gaining the patient's confidence and cooperation through explanation of the procedure and by gentle manipulation of the instruments. Painful contractions due to prostaglandin release resulting from the stretching of the myometrium during uterine dilatation can be reduced by the oral application of a prostaglandin synthetase inhibitor

2 hours before the procedure. A tranquilizer is suggested for a very apprehensive patient. Proximal tubal occlusion caused by uterotubal spasm can result from stress or from irritation of the contrast material. No medication has been successful in reducing spasm of the myosalpinx that envelops the interstitial tubal segment (World Health Organization, 1983).

The time in the cycle for the HSG varies according to the patient's clinical condition, although most procedures are done in the first week after menses. (The search for an incompetent cervical isthmus should probably be done with a premenstrual HSG when physiological contraction of the lower uterine segment is greatest.) The cannula is filled with contrast material to flush out the air because artifacts in the uterine cavity can be caused by air bubbles. After a tenaculum is fixed on the anterior cervical lip, the cannula is inserted into the external cervical os and the two instruments are held together by the properly gowned (lead apron, neck collar) physician. A scout film is suggested if a previous pelvic radiographic study was done in which contrast material was used. Small increments of contrast material are instilled as spot films are taken at propitious intervals during television fluoroscopy. Four exposures can be recorded on one 10 × 12 film. If the corpus appears displaced, traction on the tenaculum should correct the abnormal position that can prevent adequate examination of the lower uterine segment and proper evaluation of the uterine cavity (*Figure 5.2*). Manometric control is not necessary. The end points of the examination are the observations of tubal filling and spilling (*Figure 5.3*) or the complaint of increasing abdominal pain during the injection. A follow-up or drainage radiograph is essential to observe dispersion of the media. It should be taken about 30 minutes after removal of the instruments if WBCM is used. With OBCM, the drainage radiograph is taken the following day because these media do not disperse as rapidly in the peritoneal cavity (Bateman et al, 1987). To improve on the accuracy of spot films, assembled pressure registration devices were used (Karande et al, 1995). The authors found elevated tubal perfusion pressures were an ominous sign with regard to future fertility potential. Normal perfusion pressures reduced the need for a diagnostic laparoscopy as a first stage procedure.

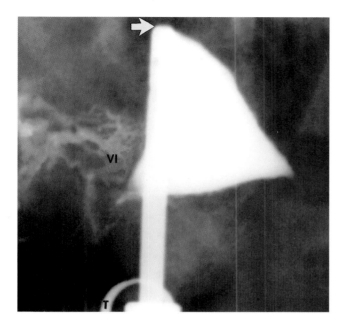

5.2a

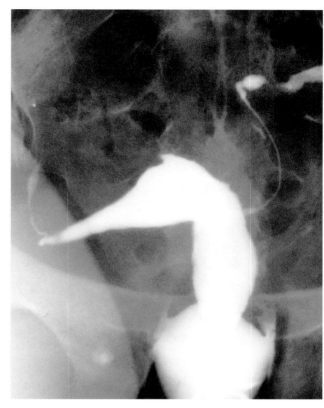

5.2c

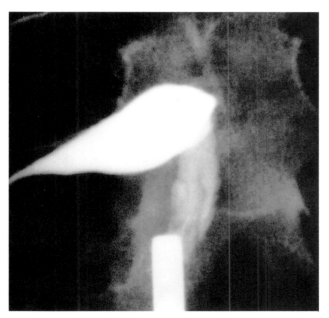

5.2b

Figure 5.2: *A failure to exert sufficient traction on the cervix prevents proper evaluation of these hysterosalpingograms. (a) Arrow indicates tip of cannula almost through the lower uterine segment. Vascular intravasation (VI) is also noted. (b) The endocervical canal is seen clearly but the uterine cavity appears on end. (c) The contrast material is seen initially in the vagina, then the endocervical canal, and fills the uterine cavity and parts of both Fallopian tubes. All three hysterosalpingograms are inadequate for proper interpretation. T, tenaculum.*

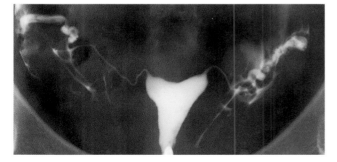

Figure 5.3: *Complete filling of a normal uterine cavity and Fallopian tubes, with spillage.*

Excessive amounts of media expose the patient needlessly to the risk of mucosal or peritoneal irritation and prevent proper interpretation of the films whereas insufficient fluid results in an incomplete study.

THERAPEUTIC EFFECTS OF HYSTEROSALPINGOGRAPHY

The HSG has often been claimed to have a therapeutic as well as a diagnostic function in infertility. A few investigators have purported to show a fertility-enhancing effect of OBCM in a group of patients with infertility of unknown cause (Soules and Spadoni, 1982; Schwabe et al, 1983; Watson et al, 1994). Some beneficial effects attributed to the HSG include:

- expulsion of inspissated mucus or blood from the tubal lumen;
- the ability to straighten kinks at the uterotubal junction or to stretch peritubal adhesions;
- dilatation of tubes in patients with fimbrial phimosis;
- creation of a favorable effect on the tubal epithelium because of the iodine content of the contrast material;
- stimulation of tubal contractibility from a bolus of fluid;
- effects on the immune milieu in the posterior cul-de-sac.

While Alper et al (1986) reported data of a prospective, randomized study that showed no difference in pregnancy rates between OBCM and WBCM, other retrospective studies suggested that OBCM may enhance fertility in that group of patients with idiopathic or unexplained infertility. The occurrence of pregnancy within 6 months of such a treatment might be considered as treatment dependent and suggested a beneficial effect of OBCM. The results of a study by Cundiff and co-authors (1995) offer some guidelines for the timing of diagnostic laparoscopy (LSC) after a normal HSG. Based on their findings it seemed prudent to wait at least 3 months after a normal HSG before proceeding with an LSC. In women who did not conceive within one year after HSG, LSC is indicated because a high incidence of pelvic abnormalities was found.

■ RISKS, COMPLICATIONS AND SIDE EFFECTS

Some lower abdominal pain and discomfort caused by the placement of the tenaculum, the insertion of the cannula, and the instillation of the contrast material are not uncommon. These symptoms are often related to the skill and patience of the physician.

Morbidity and sequelae occasionally result despite careful use (Hunt and Siegler, 1990). Some adverse effects from HSG are caused by selection of inappropriate patients or an improper technique. HSG can exacerbate pelvic inflammatory disease (PID), lead to peritonitis, a pelvic abscess, and occasionally the need for a laparotomy to solve the problem. The patients at increased risk for such an infection are those with a his-

tory of PID. The incidence and severity of the pelvic peritonitis are not influenced by the type of medium and no protective effects from prophylactic antibiotics has been shown.

The potential for hypersensitivity reactions to iodine exists with any of the HSG media but allergic reactions are rare. Uterine perforation and postexamination hemorrhage are also possibilities. Other types of complications include granuloma formation and vascular intravasation. The effects of the latter are reduced by observation of the onset of the event during the fluoroscopic examination and promptly stopping the procedure.

To reduce the exposure to radiation, other HSG methods have been described, including 100 mm fluorography, low dose, scanning-beam HSG, and color Doppler ultrasound HSG. With the latter technique sterile saline solution is used as the 'contrast material' (Battaglia et al, 1996). The risk from pelvic radiation is small. The total radiation dose to the ovaries depends on the:

- radiation output from the particular radiological equipment;
- size and shape of the patient and the composition of her tissues;
- fluoroscopic dose plus the dose from the permanent radiographs;
- number of radiographic exposures made per patient, the range being between two and six exposures per study. The objective is to reduce the radiation exposure with all diagnostic radiographic procedures.

■ NORMAL APPEARANCES

Uterine cavity

The HSG is a screening procedure that gives the initial clue to the possibility of a uterine anomaly, submucous tumors, or significant intrauterine adhesions. Since the types of abnormalities cause different reproductive outcomes and require different clinical management, a precise diagnosis is important. It is necessary to know the shape of the uterine serosal surface and of the uterine cavity. US and MRI also have been used for this purpose.

Always begin the evaluation of the HSG by viewing the endocervical canal. Its serrated borders are caused by anatomical plicae palmatae (*Figure 5.4*). Abnormalities of the endocervical canal detectable by the HSG include polyps and adhesions that cause filling defects.

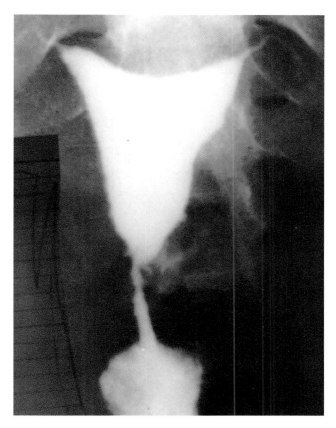

Figure 5.4: A normal uterine shadow ideally shows the endocervical canal with plicae, a narrow lower uterine segment and triangular-shaped uterine cavity.

The normal lower uterine segment has smooth parallel borders. This segment may be unusually wide, more than 1 cm in an incompetent os. Outpouchings, spicular or wedge-shaped diverticula can occur from a previous cesarean operation. The normal uterine cavity has a triangular appearance with smooth borders. The upper border, the fundus, may be convex or saddle-shaped, and the cornua are generally pointed. Physiological alterations may cause various indentations along the lateral borders of the uterine shadow but their persistence on sequential radiographs suggests an organic defect rather than a contraction.

FALLOPIAN TUBES

The HSG is an important procedure for evaluating the Fallopian tubes and, occasionally, peritoneal causes of infertility. Its advantages include the ability to show proximal and distal occlusion and some cornual lesions, and to assess the intratubal architecture. The limitations

of HSG are its inability to reveal endometriosis and significant periadnexal adhesions can escape detection; instances of false positive diagnoses of proximal tubal obstruction occur. The HSG and laparoscopy should therefore be complementary, not competitive investigative procedures.

In the search for tubal patency, the end of the HSG is either tubal filling and spill or increasing abdominal pain. If the tubes are not opacified on the HSG it is important to know:

- if the cervix was occluded adequately;
- the amount of contrast material used;
- the reason for discontinuation of the procedure before tubal filling.

Peritoneal spill from a normal HSG is identified easily. The dispersion of the agent in the pelvis depends upon:

- the type and amount of medium used;
- the degree of tubal patency;
- the presence and extent of significant periadnexal adhesions.

Collections of medium in the lateral pelves should not be mistaken for centrally placed fluid retained within the uterine canal or wall. The interpretation of small, localized pelvic collections of contrast material caused by significant peritubal adhesions, fimbrial phimosis, or even hydrosalpinges can be difficult. Contrast material coming from one patent tube may obscure the pattern of the contralateral oviduct. When an oily material is used, it may be difficult to be certain whether the 'pearly clusters' are in the cul-de-sac fluid or if they are enclosed in a hydrosalpinx. Some tubal forms look normal initially, but the follow-up or drainage radiograph may show localization of the contrast material. Sharply defined borders suggest that the contrast medium is confined within the tube. A 'halo' configuration indicates periadnexal adhesions that allow some of the fluid to surround and outline the tubal wall.

PROXIMAL TUBAL OBSTRUCTION

To differentiate cornual spasm from organic disease the intramural segment should appear filled. It is uncommon to see proximal tubal obstruction caused by organic disease in the intramural segment. The radiological differentiation of isthmic from intramural obstruction on

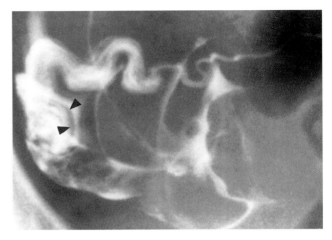

Figure 5.6: The normal outline of the tubal lumen is seen with water soluble contrast medium; arrowheads indicate dark lines caused by rugal folds.

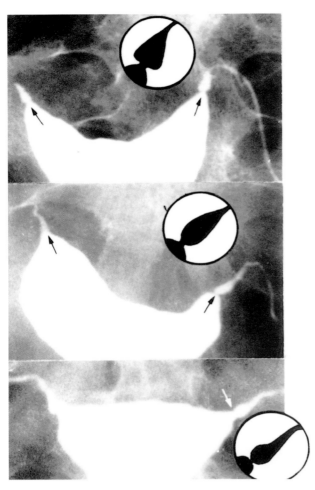

Figure 5.5: Arrows point to a pretubal bulge caused by a membrane that separates the intramural segment from the uterine cavity. Insets illustrate the most common types of pretubal bulge.

HSG can be difficult because the myometrial width cannot be discerned radiographically. The intramural section originates from the uterine cornu and extends as a fine line for about 1.5–2 cm, sometimes containing an ampulla-like dilatation, a pretubal bulge (*Figure 5.5*). It may be helpful to remember the so-called 'thumb' sign: the width of the thumb placed at the cornu will approximate that of the myometrium, the tubal shadow underneath the thumb representing the intramural segment. Ostial or selective salpingography and tubal cannulation is a technique used in patients who have a diagnosis of proximal tubal obstruction.

DISTAL TUBAL OBSTRUCTION

Ampullary opacification suggests that the proximal tube is patent, although not necessarily normal. Although distally obstructed tubes sometimes have small club-shaped ends, they can reach as much as 4–5 cm in diameter, holding large amounts of fluid. Linear dark shadows seen within the lumen, obtained with WBCM, are formed by the rugae and their presence portends a better prognosis following neosalpingostomy than if they are not evident (*Figure 5.6*). Distal tubal obstructions have been classified into four groups based on the HSG findings varying from Degree I, fimbrial phimosis, to Degree IV, occlusion with ampullary diameter more than 25 mm. One of the prognostic factors following neosalpingostomy besides thickness of the tubal wall, the percentage of ciliated cells, and the morphological condition of the tube is the degree of ampullary dilatation ascertained with HSG.

Many studies have described and compared the findings of laparoscopy and the HSG. The radiological study seems to overdiagnose proximal tubal obstruction and miss significant periadnexal adhesions. With proper technique and careful interpretation concordant results should be obtained in 70% of cases. However, the newer methods of hysteroscopy and transvaginal sonography may also be used in the evaluation of tubal patency in the infertile woman. Indeed in women whose tubes appear blocked, these methods of investigation may enhance the accuracy of tubal patency (Mitri et al, 1991). It is more usual to have a normal HSG followed by significant peritubal adhesions than to have an abnormal HSG followed by a normal laparoscopic examination. Other techniques used to detect tubal patency include the use of human serum microspheres labeled with technetium-

99m applied directly to the cervical mucosa (McCalley et al, 1985). These spheres will migrate from the vagina to the ovaries when the tubes are patent. Transvaginal high frequency transducer probes can produce pictures of a high resolution, thus enabling imaging of the Fallopian tube. Timor-Tritsch and Rottem (1987) reported on sonographic pictures of the normal and abnormal tube by this method and these authors could delineate the tubal lumen, its walls and content, and also location and mobility. In the future, transvaginal sonography (TVS) may replace HSG and limit the need for laparoscopic chromopertubation which still seem to be the 'gold standards' for the assessment of tubal patency. It appears to be a new, promising, low cost, reliable, safe and relatively painless method in which air and saline are used as the contrast medium (Heikkinen et al, 1995).

■ SUMMARY

HSG is a basic part of the infertility investigation and often the results give the physician the first clue to the presence of an intrauterine or tubal abnormality. Technically unsatisfactory or poorly interpreted HSGs are not uncommon, so that it appears justified to offer suggestions to improve skills in performance and interpretation.

REFERENCES

Alper MM, Garner PR, Spence JEH et al (1986) Pregnancy rates after hysterosalpingography with oil- and water-soluble contrast media. *Obstet Gynecol* **68**: 6–9.

Andrew E, Dahlstrom K, Sveen K et al (1981) Amipaque (metrizamide) in vascular use and use in body cavities: a survey of the initial clinical trials. *Invest Radiol* **16**: 455–465.

Bateman BG, Nunley WC Jr, Kitchin JD et al (1987) Utility of the 24 hour delay hysterosalpingogram film. *Fertil Steril* **47**: 613–617.

Battaglia C, Artini PG, D'Ambrogio G et al (1996) Color doppler hysterosalpingography in the diagnosis of tubal patency. *Fertil Steril* **65**: 317–322.

Cundiff G, Carr BR & Marshburm PB (1995) Infertile couples with a normal hysterosalpingogram: reproductive outcome and its relationship to clinical and laparoscopic findings. *J Reprod Med* **40**: 19-24.

Heikkinen H, Tekay A, Volpi E et al (1995) Transvaginal sonography for the assessment of tubal patency in infertile women: methodogical and clinical experiences. *Fertil Steril* **64**: 293-298.

Hunt RB & Siegler AM (1990) *Hysterosalpingography: Techniques and Interpretation*, pp 25–46. Chicago: Year Book Medical.

Karande V, Pratt DE, Rabin DS et al (1995) The limited value of hysterosalpingography in assessing tubal status and fertility potential. *Fertil Steril* **63**: 1167-1171.

McCalley MG, Braunstein P, Stone S et al (1985) Radionuclide hysterosalpingography for evaluation of fallopian tube patency. *J Nucl Med* **26**: 868–874.

Malstrom T (1961) A vacuum uterine cannula. *Obstet Gynecol* **18**: 773–776.

Mitri FF, Andronikou AD, Cheatwood M et al (1991) A clinical comparison of sonographic hydrotubation and hysterosalpingography. *Br J Obset Gynaecol* **98**:1031-1036.

Rappaport S, Bookstein JJ, Higgins CB et al (1982) Experience with metrizamide in patients with severe anaphylactoid reactions to ionic contrast agents. *Radiology* **143**: 321–325.

Rindfleisch W (1910) Darstellung des Cavum Uteri (Tubargraviditat). *Klin Wochenschr* **4**: 780–781.

Schwabe MG, Shapiro SS & Haning RV Jr (1983) Hysterosalpingography with oil contrast medium enhances fertility in patients with infertility of unknown etiology. *Fertil Steril* **40**: 604–606.

Soules MR & Spadoni LR (1982) Oil versus aqueous media for hysterosalpingography: a continuing debate based on many opinions and few facts. *Fertil Steril* **38**: 1–11.

Timor-Tritsch IE & Rottem S (1987) Transvaginal ultrasonographic study of the fallopian tube. *Obstet Gynecol* **70**: 424–428.

Watson A, Vandekerckhove P, Lilford R et al (1994) A meta-analysis of the therapeutic role of oil soluble contrast media at hysterosalpingography: a surprising result? *Fertil Steril* **61**: 470–477.

World Health Organization (1983) A new hysterographic approach to the evaluation of tubal spasm and spasmolytic agents. *Fertil Steril* **39**: 105–107.

Yoder IC (1988) *Hysterosalpingography and Pelvic Ultrasound in Infertility and Gynecology*. Boston: Little, Brown.

6 Lymphography and arteriography
A Kolbenstvedt

LYMPHOGRAPHY

■ INTRODUCTION

Lymphography is the best imaging method for visualization of the lymph vessels and the internal architecture of the inguinal, pelvic and lumbar nodes. Before the introduction of modern methods, such as ultrasonography, computed tomography (CT) and magnetic resonance imaging (MRI), lymphography was extensively used in oncological imaging. The first lymphangiography of lymph vessels was reported by Kinmonth (1954) and the first lymphadenography of nodes by Bruun and Engeset (1956). The visceral internal iliac lymph nodes, the nodes of the mesentery and nodes cranial to the diaphragm are not demonstrated by pedal lymphography. This fact, combined with the somewhat tedious procedure, prompted a gradual decline of lymphography for most clinical purposes during the late 1970s and early 1980s. The main literature describing normal lymphographic variations is found in publications from the 1960s and early 1970s. Recent research has dealt with methods for indirect lymphography with subcutaneous contrast medium injection and CT or MRI (Wolf et al, 1994). Knowledge of normal variations of lymph vessel anatomy is necessary for diagnostic considerations. Obstruction of lymph flow and formation of collateral flow is one of the signs of tumor spread to the lymphatic system. The difference between pathological collaterals and normally occurring loops should therefore be known. Additionally, knowledge of normal variations in the lymphographic appearance of the nodes is a prerequisite for any serious attempt to diagnose nodal disease. To assist the surgeon in an attempt to achieve a complete pelvic nodal dissection, the radiologist must be able to interpret an intraoperative radiograph in frontal projection and advise the surgeon where to look for the remaining nodes.

■ TECHNIQUE

After injection of 0.2 ml patent blue violet 11% intradermally in the first interdigital space of each foot, a lymph vessel is exposed through a small longitudinal incision on the dorsum of the foot. The vessel is cannulated with the aid of an operation microscope and an oil based contrast medium (Lipiodol Ultra Fluid 0.48 g iodine/ml; Guerbet, France) is injected by an electrically driven pump. The speed of injection is 3 ml/h on each side. As soon as contrast medium can be demonstrated in the thoracic duct by fluoroscopy, the injection is discontinued and the incisions on the feet sutured. Radiographs are exposed immediately to visualize the lymph vessels (lymphangiograms), and the following day to visualize the lymph nodes (lymphadenograms).

■ BENEFITS AND LIMITATIONS

Lymphography from the foot allows the vast majority of both the normal and metastatic pelvic lymph nodes to be visualized. Using the above technique, it was possible to visualize radiologically 98.1% of 9187 lymph nodes later removed by pelvic lymph node dissection from 300 consecutive patients with carcinoma of the uterine cervix (Kolbenstvedt, 1974a). Of 209 lymph nodes with metastases removed from these patients, 7.7% contained no contrast medium. Another 7.7% contained small amounts, while 84.6% were well filled with medium.

Filling defects combined with abnormal lymph vessel collaterals and filling defects which appear or grow during a 6 week observation period are reliable signs of metastasis. The number and size of lymph vessels and nodes allow diagnosis of other conditions, such as lymphatic hypoplasia, and also show regenerated lymph vessels and nodes and pooling of contrast medium in lymphoceles after pelvic lymph node dissection. The contrast medium stays within the nodes long enough to permit intraoperative radiography during the pelvic lymph node dissection, which in these patients is performed approximately 6 weeks after lymphography.

Preoperative lymphography with intraoperative radiographic control may be used to insure nearly complete and uniform lymph node dissection in institutions where patients with carcinoma of the uterine cervix stages Ib and II are treated surgically (Kolbenstvedt and Kolstad, 1974). This procedure also allows additional lymph node metastases to be removed with the aid of the intraoperatively exposed radiograph. The limitations of lymphography are related to the fact that very small (microscopic) metastases cannot be detected, and that, occasionally, fairly large metastatic foci may also be overlooked. Although lymphography and intraoperative radiography have a proven effect on the completeness of a pelvic lymph node dissection, a definite effect on the survival of cancer patients remains to be proven.

■ COMPLICATIONS, SIDE EFFECTS AND CONTRAINDICATIONS

The main risk of lymphography is related to the fact that the surplus contrast medium, which is not retained in the lymph nodes, is carried to the lungs through the thoracic duct, major veins and pulmonary artery. If the injection is not discontinued at the right time, the examination will cause a temporary reduction of the diffusing capacity of the lungs. Major surgery under general anesthesia immediately after lymphography may have a fatal outcome. Allergic reactions to dye or contrast medium may also occur (Lossef and Barth, 1993). Inadvertent injection into a small vein instead of a lymph vessel may be disclosed by fluoroscopy of the legs and pelvis: in veins the fat soluble contrast medium appears as round droplets (caviar sign). To prevent complications a prelymphography chest radiograph and an interview regarding chest disease is important. Lymphography should be avoided in patients with impaired lung function or pulmonary arteriovenous malformations. Previous serious reactions to contrast media are also considered as contraindications, as well as infectious skin conditions in the

region of the cut-down on the dorsum of the feet. These precautions, combined with meticulous fluoroscopy during the infusion period and avoidance of immediate surgery, make the procedure a safe one.

■ NORMAL APPEARANCES

LYMPH VESSELS

The lymphangiogram exposed immediately after injection demonstrates the femoral, inguinal, iliac and lumbar vessels.

In the upper aspect of the femoral region 5–15 lymph vessels enter inguinal nodes at the convex border (*Figure 6.1*). From the nodal hili fewer efferent inguinal vessels

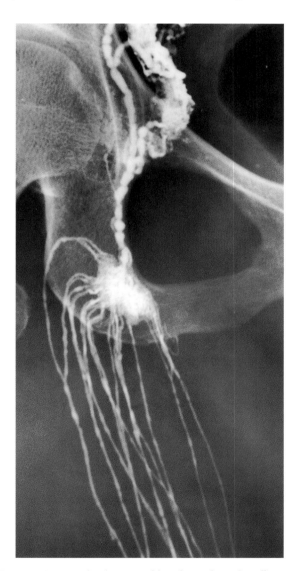

Figure 6.1*: Normal right inguinal lymph vessels: twelve afferent vessels to convexity of node; one efferent vessel from nodal hilum.*

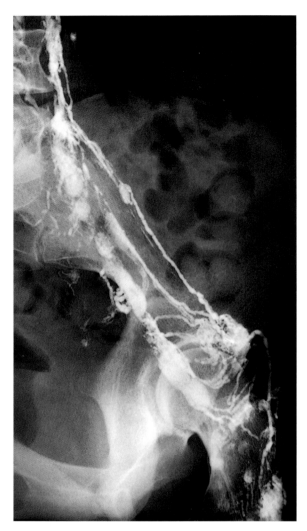

Figure 6.2: Left iliac lymph vessels in three chains: lateral, inter-mediate and medial.

enter into the external iliac region. Here the lymphatics are divided into three chains according to the classic descriptions by Cunéo and Marcille (1901) and Rouvière (1932). They run on either side of and between the external iliac artery and vein. The lateral, intermediate and medial chains are clearly demonstrated at lymphography (*Figure 6.2*) in about 40% of normal cases; more often the vessels have a disorderly and unsystematic appearance where the three main trunks cannot be discerned.

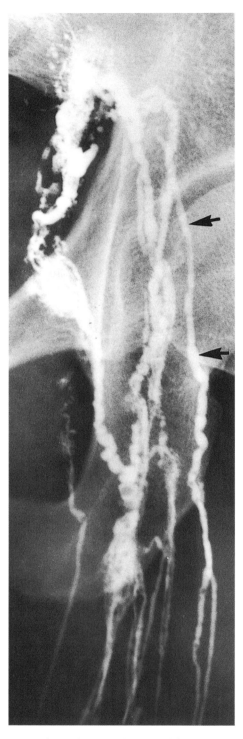

Figure 6.3: Lymph vessel (arrows) bypassing left inguinal region to lower iliac nodes. From Kolbenstvedt (1974b) with permission.

BYPASSES

All nodal groups may be bypassed. An inguinal bypass with a femoral lymph vessel passing directly into an iliac node is illustrated in *Figure 6.3*. The inguinal bypass usually ends in the most distally situated lateral external iliac node – the lateral lacunar node. The lateral lacunar node may thus often be functionally regarded as an inguinal node, although anatomically belonging to the iliac group. External iliac bypasses (*Figure 6.4*) occur in 3.5% (Kolbenstvedt, 1974b). As a rule these vessels pass by the external iliac and the lower part of the common iliac region to small nodes along the iliac crest. Common iliac bypasses are observed in about 1% of normal lymphangiograms (*Figure 6.5*). Nodes along the iliac crest may be filled through these vessels. Lumbar bypasses have been described on the right side (*Figure 6.6*).

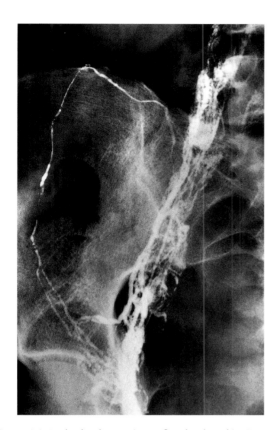

Figure 6.4: *Right iliac bypass (circumflex iliac branch). From Kolbenstvedt (1974b) with permission.*

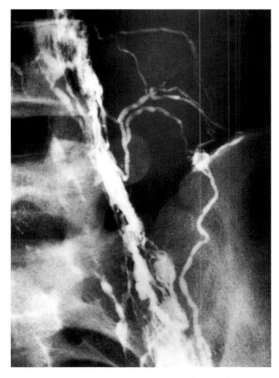

Figure 6.5: *Left common iliac bypasses with filling of node along iliac crest. From Kolbenstvedt (1974b) with permission.*

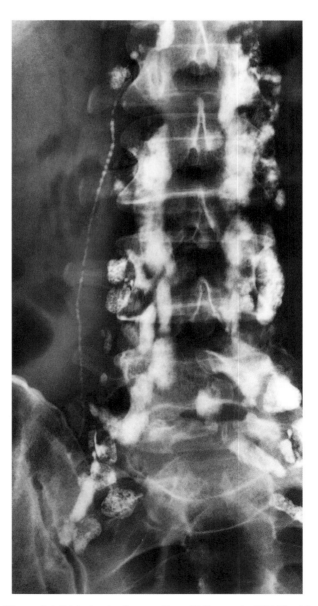

Figure 6.6: *Right lumbar bypass. From Kolbenstvedt (1974b) with permission.*

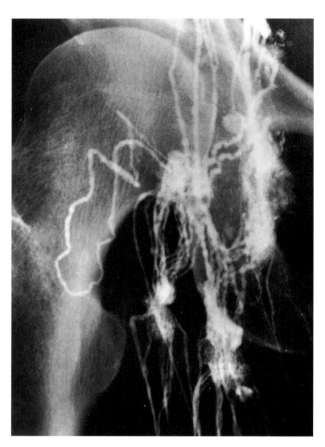

Figure 6.7: Lateral inguinal loop. From Kolbenstvedt (1974b) with permission.

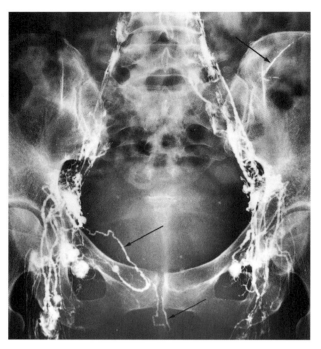

Figure 6.8: Pubic loop (arrows) to subpubic area. Filling of right obturator node. Also left iliac bypass (arrow).

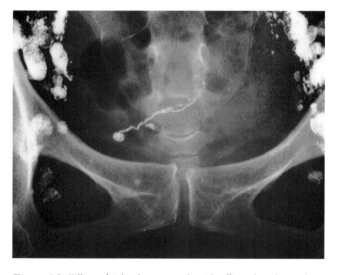

Figure 6.9: Filling of right obturator node with afferent lymph vessel.

BLIND LOOPS

Lateral inguinal loops occur in about 1% of cases (*Figure 6.7*). Pubic loops occur occasionally and may fill the so-called 'obturator node' (*Figure 6.8*). Further cranially, blind intercostal loops may appear.

LYMPH VESSELS TO THE OBTURATOR NODE

The name 'obturator node' is reserved for one or a few small internal iliac nodes along the peripheral branches of the obturator artery cranial to the obturator foramen. Visualization of this node occurs in 2–3%, and unusual lymph vessels to the nodes in 1–2% of normal cases (*Figures 6.8* and *6.9*).

PRESACRAL ANASTOMOSIS

Transverse presacral anastomosis appear in 3% of cases (*Figure 6.10*), while the lateral sacral lymph nodes are seen in nearly half of the patients.

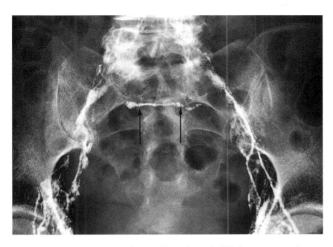

Figure 6.10: Right lateral sacral lymph node filled via presacral anastomoses (arrows).

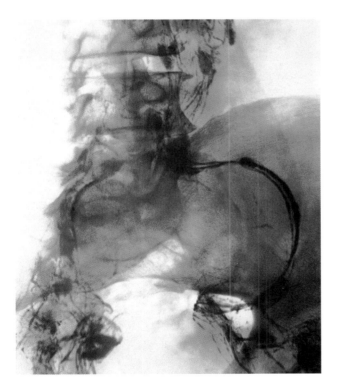

Figure 6.11: Displaced left iliac lymph vessel due to arterial tortuosity.

LYMPH VESSEL DISPLACEMENT

Tortuous arteries often displace lumbar and iliac lymph nodes and vessels (*Figure 6.11*), giving rise to differential diagnostic difficulties.

A number of additional collaterals have been reported in pathological conditions. The following abnormal

collaterals were never observed in 200 normal patients:

- dermal back flow (Kinmonth, 1972)
- uterine or rectal collaterals (Fuchs et al, 1968)
- mesenteric, splenic or hepatic collaterals (Cunningham, 1969)
- perineural sheath collaterals (Wallace et al, 1964)
- abdominal wall collaterals to the axillary region (Hartgill, 1964).

This supports the suggestion that these collaterals have a pathological significance. Trapping of oil droplets in veins through lymphovenous anastomosis was not observed in 200 normal cases (Kolbenstvedt, 1974b).

LYMPH NODES

The inguinal nodes (*Figure 6.12*) and the most distal external iliac nodes (*Figure 6.13*) often have contrast medium defects due to fibrolipomatous tissue with an upward concavity. These defects may be distinguished

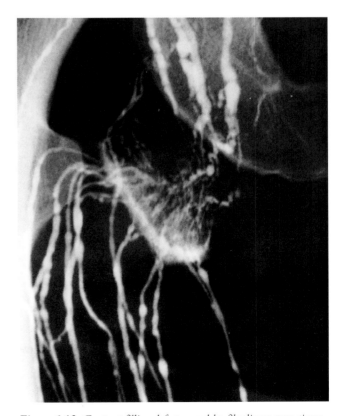

Figure 6.12: Contrast filling defect caused by fibrolipomatous tissue in right inguinal node. Defect is traversed by vessels. From Kolbenstvedt A (1975) Acta Radiol **16**: *81, with permission.*

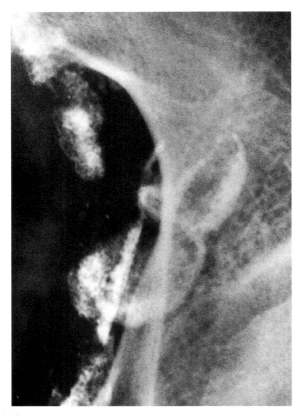

6.13a

from defects due to metastatic deposits as lymph vessels may be seen to traverse the fibrolipomatous defect (*Figure 6.12*) but not the metastatic defect. The distal external iliac nodes are called 'lacunar nodes', because they lie in the lacuna vasorum. The lateral lacunar nodes have contrast medium defects so often that they have also been named the 'semilunar nodes'. Analogous to the lymph vessels, the external iliac nodes are ranged in three columns: the external or prevascular group, the intermediate group and the medial group (*Figure 6.14*). The distal node of the medial external iliac group may lie close to, or be continuous with, the upper deep medial inguinal node (node of Cloquet).

The nodes along the parietal branches of the internal iliac artery (*Figure 6.15*) are the lateral sacral nodes, the superior and inferior gluteal nodes and the rarely seen obturator nodes. Internal iliac nodes are filled at lymphography in nearly 50% of cases. They often have defects due to fibrofatty tissue, like the inguinal and distal external iliac nodes.

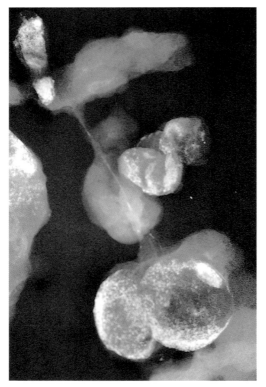

6.13b

Figure 6.13: *(a) Lower left external iliac lymph nodes with semilunar appearance due to lipomatosis. From Kolbenstvedt A (1975)* Acta Radiol *16: 81, with permission. (b) Radiograph of removed nodes with lipomatous infiltration.*

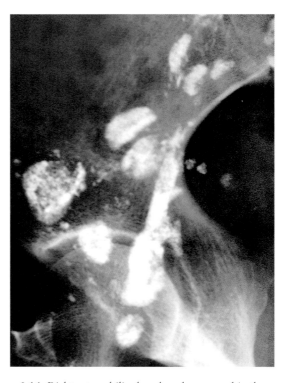

Figure 6.14: *Right external iliac lymph nodes arranged in three groups. The lowest node in the medial group often remains after lymph node dissection.*

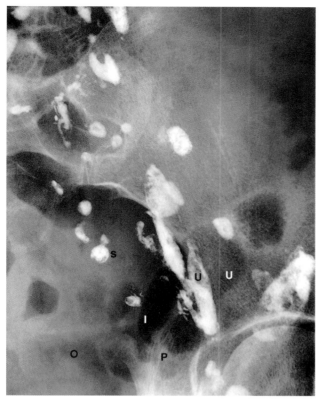

6.15a

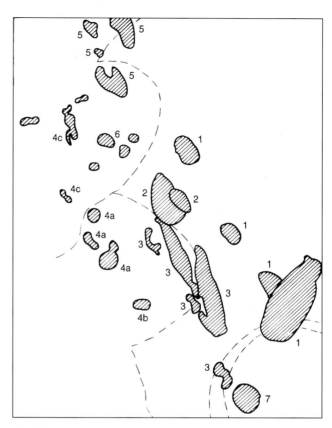

6.15b

Figure 6.15: *(a) Left external iliac nodes and left internal iliac nodes. From Kolbenstvedt (1974a) with permission. (b) Nomenclature of the left iliac lymph nodes (shown in oblique projection): 1, lateral external iliac; 2, intermediate external iliac; 3, medial external iliac; 4, internal iliac (4a, superior gluteal; 4b, inferior gluteal;*

4c, lateral sacral); 5, common iliac; 6, nodes of the iliac bifurcation (these nodes lie on the borderlines between the external, internal and common iliac regions: exact classification is difficult without arteriography); 7, deep inguinal .

During pelvic lymph node dissection certain nodes have a tendency to remain, as shown on intraoperative radiographs. These nodes are the nodes of the internal iliac chain, the distal node of the medial external iliac group, and the intermediate nodes in the common iliac region (Kolbenstvedt and Kolstad, 1976). Here, the intermediate nodes are lying in a retrovascular position in the fossa between the psoas muscle and the body of

the fifth lumbar vertebra (Cunéo and Marcille's fossa).

Since the most important signs of metastatic infiltration are contrast medium defects in the lymph nodes combined with abnormal lymphatic collaterals due to obstruction, it is a prerequisite for correct interpretation to be familiar with the normally occurring nodal defects and the normal variation of lymph vessels.

ARTERIOGRAPHY

■ TECHNIQUE

Catheterization of a femoral artery using the Seldinger technique is the preferred approach. Bilateral simultaneous visualization of the internal iliac arteries (*Figure*

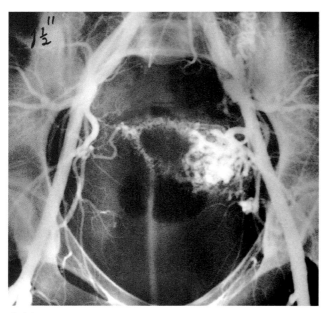

6.16a

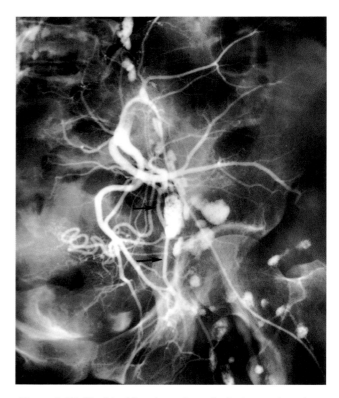

Figure 6.17: Combined lymphography and selective arteriography of the internal iliac artery. The nodes in the medial external iliac group lie between the external iliac artery (catheter) and the obturator artery (arrows). From Kolbenstvedt (1974a) with permission.

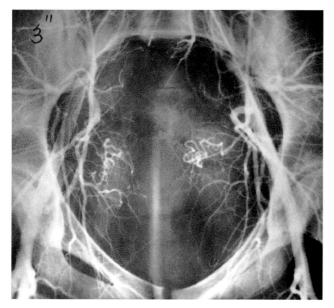

6.16b

*Figure 6.16: Pelvic arteriography in malignant trophoblastic disease. (a) Before treatment: vascular tumor in the left side of the uterus. (b) Normal arteriogram 6 weeks after methotrexate treatment. From Kolstad P & Liverud K (1969) Pelvic arteriography in malignant trophoblastic neoplasia. Am J Obstet Gynecol **105**: 175.*

6.16) can be obtained with contrast medium injection above the aortic bifurcation combined with compression of both femoral arteries. In the frontal projection there is much superimposition of the individual branches of pelvic arteries. These are better visualized in oblique projections after selective catheterization of the internal iliac artery. This may be performed from ipsilateral (*Figure 6.17*) or contralateral puncture (crossover technique). The female genital organs have a double arterial blood supply from the ovarian and uterine arteries. The ovarian arteries generally arise from the frontal aspect of the aorta on a level with the second lumbar vertebra. They can be visualized by aortic or selective injection (Lathrop and Frates, 1970).

■ BENEFITS AND LIMITATIONS

Arteriography for diagnostic purposes in oncology has largely been replaced by noninvasive methods. The exception is malignant trophoblastic neoplasia (*Figure 6.16*), in which several authors have reported the value of arterial visualization (Kolstad and Liverud, 1969; Hata et al, 1987). Other indications are pelvic angiodysplasia and arterial fistulas to intestinal (Hirakata et al, 1991) or lower urinary (Gelder et al, 1993) tract. In addition, arterial catheterization is mandatory for interventional procedures such as embolization in trauma or angiodysplasia or arterial drug infusion.

■ COMPLICATIONS AND SIDE EFFECTS

Arterial catheterization in experienced hands is considered a relatively safe procedure. In elderly individuals with arteriosclerosis and arterial wall calcifications the risk of intimal damage and dissection increases. Hematomas at the puncture site occur, especially in patients on anticoagulant medication or with bleeding disorders. Gentle catheterization techniques and careful surveillance of the puncture site are important in the prevention of risk.

It may be difficult to trace the bleeding artery in patients with bleeding from gynecological neoplasia. Embolization of the internal iliac trunk may imply inadvertent occlusion of vesical and hemorrhoidal arteries and necrosis due to ischemia. Tracing of the bleeding artery and use of embolizing agents that occlude the arterial tree at the level of the arterioles will reduce the risk of necrosis because the capillary bed will be preserved from collateral circulation.

■ NORMAL APPEARANCES

Traditionally the internal iliac artery has been described as branching into an anterior group of vessels comprising the vesical, hemorrhoidal, uterine, obturator, pudendal and inferior gluteal arteries, and a posterior group comprising the iliolumbar, lateral sacral and superior gluteal arteries. In the anterior group, the pudendal and inferior gluteal artery first curve posteriorly behind the coccygeus muscle.

In his study of cadaveric angiograms, Nilsson (1967) found that subdivision into a posterior and an anterior

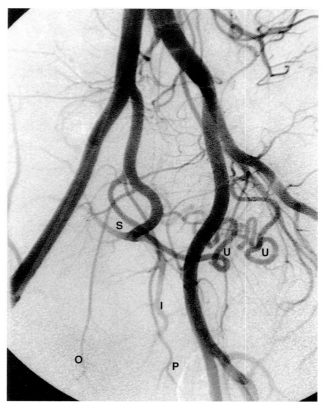

6.18a

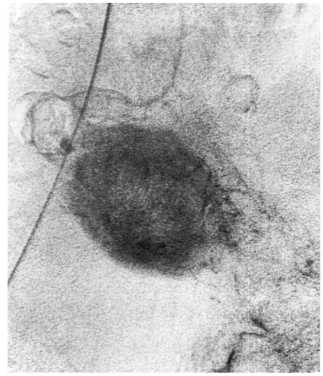

6.18b

Figure 6.18: *(a) Digital subtraction angiography of normal pelvic arteries in right anterior oblique projection. The obturator artery (O) runs more anteriorly than the pubic artery (P). U, uterine arteries; I, inferior gluteal artery; S, superior gluteal artery. (b) Parenchymal phase with much staining of the uterus (premenstrual period).*

main branch system with various sub-branches was insufficient. The wide variations make it difficult to trace the individual arteries at their origin. The superior and inferior gluteal arteries and the internal pudendal artery constituted three main identifiable trunks serving as basic landmarks. To facilitate identification of the other branches one may identify the peripheral branching and trace arteries proximally. The first part of the uterine artery runs downwards and forwards along the lateral pelvic wall. The second part runs medially in the parametrium in front of the ureter, giving off a cervicovaginal branch. The third part runs along the lateral margin of the uterus towards the cornu where it divides into fundal, ovarian and tubal branches (Borell and Fernström 1953, 1954). The course is straighter in nulliparae, more tortuous in multiparae because of reduction of the uterine size after pregnancy. The number of intramural vessels and the staining of the uterine wall (*Figure 6.18*) vary during the phases of the menstrual cycle with a larger number of visible branches shortly before an expected menstruation. The inferior gluteal artery may continue downwards (persistent sciatic artery) and supply the limb from the popliteal artery downwards. An extensive description of all branches of the internal iliac artery is given by Merland and Chiras (1981).

REFERENCES

Borell U & Fernström I (1953) The adnexal branches of the uterine artery. An arteriographic study in human subjects. *Acta Radiol (Diagn)* **40**: 561–582.

Borell U & Fernström I (1954) The ovarian artery. An angiographic study in human subjects. *Acta Radiol (Diagn)* **42**: 253–265.

Bruun S & Engeset A (1956) Lymphadenography. A new method for the visualization of enlarged lymph nodes and lymphatic vessels (preliminary report). *Acta Radiol* **45**: 389–395.

Cunéo B & Marcille M (1901) Topographie des ganglions ilio-pelviens. *Bull Soc Anat (Paris)* **3**: 653–663.

Cunningham JB (1969) The demonstration of an unusual combination of collateral channels during lymphography: a case report. *J Can Assoc Radiol* **20**: 189–191.

Fuchs WA, Davidson JW & Fischer HW (eds) (1968) *Lymphography in Cancer*, p 105. Berlin: Springer.

Gelder MS, Alvarez RD & Partridge EE (1993) Ureteroarterial fistula in exenteration of patients with indwelling ureteral stents. *Gynecol Oncol* **50**: 365–370.

Hartgill JC (1964) Lymphography in the management of pelvic malignant disease. *J Obstet Gynaecol Br Commonw* **71**: 835–853.

Hata H, Sasaki K & Nakano R (1987) Pelvic angiography in malignant trophoblastic disease. *Gynecol Obstet Invest* **23**: 28–33.

Hirakata R, Hasuo K, Yasumori K et al (1991) Arterioenteric fistulae: diagnosis and treatment by angiography. *Clin Radiol* **43**: 328–330.

Kinmonth JB (1954) Lymphangiography in clinical surgery and particularly in the treatment of lymphoedema. *Ann R Coll Surg Engl* **15**: 300–306.

Kinmonth JB (1972) *The Lymphatics. Disease, Lymphography and Surgery*, p 108. London: Edward Arnold.

Kolbenstvedt A (1974a) A critical evaluation of foot lymphography in the demonstration of the regional lymph nodes of the uterine cervix. *Gynecol Oncol* **2**: 24–38.

Kolbenstvedt A (1974b) Normal lymphographic variations of lumbar, iliac and inguinal lymph vessels. *Acta Radiol* **15**: 662–669.

Kolbenstvedt A & Kolstad P (1974) Pelvic lymph node dissection under peroperative lymphographic control. *Gynecol Oncol* **2**: 39–59.

Kolbenstvedt A & Kolstad P (1976) The difficulties of complete lymph node dissection in radical hysterectomy for carcinoma of the cervix. *Gynecol Oncol* **4**: 244–254.

Kolstad P & Liverud K (1969) Pelvic arteriography in malignant trophoblastic neoplasia. *Am J Obstet Gynecol* **105**: 175–182.

Lathrop JC & Frates RE (1970) Selective ovarian angiography in trophoblastic disease. *Obstet Gynecol* **35**: 844–851.

Lossef SV & Barth KH (1993) Severe delayed hypotensive reaction after ethiodol lymphangiography despite premedication. *AJR* **161**: 417–418.

Merland JJ & Chiras J (1981) *Arteriography of the Pelvis*. Berlin: Springer.

Nilsson JC (1967) Angiography in tumors of the urinary bladder. *Acta Radiol Suppl* **263**.

Rouvière H (1932) *Anatomie des Lymphatiques de l'Homme*. Paris: Masson.

Wallace S, Jackson L, Dopp GD et al (1964) Lymphatic dynamics in certain abnormal states. *AJR* **91**: 187–196.

Wolf GL, Rogowska J, Hanna GK et al (1994) Percutaneous CT lymphography with perflubron: imaging efficacy in rabbits and monkeys. *Radiology* **191**: 501–505.

7 CT scanning of the female pelvis
L Van Hoe, S Gryspeerdt and AL Baert

■ EQUIPMENT

PRINCIPLES OF COMPUTED TOMOGRAPHY

Computed tomography (CT) is a cross-sectional imaging technique that uses ionizing radiation. The patient is positioned in the gantry and X-rays are emitted by the X-ray tube. The radiation beam passes through the patient and is attenuated to a degree that depends on the tissues traversed. The amount of residual radiation is measured behind the patient by an array of detectors. The same procedure is then repeated, this time in a slightly different angular projection and a second measurement is made. After several repetitions, the two-dimensional image of a section (slice) can be calculated from the data obtained. The patient is then translated relative to the X-ray tube and the detectors and the same series of measurements is obtained in order to calculate a second cross-sectional image (Barnes and Lakshminarayanan, 1989).

The gray scale value (or CT number) of a picture element (pixel) in a CT image is related to the linear attenuation coefficient of the tissue contained in the corresponding volume element (voxel) and is expressed in Hounsfield units (HU). Most soft tissues have a CT number between 0 and 100 HU, 0 being the CT number allocated to water. Because the different structures located in the female pelvis have comparable attenuation coefficients, they have comparable CT numbers, and contrast on an 'unenhanced' CT image is relatively poor. For this reason, intravenous contrast material is routinely administered in most centers when a CT scan of the pelvis is obtained.

TECHNICAL DEVELOPMENTS

There have been many technical innovations in CT since the installation of the first CT scanner in 1972.

The current generation of scanners use slip ring technology, which means that sliding contacts connect the stationary and rotating parts of the gantry. This technology allows continuous rotation of the X-ray tube and detectors. Furthermore, there have been substantial improvements in detector efficiency and X-ray tube cooling capability. Helical or spiral CT was introduced in 1989 (Kalender et al, 1990) and is considered as the state of the art CT technique (Zeman et al, 1993). In helical CT, continuous rotation of the X-ray tube is combined with continuous translation of the patient. The improved scan speed in helical CT leads to shortened examination times, better image quality and more efficient use of intravenous contrast media. Another advantage of helical CT is that overlapping images can be reconstructed a posteriori from the obtained raw data set whenever required; these images can be used for calculation of coronal or sagittal reformattings (*Figure 7.1*).

■ TECHNIQUE

PATIENT PREPARATION

Adequate opacification of the distal small bowel is essential in pelvic CT; a dilute solution of contrast medium (Gastrografin) is therefore administered approximately 60 minutes before the examination. In certain clinical situations (for instance, staging of gynecological neoplasms), adequate opacification of the colon is also important. This can be obtained by retrograde administration of a dilute Gastrografin solution (*Figure 7.2*). A vaginal tampon is inserted whenever adequate visualization of the vagina is required (Cohen et al, 1977).

SCAN PARAMETERS

The slice thickness (collimation) for a pelvic CT study is usually between 5 and 10 mm, depending on the

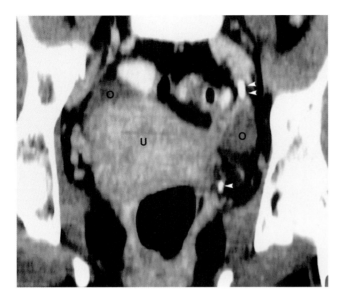

7.1a

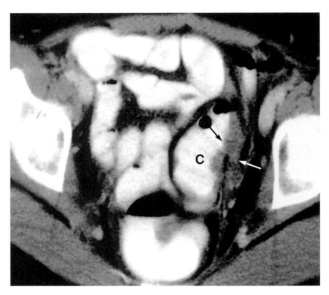

Figure 7.2: *Importance of adequate opacification of the colon. Soft tissue mass between the lateral pelvic wall and the colon (C), representing recurrent ovarian carcinoma (arrows). This relatively small mass is well seen because it has a much lower density than the contrast filled colonic lumen.*

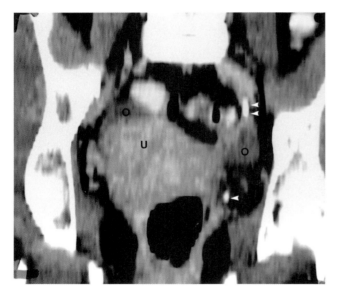

7.1b

Figure 7.1: *Influence of image reconstruction interval on quality of reformatted images. The coronal images shown in (a) and (b) are calculated from the same raw data set (collimation 5 mm). Axial images were calculated at 2 mm table increments in (a) and 5 mm increments in (b). The uterus (U), right and left ovary (O), the left ureter (arrowheads) are well seen. Note suboptimal image quality in (b).*

specific purpose of the study. The tube voltage and tube current are adjusted for each individual patient, in order to find the optimal compromise between radiation dose and image noise. An additional parameter to be selected in helical CT is the table feed, which is the speed of translation of the examination table in millimeters per second. Typically the table feed is 1 to 1.5 times the collimation. Selection of higher table feed values improves

the scan speed but negatively influences the spatial resolution in the longitudinal direction, and thus the quality of reformatted images.

INTRAVENOUS CONTRAST ADMINISTRATION

Administration of iodinated contrast material improves the contrast between different organs and structures in the female pelvis. Parameters to be selected are the total amount of contrast medium administered, the injection rate and the scan delay time (that is, the time interval between the start of the administration of contrast material and scanning). There is little consensus in the literature concerning the optimal technique for contrast administration in CT scanning of the pelvis, basically because of the lack of dedicated studies comparing different methods. When the upper abdomen is included in the CT study (which is the case in the majority of patients), upper abdominal organs such as the liver should be scanned during the phase of peak parenchymal enhancement. When helical CT is available, the entire abdomen can be scanned with two or three consecutive helical scans, each performed during breath-hold. Rapid injection of contrast material (2–3 ml/s) is preferred whenever technically possible. Typical delay times

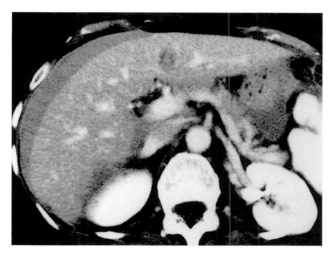

7.3a

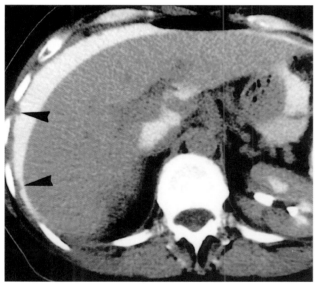

7.3b

Figure 7.3: *Detection of small peritoneal metastases with CT peritoneography in a patient with serous cystadenocarcinoma of right ovary. (a) Contrast enhanced CT shows ascites but fails to show peritoneal implants. (b) CT performed after intraperitoneal injection of contrast material shows several small metastatic lesions (arrows).*

between contrast injection and scanning are 70–80 s for the upper abdomen and 1.5–3 min for the pelvis. More delayed scans of the pelvis are obtained when opacification of the ureters and/or the bladder is required (Walsh et al, 1992).

NOTE: CT PERITONEOGRAPHY

In CT peritoneography a water soluble contrast agent is injected in the peritoneal cavity before scanning. Typically 60 ml of a low osmolality contrast agent is instilled

into the peritoneal cavity together with at least 1 liter of normal saline. This technique has been used for detection of peritoneal metastases in patients with suspected primary or recurrent ovarian cancer (*Figure 7.3*) (Giunta et al, 1990; Fraski et al, 1994).

■ BENEFITS AND LIMITATIONS

GENERAL

Advantages of CT are its excellent spatial resolution and its ability to differentiate between fluid, fat, solid lesions and calcifications, based on analysis of gray scale values. Furthermore, the diagnostic performance of the technique is relatively operator independent and is not negatively influenced by the presence of anatomical conditions such as bowel distension or obesity. Disadvantages are the relatively high cost (compared to ultrasonography), the exposure of the patient to ionizing radiation, and the need for administration of contrast material.

NEOPLASTIC LESIONS: DETECTION, CHARACTERIZATION AND LOCAL STAGING

CERVICAL CANCER

While CT has no role in the early detection of cervical cancer, the technique can be used for evaluation of tumor size and local extension. Pelvic side wall invasion, ureteral obstruction and invasion of the bladder or rectum can be demonstrated. The accuracy for staging varied between 58 and 88% in different reports (Walsh, 1992). Of critical importance in patients with cervical carcinoma is the diagnosis of parametrial invasion. CT findings described as being suggestive of parametrial involvement are: (1) irregularity or poor definition of the lateral cervical margins; (2) prominent parametrial soft tissue strands (*Figure 7.4*); (3) obliteration of the periureteral fat plane; and (4) an eccentric parametrial soft tissue mass (Vick et al, 1984). Although the last two findings are only seen in neoplastic involvement of the parametria, the first two findings can also be seen with parametrial inflammation. CT therefore often overestimates the extent of disease (Walsh, 1992). Helical CT might improve the differentiation between normal

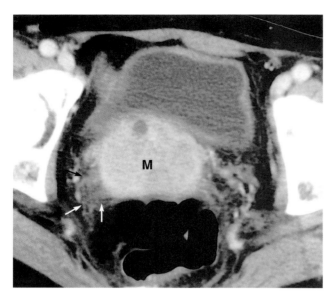

Figure 7.4: Cervical carcinoma with parametrial invasion (stage IIb disease). Large soft tissue mass (M) in the cervix, representing cervical cancer. Infiltration of the parametrial fat (arrows) suggests parametrial invasion.

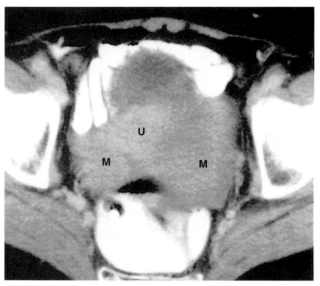

7.6a

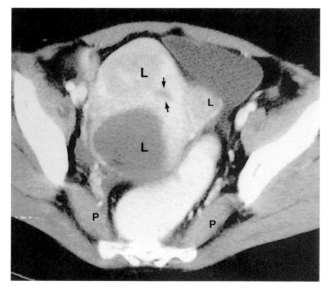

Figure 7.5: Variable appearance of leiomyomas. Three leiomyomas (L) are seen as hypodense structures surrounded by well enhanced myometrial tissue. Note that the posteriorly located mass has a very low density (fluid density), which is most likely to be related to necrosis and/or hemorrhage. Arrows, uterine cavity; P, piriformis muscle.

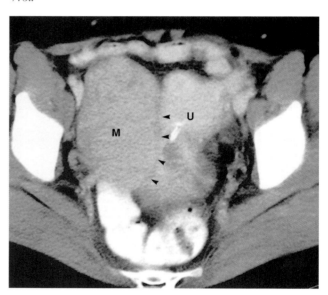

7.6b

Figure 7.6: Limitations of CT in distinguishing extrauterine leiomyomas and solid ovarian tumors. (a) CT shows bilateral soft tissue mass (M) that cannot be separated from the uterus (U): histologically proved bilateral ovarian adenofibroma. (b) In this patient, CT shows a solid mass (M) that displaces the uterus (U) to the left. This mass seems to be separated from the uterine wall by a thin fat plane (arrowheads). Final diagnosis: sessile leiomyoma.

UTERINE TUMORS

parametrial vessels and ligaments from adenopathy and tumor extension (Urban and Fishman, 1995).

CT has a high sensitivity and specificity rate in the detection of recurrent disease (Walsh et al, 1981). The differentiation of therapy-related fibrosis and recurrent tumor may, however, remain difficult.

Transvaginal ultrasonography (TVS) and magnetic resonance imaging (MRI) are the methods of choice for the detection and specific diagnosis of leiomyomas. The CT appearances of uterine leiomyomas are protean, and leiomyomas should therefore be included in the differential diagnosis of all cervical and uterine masses (*Figure 7.5*). The differentiation between sessile leiomyomas

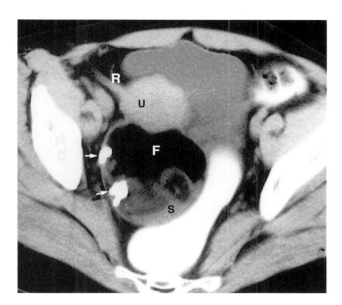

Figure 7.7: *Typical appearance of benign teratoma. CT shows a retrouterine mass that contains fat (F), a solid component (S) and teeth-like structures (arrows). U, uterus; R, round ligament.*

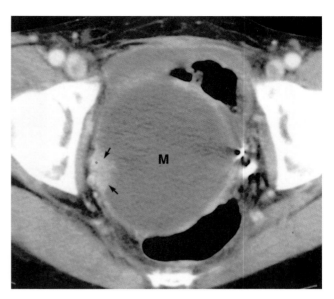

Figure 7.8: *Malignant ovarian tumor. CT shows a predominantly cystic mass (M) with a relatively small solid component (arrows): serous cystadenocarcinoma.*

and solid ovarian tumors may be difficult (*Figure 7.6*). Conventional CT has not proved accurate in the determination of myometrial invasion in patients with endometrial carcinoma, and the role of spiral CT is not yet established (Urban and Fishman, 1995). In any case, MRI is the technique of choice for demonstration of cervical extension and assessment of myometrial invasion depth (stage I and II endometrial cancer). The accuracy of CT staging in patients with stage III–IV disease is 83–86% (Walsh, 1992). The absence of fat planes between a uterine tumor and rectum or bladder does not necessarily indicate local extension as these fat planes may be absent in normal patients (Li and Mastin, 1990).

OVARIAN TUMORS

CT detection of fat and calcification in an adnexal mass is virtually diagnostic of benign teratoma (*Figure 7.7*) (Buy et al, 1989; Urban and Fishman, 1995). The presence of a thick wall, thick septa, papillary projections and/or solid portions in a predominantly cystic adnexal mass suggests malignancy (*Figure 7.8*). Unilocular or multilocular masses with thin septa and a thin wall are usually benign, even if they are large (*Figure 7.9*). False positive and negative CT diagnoses of malignancy occur (as in other imaging studies), firstly because benign lesions may contain solid components (false positive diagnosis of malignancy),

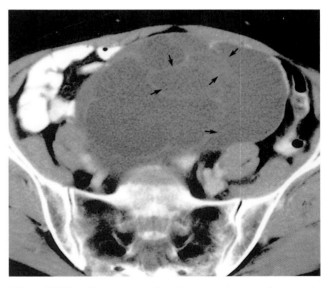

Figure 7.9: *Typical appearance of mucinous cystadenoma. Large cystic mass with multiple thin septa (arrows) but without solid component.*

and secondly because apparently benign lesions may contain small foci of malignant degeneration.

Spread of ovarian carcinoma is primarily in the peritoneal cavity. It is well known that the CT sensitivity for detection of small peritoneal implants is low. Furthermore, the presence of ascites, which is commonly associated with advanced peritoneal tumor spread, is an aspecific finding (Outwater and Schiebler, 1994); however, larger peritoneal implants inside or outside the pelvis are usually well visible (*Figure 7.10a*). Similarly,

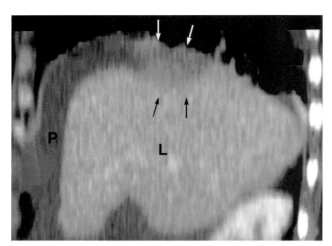

7.10a

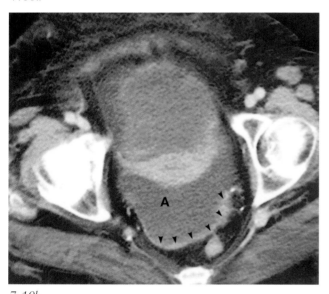

7.10b

Figure 7.10: *Demonstration of peritoneal metastases in ovarian cancer. (a) Sagittal CT through the liver shows metastatic implant in the right subdiaphragmatic space (arrows). L, liver; P, peritoneal space. (b) CT at the level of the uterus of another patient shows ascites (A) and diffuse peritoneal thickening (arrowheads).*

diffuse peritoneal thickening may be observed in patients with ascites (*Figure 7.10b*). Preliminary studies have shown that CT peritoneography is much more sensitive than standard CT for detection of metastatic peritoneal disease in patients with primary or recurrent ovarian carcinoma (*Figure 7.3*) (Giunta et al, 1990; Fraski et al, 1994). While it is clear that CT cannot replace second-look laparotomy for demonstration of complete remission of disease (Goldhirsch et al, 1983; Megibow et al, 1988), it appears that CT and CT peritoneography can be used to avoid this procedure in certain patients by demonstrating macroscopic peritoneal implants.

NEOPLASTIC LESIONS: EVALUATION OF DISTANT METASTASES

Demonstration of metastases in lymph nodes, liver or lungs is an important task for CT in the assessment of gynecological tumors. The reported accuracy for detection of pelvic and para-aortic lymph nodes by CT varies between 65–80% and 80–98%, respectively (Walsh et al, 1992). False positive or negative CT studies can occur because (1) microscopic lymph node invasion cannot be detected, and (2) inflammation may result in lymph node enlargement. The accuracy of CT increases significantly when CT guided fine needle aspiration biopsy of lymph nodes is routinely used (Oyen et al, 1994).

INFLAMMATORY DISEASE

CT can be helpful in selected cases of suspected inflammatory disease. The characteristic tubular shape of a hydrosalpinx or pyosalpinx is regularly recognized on axial and reformatted CT images (*Figure 7.11*). Furthermore, CT may be helpful in patients with unexplained fever in the postpartum by demonstrating hematomas, abscesses and/or thrombophlebitis of deep pelvic veins (Brown et al, 1991; Van Hoe et al, 1994).

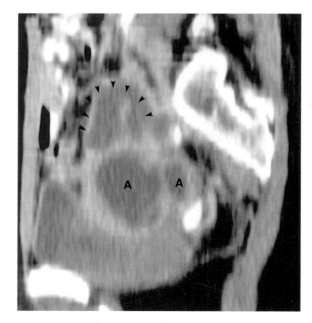

Figure 7.11: *Pyosalpinx. Sagittal CT shows a fluid-containing tubular structure (arrowheads) above two thick-walled fluid collections (A): pyosalpinx with tubo-ovarian abscess.*

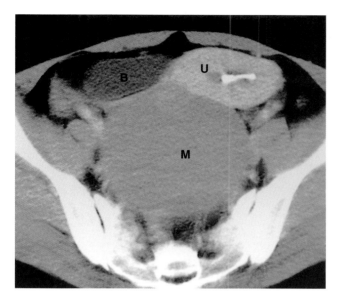

Figure 7.12: Endometrioma. Image obtained at the level of the uterus shows a large homogeneous 'mass' (M) with CT density that is intermediate between fluid and soft tissue: typical CT appearance of blood. U, uterus; B, bladder.

OTHER APPLICATIONS

There is no role for CT in the evaluation of congenital uterine anomalies. Endometriomas are commonly confused with other ovarian lesions at CT (Fishman et al, 1983); however, their appearance may occasionally be quite suggestive (*Figure 7.12*).

Tubo-ovarian torsion is another entity that can be diagnosed by CT (Ghossein et al, 1994; Kimura et al, 1994).

■ COMPLICATIONS AND SIDE EFFECTS

RADIATION EXPOSURE

Because CT uses ionizing radiation, the technique is only justified when the information provided by the CT study is of sufficient importance to the health of the person being imaged. Dose values within a specific section are determined by factors such as voltage, tube current, scan time, scan field, collimation and spacing. When compared with conventional CT, helical CT has the advantage of allowing retrospective calculation of overlapping slices without increasing the radiation dose (Zeman et al, 1993).

Most of the concern regarding body CT radiation doses is based on the risk of somatic effects. First trimester pregnancy is a contraindication to CT imaging because of the risk of inducing serious deleterious fetal effects.

For typical scanning sequences over the pelvic region of a pregnant woman, the conceptus dose (being the dose delivered to the fetus or embryo) may range from 30 to 100 mGy (Rothenberg and Pentlow, 1992).

CONTRAST MEDIA

Side effects of iodinated contrast media are allergic reaction, nephrotoxicity and cardiovascular stress. It is well known that nonionic contrast media have less allergic potential and fewer adverse effects on the cardiovascular system in comparison with ionic contrast media (Katayama and Tanako, 1988). Whether nonionic contrast media also cause less nephrotoxicity is still a matter for debate. Certain conditions, such as diabetes, proteinuria and multiple myeloma, predispose to renal complications after contrast medium administration and can therefore be considered as relative contraindications (Lautin et al, 1991). Emergency treatment of severe allergic reactions consists of intravenous or intramuscular administration of epinephrine (adrenaline) (1 mg). In patients with known allergy, the risk of an allergic reaction can be significantly reduced by the administration of corticosteroids and antihistaminics before the injection of contrast medium.

■ NORMAL APPEARANCES

UTERINE BODY AND CERVIX

The *normal uterus* is typically in the midline between the bladder and the rectum, depending on the degree of bladder and rectal distension and on normal anatomical variation. The myometrium is significantly enhanced after introduction of a contrast medium (*Figure 7.13*). The normal uterine cavity and cervical canal are seen as fluid-containing areas on contrast enhanced studies. The different layers of the uterine wall cannot be distinguished at CT.

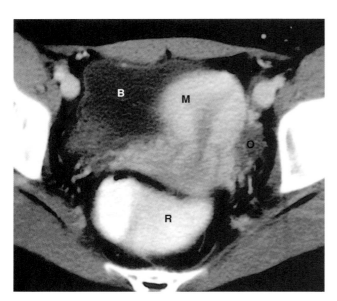

Figure 7.13: Normal uterus in anteversion. Note significant enhancement of the myometrium (M). The uterine cavity is seen as a hypodense central stripe. B, bladder; R, rectum; O, left ovary.

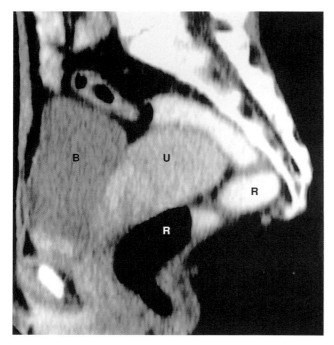

Figure 7.14: Midline sagittal CT image through a normal uterus. The uterus (U) is seen between the bladder (B) and rectosigmoid (R).

Accurate determination of the size of the uterus by CT may be difficult, particularly in cases of anteversion or retroversion. Sagittal images may be useful for demonstration of the anatomical relationship between the uterus and surrounding organs such as the bladder and rectum (*Figure 7.14*) (Constant et al, 1989).

The location and/or appearance of the uterus may be altered after pelvic surgery and after cesarean section or vaginal delivery. Posterior displacement is common after surgery for rectal carcinoma (Kelvin et al, 1983). The following changes are normal after uncomplicated delivery: increased uterine size, presence of blood in the uterine cavity, and presence of intrauterine gas (Garagiola et al, 1989). After cesarean section, CT may demonstrate apparent myometrial defects at the incision site, particularly in the case of low transverse incision. These defects should be recognized as normal postoperative anatomy, so that unnecessary surgery or additional treatment can be avoided (Twickler et al, 1991).

Developmental variants of the uterus cannot be directly visualized with CT. They can be detected, however, in cases of associated hematometra (Petrich and Cory, 1986).

The *normal cervix* is seen as an oval or round structure of soft tissue attenuation. The junction of the cervix and the vagina can be estimated when an air-containing tampon is inserted into the vagina. Three layers are commonly seen on contrast enhanced CT scans: a thin enhancing inner layer (probably representing the cervical mucosa and plicae palmatae), a relatively hypodense middle layer (cervical stroma), and a thin enhancing outer layer (*Figure 7.15*). The cervical

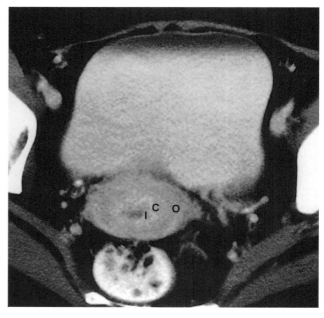

Figure 7.15: Normal cervix. Three different cervical layers can be distinguished on this contrast enhanced image: a thin enhancing inner layer (I), a more hypodense central layer (C), and a thin enhancing outer layer (O).

canal is often seen as a hypodense central area, which is probably related to the presence of secretions. Normal CT size criteria for the cervix are not precisely known, but in general the cervix is about 2 cm long and less than 3 cm in transverse diameter (Vick et al, 1984).

OVARIES AND FALLOPIAN TUBES

The normal Fallopian tube is not visible on CT.

The ovaries are located in the ovarian fossae on the posterior floor of the true pelvis (posterior pelvic peritoneal space) (*Figure 7.16*). They are bordered anteriorly by the broad ligament (*Figure 7.16a*), the mesovarium and the ovarian vessels, superiorly by the external iliac vessels, and posteriorly or posterolaterally by the ureter and the internal iliac vessels (*Figure 7.16b*).

The ovaries may be located in unusual positions. Normal ovaries (and ovarian tumors) may be found in the anterior paravesical space. An ectopic position of the ovaries is common in patients with congenital absence of the uterus, probably because of absent fixation by the round ligament (Reed et al, 1990). Furthermore, ovaries may be located in the iliac fossa, in the paracolic gutter, or close to the iliopsoas muscle after surgical transposition of the ovary in patients who have undergone hysterectomy (Bashist et al, 1989).

It can be difficult to identify normal ovaries on CT images, particularly in pediatric and postmenopausal women (Gross et al, 1983). This is not surprising if one considers the normal size of postmenopausal ovaries. In a sonographic study, Tepper et al (1995) found a mean ovarian volume of 8.6 cm³ in the first menopausal year, 4 cm³ in the fifth menopausal year, and only 2.8 cm³ in the tenth menopausal year.

Small cystic structures, corresponding to follicular cysts, can often be detected in normal ovaries. While most functional cysts have a diameter of less than 1 cm, diameters up to 4 cm have been observed. Diagnosis of a functional ovarian cyst can be made confidently by demonstration of diminished size on follow-up imaging studies.

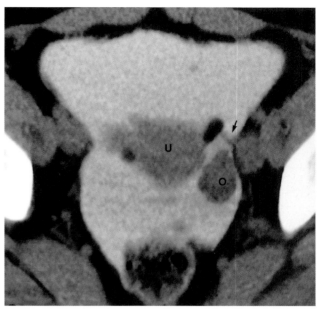

7.16a

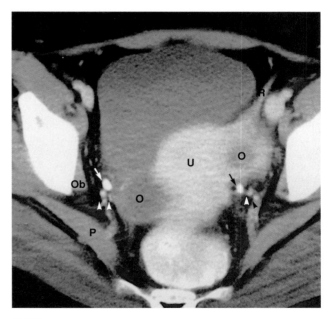

7.16b

Figure 7.16: Normal ovaries. (a) Image obtained after intraperitoneal injection of iodinated contrast material. Note location of the left ovary (O) in the ovarian fossa, posteriorly to the broad ligament (arrow). U, uterus. (b) Typical position of both ovaries (O), close to the ureter (arrows) and internal iliac vessels (arrowheads). U, uterus; R, round ligament; Ob, obturator muscle; P, piriformis muscle.

PELVIC LIGAMENTS

The broad ligament is formed by two layers of peritoneum and extends laterally from the uterus to the pelvic side wall (Forshager and Walsh, 1994). Its superior or free border is formed by the Fallopian tube medially and the suspensory ligament of the ovary laterally. The lower margin of the broad ligament ends at the cardinal ligament. While the broad ligament is not seen in normal patients, it can be identified when ascites is present and after intraperitoneal injection of contrast material (*Figure 7.17*).

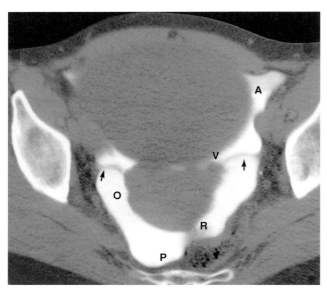

Figure 7.17: *Broad ligament and pelvic peritoneal spaces. CT image obtained after intraperitoneal injection of contrast material. The broad ligament is well visible at both sides of the uterus (arrows). A, anterior pelvic peritoneal space; V, vesicouterine fossa; R, rectouterine fossa; O, right ovarian fossa; P, right pararectal fossa.*

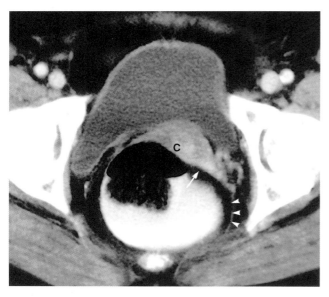

Figure 7.18: *Cardinal and uterosacral ligaments. Axial image through the cervix (C). Both the cardinal ligament (arrows) and the thin uterosacral ligament (arrowheads) are well seen at the left.*

The cardinal ligament is usually seen on a CT scan as a triangular soft tissue structure, with the base of the triangle abutting the cervix and the apex tapering toward the pelvic side wall (*Figure 7.18*). The ligament exhibits wide variations in thickness, contour and shape.

The round ligament attaches to the anterolateral uterine fundus and runs in a curved course within the broad ligament to enter the internal inguinal ring. It is frequently seen on CT scans as a thin, soft tissue band (*Figure 7.16*).

The uterosacral ligaments extend posteriorly from the lateral cervix to the sacral body, and are also commonly seen on CT (*Figure 7.18*).

The suspensory ligament is only rarely visible on CT images.

PELVIC CAVITY

The pelvic peritoneal space can be subdivided into an anterior and a posterior space. These spaces are normally invisible on CT but can be distinguished when intraperitoneal fluid is present (*Figure 7.17*). The ovaries and the ampullary portions of the Fallopian tubes are occasionally located in the anterior pelvic space. The posterior space is subdivided into the vesicouterine space, the rectouterine pouch, the ovarian fossae and the pararectal fossae (*Figure 7.17*) (Auh et al, 1986).

PELVIC LYMPH NODES

Demonstration of normal lymph nodes by CT depends on several factors, such as the amount of retroperitoneal fat, slice thickness and administration of intravenous contrast material. Pelvic lymph nodes are divided into common iliac lymph nodes, internal iliac lymph nodes (including obturator and presacral nodes) and external iliac nodes (lateral, middle and medial groups) (*Figure 7.19*). Recent studies in normal patients have shown that the large majority of normal lymph nodes in the pelvis have a maximum short axis diameter that is less than 10 mm. Vinnicombe et al (1995) suggest the following upper limits of normal for maximum short axis diameter in pelvic lymph nodes: 7 mm for internal iliac nodes, 8 mm for obturator nodes, 9 mm for common iliac nodes and 10 mm for external iliac location.

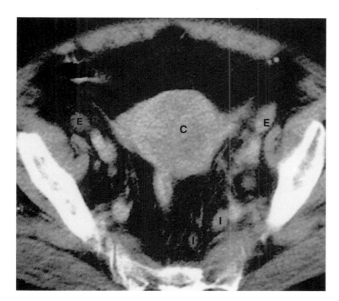

Figure 7.19: Enlarged pelvic lymph nodes. Patient with cervical carcinoma (C). Note enlarged nodes in the internal (I) and external (E) iliac nodal chains.

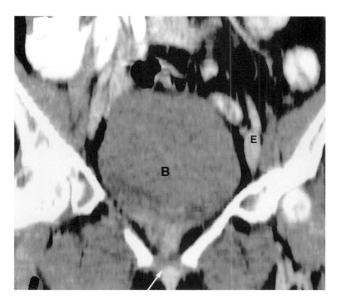

Figure 7.20: Urogenital diaphragm. On this coronal image, the urogenital diaphragm is seen as a structure with soft tissue density between the ischiopubic rami (arrow). B, urinary bladder; E, external iliac vessels.

PELVIC FLOOR

The levator ani muscle, which represents the medial boundary of the triangular ischiorectal fossa, extends from the lateral pelvic walls downward and medially, and provides support for the pelvic organs (Tisnado et al, 1981). The urogenital diaphragm is best seen on reformatted images and is depicted as a soft tissue structure between the ischiopubic rami (*Figure 7.20*). Both the

piriformis and obturator internus muscles are clearly identifiable on axial and reformatted CT images (*Figures 7.5* and *7.16b*).

REFERENCES

Auh YH, Rubenstein WA & Markisz JA (1986) Intraperitoneal paravesical spaces: CT delineation with US correlation. *Radiology* **159**: 311–317.

Barnes GT & Lakshminarayanan AV (1989) Computed tomography: physical principles and image quality considerations. In Lee KT, Sagell SS & Stanley RJ (eds) *Computed Body Tomography with MRI Correlation*, 2nd edn, pp 1–22. New York: Raven Press.

Bashist B, Friedman WN & Killackey MA (1989) Surgical transposition of the ovary: radiologic appearance. *Radiology* **173**: 857–860.

Brown CEL, Dunn DH & Harrell R (1991) Computed tomography for evaluation of puerperal infections. *Surg Gynecol Obstet* **172**: 285–289.

Buy J, Ghossain MA, Moss AA et al (1989) Cystic teratoma of the ovary: CT detection. *Radiology* **171**: 697–701.

Cohen WN, Seidelmann FE & Bryan PJ (1977) Use of a tampon to enhance vaginal localization in CT. *AJR* **128**: 1064–1065.

Constant O, Cooke J & Parsons CA (1989) Reformatted computed tomography of the female pelvis: normal anatomy. *Br J Obstet Gynaecol* **96**: 1047–1053.

Fishman EK, Scatarige JC & Saksouk FA (1983) Computed tomography of endometriosis. *J Comput Assist Tomogr* **7**: 257–264.

Forshager MC & Walsh JW (1994) CT anatomy of the female pelvis: a second look. *Radiographics* **14**: 51–66.

Fraski G, Contino A, Iafaioli RV et al (1994) CT of the abdomen and pelvis with peritoneal administration of soluble contrast in detection of residual disease for patients with ovarian cancer. *Gynecol Oncol* **52**: 154–160.

Garagiola DM, Tarver RD, Gibson L et al (1989) Anatomic changes in the female pelvis after uncomplicated vaginal delivery: a CT study on 14 women. *AJR* **153**: 1239–1241.

Ghossein MA, Buy JN, Bazot M et al (1994) CT in adnexal torsion with emphasis on tubal findings: correlation with US. *J Comput Assist Tomogr* **18**: 619–625.

Giunta S, Tipaldi L, Diutellevi F et al (1990) CT demonstration of peritoneal metastases after intraperitoneal injection of contrast medium. *Clin Imaging* **14**: 31–33.

Goldhirsch A, Triller JK, Greiner R et al (1983) Computed tomography prior to second-look operation in advanced ovarian cancer. *Obstet Gynecol* **62**: 630–634.

Gross BH, Moss AA, Mihara K et al (1983) Computed tomography of gynecologic diseases. *AJR* **141**: 765–773.

Kalender WA, Seisler W, Klotz E et al (1990) Spiral volumetric CT with single breath-hold technique, continuous transport, and continuous scanner rotation. *Radiology* **176**: 181–183.

Katayama H & Tanako T (1988) Clinical survey of adverse reactions to contrast media. *Invest Radiol* **23**: 88–89.

Kelvin FM, Korobkin M, Heaston DK, Grant JP & Akwari O (1983) The pelvis after surgery for rectal carcinoma: serial CT observations with emphasis on nonneoplastic features. *AJR* **141**: 959–964.

Kimura I, Togashi K, Kawakami S et al (1994) Ovarian torsion: CT and MR imaging appearances. *Radiology* **190**: 337–341.

Lautin EM, Freeman NJ, Schoenfeld AH et al (1991) Radiocontrast-associated renal dysfunction. *AJR* **157**: 49–58.

Li KCP & Mastin ST (1990) Normal variations of pelvic fat distribution: implications on CT staging of pelvic tumors. *Clin Imaging* **14**: 319–322.

Megibow AJ, Bosniak MA & Ho AG (1988) Accuracy of CT in detection of persistent or recurrent ovarian carcinoma: correlation with second-look laparotomy. *Radiology* **166**: 341–345.

Outwater EK & Schiebler ML (1994) Magnetic resonance imaging of the ovary. *MRI Clin North Am* **2**: 245–274.

Oyen RH, Van Poppel HP, Ameye FE et al (1994) Lymph node staging of localized prostatic cancer with CT and CT guided fine needle aspiration biopsy: prospective study of 285 patients. *Radiology* **190**: 315–322.

Petrich LA & Cory DA (1986) Unilateral obstruction of septate uterus: computed tomography and ultrasound appearances. *Br J Radiol* **59**: 1225–1226.

Reed DH, Dixon AK & Braude PR (1990) Ectopic ovaries associated with absent uterus and pelvic kidney: CT findings. *J Comput Assist Tomogr* **14**: 157–158.

Rothenberg LN & Pentlow KS (1992) Radiation dose in CT. *Radiographics* **12**: 1225–1243.

Tepper R, Zalel Y, Markov S et al (1995) Ovarian volume in post-menopausal women: suggestions to an ovarian size normogram for postmenopausal age. *Acta Obstet Gynecol Scand* **74**: 208–211.

Tisnado JT, Amendola MA, Walsh JW et al (1981) Computed tomography of the perineum. *AJR* **136**: 475–481.

Twickler DM, Setiawan AT, Harrell RS et al (1991) CT appearance of the pelvis after cesarean section. *AJR* **156**: 523–526.

Urban BA & Fishman EK (1995) Spiral CT of the female pelvis: clinical applications. *Abdom Imaging* **20**: 9–14.

Van Hoe L, Baert AL, Marchal G, Spitz B & Penninckx F (1994) Thrombosed ovarian vein collateral mimicking acute appendicitis on CT. *J Comput Assist Tomogr* **18**: 643–646.

Vick CW, Walsh JW, Wheelock JB & Brewer WH (1984) CT of the normal and abnormal parametria in cervical cancer. *AJR* **143**: 597–603.

Vinnicombe SJ, Norman AR, Nicolson V et al (1995) Normal pelvic lymph nodes: evaluation with CT after bipedal lymphangiography. *Radiology* **194**: 349–355.

Walsh JW (1992) Computed tomography of gynecologic neoplasms. *Radiol Clin North Am* **30**: 817–830.

Walsh JW, Amendola MA, Hall DJ et al (1981) Recurrent carcinoma of the cervix: CT diagnosis. *AJR* **136**: 117–122.

Zeman RK, Fox SH, Silverman PM et al (1993) Helical (spiral) CT of the abdomen. *AJR* **160**: 917–925.

8 *Magnetic resonance imaging of the female pelvis*
DM Chernoff and H Hricak

◼ INTRODUCTION

Magnetic resonance imaging (MRI) has undergone considerable technological development since the first reports of its clinical use in the female pelvis in 1983 (Bryan et al, 1983; Hricak et al, 1983). This chapter will provide an overview of current pelvic MRI techniques and a survey of normal female pelvic anatomy as viewed at MRI.

◼ EQUIPMENT

MAGNET DESIGN

MRI of the female pelvis may be performed in imaging systems of widely varying configurations and magnetic field strengths. High field systems (>1 T, 1 T = 10 000 times the earth's magnetic field strength) in principle have better signal-to-noise properties than lower field systems, permitting faster imaging and/or higher spatial resolution. High field systems, however, are generally more expensive to purchase and maintain than their low or midfield counterparts, and cost considerations may play a role in the choice of MRI equipment. The current standard imaging system configuration places the patient within the center of a hollow cylindrical magnet, having the appearance of a tunnel or bore. This configuration simplifies magnet design but limits access to the patient during imaging and may produce claustrophobia. Alternative magnet designs with a more open configuration are in development but have yet to replace conventional systems for routine clinical use.

RECEIVER COILS

Either body coil or local receiver coils can be used for imaging the pelvis. The use of multiple surface coils (small coils closely applied to the body region of inter-est), arranged as a so-called phased array, has been shown to improve the signal-to-noise (S:N) ratio of pelvic magnetic resonance (MR) images (Reiman et al, 1988; Hayes et al, 1991, 1992; McCauley et al, 1992a). The improved S:N ratio derived from use of local coils can be exchanged for improved spatial resolution and/or decreased imaging time (Hayes et al, 1992). If a phased array coil is available, it should be used routinely for pelvic imaging, reserving the whole volume body coil for use in very obese patients, in whom local coils may show decreased sensitivity in the center of the pelvis.

◼ TECHNIQUE

TISSUE CONTRAST

Unlike computed tomography (CT) and sonography, in which contrast is largely determined by differences in electron density and acoustic impedance, respectively, tissue contrast in MRI is a complex function of intrinsic tissue properties and imaging parameters (the 'pulse sequence'). The primary tissue properties determining contrast in MRI are T_1, T_2, and proton density. T_1 and T_2 are exponential time constants describing certain recovery processes of tissue magnetization following a disturbance of equilibrium. Tissue contrast depends both on these intrinsic properties of tissue and on the precise pulse sequence used. Most imaging sequences lead to images that are either T_1-weighted, proton density weighted, or T_2-weighted.

PULSE SEQUENCES

Both T_1- and T_2-weighted images are required to evaluate the female pelvis. T_2-weighted images reveal the zonal architecture of the uterus, cervix, vagina and urethra, and demonstrate ovarian cysts and follicles. T_1-weighted images are an important complement to

T_2-weighted images in characterizing hemorrhagic or fat-containing lesions. T_1-weighted images are also more sensitive than T_2-weighted images in detecting lymph node enlargement. T_1-weighted images obtained after injection of intravenous contrast media may improve delineation of inflammatory and neoplastic lesions.

Both T_1- and T_2-weighted images are most commonly obtained via 'spin echo' (SE) sequences. Fast spin echo (FSE) is a recent advance that produces T_2-weighted images in a fraction of the time required by conventional SE. FSE images are generally superior to conventional SE for pelvic T_2-weighted imaging (Smith et al, 1992a, 1992b). Gradient echo (GRE) is an imaging sequence in which flowing blood demonstrates very high signal intensity, creating an angiographic effect. In pelvic imaging, GRE sequences are used to document blood flow, distinguish lymph nodes from blood vessels in questionable cases, and to follow the time course of tissue enhancement after bolus intravenous administration of MR contrast media.

FAT SATURATION

Fat saturation is a technique that can be added to most pelvic imaging sequences. Fat saturation selectively reduces the signal from fat, which may improve contrast between fat (normally high in signal intensity on both T_1- and T_2-weighted images) and enhancing either hemorrhagic lesions (on T_1-weighted images) or inflammation (on T_2-weighted images). Fat-suppressed MRI may improve sensitivity in detection of pelvic endometriosis (Sugimura et al, 1993; Ha et al, 1994; Takahashi et al, 1994), and may be more effective than sonography in differentiating a benign mature teratoma (dermoid) from an endometrioma (Stevens et al, 1993; Jain and Jeffrey, 1994).

IMAGING PLANES

Unlike CT, MRI can be performed in any plane of section. Pelvic imaging in the axial and sagittal planes are routine. Additional imaging in the coronal plane is often obtained; the sagittal and coronal planes are often useful and sometimes essential in delineating the extent of pathology. An oblique imaging plane along a principal axis of an organ such as the uterus may be helpful in optimizing anatomical depiction (Baumgartner and Bernardino, 1989).

PATIENT PREPARATION

Patient preparation is focused primarily on reduction of motion artifact. Motion artifact from bowel is minimized if the patient fasts for at least 6 hours before the study (Winkler and Hricak, 1986). A 1 mg intramuscular injection of glucagon will further reduce artifacts by causing temporary cessation of bowel peristalsis; glucagon is suggested for all pelvic MRI studies unless medically contraindicated (Winkler and Hricak, 1986). The patient should void before the study to reduce motion artifacts related to a distended bladder. Prone positioning (to reduce pelvic motion and relieve claustrophobia) has been examined but does not offer advantages (McCauley et al, 1992b).

CONTRAST AGENTS

INTRAVENOUS AGENTS

Intravenous MR contrast agents are used to improve tissue contrast based on differences in delivery and retention of the agent. The most widely used MR contrast agents are chelated complexes of gadolinium. In the usual dose range, these agents produce their greatest effect on T_1-weighted images, in a manner roughly analogous to the effect of iodinated contrast in CT. In the female pelvis, contrast agents are useful in the characterization and staging of endometrial, vaginal, bladder and ovarian neoplasms, in differentiating recurrent tumor from fibrosis, and in infectious or inflammatory disease. Intravenous contrast is rarely used in evaluating cervical cancer or benign tumors of the uterus.

GASTROINTESTINAL AGENTS

Oral and/or rectal administration of contrast agents may improve overall MR image quality (Panaccione et al, 1991; Ros et al, 1991; Patten et al, 1992; Mattrey et al, 1994). The most promising agents produce negative contrast (darkening of bowel contents), which decreases peristalsis-related imaging artifact. The efficacy of these agents and their side effects are currently under investigation.

■ BENEFITS AND LIMITATIONS

The benefits of pelvic MRI accrue from its excellent tissue contrast, multiplanar imaging capability and absence of ionizing radiation. In these respects, MRI is similar to sonography. Unlike sonography, however, there are no 'blind spots' due to intervening bowel gas, calcifications and fatty tissue. MRI provides a larger field of view than sonography, often providing better depiction of anatomical relationships. Furthermore, as MRI sections are obtained in a systematic, volumetric fashion, the examination is much less operator dependent than is sonography.

Potential limitations of MRI stem from:

- prolonged imaging time relative to both CT and sonography;
- greater vulnerability to motion-related image artifacts;
- high imaging costs;
- incompatibility with some implanted metallic and electronic devices (see below);
- potential for claustrophobia.

IMAGING TIME AND MOTION ARTIFACTS

A typical MRI session lasts 30 minutes or longer, and each sequence takes several minutes to perform. Because data used to create individual sections within an imaged volume are usually acquired simultaneously, rather than one section at a time, motion artifacts can affect every image in the sequence. Sources of motion include breathing, bowel peristalsis and/or gross patient movements. Standard steps to reduce these sources of artifact include: fasting for 6 hours before examination and injection of 1 mg glucagon intramuscularly to minimize bowel peristalsis (Winkler and Hricak, 1986); instructing the patient to lie still and breathe evenly and shallowly during acquisition of each imaging sequence; and using respiratory motion compensation algorithms (Bailes et al, 1985).

COSTS AND COST EFFECTIVENESS

The cost of pelvic MRI varies widely, and comparison with the cost of other imaging modalities is therefore dif-ficult. It is generally true that the technical costs of MRI are greater than those of CT and sonography, in large part as a result of lower patient throughput and higher equipment costs. Rather than focusing solely on cost, it is perhaps more appropriate to ascertain the cost effectiveness of MRI relative to other diagnostic tests. The greater availability, lower cost and excellent diagnostic capability of sonography make it the most cost effective imaging modality in benign pelvic disease. In the evaluation of pelvic malignancy or in cases where sonography findings are not clearly benign, however, MRI may be the most cost effective imaging modality (Schwartz et al, 1994). In comparing the cost effectiveness of CT with MRI in the female pelvis, consideration must also be given to the risks of intravenous contrast agents and cost of treatment of adverse events; in patients at high risk for contrast induced nephrotoxicity, MRI may be more cost effective than CT (Lessler et al, 1994). Further cost effectiveness studies will be required to establish the appropriate role of MRI for other indications.

■ CONTRAINDICATIONS, COMPLICATIONS AND SIDE EFFECTS

METALLIC/ELECTRONIC IMPLANTS

Any metallic foreign body or electronic device within a patient represents a source of imaging artifact as well as a potential hazard. Metallic devices, such as orthopedic implants and surgical clips, cause local image artifacts due to magnetic field distortion, but do not generally represent a safety hazard. Intrauterine devices do not pose a hazard and cause minimal artifacts. Other metallic foreign bodies, e.g. projectile fragments, may be unsafe, depending on location – for example, migration of an intraocular metallic fragment during MR examination, causing unilateral blindness, has been reported (Kelly et al, 1986). Older ferromagnetic cerebral aneurysm clips, cardiac pacemakers, nerve stimulators and other implanted electronic devices may present a health hazard, due to torque exerted on the object by the magnetic field, heating by radiofrequency energy or electromagnetic interference, and should be considered absolute contraindications to imaging. For a comprehensive list of compatibility of electronic and metallic devices with MRI, the reader is referred to recent reviews (Shellock and Kanal, 1991; Shellock, 1992).

MRI AND THE UNSTABLE PATIENT

The relative inaccessibility of the patient during MR examination and difficulties in using standard resuscitation equipment in the MR scanning room (due to ferromagnetic effects and electrical interference) justify considerable caution in MRI of medically unstable patients. Prudence dictates that these patients should not undergo MRI unless there is a strong medical indication to do so and provisions are made to remove the patient quickly from the scan room in the event that resuscitation is required. A number of MRI-compatible physiological monitoring systems are commercially available to permit intubated, unstable or anesthetized patients to undergo MR examination more safely (Shellock, 1992).

MRI CONTRAST SAFETY

MR contrast agents have proved to be extremely safe in clinical practice (Goldstein et al, 1990), with a rate of severe adverse reactions approximating 1:400 000 for the most widely used agent, gadopentetate dimeglumine. Excretion of gadolinium chelates is predominantly via renal glomerular filtration (Weinmann et al, 1983). Unlike iodinated contrast agents, side effects of intravenously administered gadolinium chelates are rare and nephrotoxic effects are minimal (Carr, 1994). These agents readily cross the blood–placental barrier and are excreted in breast milk; their safety in pregnancy and breast feeding has not been firmly established (Kanal, 1994).

MRI DURING PREGNANCY

The absolute safety of MRI during pregnancy has not been established (Kanal, 1994). There is currently no evidence that MRI is hazardous to the developing fetus, and no mutagenic or other adverse effects have been detected in experimental and clinical studies (Schwartz and Crooks, 1982; McRobbie and Foster, 1985). Fur-

ther studies, however, are needed. MRI offers an alternative to sonography in the evaluation of diseases of the female pelvis and abdomen coincident with pregnancy and in evaluation of the pregnancy itself (McCarthy et al, 1985; Powell et al, 1986, 1988; Benson et al, 1991). The absence of ionizing radiation renders MRI potentially safer for the fetus than CT; however, there should be discretionary use of MRI during pregnancy, reserving its use for cases where sonography is not adequate and where CT would otherwise be required (Colletti and Platt, 1989; Hricak, 1989).

■ NORMAL APPEARANCES

CLINICAL ROLE

MRI currently has five major roles in gynecological imaging:

1 staging of malignant endometrial, cervical, and vaginal neoplasms (Bragg and Hricak, 1993);

2 detection of recurrent or residual tumor after cancer surgery or radiation therapy (Hricak, 1990; Hricak et al, 1993);

3 characterizing pelvic masses when sonography or CT is not definitive;

4 staging ovarian cancer when CT is inconclusive or iodinated contrast is contraindicated;

5 imaging of congenital anomalies (Forstner and Hricak, 1994; Secaf et al, 1994).

Further details of the role of MRI in evaluating specific diseases are presented in Section 2. MRI may be useful in dynamic evaluation of pelvic floor relaxation (Yang et al, 1991; Brubaker and Heit, 1993; Goodrich et al, 1993; Kirschner-Hermanns et al, 1993). In obstetrics, MRI has seen limited use in evaluation of placenta previa (Powell et al, 1986; Kay and Spritzer, 1991) and pelvimetry (Stark et al, 1985; Wright et al, 1992).

UTERUS, PARAMETRIUM AND VAGINA

Uterine and vaginal anatomy are well visualized by MRI. The normal morphological features of these organs at MRI are governed by patient age and hormonal status (Demas et al, 1986; Haynor et al, 1986; McCarthy et al, 1986).

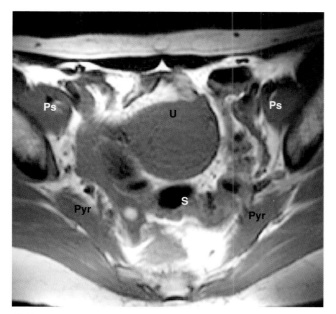

8.1a

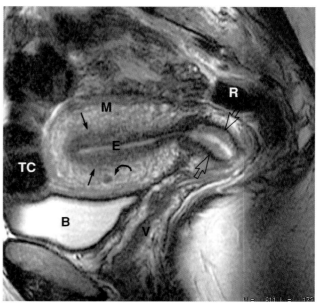

8.2a

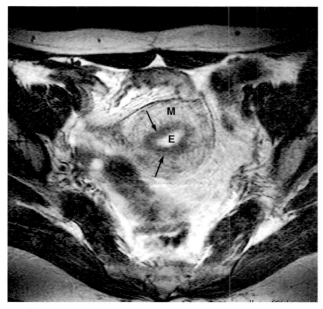

8.1b

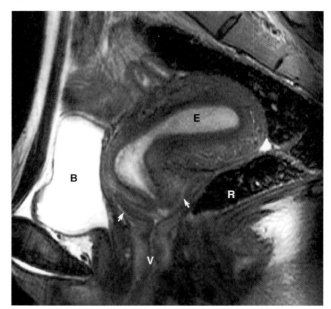

8.2b

Figure 8.1: *Normal uterine anatomy. (a) Axial T₁-weighted spin echo image of the uterine corpus. Differentiation between myometrium and endometrium is indistinct. U, uterus; S, sigmoid colon; Ps, psoas muscle; Pyr, piriformis muscle. (b) Corresponding T₂-weighted fast spin echo section shows three zones of the uterus: endometrium (E), junctional zone (arrows), and myometrium (M).*

UTERUS

Corpus

In women of reproductive age, the uterus normally measures 6–9 cm in length (Langlois, 1970). On T₁-weighted images, the uterus demonstrates homogeneous intermediate signal intensity (*Figure 8.1a*). On T₂-

Figure 8.2: *Midline sagittal pelvic anatomy and normal variation. T₂-weighted fast spin echo midline images obtained in two different adult females demonstrate (a) anteversion and (b) retroflexion of the uterus. The midline sagittal view offers superb detail of the uterus, cervix, vagina and adjacent midline structures. E, endometrium; M, myometrium; V, vagina; B, bladder; R, rectum; TC, transverse colon; long arrows, junctional zone; open arrows, low intensity cervical stroma and medium to high intensity cervical mucosa; short arrows, vaginal fornices; curved arrow, small leiomyoma.*

weighted images, three distinct uterine layers are seen: endometrium, junctional zone and myometrium (Hricak et al, 1983; Lee et al, 1985) (*Figures 8.1b* and *8.2*). Although three uterine zones can also be identified by

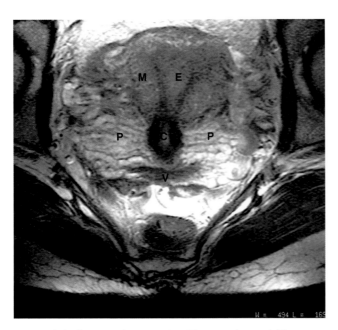

Figure 8.3: Cervix and parametria. Transverse long axis T_2-weighted fast spin echo section demonstrates excellent delineation of the cervix, uterus and parametria. E, endometrial cavity; M, myometrium; C, cervix; V, posterior vaginal fornix; P, parametria.

sonography, they differ in width from those identified by MRI and are not directly comparable (Mitchell et al, 1990).

The endometrium, which comprises the inner lining of the uterus, has high signal intensity on T_2-weighted images. Endometrial thickness varies with the menstrual cycle. The normal endometrial thickness on MRI ranges from 1–3 mm during the early proliferative phase to 5–7 mm during the midsecretory phase (Demas et al, 1986; Haynor et al, 1986; McCarthy et al, 1986).

The myometrium comprises the thick muscular layer of the uterus and is of intermediate signal intensity on T_2-weighted images. Signal intensity increases slightly during the midsecretory phase (Demas et al, 1986; Haynor et al, 1986; McCarthy et al, 1986).

The myometrial and endometrial layers are separated by the low signal intensity junctional zone. The junctional zone is more likely to represent inner myometrium with a lower water content (McCarthy et al, 1989) and higher nuclear:cytoplasmic ratio (Scoutt et al, 1991) than outer myometrium. The junctional zone width is normally less than 5 mm. A widened junctional zone is seen in diffuse adenomyosis (Mark and Hricak, 1987). Localized disruption of the junctional zone

serves as a sensitive marker of myometrial invasion by endometrial cancer (Hricak et al, 1987).

Cervix

On T_2-weighted images, the normal adult cervix demonstrates an inner zone of high signal intensity, surrounded by a low signal intensity middle layer and intermediate signal intensity outer layer (*Figures 8.2 and 8.3*). The inner zone is most likely to correspond to mucous glands and secretions, while the outer two layers correspond to cervical stroma with different nuclear:cytoplasmic ratios (Scoutt et al, 1993). Nabothian cysts are a common benign finding in the cervix, representing enlarged or obstructed cervical mucus glands. On T_2-weighted images, Nabothian cysts are round or oval and have very high signal intensity (similar to urine).

PARAMETRIUM

The parametrium is a cellular connective tissue contiguous with the 'bare area' of the uterus (uncovered by peritoneum). It carries the uterine vessels and lymphatics, as well as the ureters. The parametrium has signal intensity equal to myometrium on T_1-weighted images but is distinguishable on T_2-weighted images (*Figure 8.3*). Because the parametrium may become invaded early by cervical cancer, recognition of its normal MRI appearance is important.

VARIATION WITH AGE AND HORMONAL STATUS

In the infant, the zonal anatomy of the uterus is well visualized by MRI because of the lingering influence of maternal estrogens. In the premenarchal female, the uterine corpus is small and the zonal anatomy indistinct. The cervix of the premenarchal female is similar to the adult cervix in size, but accounts for more than half the uterine length because of the arrested development of the corpus (*Figure 8.4a*).

After the menopause, involution of the cervix parallels that of the uterine corpus and zonal anatomy becomes indistinct (Demas et al, 1986) (*Figure 8.4b*). The endometrial thickness decreases to less than 3 mm. If hormonal replacement therapy is instituted, the uterus may retain its premenopausal MR signal characteristics, with preserved zonal anatomy.

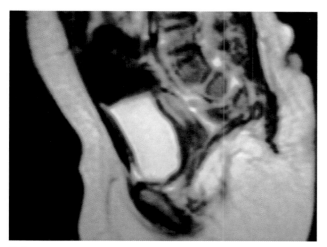

8.4a

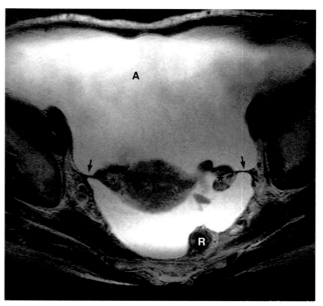

Figure 8.5: *Broad ligaments. T₂-weighted fast spin echo section shows the broad ligaments (arrows) outlined by high intensity ascites fluid (A). Fallopian tubes (asterisks) are also visualized due to the contrast with surrounding fluid. U, uterus; R, rectum.*

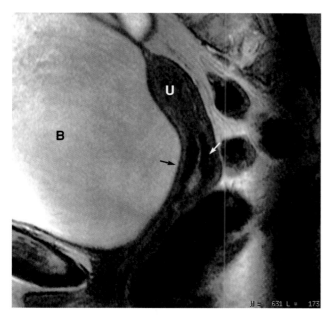

8.4b

Figure 8.4: *MRI appearance of the (a) premenarchal and (b) post-menopausal uterus is similar. Both (a) and (b) are sagittal T₂-weighted images. Age variation in MRI appearance of the uterus: sagittal T₂-weighted fast spin echo sections through the uterus in (a) a 7-year-old premenarchal female and (b) a 72-year-old post-menopausal female demonstrate a small uterine corpus with poor zonal differentiation (see Figure 8.1c for comparison with the uterus of a female of reproductive age). The cervix (arrows) maintains a relatively constant size throughout life. U, uterus; B, bladder.*

UTERINE LIGAMENTS

The broad ligaments are formed by the anterior and posterior reflections of the peritoneum as they pass over the Fallopian tubes, forming a thin sheet that is not reliably identified on MRI unless outlined by free intraperitoneal fluid (*Figure 8.5*). The round ligaments carry lymphatics which drain the fundus of the uterus into inguinal lymph nodes. They originate at the lateral angles of the uterus and course inferolaterally, passing through the inguinal canal and inserting in the labia majora. The round ligaments can be identified routinely at MRI (*Figure 8.6*). The suspensory uterine ligaments – cardinal and uterosacral – are often but not routinely visualized (*Figure 8.6b*).

VAGINA

The vagina is a fibromuscular tube extending from the vestibule to the uterus, and is located between the bladder and urethra anteriorly and the rectum posteriorly. The vagina demonstrates intermediate signal intensity on T₁-weighted images, with relatively poor contrast between rectum posteriorly and urethra anteriorly. The vagina is well visualized on contrast enhanced T₁-weighted images or on T₂-weighted images (Hricak et al, 1988) (*Figure 8.7*). Tampons in the vagina are not necessary for accurate assessment and may actually distort tissue detail.

As with the uterus, the MRI appearance of the vagina is under hormonal influence (Hricak et al, 1988). In the early proliferative phase, T₂-weighted images show high signal intensity central epithelium and mucus with a low signal intensity muscular wall. At the beginning of the secretory phase there is an increase in the thickness of

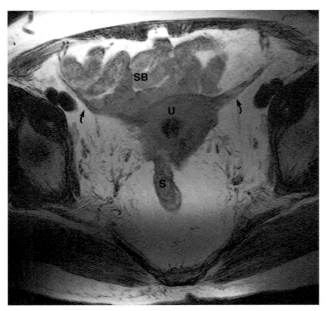

8.6a

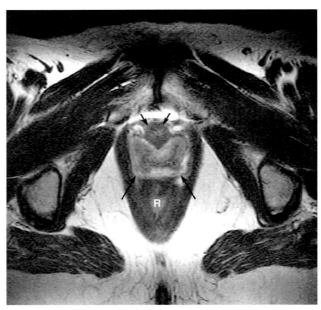

8.7a

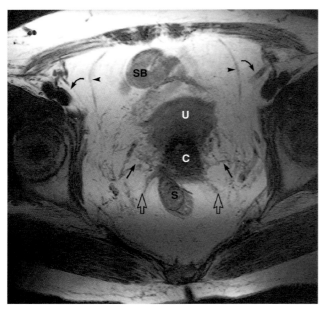

8.6b

Figure 8.6: *Uterine and pelvic ligaments. Axial T₂-weighted fast spin echo sections at adjacent levels demonstrate the round ligaments (curved arrows in (a)) as thick cords coursing anterolaterally from the uterine fundus towards the inguinal canals. The cardinal ligaments (straight arrows in (b)) extend from the cervix laterally towards the pelvic side wall, while the uterosacral ligaments (open arrows) curve posteriorly towards the sacrum. The medial and lateral umbilical ligaments (arrowheads and curved arrows, respectively) are also seen. Ligaments are unusually well demonstrated due to the presence of pelvic lipomatosis (note widened presacral space). U, uterus; C, cervix; S, sigmoid colon; SB, small bowel loops.*

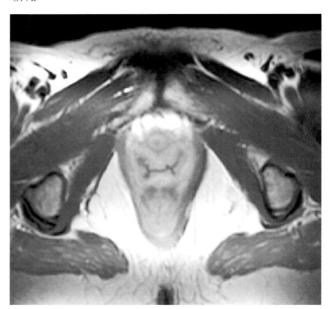

8.7b

Figure 8.7: *Cross-sectional appearance of the vagina. (a) Axial T₂-weighted fast spin echo and (b) contrast enhanced T₁-weighted spin echo sections through the midvagina show the typical H-shaped configuration of the collapsed vagina (long arrows in (a)). The vaginal epithelium and mucus form the thin inner vaginal layer (bright and dark in (a) and (b), respectively). The T₂-weighted section demonstrates the medium intensity muscular vaginal wall surrounded by high intensity vascular tissue. The vaginal wall is easily distinguishable from the rectum (R) posteriorly and the urethra (short arrows in (a)) anteriorly.*

ORAL CONTRACEPTIVE PREPARATIONS, EXOGENOUS ESTROGENS

Exogenous hormone therapy can have profound effects on the MRI appearance of the uterus and vagina. The

the central mucosa and in signal intensity of the wall, reducing zonal contrast. In late pregnancy, zonal anatomy is similarly indistinct.

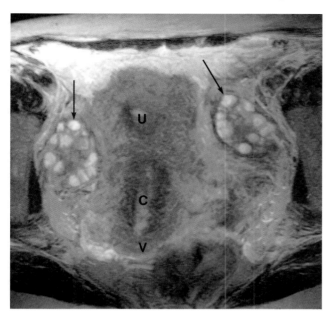

8.8a

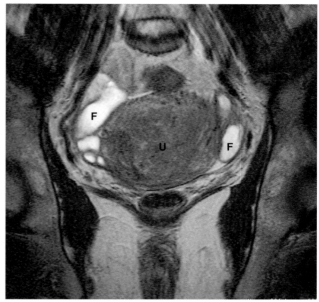

8.9a

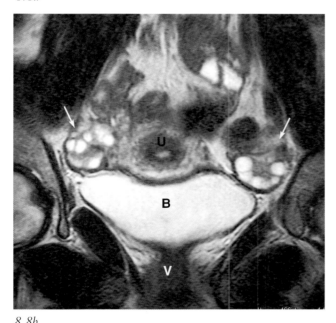

8.8b

Figure 8.8: *Ovaries. (a) Axial and (b) coronal T₂-weighted fast spin echo sections through the ovaries in a 34-year-old woman demonstrate multiple follicular cysts (rounded high intensity structures) located peripherally within the ovaries (arrows). The large number of peripheral cysts is unusual and may indicate polycystic ovarian disease. U, uterus; C, cervix; V, vagina; B, bladder.*

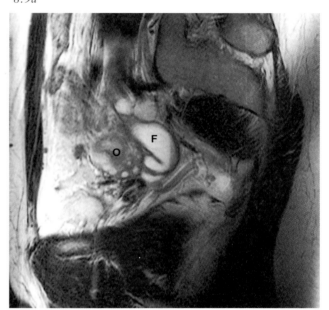

8.9b

Figure 8.9: *Fallopian tubes. (a) Coronal and (b) sagittal T₂-weighted fast spin echo sections in a female with peritubal adhesions demonstrate the typical serpiginous tubular appearance of hydrosalpinx. F, Fallopian tube; O, ovary; U, uterus.*

ADNEXA

The ovaries can be identified at MRI in at least 85% of women of reproductive age (Dooms et al, 1986). Ovaries have low to medium signal intensity on T₁-weighted images, and increase in relative signal intensity on T₂-weighted images (*Figure 8.8*). Contrast between ovaries and adjacent uterus or bowel is poor on T₁-weighted

signal intensity of the myometrium may increase on both T₁- and T₂-weighted images in women taking oral contraceptives (Demas et al, 1986). The use of exogenous estrogens after the menopause maintains an MRI appearance of the uterus and vagina similar to that of the early proliferative phase (Demas et al, 1986).

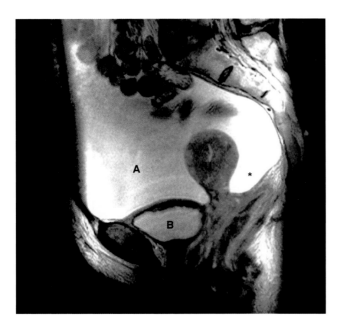

Figure 8.10: Peritoneal reflections. T_2-weighted fast spin echo mid-line sagittal section shows high intensity ascites outlining the anterior and posterior peritoneal reflections. A, ascites; asterisk, pouch of Douglas (cul-de-sac); U, uterus; B, bladder; R, rectum; SB, small bowel loops.

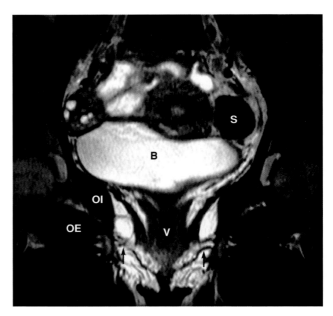

Figure 8.11: Pelvic cavity and floor. Coronal T_2-weighted fast spin echo section at the level of the femoral heads demonstrates the transversus perinei muscle (arrows) extending from the vagina to the ischium. This muscle, together with convergent tendons (central perineal tendon) forms the pelvic floor. O, ovary; U, uterus; S, sigmoid colon; B, bladder; V, vagina; OI, obturator internus muscle; OE, obturator externus muscle.

images. On T_2-weighted images, contrast between ovaries and adjacent fat may occasionally be poor (unless fat saturation is employed), but follicular cysts, which have very high signal intensity, are usually evident (*Figure 8.8*). Identification of normal ovaries at MRI in premenarchal and postmenopausal females is unreliable because the ovaries are small and follicular cysts are usually not present. Identification of normal Fallopian tubes at MRI is rare, due to their small diameter and lack of contrast with adjacent tissues. When hydrosalpinx is present, the Fallopian tubes can be identified on T_2-weighted images as serpiginous tubular structures filled with high signal intensity fluid (*Figure 8.9*).

PELVIC CAVITY AND FLOOR

Coronal and sagittal planes of section are helpful in the delineation of pelvic cavity boundaries. Localization of structures as intraperitoneal, retroperitoneal or extraperitoneal and evaluation of the pelvic floor are perhaps of greatest clinical relevance.

Peritoneal surfaces are not readily delineated by MRI unless bounded by fluid (*Figure 8.10*); however, knowledge of the compartment of normal pelvic structures

will aid in assigning a neighboring mass to the appropriate anatomical compartment.

The position of the levator ani muscle complex and the pelvic floor are of interest in the evaluation of stress incontinence and pelvic floor descent. These structures can be visualized at MRI (*Figure 8.11*). Dynamic evaluation of the pelvic floor by MRI during Valsalva maneuvers and other forms of straining shows promise as a means of accurate depiction of the severity of pelvic floor descent and of assessing the anatomical result of surgical repair (Brubaker and Heit, 1993; Goodrich et al, 1993).

REFERENCES

Bailes DR, Gilderdale DJ, Bydder GM, Collins AG & Firmin DN (1985) Respiratory ordered phase encoding (ROPE): a method for reducing respiratory motion artifacts in MR imaging. *J Comput Assist Tomogr* **9**: 838.

Baumgartner BR & Bernardino ME (1989) MR imaging of the cervix: off-axis scan to improve visualization of zonal anatomy. *AJR* **153**: 1001–1002.

Benson RC, Colletti PM, Platta LD & Rells PW (1991) MR imaging of fetal anomalies. *AJR* **156**: 1205–1207.

Bragg DG & Hricak H (1993) Imaging in gynecologic malignancies. *Cancer* **71**: 1648–1651.

Brubaker L & Heit MH (1993) Radiology of the pelvic floor. *Clin Obstet Gynecol* **36**: 952–959.

Bryan PJ, Butter HE, LiPuma JP et al (1993) NMR scanning of the pelvis: initial experience with a 0.3 T system. *AJR* **141**: 1111–1118.

Carr JJ (1994) Magnetic resonance contrast agents for neuroimaging: safety issues. *Neuroimaging Clin North Am* **4**: 43–54.

Colletti PM & Platt LD (1989) Obstetrical MRI acceptable under specific criteria. *Diagn Imaging* **5**: 32–36.

Demas BE, Hricak H & Jaffe RB (1986) Uterine MR imaging: effects of hormonal stimulation. *Radiology* **159**: 123–126.

Dooms GC, Hricak H & Tscholakoff D (1986) Adnexal structures: MR imaging. *Radiology* **158**: 639–646.

Forstner R & Hricak H (1994) Congenital malformations of uterus and vagina. *Radiologe* **34**: 397–404.

Goldstein HA, Kashamian FK, Blumetti RF, Hoyoak WI, Hugo FP & Blumsfield DM (1990) Safety assessment of gadopentetate dimeglumine in US clinical trials. *Radiology* **174**: 17–23.

Goodrich MA, Webb MJ, King BF, Bampton AE, Campeau NG & Riederer SJ (1993) Magnetic resonance imaging of pelvic floor relaxation: dynamic analysis and evaluation of patients before and after surgical repair. *Obstet Gynecol* **82**: 883–891.

Ha HK, Lim YT, Kim HS, Suh TS, Song HH & Kim SJ (1994) Diagnosis of pelvic endometriosis: fat-suppressed T1-weighted vs conventional MR images. *AJR* **163**: 127–131.

Hayes CE, Hattes N & Roemer PB (1991) Volume imaging with MR phased arrays. *Magn Reson Med* **18**: 309–319.

Hayes CE, Dietz MJ, King BF & Ehman RL (1992) Pelvic imaging with phased-array coils: quantitative assessment of signal-to-noise ratio improvement. *J Magn Reson Imaging* **2**: 321–326.

Haynor D, Mack L, Soules M et al (1986) Changing appearance of the normal uterus during the menstrual cycle: MR studies. *Radiology* **161**: 459–462.

Hricak H (1989) Guidelines for magnetic resonance imaging in obstetrics and gynecology. In *Clinical Applications of Magnetic Resonance Imaging*, pp 31–35. Reston, VA: American College of Radiology.

Hricak H (1990) Postoperative and postradiation changes in the pelvis. *Magn Reson Q* **6**: 276–297.

Hricak H, Alpers C, Crooks LE & Sheldon PE (1983) Magnetic resonance imaging of the female pelvis: initial experience. *AJR* **141**: 1119–1128.

Hricak H, Stern J & Fisher MR (1987) MRI in the evaluation of endometrial carcinoma and its staging. *Radiology* **162**: 297–305.

Hricak H, Chang YCF & Thurnher S (1988) Vagina: evaluation with MR imaging. I. Normal anatomy and congenital anomalies. *Radiology* **169**: 169–174.

Hricak H, Swift PS, Campos Z, Quivey JM, Gildengorin V & Goranson H (1993) Irradiation of the cervix uteri: value of unenhanced and contrast-enhanced MR imaging. *Radiology* **189**: 381–388.

Jain KA & Jeffrey RB Jr (1994) Evaluation of pelvic masses with magnetic resonance imaging and ultrasonography. *J Ultrasound Med* **13**: 845–853.

Kanal K (1994) Pregnancy and the safety of MRI. *MRI Clin North Am* **2**: 309–317.

Kay HH & Spritzer CE (1991) Preliminary experience with magnetic resonance imaging in patients with third-trimester bleeding. *Obstet Gynecol* **78**: 424–429.

Kelly WM, Pagle PG, Pearson A, San Diego AG & Soloman MA (1986) Ferromagnetic intraocular foreign body causes unilateral blindness after MR study. *AJNR* **7**: 243–245.

Kirschner-Hermanns R, Wein B, Niehaus S, Schaefer W & Jakse G (1993) The contribution of magnetic resonance imaging of the pelvic floor to the understanding of urinary incontinence. *Br J Urol* **72**: 715–718.

Langlois LP (1970) The size of the normal uterus. *J Reprod Med* **4**: 31–39.

Lee JKT, Gersell DJ, Balfe DM, Worthington JL, Picus D & Gapp G (1985) The uterus: in vitro MR–anatomic correlation of normal and abnormal specimens. *Radiology* **157**: 175–179.

Lessler DS, Sullivan SD & Stergachis A (1994) Cost-effectiveness of unenhanced MR imaging vs contrast-enhanced CT of the abdomen or pelvis. *AJR* **163**: 5–9.

McCarthy SM, Stark DD, Filly RA, Callen PW, Hricak H & Higgins CB (1985) Obstetrical magnetic resonance imaging: maternal anatomy. *Radiology* **154**: 421–425.

McCarthy S, Tauber C & Gore J (1986) Female pelvic anatomy: MR assessment of variations during the menstrual cycle and with use of oral contraceptives. *Radiology* **160**: 119–123.

McCarthy S, Scott G, Majumdar S et al (1989) Uterine junctional zone: MR study of water content and relaxation properties. *Radiology* **171**: 241–243.

McCauley TR, McCarthy S & Lange R (1992a) Pelvic phased array coil: image quality assessment for spin-echo MR imaging. *Magn Reson Imaging* **10**: 513–522.

McCauley TR, Wright JG, Bell SM & McCarthy S (1992b) Effect of prone versus supine patient positioning on pelvic magnetic resonance image quality. *Invest Radiol* **27**: 1005–1008.

McRobbie D & Foster MA (1985) Pulsed magnetic field exposure during pregnancy and implications for NMR foetal imaging: a study with mice. *Magn Reson Imaging* **3**: 231–234.

Mark AS & Hricak H (1987) Adenomyosis and leiomyoma: differential diagnosis by means of magnetic resonance imaging. *Radiology* **163**: 527–529.

Mattrey RF, Trambert MA, Brown JJ et al (1994) Perflubron as an oral contrast agent for MR imaging: results of a phase III clinical trial. *Radiology* **191**: 841–848.

Mitchell DG, Schonholz L, Hilpert PL, Pennell RG, Blum L & Rifkin MD (1990) Zones of the uterus: discrepancy between US and MR images. *Radiology* **174**: 827–831.

Panaccione JL, Ros PR, Torres GM & Burton SS (1991) Rectal barium in pelvic MR imaging: initial results. *J Magn Reson Imaging* **1**: 605–607.

Patten RM, Moss AA, Fenton TA & Elliott S (1992) OMR, a positive bowel contrast agent for abdominal and pelvic MR imaging: safety and imaging characteristics. *J Magn Reson Imaging* **2**: 25–34.

Powell MC, Buckley J, Price H, Worthington BS & Symonds EM (1986) Magnetic resonance imaging and placenta previa. *Am J Obstet Gynecol* **154**: 565–569.

Powell MC, Worthington BS, Buckley JM et al (1988) Magnetic resonance imaging in obstetrics. I: Maternal anatomy. *Br J Obstet Gynaecol* **95**: 31–37.

Reiman TH, Heiken JP, Totty WG & Lee JKT (1988) Clinical MR imaging with a Helmholtz-type surface coil. *Radiology* **169**: 564–566.

Ros PR, Steinman RM, Torres GM et al (1991) The value of barium as a gastrointestinal contrast agent in MR imaging: a comparison study in normal volunteers. *AJR* **157**: 761–767.

Schwartz JL & Crooks LE (1982) NMR imaging produces no observable mutations or cytotoxicity in mammalian cells. *AJR* **139**: 583–585.

Schwartz LB, Panageas E, Lange R, Rizzo J, Comite F & McCarthy S (1994) Female pelvis: impact of MR imaging on treatment decisions and net cost analysis. *Radiology* **192**: 55–60.

Scoutt LM, Flynn SD, Luthringer DJ, McCauley TR & McCarthy SM (1991) Junctional zone of the uterus: correlation of MR imaging and histologic examination of hysterectomy specimens. *Radiology* **179**: 403–407.

Scoutt LM, McCauley TR, Flynn SD, Luthringer DJ & McCarthy SM (1993) Zonal anatomy of the cervix: correlation of MR imaging and histologic examination of hysterectomy specimens. *Radiology* **186**: 159–162.

Secaf E, Hricak H, Gooding CA et al (1994) Role of MRI in the evaluation of ambiguous genitalia. *Pediatric Radiol* **24**: 231–235.

Shellock FG (1992) MRI biologic effects and safety considerations. In Higgins CB, Hricak H & Helms CA (eds) *Magnetic Resonance Imaging of the Body*, 2nd edn, pp 233–266. New York: Raven Press.

Shellock FG & Kanal E (1991) Policies, guidelines, and recommendations for MR imaging safety and patient management. *J Magn Reson Imaging* **1**: 97–101.

Smith RC, Reinhold C, Lange RC, McCauley TR, Kier R & McCarthy S (1992a) Fast spin-echo MR imaging of the female pelvis. Part I. Use of a whole-volume coil. *Radiology* **184**: 665–669.

Smith RC, Reinhold C, McCauley TR et al (1992b) Multicoil high-resolution fast spin-echo MR imaging of the female pelvis. *Radiology* **184**: 671–675.

Stark DD, McCarthy SM, Filly RA, Parer JT, Hricak H & Callen PW (1985) Pelvimetry by magnetic resonance imaging. *AJR* **144**: 947–950.

Stevens SK, Hricak H & Campos Z (1993) Teratomas versus cystic hemorrhagic adnexal lesions: differentiation with proton-selective fat-saturation MR imaging. *Radiology* **186**: 481–488.

Sugimura K, Okizuka H, Imaoka I et al (1993) Pelvic endometriosis: detection and diagnosis with chemical-shift MR imaging. *Radiology* **188**: 435–438.

Takahashi K, Okada S, Ozaki T, Kitao M & Sugimura K (1994) Diagnosis of pelvic endometriosis by magnetic resonance imaging using `fat-saturation' technique. *Fertil Steril* **62**: 973–977.

Weinmann H-J, Brasch RC, Press W-R & Wesbey GE (1983) Characteristics of gadolinium-DTPA complex: a potential NMR contrast agent. *AJR* **142**: 619–624.

Winkler M & Hricak H (1986) Pelvis imaging with MR. Technique for improvement. *Radiology* **158**: 848–849.

Wright AR, Cameron HM & Lind T (1992) Magnetic resonance imaging pelvimetry: a useful adjunct in the management of the obese patient. *Br J Obstet Gynaecol* **99**: 852–853.

Yang A, Mostwin JL, Rosenshein NB & Zerhouni EA (1991) Pelvic floor descent in women: dynamic evaluation with fast MR imaging and cinematic display. *Radiology* **179**: 25–33.

Section One:
Explorative Techniques

PART 2
NEW TECHNICAL DEVELOPMENTS:
NORMAL APPEARANCES AND PATHOLOGY

9 Ultrasonography: color Doppler flow
J Zaidi and S Campbell

■ INTRODUCTION

In 1950 Wild described for the first time the application of ultrasonic pulses for the detection of tissue density changes in the in vitro setting. This discovery led to the birth of the ultrasound era. Donald et al (1958) developed a system for assessing abdominal masses using pulsed ultrasound, but it was not until the 1960s that the potential use of pulsed ultrasound in obstetric and gynecological practice was fully realized (Campbell, 1968; Donald, 1969) and the technique hailed as a great advance because of its noninvasive nature. In gynecological practice Kratochwil (1969) reported the use of a transvaginal probe with improved resolution of imaging of the pelvic organs. Since these initial reports, ultrasound technology has undergone rapid development. The recent advent of high frequency endovaginal probes in combination with real time ultrasound has improved the image quality of the pelvic organs without the need for a full bladder. As a result, transvaginal ultrasonography has now superseded transabdominal ultrasound scanning in modern gynecological ultrasound practice.

With the arrival of Doppler ultrasound, it became possible to investigate vascular changes in a noninvasive fashion. Satomora (1959) was the first to perform blood flow studies in superficial human vessels using Doppler ultrasound. The technique soon became established in clinical practice for the assessment of vascular disease, particularly the carotid artery and leg vessels (Atkinson and Woodcock, 1972). Studies in obstetrics were initially conducted on the fetal umbilical artery using continuous wave Doppler (Fitzgerald and Drumm, 1977); however, conventional continuous wave Doppler systems were found to produce confusing signals from flow or tissue movement occurring anywhere along the entire length of the ultrasound beam and the use of this method for examining flow in specific deep vessels was therefore limited. The development of pulsed Doppler systems allowed the operator to sample signals at a chosen depth and, when combined with real time ultrasound imaging (the so-called 'duplex' method), any specific vessel could be precisely localized and studied. MacCallum et al (1978) used only pulsed Doppler to study the umbilical artery, while Eik-Nes et al (1980) used the duplex technique to detect blood flow changes in the human fetus. Furthermore, pulsed and continuous wave studies of the uteroplacental circulation were found to be reliable in the diagnosis and prediction of fetal intrauterine growth retardation (Campbell et al, 1983).

Studies of the pelvic circulation in nonpregnant women were initially performed using the transabdominal approach (Taylor et al, 1985). With the advent of the transvaginal Doppler technique and its close proximity to the pelvic vessels, it was soon possible to accurately locate and describe flow characteristics of the uterine and ovarian arteries. With the addition of color Doppler ultrasound, improved spatial evaluation, localization of blood vessels and analysis of flow velocity waveforms by pulsed Doppler were thus facilitated.

■ EQUIPMENT

All ultrasound examinations described in this chapter were performed using an Acuson XP 128/10 ultrasound system (Acuson Corp, Mountain View, California, USA) (*Figure 9.1*). This system was equipped with both EV-519 (*Figure 9.2*) and EC-7 (*Figure 9.3*) endovaginal probes. The EV-519 probe emitted an ultrasound frequency of 5 MHz for B-mode imaging, while the frequency in the EC-7 probe could be varied between 5 and 7.5 MHz. In both the color and pulsed Doppler modes, the Doppler ultrasound had a frequency of 5 MHz in the EV-519 transducer

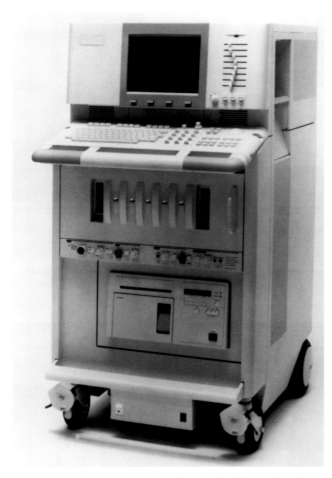

Figure 9.1: Acuson XP 128/10 color Doppler ultrasound machine.

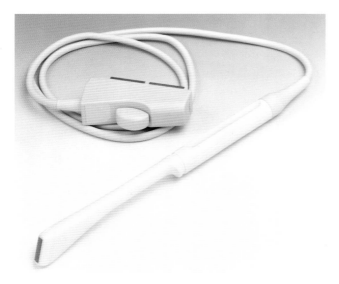

Figure 9.2: EV-519 endovaginal probe.

model, while the EC-7 probe emitted either 5 or 7.5 MHz for color Doppler and 5 MHz for pulsed Doppler ultrasound. The focal range of the transducer could be easily

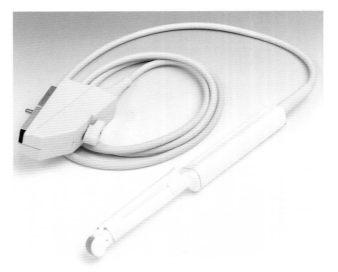

Figure 9.3: EC-7 endovaginal probe.

varied according to the depth of the organ studied. The Doppler system was equipped with a high pass filter to remove signals from vessel wall movements in the path of the Doppler ultrasound pulse. The high pass filter was set as low as possible so that low blood velocities were still detected. We used a high pass filter set at 125 Hz. In the studies described in this chapter the scans were performed using the EV-519 probe as the EC-7 probe was only recently acquired.

▪ TECHNIQUE

In medical imaging, when a Doppler transducer emits a beam of ultrasound waves into the body, wave reflection occurs at each boundary between and within tissues having different acoustic impedances. The returning echoes from stationary sites are received at the emitted frequency, but if ultrasound waves are reflected from a moving target, such as red blood cells, the movement of the target causes a frequency shift in the reflected signal. This frequency shift (f_d), also known as the Doppler shift frequency or Doppler frequency, is detected by the ultrasound receiver. The frequency shift is proportional to the velocity of the moving target and is expressed as follows:

$$f_d = 2f_t\, v \cos \theta / c$$

where f_t is the transmitted ultrasound frequency, v is the velocity of the target, c is the velocity of sound in the

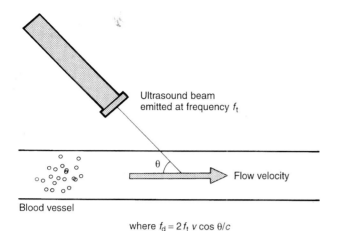

where $f_d = 2 f_t v \cos \theta / c$

Figure 9.4: *Beam/vessel angle necessary for measuring blood flow velocity. (See text for explanation.)*

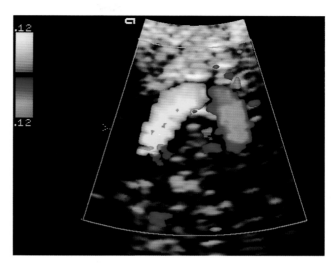

Figure 9.5: *Color Doppler imaging of a uterine artery with blood flowing away from and towards the probe (seen as a blue and red color Doppler image, respectively).*

medium and θ is the angle between the ultrasound beam and the direction of movement of the target. Flow velocity is normally assumed to be along the axis of the vessel and θ is often described as the beam/vessel angle (*Figure 9.4*). In general, the value of c for a particular tissue type will remain constant and therefore the f_d will vary by the other three factors in the equation. The magnitude of the f_d rises as the velocity of the target rises and as the magnitude of the transmitted ultrasound frequency (f_t) rises. This means that higher frequency ultrasound probes are more sensitive to lower flow velocities. Furthermore, the f_d rises as the emitted ultrasound beam becomes more aligned to the direction of flow, i.e. as θ becomes smaller or $\cos \theta$ rises. In medical imaging, if the emitted ultrasound frequency and θ are fixed, f_d will vary in direct proportion to the flow velocity. Thus the Doppler ultrasound technique can be used to measure blood flow velocity. In Doppler recordings from flowing blood, the signal received does not contain one single frequency but a spectrum of frequencies over the cardiac cycle, called the Doppler shift spectrum.

In pulsed Doppler systems short pulses of ultrasound are transmitted at regular intervals and the returning echoes are received after a short period of time. The pulsed Doppler systems allow measurement of the depth (or range) at which blood flow is observed (by measuring the time taken for the pulse to be transmitted to and reflected back from the blood cells). Furthermore, the size of the sample volume (or range gate) can be changed by altering the time over which the signal is received. As a result, the operator is able to study flow in a particular area of interest analyzing the full Doppler shift spectrum.

In practice it is necessary to guide the Doppler beam to the specific area of interest. This facility is achieved by duplex ultrasound (or image directed Doppler ultrasound) where the real time ultrasound image (or B-mode image) is used to select the location for interrogation by Doppler ultrasound. The machine is then switched to operate in the pulsed Doppler mode with the sample volume placed in the area of interest.

Using color Doppler imaging (CDI) the resultant Doppler frequency shifts can be encoded in color and superimposed in two dimensions on a real time image. Although CDI uses pulsed Doppler ultrasound, its processing is different from that used to provide the Doppler shift spectrum. CDI uses fewer, shorter pulses along each color scan line of the image to give a mean frequency shift and a variance at each small area of measurement. This frequency shift is converted into a color pixel. The scanner then repeats this for several lines to build up the color image, which is superimposed on the B-mode image. The color assigned to the frequency shifts is usually based on the direction of flow (i.e. blue for frequency shifts away from the ultrasound beam and red for shifts towards the beam) (*Figure 9.5*). As frequency shifts increase, there is an increase in color intensity. This intensity of the color Doppler image reflects the intensity weighted mean velocity of blood in the blood vessels and therefore an increase in color intensity

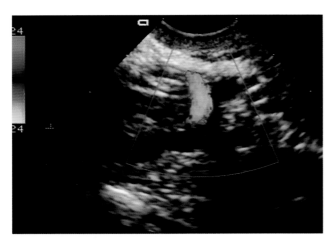

Figure 9.6: Color Doppler ultrasound can be used to identify a uterine artery easily.

should reflect an increased blood flow velocity; however, since the intensity of the color Doppler image is related to the beam/vessel angle, an area of bright color indicating high Doppler shift could reflect a low beam/vessel angle with a low blood flow velocity (Kremkau, 1990).

Modern ultrasound machines combine a high quality real time ultrasound image with color and pulsed Doppler ultrasound. The CDI facility allows easy vessel identification (*Figure 9.6*), description of the direction of flow (*Figure 9.5*) and a subjective assessment of blood circulation throughout the entire color Doppler image (*Figure 9.7*). Subsequent activation of the pulsed Doppler function produces flow velocity waveforms at the particular site within the vessel, which can be used to provide an analysis of flow velocity and impedance (*Figure 9.8*). Thus CDI and pulsed Doppler systems are complementary to each other and should be used as such.

Doppler shift information can be analyzed qualitatively, quantitatively and semiquantitatively.

QUALITATIVE ANALYSIS

Using CDI the presence or absence of flow can be determined and displayed on the gray scale image. This is one of the simplest but perhaps most useful applications of Doppler ultrasound. It may be used, for example, to exclude occlusion by thrombosis or congenital malformation. Confirming the absence of flow is a little more difficult. It is important that the lack of a Doppler signal is a consequence of a lack of flow rather than of the acoustic or electrical parameters of the system. The direction of flow can be determined, which is particularly useful in the assessment of blood

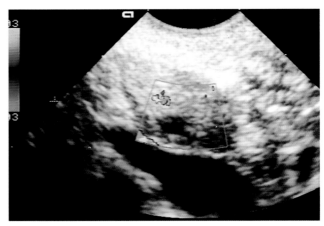

9.7a

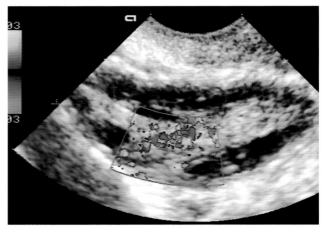

9.7b

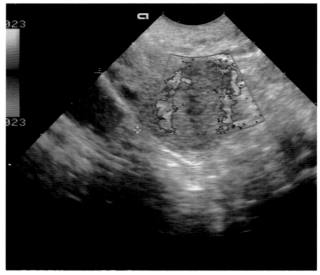

9.7c

Figure 9.7: (a) Normal ovary in the early follicular phase. Note the position of the color Doppler box over the ovarian stroma and the small amount of color representing a small frequency shift. (b) Example of a polycystic ovary with subjectively increased vascularity within the ovarian stroma. (c) Example of a corpus luteum with an intense ring of color in its wall, denoting increased vascularity.

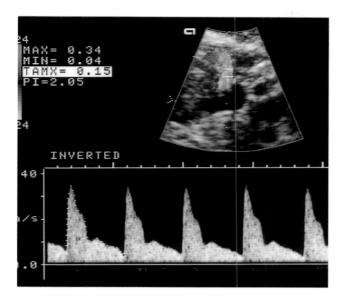

Figure 9.8: *Flow velocity waveform of a uterine artery.*
$V_{max} = 0.34 \ m/s; \ PI = 2.05.$

flow in fetal vessels and in elucidating vascular abnormalities such as the twin–twin transfusion syndrome. Furthermore, arterial blood flow in various parts of the pelvic circulation has characteristic waveforms; these are described later.

QUANTITATIVE ANALYSIS

Using Doppler ultrasound it is possible to estimate the absolute velocity (cm/s) and volume flow rate (ml/min) of blood in large vessels. To estimate velocity it is essential to know the beam/vessel angle of the vessel insonated, keeping the magnitude of the insonation angle to a minimum, thus minimizing error. For angles less than 30° the error in velocity estimation will be insignificant, while larger angles will be associated with greater error. The velocity measurements that can be made include peak systolic blood flow velocity, time averaged maximum velocity and time averaged mean velocity. For larger vessels flow velocity estimations are possible but, if vessels are small and tortuous, measurement of the beam/vessel angle is difficult and true blood flow velocity estimation may be inaccurate. This is especially the case with angiogenesis where there are many small, tortuous vessels. In practice, however, it may be assumed that at least one vessel in the vascular bed will be located at a low angle, so maximum peak systolic velocities can be measured with minimum error (Campbell et al, 1993; Sladkevicius et al, 1993).

Most duplex scanners now have a cursor to measure this angle directly and automatically calculate the cor-

rected velocity. Volume flow rate measurement by Doppler ultrasound is fraught with difficulties. The vessel cross-sectional area must be calculated and flow velocity estimated. In practice the vessel diameter needs to be measured and the area calculated; however, inaccuracy arises because even a tiny error in diameter measurement (e.g. 0.5 mm) would result in a large percentage error in volume flow.

SEMIQUANTITATIVE ANALYSIS

Since measurements of flow velocity and volume flow are complex and may not be suitable for routine clinical use, simpler Doppler measurements that are only semiquantitative are proving to be of diagnostic interest. These simpler measurements are based on the analysis of the Doppler spectral display, known as the time velocity waveform or flow velocity waveform. The maximum Doppler shift frequency is proportional to the velocity of the fastest moving blood within the sample volume, and characterization of the variation of this quantity with time can provide information regarding both the condition of the proximal circulation and the resistance of the distal vasculature. For a given pressure waveform, the relative flow in diastole will change with the impedance to flow caused by the resistance of the downstream vasculature. Thus flow velocity waveforms with high flow in diastole are associated with low impedance (*Figure 9.9*), while waveforms with little or reverse flow in diastole are associated with high impedance (*Figure 9.10*).

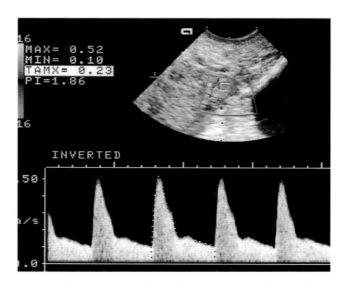

Figure 9.9: *Uterine artery flow velocity waveform with increased flow in diastole in a patient undergoing in vitro fertilization treatment.* $V_{max} = 0.52 \ m/s; \ PI = 1.86.$

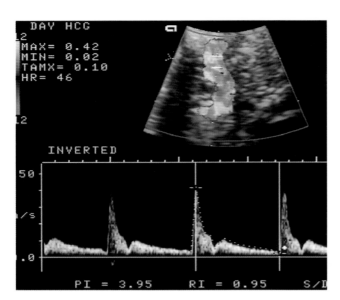

Figure 9.10: *Uterine artery flow velocity waveform with reduced flow in diastole in a patient undergoing in vitro fertilization treatment. Note the presence of a notch in both Figures 9.9 and 9.10. $V_{max} = 0.42$ m/s; PI = 3.95.*

Since the Doppler frequency shift is directly proportional to the flow velocity, with the constant of proportionality determined by the beam/vessel angle, the ratio of two Doppler shifted frequencies is independent of this angle. As a result it is possible to use such ratios as an index of pulsatility of the waveform and a measure of distal impedance. A number of indices based on the maximum Doppler shift waveform (i.e. the envelope of the flow velocity waveform) have been described as a measure of this impedance.

- The pulsatility index (PI) was originally described by Gosling and King in 1969 (Gosling and King, 1975) and is defined as:

  PI = $(S − D)$/mean

  where S is the maximum Doppler shifted frequency, D is the minimum Doppler shifted frequency and mean is the mean of the maximum Doppler shifted frequencies over the cardiac cycle.
- The resistance index (RI) described by Pourcelot (1974) is defined as:

  RI = $(S − D)$/S

  where S is the peak systolic and D is the end diastolic frequency.
- Systolic:diastolic ratio (S:D) is calculated by dividing the peak systolic frequency by the end diastolic frequency.

Each of these indices is independent of the beam/vessel angle but the PI appears most accurately to reflect

blood impedance from a comparison of blood flow in neonatal cerebral arteries using an in vitro model (Miles et al, 1987).

TECHNIQUE OF COLOR DOPPLER MEASUREMENT

UTERINE ARTERY

The uterine artery may be visualized by color Doppler imaging lateral to the internal cervical os. If the transducer is held in the longitudinal plane and the tip of the probe gently moved into each vaginal fornix, the uterine artery can be seen ascending up the lateral aspect of the uterus. A pulsed Doppler range gate can then be applied across the vessel, ensuring that the angle between the Doppler beam and the vessel is close to zero. Flow velocity waveforms illustrating the shifted Doppler frequencies can thus be demonstrated (*Figures 9.9* and *9.10*). The uterine artery has a characteristic early diastolic notch.

SUBENDOMETRIAL VESSELS

Vessels in the endometrial region can be evaluated using color Doppler ultrasound. Initially a subjective assessment of the presence or absence of color flow in the endometrial and subendometrial region can be described by placing the color Doppler box across the area of interest. The depth of vascular penetration of the endometrium can be assessed by determining the innermost part of the endometrium with pulsatile vessels. Vascular penetration of the 'triple' line endometrium can be classified as proposed by Applebaum (1993):

- zone 1, vessels penetrating the outer hypoechogenic area surrounding the endometrium but not entering the hyperechogenic outer margin of the endometrium (*Figure 9.11*);
- zone 2, vessels penetrating the hyperechogenic outer margin of the endometrium (*Figure 9.12*);
- zone 3, vessels entering the hypoechogenic inner area between the hyperechogenic outer margin of the endometrium and the endometrial canal (*Figure 9.13*);
- zone 4, vessels reaching the endometrial cavity.

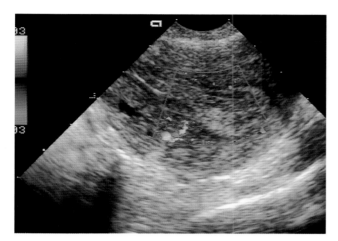

Figure 9.11: Zone 1 vascular penetration. Vessels are seen penetrating the periendometrial hypoechogenic region but not entering the outer hyperechogenic region of the endometrium.

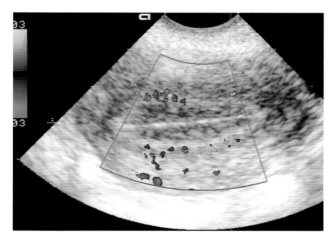

Figure 9.12: Zone 2 vascular penetration. Vessels are seen penetrating the hyperechogenic outer margin of the endometrium.

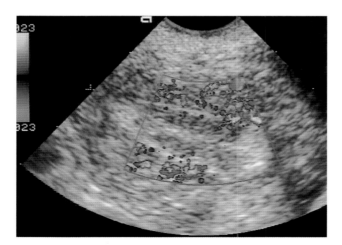

Figure 9.13: Zone 3 vascular penetration. Vessels are seen penetrating the hypoechogenic inner area between the hyperechogenic outer margin of the endometrium and the endometrial canal.

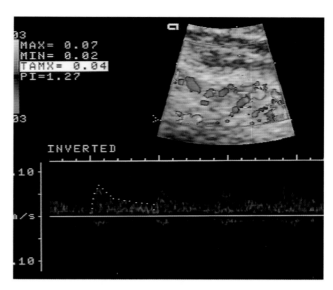

Figure 9.14: Flow velocity waveforms obtained from the subendometrial region or zone 1. $V_{max} = 0.07$ m/s; PI = 1.27.

Finally, subendometrial (zone 1) Doppler blood flow velocimetry can be determined by using the color Doppler technique. Having selected areas of maximum color intensity, a Doppler range gate can be applied and the pulsed Doppler function activated to assess blood flow velocity. Peak systolic blood flow velocity waveforms are thus detected and measurements repeated until optimal flow velocity waveforms (i.e. those with the maximum Doppler shifted frequencies) are obtained (*Figure 9.14*).

OVARIAN STROMAL VESSELS

The intraovarian blood flow of each ovary can be assessed by color Doppler ultrasound. The color Doppler box can be placed over the ovarian stroma and blood vessels clearly visualized. An ovarian stromal artery may be defined as any small artery in the ovarian stroma not close to the surface of the ovary or near the wall of a follicle. Areas of maximum color intensity, representing the greatest Doppler frequency shifts, can be selected for pulsed Doppler examination. The resultant flow velocity waveforms produced can be selected for analysis. As for the subendometrial vessels, the optimal flow velocity waveforms (i.e. those with the largest Doppler shifts) can be analyzed (*Figure 9.15*).

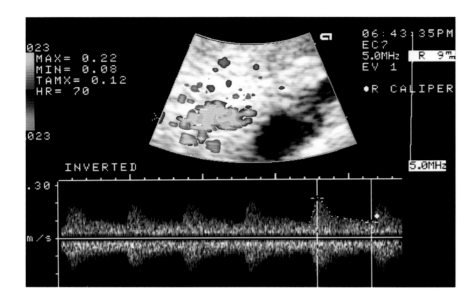

Figure 9.15: Flow velocity waveforms from the ovarian stroma. Note the position of the pulsed Doppler range gate over the ovarian stroma and not near the surface of the ovary or near a follicle. $V_{max} = 0.22$ m/s; PI = 1.13.

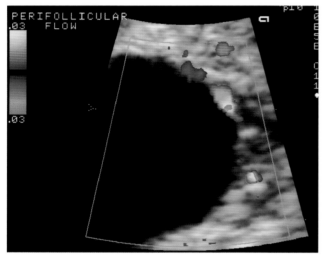

9.16a

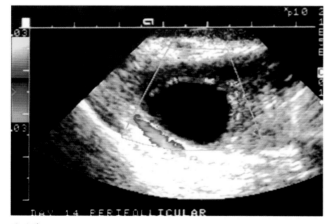

9.16b

Figure 9.16: (a) Follicular vessels can be seen developing circumferentially around a dominant ovarian follicle on day 11 of the menstrual cycle. (b) An intense ring of vessels around a dominant ovarian follicle on the day of the LH surge.

FOLLICULAR VESSELS

Ovarian stromal arteries terminate as vascular arcades around the wall of the developing ovarian follicles. Using color Doppler ultrasound, vessels in the follicular wall may be seen developing circumferentially around a developing ovarian follicle (*Figure 9.16*). These vessels probably represent an anastomotic network of capillaries surrounding the avascular granulosa cell layer. After activating the pulsed Doppler function the flow velocity waveforms in the region sampled may be demonstrated (*Figure 9.17*).

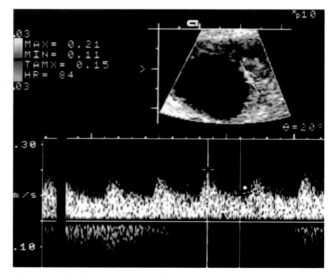

Figure 9.17: Flow velocity waveforms from the follicular vessels on the day of the LH surge. $V_{max} = 0.21$ m/s; PI = 0.67.

■ BENEFITS AND LIMITATIONS

Transvaginal color Doppler ultrasonography allows the operator to assess the vascular changes to the pelvic organs in a noninvasive fashion. B-mode ultrasonography using the transvaginal approach is now accepted as the optimal method for examining the female pelvis. The combination of high frequency Doppler transducers and endovaginal probes allows excellent conventional gray scale imaging, clear color Doppler sonograms allowing accurate location of vessels (Kurjak et al, 1989; Steer et al, 1990) and improved resolution of flow velocity waveforms.

The technique may thus be used to evaluate vascular changes to the female pelvic organs during the normal menstrual cycle (Scholtes et al, 1989; Steer et al, 1990; Campbell et al, 1993; Sladkevicius et al, 1993). This information can improve our understanding of reproductive physiology and provide a rational basis for investigating blood flow changes in pathological conditions such as the polycystic ovary syndrome (Battaglia et al, 1995; Zaidi et al, 1995c, 1995d) and the luteinized unruptured follicle (Zaidi et al, 1995a). Color Doppler ultrasound may also be used to assist in the diagnosis of ovarian and uterine malignancy (Bourne et al, 1989, 1990; Kurjak et al, 1989), study uterine receptivity in women undergoing in vitro fertilization (Steer et al, 1992; Favre et al, 1993; Zaidi et al, 1995e) and investigate vascularity of ectopic pregnancies (Jurkovic et al, 1992; Tekay and Joupplia, 1992).

Although transvaginal color Doppler ultrasound is practiced in large centers, the equipment tends to be expensive and is thus not available to all gynecological units. Furthermore, since there are no prospective randomized trials assessing the clinical use of this technology, there is still much debate regarding the usefulness of color Doppler ultrasound over conventional B-mode imaging. However, it is hoped that as a greater understanding of the normal physiological changes is developed, rigorous prospective studies of the clinical application of this technology in gynecological practice will occur.

■ COMPLICATIONS AND SIDE EFFECTS

Over the last few years there has been much debate regarding the safety of diagnostic ultrasound in obstetric and gynecological practice. Although the emitted ultrasound waves are converted into heat energy and absorbed by the surrounding tissues, to date there is no evidence of any detrimental effects in humans. The power output of pulsed Doppler ultrasound is, however, many times greater than that of standard B-mode imaging and is therefore more likely to cause a greater transfer of heat energy. As a result of these concerns the World Federation for Ultrasound in Medicine and Biology (WFUMB, 1992) drew up guidelines and recommendations regarding the thermal effects of diagnostic ultrasound examination and recommended that ultrasound exposures resulting in a maximum temperature rise of $1.5°C$ were acceptable in clinical practice.

The United States Food and Drug Administration (FDA) have also produced guidelines regarding the maximum power output of ultrasound in different clinical situations. The power output, more commonly known as the spatial peak temporal average intensity (SPTA), can be adjusted by the operator on the ultrasound machine. A maximum value of SPTA < 94 mW/cm^2 has been recommended by the FDA for obstetric ultrasound. Although most ultrasound machines automatically set SPTA well below these recommendations, it is also prudent to keep the ultrasound examination time or the exposure time to a minimum, thereby minimizing the delivery of ultrasound energy.

The following guidelines are suggested as measures to minimize the exposure of ultrasound energy.

- First perform the standard B-mode ultrasound scan. Once the appropriate region for Doppler examination is visualized, the color Doppler function can be activated. Color Doppler (CDI) does not significantly increase the delivery of ultrasound energy but allows easy vessel identification before activating pulsed Doppler ultrasound. Using CDI in this way the exposure to pulsed Doppler ultrasound can be restricted to a few seconds.

- When Doppler ultrasound is not required, the Doppler functions should be switched off. One often needs to alternate between

B-mode imaging with CDI and CDI with pulsed Doppler ultrasound. In this situation only activate the pulsed Doppler function when absolutely necessary.

▪ The power output for color and pulsed Doppler ultrasound should be kept at the lowest level necessary to obtain an adequate signal.

▪ Keep the ultrasound exposure time to a minimum.

▪ NORMAL APPEARANCES

The documentation of hemodynamic changes in the ovarian and uterine arteries during the normal menstrual cycle is essential to improve our understanding of reproductive physiology and forms the foundation for studies of the pelvic circulation in pathological conditions.

UTERINE ARTERY

A number of studies have been published on the uterine circulation during the spontaneous menstrual cycle (Taylor et al, 1985; Goswamy and Steptoe, 1988; Scholtes et al, 1989; Battaglia et al, 1990; Steer et al, 1990; Collins et al, 1991; Sladkevicius et al, 1993). All the previous studies differed in study design and methodology and reported different results; however, a number of conclusions regarding uterine artery blood flow changes during the menstrual cycle have evolved. Uterine artery PI has been reported to peak on day 1 of menstruation, thereafter declining (Steer et al, 1990) and to rise again in the late follicular phase or at the time of ovulation (Goswamy and Steptoe, 1988; Scholtes et al, 1989; Battaglia et al, 1990; Steer et al, 1990); however, Collins et al (1991) did not notice any significant daily change in uterine PI over the periovulatory period, whereas Sladkevicius et al (1993) demonstrated a significantly higher uterine artery PI 2 days after ovulation. During the luteal phase there does appear to be general agreement that uterine artery PI or RI appears to decline (Battaglia et al, 1990; Steer et al, 1990; Sladkevicius et al, 1993; Zaidi et al, 1994a).

Recently, we have studied prospectively the hemodynamic changes in the uterine arteries during the menstrual cycle in normal healthy women, using both hormonally derived and fixed time points. The results suggest that there is a circadian rhythm in uterine artery PI and time averaged maximum velocity (TAMX) over

the periovulatory period (Zaidi et al, 1995b). Uterine artery PI appears to be lower in the early morning and increases during the day (*Figure 9.18*), with TAMX showing the opposite effect (*Figure 9.19*). These fluctuations appear to be independent of the midcycle hormonal changes. We believe that these changes have important implications for future Doppler blood flow studies and would suggest that the interpretation of

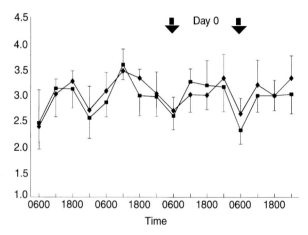

Figure 9.18: Circadian rhythm in uterine artery PI. Day 0 = day of the LH surge; values are mean ± SE. ■, Dominant uterine artery PI; ◆, nondominant uterine artery PI. From Zaidi J, Jurkovic D, Campbell S, Pittrof R, McGregor A & Tan SL (1995) Description of circadian variation in uterine artery blood flow during the peri-ovulatory period. Hum Reprod 10: 1642–1646. Reproduced with permission of Oxford University Press.

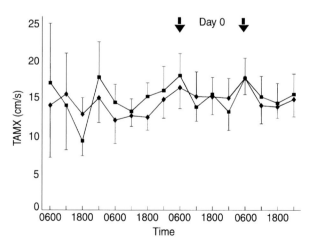

Figure 9.19: Circadian rhythm in uterine artery TAMX. Day 0 = day of the LH surge; values are mean ± SE. ■, Dominant uterine artery TAMX; ◆, nondominant uterine artery TAMX. From Zaidi J, Jurkovic D, Campbell S, Pittrof R, McGregor A & Tan SL (1995) Description of circadian variation in uterine artery blood flow during the peri-ovulatory period. Hum Reprod 10: 1642–1646. Reproduced with permission of Oxford University Press.

Doppler studies of the uterine artery must take this circadian rhythm into account.

When the longitudinal changes in uterine artery blood flow over the menstrual cycle were analyzed using the day of the luteinizing hormone (LH) surge as the reference point, there did appear to be a gradual increase in TAMX in the uterine artery on the side bearing the dominant ovarian follicle (dominant uterine artery), with no change in the contralateral vessel. Sladkevicius et al (1993) have previously reported this finding, although they used the presumed day of follicular rupture as the reference point. In contrast, we noted no significant change in PI in either uterine artery during the follicular phase, although PI reached a peak on the day of the LH surge and LH surge −1 in the dominant and nondominant uterine arteries, respectively. Dominant uterine artery PI then declined during the luteal phase of the cycle (Zaidi et al, 1994a).

SUBENDOMETRIAL VESSELS

Collins et al (1991) were unable to detect flow velocity waveforms from the endometrium until the day of ovulation. More recently, Sladkevicius et al (1993) were able to study the serial changes in Doppler velocimetry of the subendometrial vessels during the menstrual cycle and documented flow velocity waveforms in the subendometrial vessels from cycle day 4. The Doppler blood flow changes in the uterine arteries were reflected in the subendometrial vessels (Sladkevicius et al, 1993). The differences in the results between the two studies is likely to be due to differences in the sensitivity of the ultrasound equipment used. Recently, we have studied subendometrial and intraendometrial perfusion in patients undergoing in vitro fertilization treatment and have reported that there is a failure of embryo implantation if subendometrial blood flow is absent (Zaidi et al, 1995f).

INTRAOVARIAN VESSELS

Anatomically the ovary is surrounded by many vessels. The uterine artery lies inferiorly and medially to the ovary; the tubal and ovarian branches of the uterine artery lie above the ovary; the ovarian and iliac arteries lie lateral to the ovary. Since there are so many vessels surrounding the ovary, it is often difficult to identify accurately the ovarian artery by color Doppler. Although a number of researchers have described vascular changes in the ovarian artery during the menstrual cycle (Taylor et al, 1985; Scholtes et al, 1989; Hata et al, 1990), more recently the description of intraovarian hemodynamics has become more popular (Kurjak et al, 1989; Bourne et al, 1991; Collins et al, 1991; Campbell et al, 1993; Sladkevicius et al, 1993; Zaidi et al, 1994b, 1995d). The reason for this may be because the identification of intraovarian vessels by color Doppler, specifically follicular and ovarian stromal vessels (*Figures 9.15–9.17*) is far easier and may provide more useful information regarding reproductive physiology.

Collins et al (1991), using transvaginal color Doppler ultrasound, noted vessels in the granulosa–thecal cell interface at the time of the LH rise with maximum velocity (V_{max}) rising over the periovulatory period. The PI was, however, noted to remain relatively constant over the same period. Campbell et al (1993) noted similar findings, with perifollicular or follicular V_{max} rising from about 24 hours before and continuing to rise for 3 days after follicular rupture. The changes in follicular blood flow velocity appear to follow the rise in circulating LH. The authors went on to suggest that these findings may reflect an increase in blood flow around the time of ovulation, possibly reflecting neoangiogenesis.

More recently Sladkevicius et al (1993) documented vascular changes in the arteries in ovarian hilum, stroma and wall of the dominant follicle and corpus luteum during the menstrual cycle. They also noted that the ovary bearing the dominant follicle displayed a greater amount and intensity of color coded areas from 1–2 days before ovulation until formation of the corpus luteum. Blood flow velocity was also noted to be greater in the wall of the corpus luteum than in the wall of the dominant follicle.

We have studied prospectively the hemodynamic changes in the follicular and ovarian stromal vessels during the menstrual cycle in normal healthy women in relation to the onset of the LH surge. The women underwent color Doppler examination serially throughout the cycle and were scanned every 6 hours over the periovulatory period. We noted a rise in V_{max} in the wall of the dominant follicle and in the adjacent ovarian stroma during the follicular phase of the cycle. After the LH surge V_{max} rose more steeply and remained fast in the midluteal phase (*Figures 9.20* and *9.21*). The

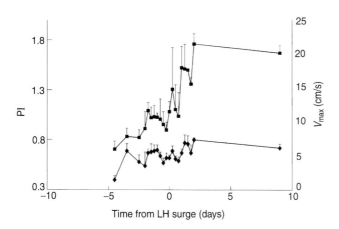

Figure 9.20: Changes in follicular V_{max} *and PI during the menstrual cycle in relation to the onset of the LH surge. Values are mean* $\pm$ *SE;* ■, *follicular* V_{max}; ◆, *follicular PI.*

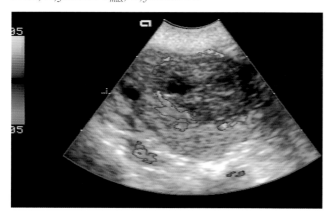

9.21a

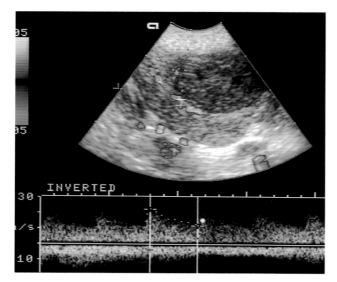

9.21b

Figure 9.21: (a) Color Doppler ultrasound of an active corpus luteum during the midluteal phase. (b) Flow velocity waveform from the wall of the corpus luteum showing high blood flow velocity. $V_{max} = 0.22$ m/s; PI = 0.60.

changes in V_{max} correlated significantly with the changes in serum concentration of LH (Zaidi et al, 1994c). There was no significant change in PI in the wall of the dominant follicle or in its adjacent stroma, and similarly there was no significant change in either V_{max} or PI in the contralateral ovary. These findings are similar to the previous studies cited, with the hemodynamic changes possibly reflecting a process of angiogenesis occurring during follicular development, ovulation and formation of the corpus luteum. It is possible that the changes in LH may be the trigger for this angiogenic process.

In conclusion, color Doppler studies of the uterine artery show a decline in impedance during the luteal phase of the menstrual cycle, suggesting that there is an increase in perfusion at the time of embryo implantation. This may be of clinical importance in the assessment of the infertile couple (Steer et al, 1994). Color Doppler studies of the follicular and ovarian stromal vessels in the ovary bearing the dominant ovarian follicle have shown an increase in blood flow velocity during the periovulatory period, particularly around the time of the LH surge. These observations indicate a process of angiogenesis occurring at the time of ovulation. Knowledge of this angiogenic process may be clinically important in the investigation of conditions such as the luteinized unruptured follicle and the polycystic ovary syndrome.

■ ACKNOWLEDGEMENTS

We would like to thank Ms Debbie Sheddon and Mr Keith White of Acuson UK for technical assistance and loan of their ultrasound equipment.

REFERENCES

Applebaum M (1993) The 'steel' or 'teflon' endometrium: ultrasound visualization of endometrial vascularity in IVF patients and outcome. *Ultrasound Obstet Gynecol* **3** (**suppl 2**): 10.

Atkinson P & Woodcock JP (1972) In *Doppler Ultrasound and its Use in Clinical Measurement,* pp 134–137. London: Academic Press.

Battaglia C, Larocca E, Lanzani A, Valentini M & Genazzani AR (1990) Doppler ultrasound studies of the uterine arteries in spontaneous and IVF stimulated ovarian cycles. *Gynecol Endocrinol* **4**: 245–250.

Battaglia C, Artini PG, D'Ambrogio G, Genazzani A & Genazzani A (1995) The role of color Doppler imaging in the diagnosis of polycystic ovary syndrome. *Am J Obstet Gynecol* **172**: 108–113.

Bourne T, Campbell S, Steer C, Whitehead MI & Collins WP (1989) Transvaginal color flow imaging: a possible new screening test for ovarian cancer. *BMJ* **299**: 1367–1370.

Bourne T, Campbell S, Whitehead MI, Royston P, Steer CV & Collins WP (1990) Detection of endometrial cancer in postmenopausal women by transvaginal ultrasonography and colour flow imaging. *BMJ* **301**: 369.

Bourne TH, Jurkovic D, Waterstone J, Campbell S & Collins WP (1991) Intrafollicular blood flow during human ovulation. *Ultrasound Obstet Gynecol* **1**: 53–59.

Campbell S (1968) An improved method of fetal cephalometry by ultrasound. *J Obstet Gynaecol Br Commonw* **75**: 568–576.

Campbell S, Diaz-Recasens J, Griffin DR et al (1983) New Doppler technique for assessing utero-placental blood flow. *Lancet* **i**: 675–677.

Campbell S, Bourne TH, Waterstone J et al (1993) Transvaginal color flow imaging of the periovulatory follicle. *Fertil Steril* **60**: 433–438.

Collins W, Jurkovic D, Bourne T, Kurjak A & Campbell S (1991) Ovarian morphology, endocrine function and intra-follicular blood flow during the periovulatory period. *Human Reprod* **6**: 319–324.

Donald I (1969) On launching a new diagnostic science. *Am J Obstet Gynecol* **103**: 609.

Donald I, MacVicar J & Brown TG (1958) Investigations of abdominal masses: pulsed ultrasound. *Lancet* **i**: 1188–1194.

Eik-Nes SH, Brubakk AO & Ulstein MK (1980) Measurement of human foetal blood flow. *Lancet* **i**: 283–285.

Favre R, Bettahar K, Grange G et al (1993) Predictive value of transvaginal uterine Doppler assessment in an in vitro fertilization program. *Ultrasound Obstet Gynecol* **3**: 350–353.

Fitzgerald DE & Drumm JE (1977) Non-invasive measurement of the foetal circulation using ultrasound: a new method. *BMJ* **ii**: 1450–1451.

Gosling RG & King DH (1975) Ultrasonic angiology. In Harens AW & Adamson L (eds) *Arteries and Veins*, pp 61–98. Edinburgh: Churchill Livingstone.

Goswamy RK & Steptoe PC (1988) Doppler ultrasound studies of the uterine artery in spontaneous ovarian cycles. *Hum Reprod* **3**: 721–726.

Hata K, Hata T, Senoh D et al (1990) Change in ovarian arterial compliance during the human menstrual cycle assessed by Doppler ultrasound. *Br J Obstet Gynaecol* **97**: 163–166.

Jurkovic D, Bourne T, Jauniaux E, Campbell S & Collins WP (1992) Transvaginal color Doppler study of blood flow in ectopic pregnancies. *Fertil Steril* **57**: 68–73.

Kratochwil A (1969) Ein neues vaginales schnittbildverfahren. *Geburtshilfe Frauenheilkd* **29**: 379–385.

Kremkau FW (1990) *Doppler Ultrasound. Principles and Instruments.* Philadelphia: WB Saunders.

Kurjak A, Zalud I, Jurkovic D, Alfirovic Z & Miljan M (1989) Transvaginal color Doppler assessment of pelvic circulation. *Acta Obstet Gynecol Scand* **68**: 131–135.

MacCallum WD, William CS, Napel S & Daigle RE (1978) Fetal blood velocity waveforms. *Am J Obstet Gynecol* **132**: 425–429

Miles RD, Menke JA, Bashiru M & Colliver JA (1987) Relationships of five Doppler measures with flow in an in vitro model and clinical findings in newborn infants. *J Ultrasound Med* **6**: 597–599.

Pourcelot L (1974) Applications clinique de l'examen Doppler transcutane. In Peronneau P (ed.) *Velocimetric Ultrasonore Doppler*, pp 213–240. Paris: Inserm.

Satomora A (1959) Study of the flow pattern in peripheral arteries by ultrasonics. *J Acoust Soc Jpn* **15**: 151–158.

Scholtes MCW, Wladimiroff JW, van Rijen HJM & Hop WCJ (1989) Uterine and ovarian flow velocity waveforms in the normal menstrual cycle: a transvaginal study. *Fertil Steril* **52**: 981–985.

Sladkevicius P, Valentin L & Marsal K (1993) Blood flow in the uterine and ovarian arteries during the normal menstrual cycle. *Ultrasound Obstet Gynecol* **3**: 199–208.

Steer CV, Campbell S, Pampiglione J, Mason BA & Collins WP (1990) Transvaginal colour flow imaging of the uterine arteries during the ovarian and menstrual cycles. *Hum Repord* **5**: 391–395.

Steer CV, Campbell S, Tan SL et al (1992) The use of transvaginal color flow imaging after in vitro fertilization to identify optimum uterine conditions before embryo transfer. *Fertil Steril* **57**: 372–376.

Steer CV, Tan SL, Mason BL & Campbell S (1994) Midluteal-phase vaginal color Doppler assessment of uterine artery impedance in a subfertile population. *Fertil Steril* **61**: 53–58.

Taylor KJW, Burns PN, Wells PNT, Conway DI & Hull MJR (1985) Ultrasound Doppler flow studies of the ovarian and uterine arteries. *Br J Obstet Gynaecol* **92**: 240–246.

Tekay A & Jouppila P (1992) Color Doppler flow as an indicator of trophoblastic activity in tubal pregnancies detected by transvaginal ultrasound. *Obstet Gynecol* **80**: 995–999.

WFUMB (1992) Report on WFUMB symposium on safety and standardisation in medical ultrasound. *Ultrasound Med Biol* **18**: 731–809.

Wild J (1950) The use of ultrasonic pulse for the measurement of biological tissues and the detection of tissue density changes. *Surgery* **27**: 161.

Zaidi J, Campbell S, Pittrof R et al (1994a) Blood flow changes in the subendometrial and uterine arteries during the normal menstrual cycle. *Ultrasound Obstet Gynecol* **4** (**suppl 1**): 117.

Zaidi J, Campbell S, Pittrof R, Okokon E, Collins WP & Tan SL (1994b) Blood flow changes in the follicular wall and ovarian stroma during the normal menstrual cycle. *Ultrasound Obstet Gynecol* **4** (**suppl 1**): 118.

Zaidi J, Campbell S, Pittrof R, Okokon E, Collins WP & Tan SL (1994c) Endocrine changes during the menstrual cycle: correlations with blood flow changes in the wall of the dominant follicle and ovarian stroma. *J Endocrinol* **143** (**suppl**) (abstract 022).

Zaidi J, Jurkovic D, Campbell S, Collins W, McGregor A & Tan SL (1995a) Luteinized unruptured follicle: morphology, endocrine function and blood flow changes during the menstrual cycle. *Human Reprod* **10**: 44–49.

Zaidi J, Jurkovic D, Campbell S, Pittrof R, McGregor A & Tan SL (1995b) Description of circadian variation in uterine artery blood flow during the peri-ovulatory period. *Hum Reprod* **10**: 1642–1646.

Zaidi J, Pittrof R, Campbell S, Okokon E & Tan SL (1995c) A longitudinal study of the blood flow changes in the follicular wall and ovarian stroma during the menstrual cycle in women with the polycystic ovarian syndrome. *Hum Reprod* **10** (abstract book 2, no. 330).

Zaidi J, Campbell S, Pittrof R et al (1995d) Ovarian stromal blood flow in women with polycystic ovaries. A possible new marker for ultrasound diagnosis? *Hum Reprod* **10**: 1992–1996.

Zaidi J, Pittrof R, Shaker A, Kyei-Mensah A, Campbell S & Tan SL (1995e) Assessment of uterine artery blood flow on the day of human chorionic gonadotropin administration by transvaginal color Doppler ultrasound in an in vitro fertilization program. *Fertil Steril* **65**: 377–381.

Zaidi J, Campbell S, Pittrof R & Tan SL (1995f) Assessment of endometrial thickness, morphology, endometrial vascular penetration and velocimetry in predicting implantation in an in vitro fertilization program. *Ultrasound Obstet Gynecol* **6**: 191–198.

10 Endoscopy: salpingoscopy
I Brosens

■ INTRODUCTION

Salpingoscopy is an endoscopic technique designed for the inspection of the tubal ampullary mucosa at the time of laparotomy or laparoscopy. Recent studies have shown that tubal mucosal adhesions are more significantly related to pregnancy outcome than pelvic adhesions (Heylen et al, 1995; Marana et al, 1995b; Vasquez et al, 1995a). The mucosal adhesions are underestimated by hysterosalpingography, while they are overestimated when compared with the presence of pelvic adhesions found at laparoscopy or laparotomy. Direct visualization of the tubal ampullary mucosa by transabdominal endoscopic techniques has been described as salpingoscopy or tuboscopy.

■ EQUIPMENT

A variety of telescopes, such as a modified hysteroscope and flexible bronchoscope, have been used to gain access to the tubal lumen at laparotomy or laparoscopy. Currently, a specially designed rigid salpingoscope has been developed to allow salpingoscopy to become a standard endoscopic procedure in the investigation of infertility (Brosens et al, 1987).

■ TECHNIQUE

The technique is based on the visualization of the ampullary segment after distension by a saline drip. The instruments include the salpingoscope, which is similar to the ureterocystoscope and has an outer diameter of 2.8 mm, the salpingoscope sheath with a connection for a saline drip, the obturator and an atraumatic tubal grasping forceps (*Figure 10.1*). The sheath with the obturator is introduced into the tube and once in place the tube is

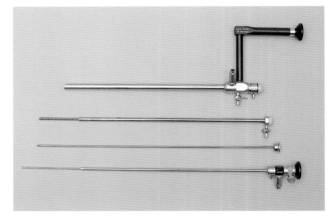

10.1a

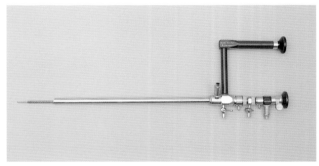

10.1b

Figure 10.1: *(a) The salpingoscope comprises three parts: the telescope (bottom), the obturator and the sheath with connection for a saline drip. The system is used in combination with the laparoscope. (b) The salpingoscope is introduced into the operation channel of the laparoscope.*

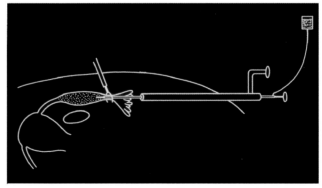

Figure 10.2: *Distension of the ampullary segment is obtained by a saline drip after clamping the tube using an atraumatic rounded grasping forceps at the level of the infundibulum.*

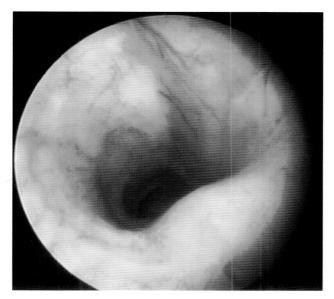

10.3a

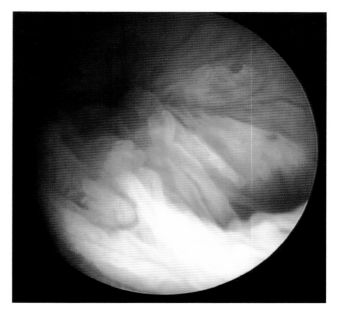

10.3c

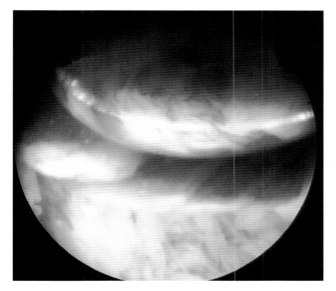

10.3b

Figure 10.3: *At salpingoscopy no folds are seen (a) but on withdrawal from the air bubble (b) the folds become visible in the saline (c).*

clamped with an atraumatic rounded tubal forceps at the level of the infundibulum. The obturator is then replaced by the endoscope and the saline drip connected to the sheath is opened to distend the ampullary segment (*Figure 10.2*). Air bubbles should be allowed to escape before the salpingoscope is introduced because they compress the folds against the wall.

The following technical problems can occur during salpingoscopy.

- The telescope is introduced into the tube but there is no visibility when the optic is advanced against the tubal wall. The problem is solved by slight withdrawal of the scope or by stretching the tube using the tubal forceps.

- When air bubbles have not been removed they can compress the folds and no folds are seen. By moving the scope slowly back or forward the optic can escape from the air bubble (*Figure 10.3*).

- The telescope has inadvertently perforated the tubal wall and the interstitial connective tissue of the mesosalpinx is identified as adhesions (*Figure 10.4a*). Careful withdrawal of the scope under direct visualization allows identification of the site of perforation (*Figure 10.4b*).

- Edematous swelling of the mesosalpinx can occur in the absence of perforation and is suggestive of an abnormal tubal mucosa with areas of epithelial desquamation. The tube should be investigated for chronic salpingitis.

- The tortuous or convoluted tube presents a problem as herniation of the mucosa makes cannulation and progression of the telescope in the tube difficult (*Figure 10.5*).

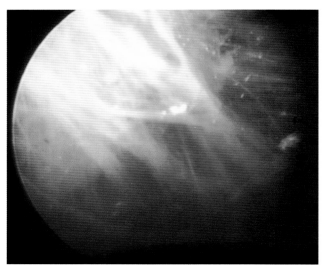

10.4a

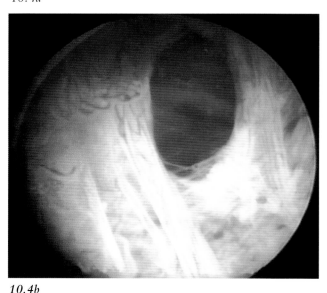

10.4b

Figure 10.4: *(a) Interstitial tissue of the mesosalpinx; (b) on withdrawal the perforation is seen.*

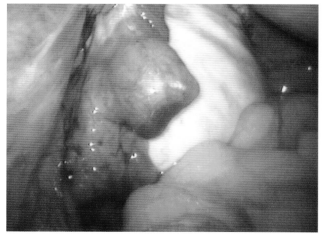

Figure 10.5: *A tortuous tube makes access difficult beyond the distended zone.*

▪ BENEFITS AND LIMITATIONS

The detection and identification of tubal mucosal lesions require good visibility. The benefits of salpingoscopy are the easy application of the technique at the time of abdominal surgery and the excellent visualization of the tubal mucosa. Tubal mucosal adhesions have been shown to provide the most critical parameter for the outcome of pregnancy and the risk of ectopic pregnancy in pelvic inflammatory disease. The correlation of salpingoscopy with hysterosalpingography shows that tubal mucosal lesions are underdiagnosed by hysterosalpingography in 48–55% of cases (Henry-Suchet et al, 1985; Puttemans et al, 1987). On the other hand, pelvic serosal adhesions detected at laparoscopy show no good correlation with tubal mucosal adhesions (Heylen et al, 1995; Marana et al, 1995b; Vasquez et al, 1995b). Visual inspection of the fimbriae is important to detect sequelae of tubal infection but is discordant with salpingoscopy in 23–38% of cases (Henry-Suchet et al, 1985; Shapiro et al, 1988).

Salpingoscopy is limited to the inspection of the complex mucosal fold system of the ampullary segment. The rigid telescope with its rod lens gives a clear and bright image with a wide and deep field of view in this segment but cannot enter the isthmic segment. The lumen of the isthmus averages 0.5 mm and the mucosal folds, usually four or five in number, are low and slightly rounded. Falloposcopy has been described as the microendoscopic technique for the visual exploration of the human Fallopian tube from the uterotubal ostium up to the fimbria, using the transvaginal approach (Kerin et al, 1990). Falloposcopy and salpingoscopy should be seen as complementary procedures in the exploration of the Fallopian tube. The potential of falloposcopy needs further evaluation with respect to its reproducibility of observations in the different tubal segments and clinical validation (Kerin et al, 1992).

▪ COMPLICATIONS

Complications from salpingoscopy are rare. It is possible to damage the fimbriae with the tubal grasping forceps and to cause minor bleeding. It is preferable to introduce the sheath without grasping the fimbriae but by stabilizing the tube at the infundibulum, and to use an atraumatic rounded tube-holding forceps.

The most serious complication is damage to the tubal mucosa and perforation of the tubal wall, which can occur when the sheath is introduced but is more likely if the telescope is advanced blindly or if there are rough movements of the scope. The need for very gentle handling of the tube and the instruments cannot be stressed too strongly. With these safeguards there should be no significant complications from salpingoscopy.

■ NORMAL APPEARANCES

The infundibulum has a concentric structure consisting of large folds and an opening which can be easily cannulated with a probe of 3–5 mm (*Figure 10.6a*). The ampulla is composed of four or five large parallel folds with accessory folds on the lateral sides and three or four small rounded folds between them (*Figure 10.6b*). A fine capillary vascularization can be seen in the transparent mucosa of the folds (*Figure 10.6c*). At the

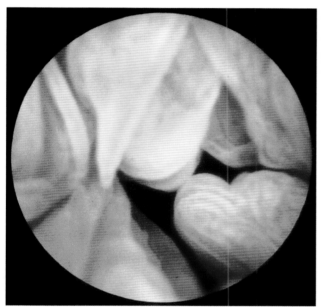

10.6a

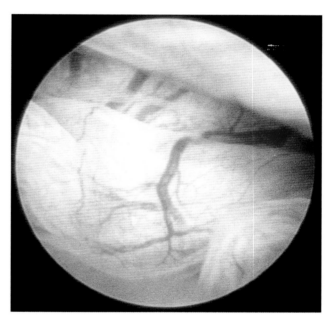

10.6c

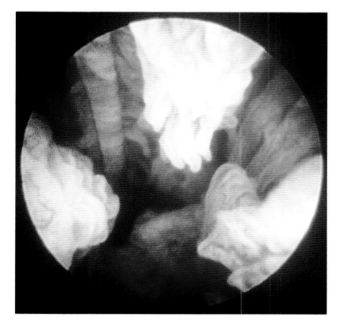

10.6b

Figure 10.6: Salpingoscopy of normal Fallopian tube.
(a) Concentric large folds at the infundibulum. (b) Large parallel folds with accessory folds and small rounded folds between them line the ampullary segment. (c) A fine capillary network is seen in the thin mucosal fold.

isthmic–ampullary junction the large ampullary folds abruptly become small and join together to continue in the isthmic segment as small, rounded folds. These junctions should not be confused with adhesions. Variations from the normal occur. Abnormalities of the large folds, such as an increased frondosal structure, varicosities of the subepithelial capillaries and small white or opaque deposits on the folds can be observed (*Figure 10.7*).

The wall can show abnormalities such as distension and flattening in the tortuous tube (*Figure 10.8*) or accessory ostia (*Figure 10.9*).

■ CLINICAL INDICATIONS

Salpingoscopy is indicated when tubal pathology is present or suspected.

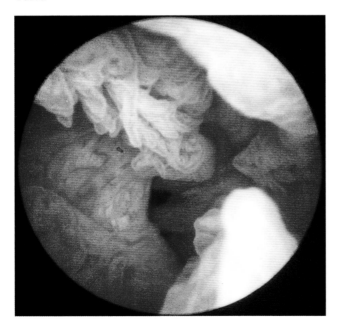

10.7a

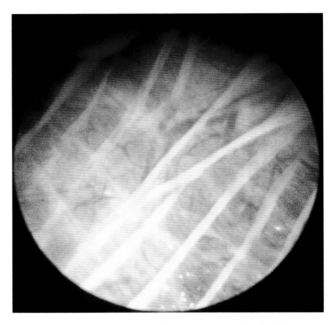

Figure 10.8: *Flattening of the folds, not to be confused with a hydrosalpinx, in a tortuous tube.*

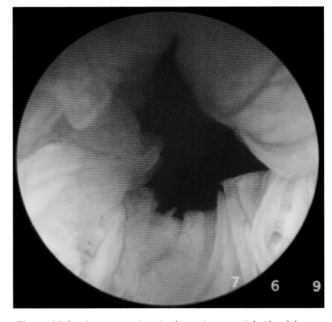

10.7b

Figure 10.7: *Prominent frondosal appearance of ampullary folds at (a) the infundibulum and (b) ampullary segment.*

Figure 10.9: *Accessory ostium in the antimesenterial side of the ampullary segment.*

In *proximal tubal block* transabdominal salpingoscopy is the only technique that allows exploration of the ampullary tubal mucosa. In these cases the ampullary mucosa is normal in 80% of cases (Gürgan et al, 1994).

Pelvic inflammatory disease (PID) is the most frequent cause of distal tubal pathology, but causes serosal adhesions more frequently than mucosal adhesions. There is no doubt that microscopic tubal lesions can be seen at microscopy in the absence of mucosal adhesions, but at present the mucosal adhesions are the most reliable parameter for the detection of severe sequelae of infection at the time of endoscopy. In addition, there is poor correlation between the presence and extent of serosal and mucosal adhesions in PID as mild pelvic adhesions can be associated with severe mucosal adhesions. Mucosal adhesions are present in 57% of PID patients with hydrosalpinx and in 22% with pelvic adhesions (De Bruyne et al, 1989; Heylen et al, 1995).

Endometriosis can be associated with an extensive degree of pelvic adhesions and the tube is frequently involved in severe endometriosis. Hydrosalpinx can be caused by compression or serosal structure rather than by mucosal adhesions and occlusion. Salpingoscopy in these cases almost always reveals the absence of adhesions in the ampullary mucosa (Nezhat et al, 1990; Heylen et al, 1995).

Ectopic pregnancy is frequently associated with tubal mucosal lesions (Vasquez et al, 1983). There is now increasing evidence that after conservative surgery the recurrence of ectopic pregnancy depends on the underlying disease rather than on the operating technique or the damage to the site of implantation. Salpingoscopy is becoming a powerful tool for predicting the risk of recurrent ectopic pregnancy (Marana et al, 1991, 1995a). This is of no surprise as surgery and placentation within the ampullary segment usually affect one or two folds only, while in the absence of underlying mucosal lesions the other folds can remain unaffected and secure normal ovum transport. Salpingoscopy can also be useful in detecting early tubal pregnancy and recognizing tubal abortion.

Unexplained infertility: tubal mucosal adhesions can be detected at salpingoscopy in up to 5% of infertile patients with normal findings at laparoscopy (Heylen et al, 1995).

In conclusion salpingoscopy is indicated in the conditions in which involvement of the tubal mucosa is suspected as a cause of infertility:

- history of PID or other pelvic infections
- history of ectopic pregnancy
- elevated *Chlamydia trachomatis* antibody titer
- pelvic and perihepatic adhesions, tubal phimosis and hydrosalpinx
- presence of ectopic pregnancy.

REFERENCES

Brosens I, Boeckx W, Delattin P, Puttemans P & Vasquez G (1987) Salpingoscopy: a new pre-operative diagnostic tool in tubal infertility. *Br J Obstet Gynaecol* **94**: 768–773.

De Bruyne F, Puttemans P, Boeckx W & Brosens I (1989) The clinical value of salpingoscopy in tubal infertility. *Fertil Steril* **53**: 339–340.

Gürgan T, Urman B, Yarali H, Aksu T & Kisnisci HA (1994) Salpingoscopic findings in women with occlusive and nonocclusive salpingitis isthmica nodosa. *Fertil Steril* **61**: 461–463.

Henry-Suchet J, Loffredo V, Tesquier L & Pez JP (1985) Endoscopy of the tube (tuboscopy): its prognostic value for tuboplasties. *Acta Eur Fertil* **16**: 139–145.

Heylen SM, Brosens IA & Puttemans P (1995) Clinical value and cumulative pregnancy rates following salpingoscopy during laparoscopy in infertility. *Hum Reprod* **10**: 2913–2916.

Kerin J, Daykhovsky L, Segalowitz J et al (1990) Falloposcopy: a microendoscopic technique for visual exploration of the human fallopian tube from the uterotubal ostium to the fimbria using a transvaginal approach. *Fertil Steril* **54**: 390–400.

Kerin JF, Williams DB, San Roman GA, Pearlstone AC, Grundfest WS & Surrey ES (1992) Falloposcopic classification and treatment of fallopian tube lumen disease. *Fertil Steril* **57**: 731–741.

Marana R, Muzii L, Rizzi M, Luciano A, Dell'Acqua S & Mancuso S (1991) Salpingoscopy in patients with contralateral ectopic pregnancy. *Fertil Steril* **55**: 838–840.

Marana R, Muzii L, Rizzi M, Dell'Acqua S & Mancuso S (1995a) Prognostic role of laparoscopic salpingoscopy of the only remaining tube after contralateral ectopic pregnancy. *Fertil Steril* **63**: 303–306.

Marana R, Rizzi M, Muzii L, Catalano GF, Caruana P & Mancuso S (1995b) Correlation between the American Fertility Society classifications of adnexal adhesions and distal tubal occlusion, salpingoscopy and reproductive outcome in tubal surgery. *Fertil Steril* **64**: 924–929.

Nezhat F, Winer WK & Nezhat C (1990) Fimbrioscopy and salpingoscopy in patients with minimal to moderate pelvic endometriosis. *Obstet Gynecol* **75**: 15–17.

Puttemans P, Brosens I, Delattin P, Vasquez G & Boeckx W (1987) Salpingoscopy versus hysterosalpingography in hydrosalpinges. *Hum Reprod* **2**: 535–540.

Shapiro BS, Diamond MP & DeCherney AH (1988) Salpingoscopy: an adjunctive technique for evaluation of the fallopian tube. *Fertil Steril* **49**: 1076–1079.

Vasquez G, Winston RML, Boeckx W, Gordts S & Brosens I (1983) Tubal mucosa and ectopic pregnancy. *Br J Obstet Gynaecol* **90**: 468–474.

Vasquez G, Boeckx W & Brosens I (1995a) Prospective study of tubal lesions and fertility in hydrosalpinges. *Hum Reprod* **10**: 1075–1078.

Vasquez G, Boeckx W & Brosens I (1995b) No correlation between peritubal and mucosal adhesions in hydrosalpinges. *Fertil Steril* **5**: 1032–1033.

11 *Endoscopy: falloposcopy*
IW Scudamore and ID Cooke

■ INTRODUCTION

As has been indicated in the previous chapter, the condition of the epithelium of the lumen of the Fallopian tube is fundamental to its function (Henry-Suchet et al, 1985, 1989; Boer-Meisel et al, 1986; De Bruyne et al, 1989). Direct visualization of the tubal lumen may contribute to assessment of endotubal epithelial health, yielding information that directly relates to the prospect of successful pregnancy after tubal surgery (Henry-Suchet et al, 1985). Furthermore, such a tool may be useful in both clinical and research practice, allowing sampling of the luminal environment and delivery of material into specific sections of the tube in an atraumatic and reliable way. Chapter 10 described the technique of salpingoscopy and its application for the assessment of tubal condition. In this chapter the technique of transcervical Fallopian tube endoscopy, termed falloposcopy, will be discussed.

■ EQUIPMENT

As long ago as 1849 (Tyler-Smith, 1849), descriptions of attempted transcervical tubal cannulation were published. In 1970, Mohri et al used advances in glass fiber optics to attempt transcervical tubal endoscopy. They developed a glass fiber endoscope with an outer diameter of 2.4 mm, containing a light-supplying cord and an image-transmitting cord. Hysteroscopically directed and 'blind' tactile methods of tubal cannulation were used to obtain images from inside the tube in 17 cases reported. Technical limitations and the thickness of the endoscope prevented cannulation beyond 3.0 cm in all but four cases, lending weight to the previous assertion that attempts to cannulate the proximal part of the tube would inevitably prove futile (Sweeney, 1962).

Advances in fiberoptic and light-source technology enabled development of endoscopes with greatly improved optical properties, yet with outer diameters of as little as 0.5 mm (Kerin et al, 1990a, 1990b). Modern video technology enables image processing and display with real-time recording. Kerin et al (1990a, 1990b) described the original coaxial system of falloposcopy. Hysteroscopically directed tubal cannulation with a flexible guidewire (outside diameter (OD) 0.3–0.8 mm) was performed under general anesthetic with concurrent laparoscopy. A Teflon cannula (OD up to 1.3 mm) was passed over the guidewire, the guidewire was removed and the falloposcope passed down the lumen of the Teflon cannula. Irrigation with crystalloid solution facilitated movement of the endoscope within the cannula and improved visualization by lifting the tubal epithelium off the endoscope lens. The best imaging of the tubal lumen was obtained by visualization during withdrawal of the endoscope and cannula together, keeping the lens of the endoscope at the end of the cannula while irrigating to lift the epithelium off the lens.

The Linear Eversion Catheter (LEC) system (Imagyn Medical Inc.) utilizes the principle of hydraulic pressurized propagation of a polyethylene balloon for atraumatic tubal cannulation and delivery of the endoscope into the tubal lumen. This improves the prospect of reliable cannulation as, with appropriate placement, the balloon will enter the tube along the path of least resistance. The design of the LEC system for falloposcopy (Bauer et al, 1992) gives it characteristics that allow it to be used without hysteroscopic guidance. The catheter has a plastic polymer body of 2.8 mm diameter and a sliding stainless steel inner body of 0.8 mm diameter. These are connected at their tips by a polyethylene membrane or balloon some 20 cm long and 50 μm thick. There is a closed space, confined by the outer and inner bodies and the membrane ('the balloon space'), to which access is gained via a Luer-Lok tap near the rear of the outer body. Instillation of fluid to increase the pressure in the balloon space, together with movement

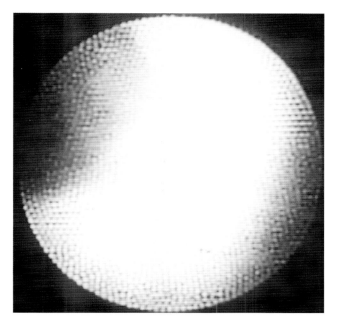

Figure 11.1: *Tubal ostium and uterotubal gutter. Catheter tip from 12 o'clock to 6 o'clock. Tubal ostium at 10 o'clock. From* Atlas of Gynecological Endoscopy, *Second Edition by Gordon et al (1995), Mosby–Wolfe Limited, London, UK.*

forward of the steel inner body within the catheter, results in the membrane unrolling from the catheter tip as a double layer balloon with the endoscope within its lumen. The balloon lifts the tissues in front of it without exerting shear forces and hence will follow curvatures within the tube with minimal risk of tubal damage.

▪ TECHNIQUE

The LEC technique is the one primarily used by these authors and so will be described in more detail.

After passage through the cervix the catheter tip is approximated to the uterotubal ostium. The tubal ostium or uterotubal gutter is identified, appearing as an ellipse or 'tunnel' depending on how far into the cornu the catheter has been advanced (*Figure 11.1*). This is achieved with the falloposcope by advancing it to the tip of the catheter, which has a crescentic appearance (*Figure 11.1*). The falloposcope is then withdrawn into the catheter behind the attachment of the balloon membrane as it must always be within the balloon during all stages of eversion. This protects the endoscope tip from direct epithelial impact, which could impair eversion

and lead to damage of the tube and/or endoscope. Pressure is introduced into the balloon space and then the steel inner body is advanced within the catheter, resulting in propagation of the balloon tip beyond the catheter and into the tubal ostium. After advancing the balloon 1–2 cm the endoscope can be used to confirm the position in the proximal tube. Continued eversion requires incremental steps as the endoscope moves forward at twice the speed of the balloon tip because the balloon membrane has to lay down a double layered wall. The endoscope tip must be kept inside the balloon but within 1 cm of the balloon tip. This requires the endoscope to be withdrawn 1–2 cm each time it reaches the balloon tip. Movement forward of the balloon tip occurs when the pressure in the balloon is increased. Raised pressure prevents movement of the endoscope independent of the balloon. Reducing the pressure allows withdrawal or advancement of the endoscope within the balloon. This is also assisted by lubrication of the balloon lumen with saline flush during movement of the endoscope.

When there are difficulties with eversion it is important to identify the balloon tip and confirm the positioning of the endoscope tip behind but close to the balloon tip. Eversion of the balloon can often be assisted by supporting the balloon with the endoscope near to its tip and advancing in shorter increments. Occasionally higher pressure may assist in propagation of the balloon tip. Forcing the advancement of the balloon/endoscope may damage the balloon, tube or endoscope. The basis of the technique is continual understanding of the relationship of the endoscope tip to the tip of the balloon. If performed properly, cannulation can be performed to a distance of 10 cm (*Figures 11.2* and *11.3*). Tubal damage is unlikely unless the endoscope is allowed to project beyond the balloon during eversion.

Retrograde imaging during withdrawal of the endoscope provides the best visualization. This requires that the endoscope tip is kept close to the balloon tip during withdrawal. As the balloon tip will move at twice the rate of the endoscope, the operator has constantly to move the endoscope forward in relation to the balloon to maintain their relationship. This is possible because lower pressure in the balloon is needed during withdrawal and, together with simultaneous flush, it is

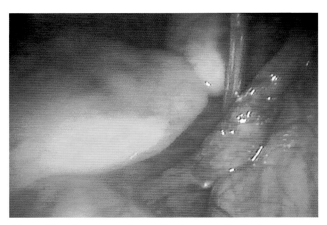

Figure 11.2: Laparoscopic image of endoscope in distal tube. Ovary and palpiteur above tube. Light from endoscope visible near fimbriae.

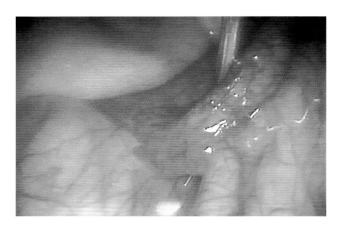

Figure 11.3: Laparoscopic image of endoscope protruding from distal tube. Ovary and palpiteur above tube. Endoscope tip visible beneath fimbriae with light shining on peritoneum.

possible to constantly 'wind forward' the endoscope during withdrawal until the balloon and endoscope re-enter the catheter. Flushing with crystalloid is also important to enable better imaging of the tubal epithelium.

▪ OUTPATIENT FALLOPOSCOPY

One of the great potential advantages of falloposcopy is that it can be performed without anesthesia as an outpatient procedure (Scudamore et al, 1992). This makes the procedure more accessible because it avoids the need for anesthesia and inpatient care, which require many specialist personnel and involve considerable morbidity and inconvenience to the patient. Costs are reduced as well. Furthermore, the patient and her partner can be involved

in the procedure. She is able to provide useful information during the procedure by indicating the site and degree of discomfort. The pain will be lateralized to the side being examined. This is a valuable aid to successful eversion and limits the risk of perforation. The degree of pain may reflect the presence and type of pathology: an occluded tube causes severe discomfort when distended by flush. The couple are able to see the images, which can be explained to them. This is an aid to their understanding of the counseling that can be given to them after the investigation. As the patient has not had an anesthetic this counseling can be given immediately after the procedure and then she can go home.

There is no doubt that the LEC method of falloposcopy can be reliably performed as an outpatient procedure (Scudamore et al, 1992; Dunphy, 1994; Dunphy and Pattinson, 1994). In our series of 192 tubes examined, cannulation and eversion sufficient to provide clinically valuable assessment was achieved in 187 (97%) (unpublished data). The bulk of these patients were given an analgesia mixture of the nonsteroidal analgesic naproxen (1 g 90 minutes before the procedure), the benzodiazepine temazepam (20 mg 20 minutes before the procedure), 5 ml of 1% lidocaine (lignocaine) in each uterosacral ligament immediately before passing the catheter through the cervix, and 50:50 O_2:N_2O mixture (Entonox) to inhale during the procedure. This combination causes minimal residual effect after the procedure and carries no risk of respiratory depression or excessive hypnotic effect during the falloposcopy. Using a visual analogue scale for questionnaire follow-up to assess the pain experienced by comparison with other stimuli (including hysterosalpingography (HSG) and laparoscopy), we have found that the degree of pain from falloposcopy using this method is marginally greater than that with HSG. Despite this, 71.3% of patients expressed a preference for avoiding general anesthesia and almost 50% of patients preferred falloposcopy to HSG or laparoscopy (Scudamore and Cooke, 1995). More powerful combinations of analgesics and hypnotics have been used (Dunphy, 1995) and probably decrease the discomfort experienced. They also increase the risks of respiratory depression and impair the ability of the patient to interact during the falloposcopy or to go home soon after.

Outpatient falloposcopy requires a dedicated setup with a gynecological couch and space for the operator, the assisting nurse (who operates the pressure device and monitors the patient s blood pressure) and the patient's partner. The falloposcopy system needs to be organized on a trolley and prepared before the patient is placed on the couch so that the procedure can be started immediately.

■ BENEFITS, LIMITATIONS AND COMPLICATIONS

Endoscopy of the tubal lumen with assessment of the state of the endotubal epithelium is likely to be of value in predicting tubal function. This is an aid to the selection of treatment modalities in reproductive medicine. If the tubal lumen appears healthy, treatment options utilizing the tube may be appropriate. These may include tubal surgery, gamete or early embryo tubal transfer, tubal or intrauterine insemination and ovulation induction. If it appears damaged, these methods of treatment may be inappropriate and assisted reproduction utilizing intrauterine transfer techniques may be preferred. In the presence of potential proximal disease falloposcopy enables assessment of the proximal segment and may even provide therapeutic tuboplasty.

General anesthesia is required for laparoscopy and salpingoscopy and often a significant component of a surgical procedure is necessary to gain access to the tube for salpingoscopic assessment. While such assessment helps in providing a prognosis for tubal function, falloposcopy offers the possibility of such assessment as an outpatient procedure before the need for a general anesthetic or any pelvic surgery. By this means a proportion of pointless laparoscopic assessments would be avoided; if the tubes were severely damaged direct transfer to assisted reproduction would be appropriate. This has obvious cost savings in preventing wasted operating theatre time, let alone the patient morbidity and social disruption of inpatient laparoscopic assessment. Added to this, improved selection of patients for particular treatment methods ought to improve rates of successful treatment and avoid the morbidity and cost of ineffective treatment choices.

Falloposcopy, particularly the LEC technique, does use expensive disposable equipment; however, if performed as an outpatient procedure in the awake patient, this is offset by the savings made in lieu of inpatient care. The endoscopes are expensive and potentially fragile but, if handled carefully, it should be possible to use them for more than 50–75 cases. Damage to the endoscopes is most likely in inexperienced hands and places a premium on proper training in the understanding of the system being used for falloposcopy. The image obtained is limited by the width of field and the fact that the direction of imaging cannot be altered within the tube. Provided that representative images of the tube are obtained, these factors probably do not affect the value of the assessment because focal pathology is not a characteristic of severely damaged tubes. The quality of the image cannot compare with that of rigid endoscopy as it is somewhat limited by the extreme narrowness of the fiberoptic endoscope. The image is best seen in real time: still images can only give an impression of characteristic appearances. This is important to remember when viewing the images presented in this chapter.

While falloposcopy has the potential for examination of the proximal and distal tube, proximal occlusion may prevent assessment of the distal tubal segments. If proximal surgery is to be considered, distal assessment by laparoscopy and salpingoscopy will be necessary. Tubal perforation at falloposcopy is rare if appropriate technique is used. If the patient is awake, pain will limit the likelihood of such perforation. As might be expected in view of the fine diameter of the endoscope, there have been no reported cases of significant complications after perforation during falloposcopy.

■ NORMAL APPEARANCES

There has been very little published with regard to the appearances of the tubal epithelium in fertile patients with apparently normal tubes. Kerin et al (1990b) reported falloposcopy findings in ten patients with patent tubes and no evidence of tubal disease by laparoscopic assessment. They found evidence of nonobstructive adhesions in two of these patients. There is no comment as to whether these patients had a history of infertility despite their apparent lack of tubal disease by conventional assessment; however, these authors indicate that, as for salpingoscopy, a characteristic

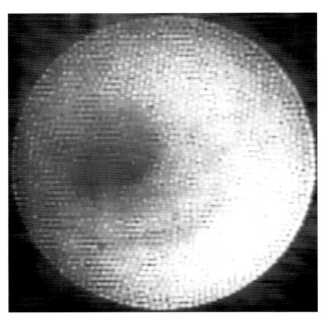

Figure 11.4: Normal proximal (intramural) appearances. Relatively smooth, regular wall with whole diameter of tube visible. From Atlas of Gynecological Endoscopy, *Second Edition by Gordon et al (1995), Mosley-Wolfe Limited, London, UK.*

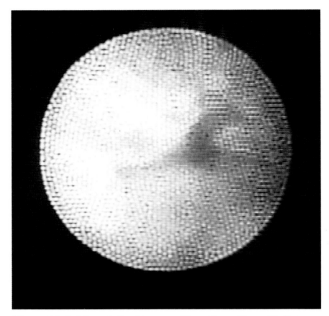

Figure 11.6: Normal distal lumen. Many finger-like epithelial folds closing down on lumen and containing vascular channels.

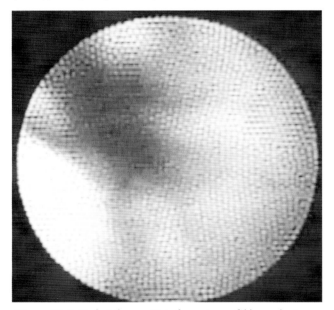

Figure 11.5: Early isthmus. Note four primary folds, regular in pattern; whole diameter of tube visible. Tubal lumen is a little dilated.

pattern of epithelial folds can be seen in the tube that is apparently healthy. In our own hands, falloposcopy has mainly been performed in patients with a suggestion of possible tubal disease and therefore neither do we have a control group of known healthy, fertile women. In 25 tubes examined personally in patients with infertility but no conventional features of tubal disease, seven (28%) appeared

damaged. We would agree that appearances that seem to indicate a lack of significant tubal damage can be identified.

The normal appearances of the tube vary depending on the segment being examined. The proximal tube is demonstrated in *Figure 11.4* and usually has the appearance of a tunnel with a flat and regular wall. The isthmic segment is characterized by the appearance of four or five longitudinal folds (*Figure 11.5*). Both of these segments can usually be seen accross their entire diameter. Beyond 5–6 cm eversion the distal segments of the tube become too wide for the entire width of the lumen to be visualized. In the distal tube the epithelium has developed its secondary folding, each of which should be freely mobile in the crystalloid flush and contains a vascular channel along its center (*Figures 11.6* and *11.7*).

▪ INDICATIONS AND ABNORMAL FINDINGS

If proximal tubal disease is suspected, falloposcopy enables direct visualization of the proximal segment and, using the LEC system, an atraumatic approach to tubal 'recanalization'. A severe narrowing of the tubal lumen indicates a stenosis, which may be 'treatable' by the tuboplasty inherent in the procedure (*Figure 11.8*). A complete occlusion appears as a blind-ending tunnel (*Figure

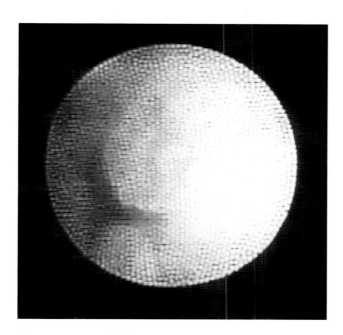

Figure 11.7: Normal fold pattern, again with healthy vascular channels.

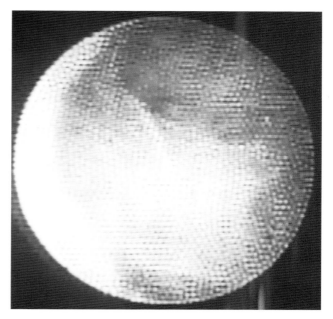

Figure 11.9: Proximal occlusion. Irregular wall of proximal segment on left of image. Debris in tube pushed up against blind-ending complete occlusion.

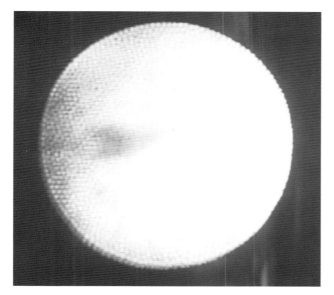

Figure 11.8: Proximal stenosis. Lumen mainly occluded with opening at 9 o'clock.

11.9), while a badly damaged but patent proximal tube has an irregular 'fibrotic' appearance with the wall sometimes appearing trabeculated. These findings have been confirmed histologically in tubal segments removed surgically after falloposcopy in our center (unpublished data). There is a high rate of tubal cannulation in patients with apparent proximal occlusion (Grow et al, 1993; Dunphy, 1994) and displaceable occlusive 'plugs' have been identified and histologically characterized

(Kerin et al, 1991; Kindermann et al, 1993). Both the tubes can be assessed in cases of unilateral or bilateral disease (Scudamore et al, 1994a), as can the distal tubal segments in most patients. A role for falloposcopy in proximal assessment and tuboplasty is therefore suggested (Confino and Radwanska, 1992; Grow et al, 1993; Lederer, 1993).

Still images taken from video recording of falloposcopy do not adequately reflect the real time image, which loses definition in lifting the still image. Interpretation of the image is influenced by the movement of the epithelial folds in the saline flush and their image definition is vastly improved in real time . In the healthy tube the folds will fall on to the endoscope lens when there is no flush. If there is distal occlusion by a phimosis or a hydrosalpinx with minimal dilatation the tubal epithelium will show fold preservation but mobility of the folds may be reduced and they may not fall back on to the lens and occlude the tubal lumen (*Figure 11.10*). If dilatation is greater and the folds are flattened there will be minimal relief perception of the tubal wall and the tubal lumen will appear as a dark cavity (*Figures 11.11* and *11.12*). The worst prognostic feature is probably the presence of intratubal adhesions (*Figures 11.13* and *11.14*).

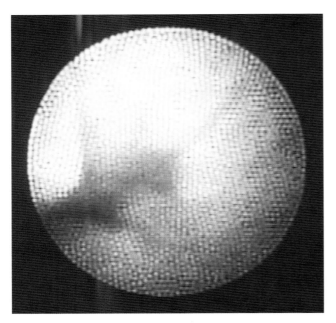

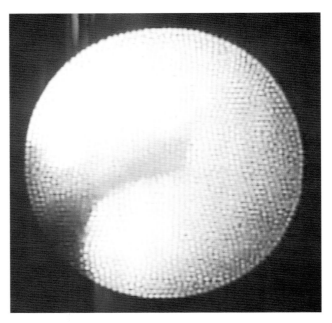

Figure 11.10: *Moderate dilatation of proximal part of ampulla. The lumen is dilated compared with normal appearances but the epithelial folds are well preserved.*

Figure 11.12: *Hydrosalpinx with fold preservation but agglutination. Tubal lumen is to bottom left. Epithelial folds are 'blunted' and do not contain normal vascular pattern.*

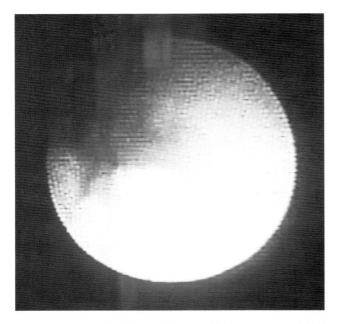

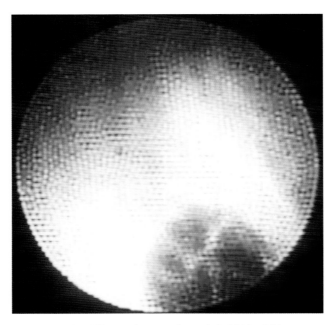

Figure 11.11: *Hydrosalpinx with minimal fold preservation. Tubal lumen is in the upper left of the image and appears dark due to distension. There are only remnant folds on the tubal wall.*

Figure 11.13: *Adhesions between the epithelial folds. Thinner type between 5 and 6 o'clock. Thicker adhesion from 12 o'clock to 4 o'clock.*

Kerin et al (1992) reported a classification of endotubal disease from examining 112 tubes from 75 women suspected of having tubal disease. They used a scoring system based on the appearances of tubal folds, vascularity, dilatation, adhesions and pallor. High scores indicated damaged tubes and they correlated these scores

inversely with subsequent pregnancy rates. The scoring system is similar to previous systems reported as being of prognostic value in treatment of distal tubal disease (Henry-Suchet et al, 1985; Boer-Meisel et al, 1986; Mage et al, 1986; American Fertility Society, 1988). Postoperative tubal function was considered to be influ-

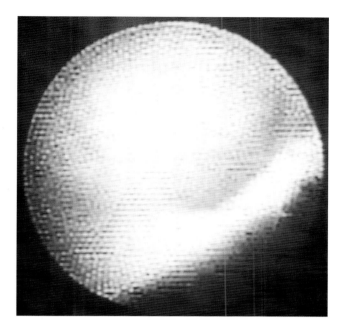

Figure 11.14: *Adhesion in a hydrosalpinx. Thick adhesion from 3 o'clock to 7 o'clock. Distended lumen to the bottom right of image. Flattened tubal wall. From* Atlas of Gynecological Endoscopy, *Second Edition by Gordon et al (1995), Mosby–Wolfe Limited, London, UK.*

enced by such factors as long ago as 1966 (Shirodkar, 1966) and they were used in perioperative classification by Hulka (1982) and Levinson (1995). A number of other series reporting the success of surgery for tubal disease emphasize that the prognosis of such treatment is strongly influenced by such appearances (Henry-Suchet et al, 1989; Winston and Margara, 1991; Dubuisson et al, 1994). Falloposcopic examination of tubes considered likely to be damaged by conventional assessment (HSG/laparoscopy) seems to assist in the identification of the tubes that really do have endotubal damage. In the series of Kerin et al (1992), 54% of tubes examined in 66 patients with conventional evidence of endotubal disease showed evidence of falloposcopic abnormality. Using the tubal score to quantify the degree of disease present, 29% showed evidence of mild/moderate disease and 25% were severely damaged. In our own series of mainly outpatient procedures in 222 Fallopian tubes of patients with suspected tubal disease from conventional tubal assessment, successful cannulation of at least the proximal segment was achieved in 217 (98%). Severe proximal disease or factors including poor patient tolerance or difficulty with balloon and endoscope eversion restricted the examination to the proximal segment in

54 (25%; 69% of these had severe proximal disease). Where both the proximal and distal segments were assessed (163 tubes; 75%), 52% had healthy appearances, while 49% showed evidence of moderate/severe damage. These data are consistent with the data from Kerin et al (1992) of 52 of 112 (46%) tubes assessed in their series as having 'normal' appearances and being considered to have a good prognosis for tubal function. Falloposcopic tubal assessment of patients with tubal disease diagnosed by conventional assessment has been compared with blinded salpingoscopic assessment of the same tubes by a different operator (Scudamore et al, 1994b). Good correlation ($P < 0.0001$) was found between the two techniques in assessing the degree of endotubal damage. Comparison with HSG has indicated that falloposcopy will identify intratubal lesions in the presence of a normal HSG as well as healthy appearances where damage was expected (Venezia et al, 1993).

∎ CONCLUSION

Falloposcopy is an endoscopic technique that complements the established techniques of HSG, laparoscopy and salpingoscopy. It allows visually directed cannulation of the proximal tube and evaluation of both the proximal and distal tubal segments in the majority of patients with suggested tubal disease. Falloposcopy can be performed as an outpatient procedure and provides a facility for assessing the degree of intratubal disease before the need for inpatient general anesthesia. The indications for falloposcopy will depend on the treatment modalities being considered. Falloposcopy may demonstrate endotubal lesions if 'unexplained' infertility is present. It may be important to consider falloposcopy if treatments requiring tubal function, such as intrauterine insemination or gamete or early embryo transfer to the tube by assisted reproduction, are being considered. Falloposcopy would appear to be indicated in both proximal and distal tubal disease. In proximal disease it will provide assessment of the proximal segment as well as potentially assessing the distal tube and having the potential for therapeutic 'recanalization' and tuboplasty. Assessment of the tubal epithelium in the presence of distal tubal disease can assist in planning subsequent management and choosing between treatment modalities such as tubal surgery or assisted reproductive techniques; however, it is a demanding procedure to learn and perform. A good understanding of the techniques and a great deal of patience are important factors in mastering the procedure.

REFERENCES

The American Fertility Society (1988) The American Fertility classifications of adnexal adhesions, distal tubal occlusion, tubal occlusion secondary to tubal ligation, tubal pregnancies, Müllerian abnormalities and intrauterine adhesions. *Fertil Steril* **49**: 944.

Bauer O, Dietrich K, Bacich S et al (1992) Transcervical access and intraluminal imaging of the fallopian tubes in the non-anaesthetized patient; preliminary results using a new fallopian access technology. *Hum Reprod* **7 (suppl 1)**: 7–11.

Boer-Meisel ME, te Velde ER, Habbema JDF & Kardaun JWPF (1986) Predicting the pregnancy outcome in patients treated for hydrosalpinges: a prospective study. *Fertil Steril* **45**: 23–29.

Confino E & Radwanska E (1992) Tubal factors in infertility. *Curr Opin Obstet Gynecol* **4**: 197–202.

De Bruyne F, Puttemans P, Boeckx W & Brosens I (1989) The clinical value of salpingoscopy in tubal infertility. *Fertil Steril* **51**: 339–340.

Dubuisson JB, Chapron C, Morice P, Aubriot FX, Foulot H & de Joliniere JB (1994) Laparoscopic salpingostomy: fertility results according to the tubal mucosal appearance. *Hum Reprod* **9**: 334–339.

Dunphy BC (1994) Office falloposcopic assessment in proximal tubal occlusive disease. *Fertil Steril* **61**: 168–170.

Dunphy BC & Pattinson HA (1994) Office falloposcopy; a tertiary level assessment for planning the management of infertile women. *Aust N Z J Obstet Gynaecol* **34**(2): 189–190.

Grow DR, Coddington CC & Flood JT (1993) Proximal tubal occlusion by hysterosalpingogram: a role for falloposcopy. *Fertil Steril* **60**: 170–174.

Henry-Suchet J, Loffredo V, Tesquier L & Pez J (1985) Endoscopy of the tube (= tuboscopy): its prognostic value for tuboplasties. *Acta Eur Fertil* **16**: 139–145.

Henry-Suchet J, Veluyre M & Pia P (1989) Statistical study of the factors influencing the prognosis in tuboplasty operations. Importance of the status of the ampullary mucosa and of chlamydial infection. [French.] *J Gynecol Obstet Biol Reprod* **18**: 571–580.

Hulka JF (1982) Adnexal adhesions: a prognostic staging and classification system. *Am J Obstet Gynecol* **144**: 141–147.

Kerin J, Surrey E, Daykhovsky L & Grundfest WS (1990a) Development and application of a falloposcope for transvaginal endoscopy of the fallopian tube. *J Laparoendosc Surg* **1**: 47–56.

Kerin J, Daykhovsky L, Segalowitz J et al (1990b) Falloposcopy: a microendoscopic technique for visual exploration of the human fallopian tube from the uterotubal ostium to the fimbria using a transvaginal approach. *Fertil Steril* **54**: 390–400.

Kerin JF, Surrey ES, Williams DB, Daykhovsky L & Grundfest WS (1991) Falloposcopic observations of endotubal isthmic plugs as a cause of reversible obstruction and their histological characterization. *J Laparoendosc Surg* **1**: 103–110.

Kerin JF, Williams DB, San Roman GA, Pearlstone AC, Grundfest WS & Surrey ES (1992) Falloposcopic classification and treatment of fallopian tube lumen disease. *Fertil Steril* **57**: 731–741.

Kindermann D, Bauer O, Fischer HP & Dietrich K (1993) Histological findings in a falloposcopically retrieved isthmic plug causing reversible proximal tubal obstruction. *Hum Reprod* **8**: 1429–1434.

Lederer KJ (1993) Transcervical tubal cannulation and salpingoscopy in the treatment of tubal infertility. *Curr Opin Obstet Gynecol* **5**: 240–244.

Levinson CJ (1995) Prognosis and results of salpingostomy: long-term follow-up. *Int J Fertil* **28**: 543–556.

Mage G, Pouly J, Bouquet de Joliniere J, Chabrand S, Riouallon A & Bruhat M (1986) A preoperative classification to predict the intrauterine and ectopic pregnancy rates after distal tubal microsurgery. *Fertil Steril* **46**: 807.

Mohri T, Mohri C & Yamadori F (1970) Flexible glass fibre endoscope for intratubal observation. *Endoscopy* **2**: 226.

Scudamore IW & Cooke ID (1995) *Can falloposcopy be performed as an outpatient procedure?* Presented at IFFS Satellite Meeting on Tubal disease, Clermont-Ferrand, 14–16 Sept.

Scudamore IW, Dunphy BC & Cooke ID (1992) Outpatient falloposcopy: intra-luminal imaging of the fallopian tube by trans-uterine fibre-optic endoscopy as an outpatient procedure. *Br J Obstet Gynaecol* **99**: 829–835.

Scudamore IW, Dunphy BC & Cooke ID (1994a) Falloposcopic comparison of unilateral and bilateral proximal tubal occlusive disease. *Hum Reprod* **9**: 340–342.

Scudamore IW, Dunphy BC, Bowman M, Jenkins J & Cooke ID (1994b) Comparison of ampullary assessment by falloposcopy and salpingoscopy. *Hum Reprod* **9**: 1516–1518.

Shirodkar VN (1966) Factors influencing the results of salpingostomy. *Int J Fertil* **11**: 361–365.

Sweeney WJ (1962) The interstitial portion of the uterine tube: its gross anatomy, course, and length. *Obstet Gynecol* **19**: 3–8.

Tyler-Smith W (1849) New method of treating sterility by the removal of obstructions of the fallopian tubes. *Lancet* **i**: 116–118.

Venezia R, Zangara C, Knight C & Cittadini E (1993) Initial experience of a new linear everting falloposcopy system in comparison with hysterosalpingography. *Fertil Steril* **60**: 771–775.

Winston RML & Margara RA (1991) Microsurgical salpingostomy is not an absolute procedure. *Br J Obstet Gynaecol* **98**: 637–642.

12 Selective salpingography
VC Karande and N Gleicher

■ INTRODUCTION

In the past few years rapid technological advances have been made available as diagnostic and therapeutic modalities that allow us to approach the Fallopian tubes (Risquez and Confino, 1993). Selective salpingography (SS), the topic of this chapter, is a minimally invasive technique that utilizes transcervically directed catheters to approach the Fallopian tubes for a variety of diagnostic and therapeutic indications (Flood and Grow, 1993).

Tubal disease is the most common etiological factor in infertility and is involved in 25–30% of patients (Confino et al, 1990). Most centers utilize hysterosalpingography (HSG) as the initial test in order to assess Fallopian tubes (Gleicher et al, 1992a). We estimate that at least 300 000 diagnostic HSGs are annually performed in the United States (Gleicher et al, 1992a). Most of these are performed using only spot radiographs with the gynecologist receiving three or four hard copies as the sole basis for interpretation. At the Center for Human Reproduction (CHR) we have replaced HSG with a so-called gynecoradiological procedure (GRP) in which HSG is only the initial step. Based on findings at HSG, we then may proceed with SS, tubal catheterization or other therapeutic procedures, as required. The entire study is documented on hard copy in split second intervals and thus provides very detailed information on the flow of contrast medium into the uterine cavity, oviducts and peritoneal cavity.

■ EQUIPMENT

GYNECORADIOLOGICAL PROCEDURE

All radiological procedures at the CHR are performed with an office based X-ray unit. This consists of a fully digitized C-arm system (presently, OEC-Diasonics

Series 9400, OEC Medical Systems, Inc., Salt Lake City, UT) (*Figure 12.1*). The X-ray image generated by the C-arm is converted to a fluoroscopic video image by an image intensifier and television camera. The fluoroscopic image is digitized and can be viewed in motion out of memory, or can be processed to enhance features of interest. It also can be saved on a hard disk to be later recalled. In the fluoroscopic mode, images can also be stored in video format on a videocassette recorder. Postprocessing can be performed on previously recorded

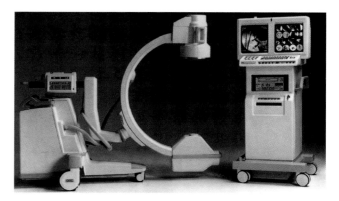

Figure 12.1: The OEC-Diasonics Series 9400 C-arm (OEC Medical Systems Inc., Salt Lake City, UT) utilized for all fluoroscopically guided procedures at the Center for Human Reproduction in Chicago.

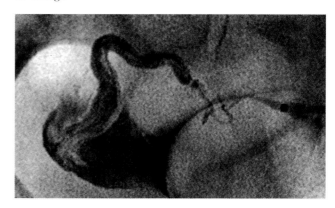

Figure 12.2: Right selective salpingography. Demonstrated is the ability to postprocess previously recorded images. In this picture, we have zoomed on the right Fallopian tube, which shows normal tubal folds. The tip of the selective salpingography catheter is seen at the proximal tubal ostium.

images. This includes the ability to zoom on a portion of an image (e.g. on one of the Fallopian tubes) or contrast enhance, which helps to better delineate abnormalities (e.g. filling defects in the uterine cavity) (*Figure 12.2*). A recorded procedure can be played back and can be processed in a manner similar to an original live image or can be slowed down for more detailed viewing.

This then allows for documentation of even the most subtle uterine abnormalities or most detailed aspects of tubal opacification, such as symmetry of fill, speed of tubal fill, tubal contour and pattern of spill (*Figure 12.3*). Relevant frames can subsequently be printed out on heat sensitive paper (Fujifilm, Thermal Imaging System FTI-500).

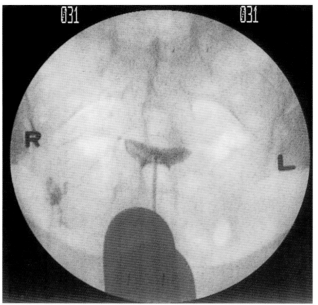

12.3a

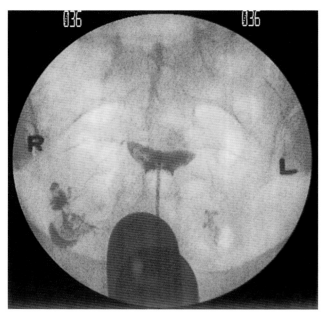

12.3c

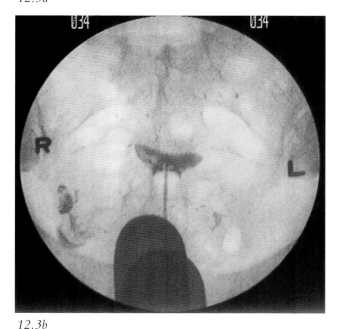

12.3b

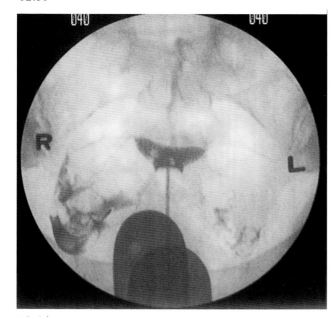

12.3d

Figure 12.3: *(a)–(d) Gynecoradiological procedure documented with printed (not X-ray film) images (Fujifilm, Thermal Imaging System FTI-500). Individual frames of any study can be recalled from memory and printed out in the desired sequence. In this case, asymmetrical tubal opacification and spill is demonstrated. The right tube* *shows prompt opacification and spill. The left tube shows delayed opacification and subsequent minimal spill. In such a situation, we would proceed with selective salpingography and the measurement of tubal perfusion pressures.*

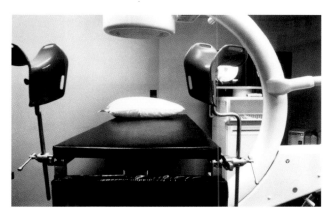

Figure 12.4: Fluoroscopic table utilized at the Center for Human Reproduction. The table is equipped with stirrups and a lap piece that can be folded to facilitate the vaginal insertion of instruments.

A specially developed gynecoradiological fluoroscopic table is used which allows placement of the patient in a dorsal lithotomy position (*Figure 12.4*). In contrast to standard fluoroscopy tables, this table is equipped with stirrups and a lap piece that can be folded, permitting placement of the patient in the standard gynecological

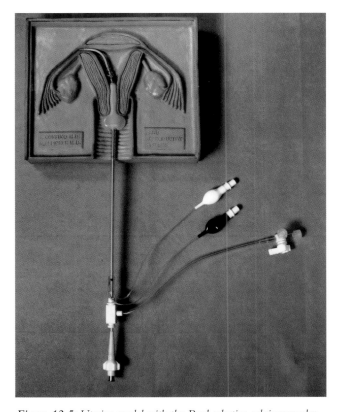

Figure 12.5: Uterine model with the Bard selective salpingography catheter (Bard Reproductive Systems, Tewksbury, MA) in place. The selective salpingography catheter is inserted through the cervical cannula. It has a curve which makes insertion into the desired uterine cornu and subsequent selective salpingography relatively easy.

dorsal lithotomy position while the GRP is performed.

Different catheter systems are available for the performance of SS. These usually utilize catheters with diameters similar to the tubal ostium (approximately 5.5 Fr). The curve of the catheter is usually preset with memory, making it easier to approach the ostia. Often an obturator can be passed through the lumen of the catheter to help negotiate its passage through the cervical canal. For many years, we utilized an excellent system manufactured by Bard Reproductive Systems (Tewksbury, MA) (*Figure 12.5*). These catheters are, however, unfortunately no longer commercially available as this company recently stopped all manufacturing activity in obstetrics and gynecology. We are therefore currently primarily using catheters manufactured by Conceptus (San Carlos, CA) and Cook Ob/Gyn (Spencer, IN), which have similar qualities to the Bard catheter shown here.

■ TECHNIQUE

During SS, the Fallopian tubes can be approached under fluoroscopic or hysteroscopic (Novy et al, 1988) guidance. We prefer the fluoroscopic approach for the following reasons (Gleicher and Pratt, 1994).

- ■ After only minimal training, the fluoroscopic guidance of catheters towards the tubal ostia and through the tubes is simpler than with any hysteroscopic technique.
- ■ Fluoroscopic control of the procedure allows instant recognition of tubal patency. In contrast, hysteroscopic guidance requires removal of the catheter apparatus and performance of an HSG or of a concomitant laparoscopy with tubal dye study to obtain the same information. Because patency is not always established on the first attempt, procedures may have to be repeated, making the hysteroscopic approach more cumbersome.
- ■ The fluoroscopic approach transfers the procedure from the operating room into an ambulatory office setting and eliminates the requirement for general anesthesia. Costs are thus significantly reduced.

Other potentially useful, though less well explored, techniques include the use of ultrasound (Confino et al, 1992) and tactile sensation (Gleicher and Pratt, 1994). They appear, however, less sensitive than either the fluoroscopic or hysteroscopic approach. In the future, as better ultrasound techniques are developed, this may change.

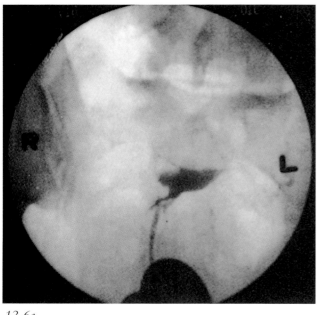

12.6a

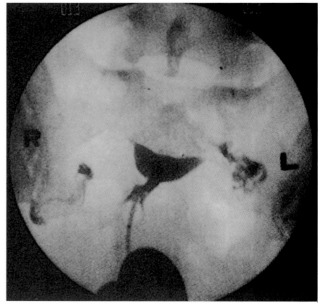

12.6c

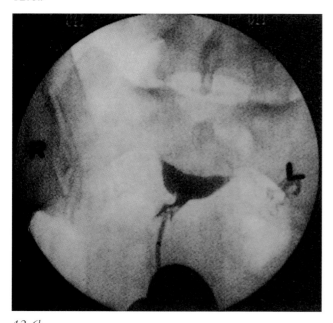

12.6b

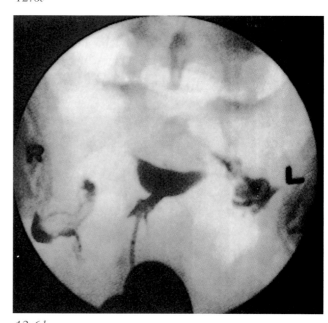

12.6d

Figure 12.6: (a)–(f) Abnormal pattern of tubal spill. In this case, there is pocketing of dye on the left, raising suspicion of the presence of peritubal adhesions. The cavity is normal and the right tube shows a normal spill pattern.

Initially, HSG is performed using a standardized technique (Gleicher et al, 1992b). Briefly, with the patient in a dorsal lithotomy position, the vagina and cervix are prepared with povidone-iodine. Analgesia is provided with a paracervical block, using 1% lidocaine (lignocaine). The HSG cannula is then inserted through the cervix and its balloon distended to hold it in place. This provides a relatively airtight uterine cavity. The distal end of the cannula is connected with polyethylene tub-ing to a preset injection pump and, by three-way stop-cock, to a pressure sensitive chip, which relays pressure information to a computer. As contrast is injected by the pump, the computer screen displays the encountered resistance in the form of a pressure curve on a screen and provides a hard copy print out. All studies are performed using water soluble contrast medium (Renografin-60, Squibb Diagnostics, Princeton, NJ) at a constant rate of 15 ml/min injection speed.

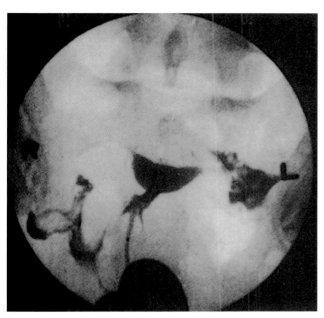

12.6e

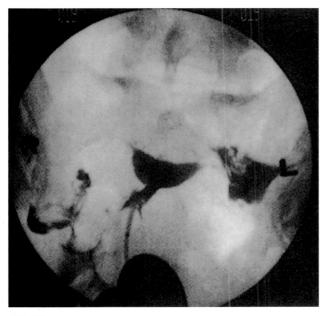

12.6f

Using the previously described digital enhancement techniques, we are consistently able to detect subtle abnormalities, such as asymmetry of tubal fill, delayed opacification, or abnormal patterns of tubal spill (*Figure 12.6*). If any of these abnormalities are diagnosed during HSG, we proceed with SS and measurement of tubal perfusion pressures, a new technique of functional tubal assessment, which will be described in more detail later in this chapter.

In 1992, for example, 152 consecutive females underwent a GRP during one series as part of their infertility workup (Karande et al, 1995a). Amongst these, 117 (77%) demonstrated apparently 'normal' findings using standard 'spot film' criteria, i.e. a normal cavity, normally appearing tubes and bilateral spill into the peritoneal cavity. Amongst these, however, a GRP detected asymmetrical tubal filling in 64 (55%), abnormal tubal spill in 32 (27%) and abnormally high tubal perfusion pressures in 55 (47%) (Karande et al, 1995a). During standard spot film HSG, most of these studies would have been considered as normal because both tubes were patent and contrast spill was observed.

SS is technically quite simple and it is possible to learn the technique in less than a day. The first step involves getting the SS catheter into the uterine cornua. With the previously used Bard system, the SS catheter was introduced through the central channel of the HSG cannula. Some currently used systems require that the HSG cannula be removed; yet others allow a double use of the cannula as both an HSG and SS catheter (Cook Ob/Gyn, Spencer, IN). If the HSG catheter needs to be removed, it is replaced by an SS catheter, which is then introduced into the cervical canal with its obturator in place. The obturator stiffens the SS catheter, making it easier to negotiate the canal. In some patients it may be easier to enter the uterine cavity without the obturator in place. Once the uterine cavity is entered, the obturator is removed, the SS catheter resumes its preset curve and is manipulated into the desired uterine cornu under fluoroscopic guidance (*Figure 12.5*). During SS, contrast is injected directly into a tube using the standardized technique described above.

▪ BENEFITS

Continuous on-line evaluation of contrast flow, as GRPs provide, is thus much superior to spot film techniques in detecting subtle abnormalities and should become a standard of care. The radiological equipment utilized at our centers is available in most radiology suites and a switch to on-line procedures should therefore be possible at most institutions without significant increase in cost. A further benefit of such greatly improved diagnostic capabilities has been a dramatic decrease in our center's need for 'diagnostic' laparoscopy.

As a consequence of better diagnosis by GRPs our utilization of laparoscopies has been reduced by as much as 60%. This is based on the fact that a GRP allows us to rule out tubal disease with virtual certainty if the study is normal and also allows us to exclude (an advanced level of) endometriosis in the presence of normal tubal perfusion pressures (see later). Laparoscopic procedures currently performed at our institution are, therefore, almost exclusively of operative nature, while diagnostic procedures have basically become extinct.

The measurement of tubal perfusion pressures (TPPs) is a newly developed technique which for the first time allows an assessment of the functional state of Fallopian tubes, i.e. their ability to result in a pregnancy. TPPs represent the Fallopian tubes' resistance to a fluid column, which is injected utilizing water soluble X-ray contrast. The technique of measuring TPPs involves the injection of contrast during SS, using a standardized and fully computerized system to record and document pressure curves, as described above. We now routinely perform SS and measure TPPs in patients with asymmetrical or delayed tubal opacification, or with an abnormal pattern of tubal spill during initial HSG (Karande et al, 1995a). Gleicher et al (1992b), using this standardized technique described above, showed that a TPP ≤ 350 mmHg is normal. Karande et al (1995a) showed elevated TPPs to be associated with decreased pregnancy rates in patients with otherwise patent tubes. The same authors investigated the possible etiology of elevated TPPs and found them to be associated with endometriosis (Karande et al, 1995b). These data provide the first suggested evidence that endometriosis may lead to tubal disease more frequently than has so far been reported in the literature.

■ COMPLICATIONS AND SIDE EFFECTS

Fluoroscopically directed SS results in irradiation of the pelvis. It is therefore prudent to consider the risks involved, not only for cancer induction but also the genetic risks to offspring and the influence on fertility. All of these risks are exceedingly low when radiation exposure time is limited and equipment is calibrated properly (Committee on the Biological Effects of Ionizing Radiation, 1980; ICRP, 1991; Gleicher and Pratt, 1994). We rigidly limit patient exposure to less than 10 minutes of radiation time. With this limit, the ovarian dose is in the order of 8.5–14 mGy (Hedgepath et al, 1991; Martensson et al, 1993). The probability for hereditary effects or cancer induction at this radiation dose is in the order of 10^{-4}. This is similar to the exposure with other radiological procedures, such as an intravenous pyelogram or a gastrointestinal series. Other precautions include the shielding of the medical team from radiation exposure with the use of lead aprons. The physician, who is closest to the X-ray tube, also wears a protective thyroid shield and eyeglasses. His or her hands are further protected by a leaded mat, placed at the foot of the X-ray table. All staff members wear radiation dosimeter badges, which are replaced monthly and sent to a radiation detection laboratory for evaluation (Gleicher and Pratt, 1994).

SS is associated with a very low complication rate. We have never had a procedure-related infection. Although it is probably unnecessary, we administer an antibiotic, such as doxycycline, for prophylaxis if the tube is entered by a catheter. This is started on the day of the procedure in a dose of 100 mg twice daily for a total of 3 days. Another potential complication is tubal or uterine perforation. The incidence of tubal perforation during tubal catheterization has been reported to be between 3 and 11% (Martensson et al, 1993). These perforations are, however, usually totally uncomplicated, heal spontaneously and require no further treatment. We also routinely counsel patients with any form of tubal disease, treated with SS or wire guides, about the possible risk of tubal pregnancy. Whether elevated TPP are associated with an increased risk of tubal pregnancy is currently under investigation.

■ INDICATIONS

Indications for SS include the following.

- *Abnormal findings during a GRP,* such as delayed or asymmetric opacification of the Fallopian tubes and pocketing of dye around the fimbrial end. In these cases, HSG is followed by SS with measurement of TPP (see below).

■ *Treatment of proximal tubal obstruction.* The use of transcervical catheters has dramatically altered the approach to proximal tubal obstruction. Previously, the only available treatment was with microsurgery. Tubal recanalization can be achieved by SS alone (Capitanio et al, 1991), by the use of wire guide with or without a coaxial catheter system (Rosch et al, 1988; Thurmond et al, 1988), or by transcervical balloon tuboplasty (Confino et al, 1990). The effectiveness of these techniques as treatment of proximal tubal obstruction has been confirmed in large populations (Gleicher et al, 1993). In fact, we reported that we were able to open at least one tube in 90% of patients with bilateral tubal cornual obstruction, and both tubes in 80%. In addition, in 68% of patients the tubes remain open at 6 months after the procedure (Confino et al, 1990). Spontaneous pregnancy rates after transcervical tubal catheterization procedures approach 40% in patients without distal tubal disease (Gleicher et al, 1993) (*Figure 12.7*) and are comparable to those achieved by the much more invasive and costly microsurgical repair of proximal tubal occlusion (Gleicher and Pratt, 1994; Das et al, 1995). Most pregnancies occur in the first few cycles after the procedure (Gleicher et al, 1993). In the United States no catheter system is specifically approved by the Food and Drug Administration for entry into Fallopian tubes. This requires the use of catheters and wire guides, which are commercially available for other purposes. Consequently, appropriate informed consents should be obtained from patients. Some catheter systems are, however, approved for use in Fallopian tubes in Europe and Japan.

■ *Early differentiation between an abnormal intrauterine and tubal pregnancy.* HSG and SS can contribute towards the differential diagnosis between an early abnormal intrauterine and an early tubal pregnancy (Gleicher et al, 1992c). The procedure is indicated in patients with abnormal serial human chorionic gonadotropin (hCG) titers that are less than 1500 miu/ml. At this early stage, transvaginal ultrasound is still unable to determine the site of an abnormal pregnancy.

The diagnosis of tubal pregnancy, using X-rays at such a point, is based on uterine as well as tubal findings. In the presence of an ectopic pregnancy, opacification of the endometrial cavity with contrast media will reveal a smooth and only mildly (if at all) enlarged cavity. Moreover, there will be no extravasation of dye. In contrast, an intrauterine pregnancy, even if early, results in significant uterine enlargement and asymmetry and will often demonstrate intramural extravasation and a filling defect (*Figure 12.8*). At present, our experience with intrauterine pregnancies is limited to missed or incomplete abortions. An intact uterine pregnancy therefore may *not* demonstrate this pattern of extravasation of contrast material.

The tubal findings on X-ray examination will vary with size and location of the tubal pregnancy. Often the tubes will not opacify during HSG and one has to proceed with SS to outline the tubes. A tubal pregnancy can appear as a circular opacification or as a diverticulum, depending on its location (*Figure 12.9*).

■ *Local instillation of a medication*, e.g. methotrexate, hyperosmolar glucose, as treatment of tubal pregnancy. Once a tubal pregnancy is diagnosed, it is possible to use SS to deliver embryotoxic medications towards the gestational sac. In a prospective multicenter study, Risquez et al (1992) treated 31 patients, who presented with a clinical diagnosis of tubal pregnancy, with SS and local injection of methotrexate (up to 50 mg). The treatment was successful in 27 (87%), but four patients required subsequent surgery. Confino et al (1994) showed similar results in a smaller series. Both studies confirmed that the Fallopian tubes remained patent after this procedure and patients subsequently had intrauterine pregnancies.

The transcervical approach, using catheters, thus appears safe, effective and relatively simple for the diagnosis as well as the treatment of tubal pregnancy. It can be performed as an office based procedure without the need for laparoscopy or general anesthesia and is therefore very cost effective.

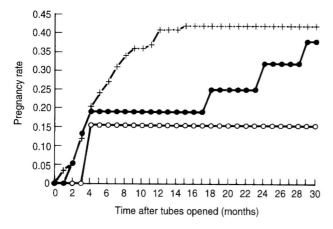

Figure 12.7: Life table analysis of pregnancy in patients who underwent successful transcervical balloon tuboplasty (+), selective salpingography (•) and hysterosalpingography (○). From Gleicher N, Confino E, Corfman R, Coulam C, DeCherney A, Haas G, Katz E, Robinson E, Tur-Kaspa I & Vermesh M (1993) The multicenter transcervical balloon tuboplasty study: conclusions and comparison to alternative technologies. Hum Reprod **8**: 1264–1271. *Reproduced with permission of Oxford University Press.*

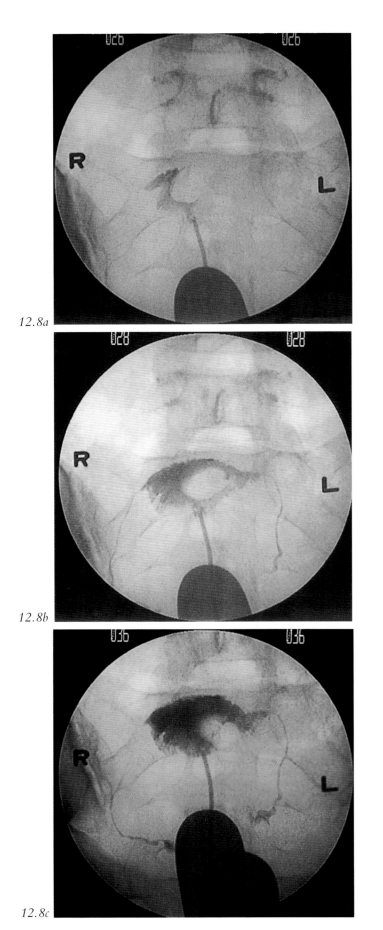

12.8a

12.8b

12.8c

Figure 12.8 (left): (a)–(c) Gynecoradiological procedure demonstrating an intrauterine filling defect which is a missed abortion. Note that both tubes are perfectly normal.

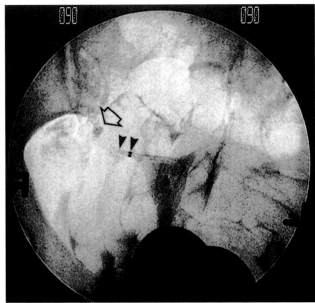

12.9a

12.9b

Figure 12.9: Diagnosis of a biochemical tubal pregnancy by selective salpingography. (a) After initial hysterosalpingography has outlined the endometrial cavity, an SS catheter is inserted in the right tubal ostium (arrowheads). A 'diverticulum' of contrast material is noted from the hysterosalpingogram (arrow), although contrast from the rest of the tube has dissipated. (b) Right SS outlines the tube and demonstrates the diverticulum (arrow) as part of the tubal contour.

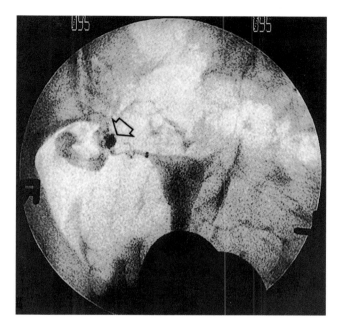

12.9c

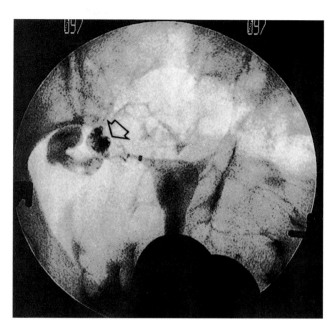

12.9e

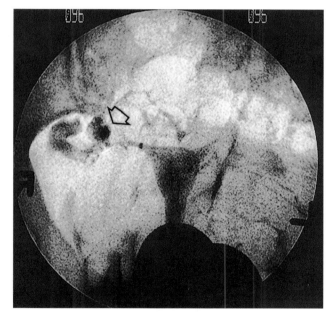

12.9d

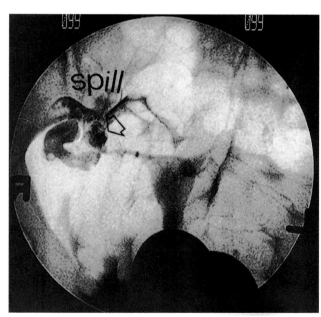

12.9f

Figure 12.9: *(cont.)(c)–(f) Subsequent instillation of dye shows increasing contrast uptake by the diverticulum, a process that continues through (f), where tubal spill is seen. The diverticulum (arrow) represents an early tubal pregnancy. Note the normal size of the uterine cavity and its sharp borders. From Gleicher N, Parrilli M & Pratt DE (1992). Hysterosalpingography and selective salpingography in the differential diagnosis of chemical intrauterine versus tubal pregnancy. Fertil Steril 57: 553–558. Reproduced with permission of the publisher, the American Society for Reproductive Medicine (The American Fertility Society).*

- *Transfer of gametes or pre-embryos during assisted reproductive technology procedures and intratubal inseminations.* The basic assumption for these indications is that any intratubal transfer is more physiological than a transfer into the uterine cavity. Since only very few randomized studies have been reported, a comparison of true pregnancy rates between gamete intrafallopian transfer, zygote intrafallopian transfer and in vitro fertilization (IVF) remains to be established. Our own experience with SS under fluoroscopic guidance for this indication remains minimal. Others have, however, used SS under ultrasound guidance (Flood and Grow, 1993), tactile sensation (Flood and Grow, 1993) or hysteroscopy (Knickerbocker et al, 1995), with pregnancy rates similar to routine IVF. The worldwide experience remains, however, limited and it is therefore not possible at this time to reach reliable conclusions about outcome in comparison with laparoscopically performed procedures.

- *Transcervical tubal sterilization.* Recently, there has been a resurgence in interest in the transcervical approach to tubal sterilization. SS is used to deliver substances, such as methyl 2-cyanoacrylate, to the tubal lumen in attempts to seal it effectively. These are, however, still experimental procedures with unacceptable failure rates. Also, the substances used often spill into the pelvis through the fimbrial end, with resultant peritoneal irritation and potential for adhesion formation. A newer system, known as the FEMCEPT device, was used by Shuber (1989) to deliver methyl 2-cyanoacrylate to the tubes. This system consists of a cannula with a distal balloon that is insufflated to prevent reflux of substances. Follow up HSG showed, however, bilateral tubal occlusion is only 88.2% of Fallopian tubes.

▪ COMPENDIUM OF ABNORMAL FINDINGS

This compendium (*Figures 12.10–12.29*) presents a collection of abnormalities that may be found during a gynecoradiological procedure. Some of these figures

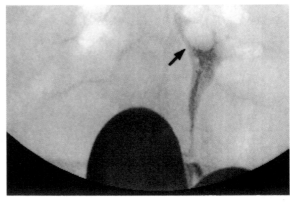

12.11a

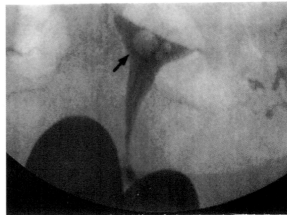

12.11b

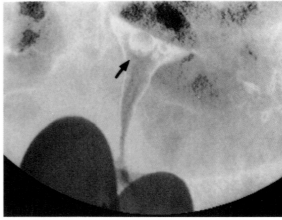

12.11c

Figure 12.11: *(a)–(c) Sequential hysterosalpingography study demonstrates filling defects in the uterine cavity; these are air bubbles (arrow). Unlike polyps or myomas, air bubbles will change position when the patient is made to rotate her hips.*

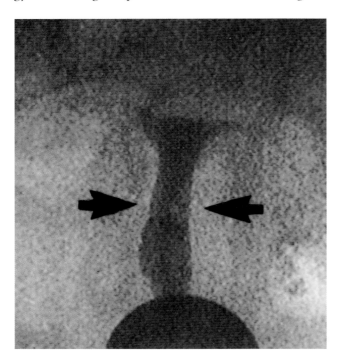

Figure 12.10: *Incompetent cervix. The arrow shows the cervix, which is wide open.*

show both positive and negative views of the same abnormality. They are easily created by manipulation of the digital images and may be useful because a negative image can sometimes give more information than a positive one.

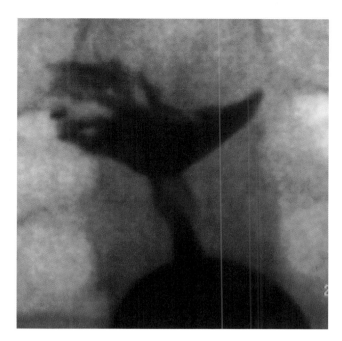

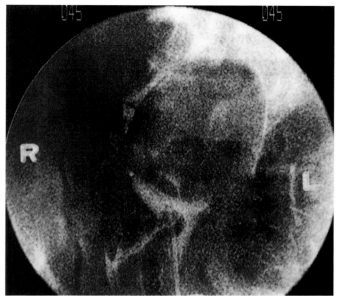

Figure 12.12: Endometrial carcinoma. Hysterosalpingography demonstrates extravasation of dye into the myometrium in the fundal region. Endometrial biopsy confirmed the presence of adenocarcinoma of the endometrium.

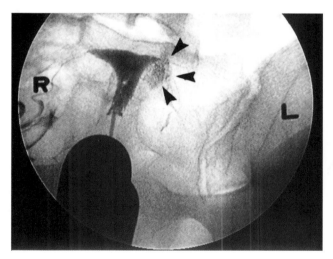

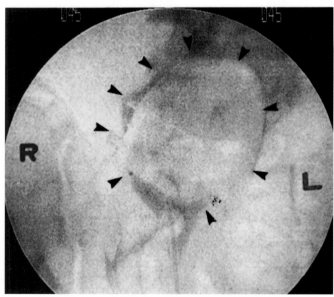

Figure 12.14: Large fundal myoma outlined by contrast medium after it has spilled into the peritoneal cavity during SS. The uterine cavity itself is normal. The SS catheter has been introduced through the central channel of a cervical cannula (with balloon) and its tip can be seen in the right uterine cornu.

Figure 12.13: Left cornual blockage. The cavity is normal and the right tube shows free spill. The left tube, however, shows cornual block with extravasation of dye into the musculature. This is an indication of severe tubal pathology, as the extravasation of contrast suggests that even high pressures do not recanalize the obstruction.

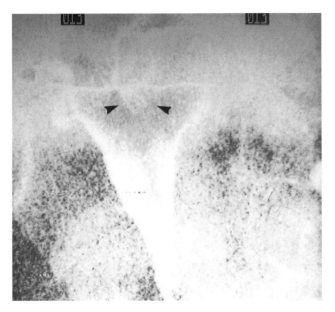

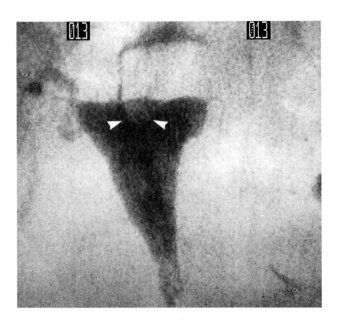

Figure 12.15: Small uterine septum. The septum is barely visible during hysterosalpingography (arrowheads). Contrast enhancement

(left) is used to delineate the septum further.

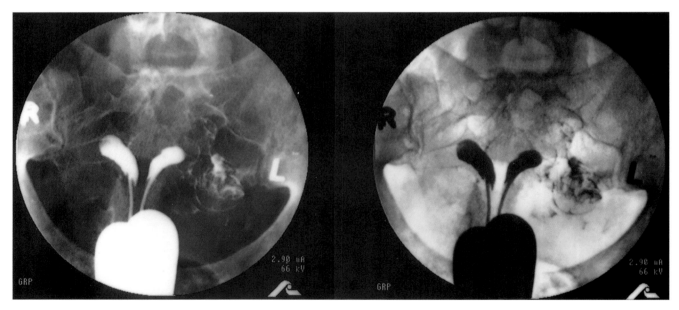

Figure 12.16: Double uterus and cervix. There is free spill of dye from the left tube, whereas the right tube shows cornual blockage.

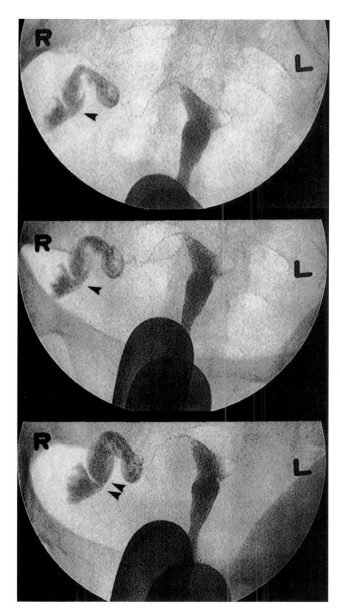

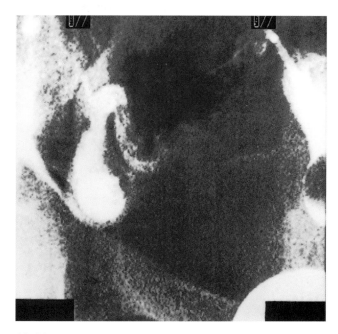

12.18a

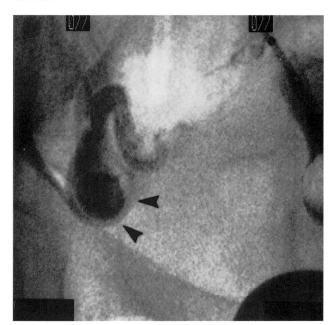

Figure 12.17: *Sequential hysterosalpingography study demonstrates fimbrial phimosis (arrowheads). The left tube is showing cornual obstruction and the filling defect in the left cornu is an air bubble.*

12.18b

Figure 12.18: *(a) and (b) Contrast and image enlargement is used for detailed evaluation of a right hydrosalpinx. The tubal rugae are clearly seen and there is thickening of the tubal walls (arrowheads).*

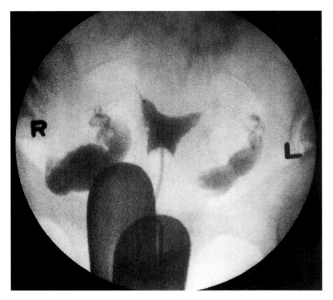

12.19a

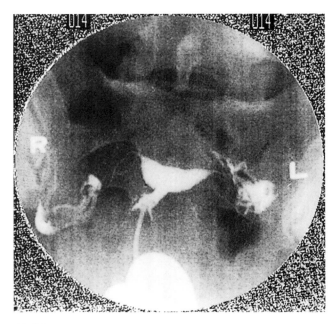

12.20a

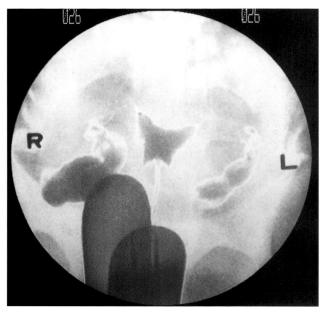

12.19b

Figure 12.19: *Bilateral hydrosalpinges with no spill in an infertile patient. The tubal rugae are absent, thus making her a poor candidate for reconstructive tubal surgery.*

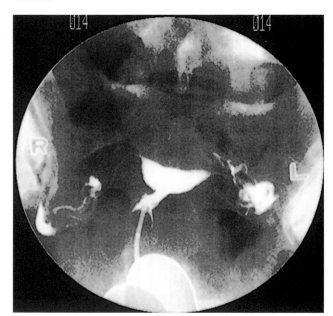

12.20b

Figure 12.20: *(a)–(f) Hysterosalpingography study demonstrating contrast and edge enhancement. The uterine cavity is normal. The*

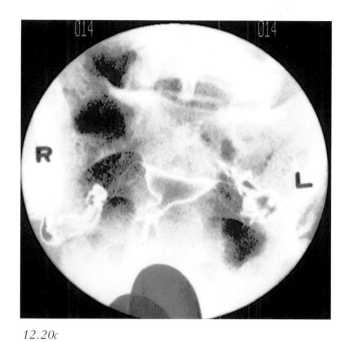

12.20c

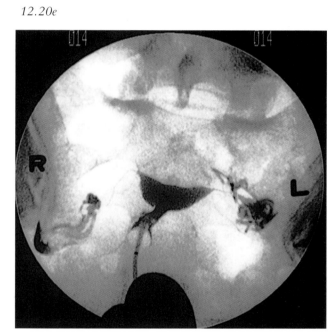

12.20e

12.20d

12.20f

right tube shows free spill, whereas the left spills into a 'pocket'.
This finding is suggestive of peritubal adhesions on the left.

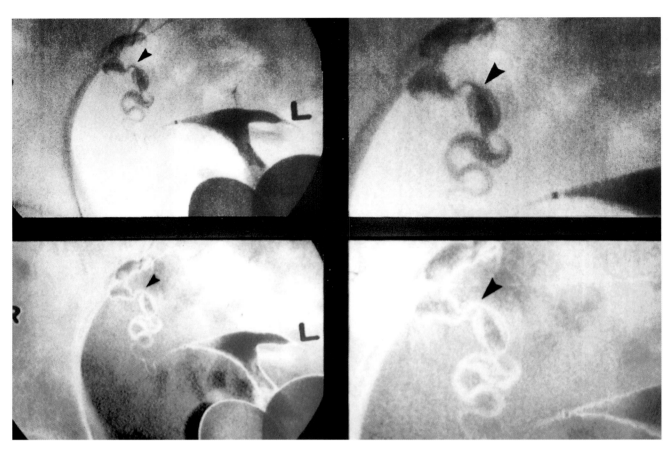

Figure 12.21: *Phimosis and side wall adhesions. SS demonstrates that the right tube is fixed to the side wall. Image enlargement (right) allows a more detailed evaluation of findings. Contrast* *enhancement (bottom) clearly demonstrates phimosis of the fimbrial end (arrowhead).*

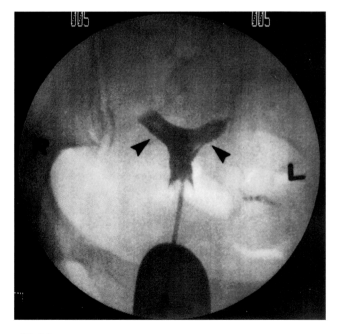

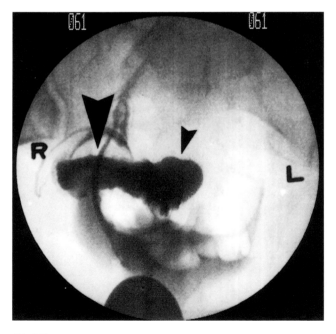

12.22a

12.22b

Figure 12.26: *Missed abortion. Frame (a) shows the presence of a bicornuate uterus. Note that both the horns are equal in size (arrowheads). Frame (b) shows the same patient with a missed* *abortion in the right horn, which is now enlarged (large arrowhead). The left cornu is relatively small (small arrowhead) (Confino et al, 1990).*

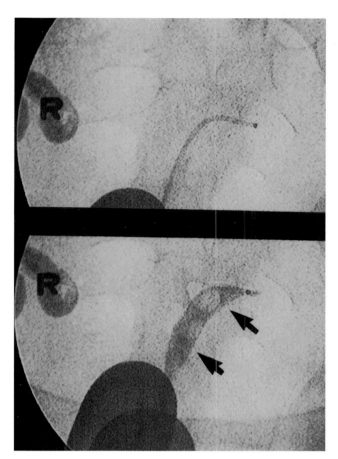

Figure 12.23: SS is being performed to treat left proximal tubal obstruction. Failure to opacify the tube leads to contrast medium flowing back into the uterine cavity (arrows), indicating the presence of a severe proximal obstruction. In such cases, one should proceed with the use of a wire guide or a balloon catheter (where available) to recanalize the tube.

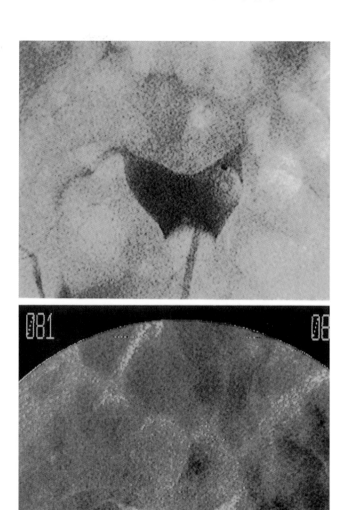

Figure 12.24: Failed selective salpingography. In this patient a cornual polyp blocks the catheter and makes access to the left tubal ostium impossible.

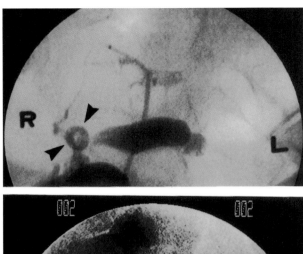

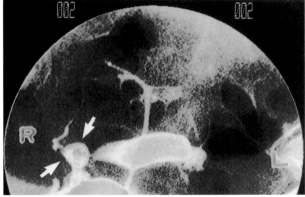

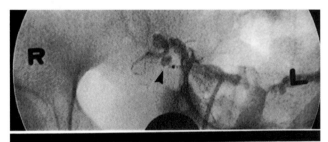

Figure 12.25: SS demonstrates the presence of a right tubal pregnancy (arrows). The fillings defect in the uterine cavity is an air bubble.

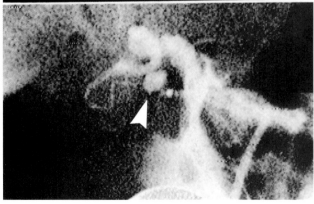

Figure 12.26: Old ectopic pregnancy. SS demonstrates the incidental finding of a circular filling defect in the right tube, which is probably an old ectopic pregnancy. Image enlargement and contrast (bottom) are used to further delineate the lesion (Confino et al, 1990).

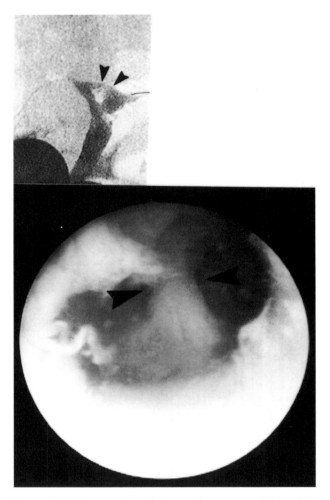

Figure 12.27: Intrauterine adhesions. The upper panel shows filling defects in the uterus, which are adhesions (arrowheads). The lower panel demonstrates a hysteroscopic view of the same adhesion (arrowheads).

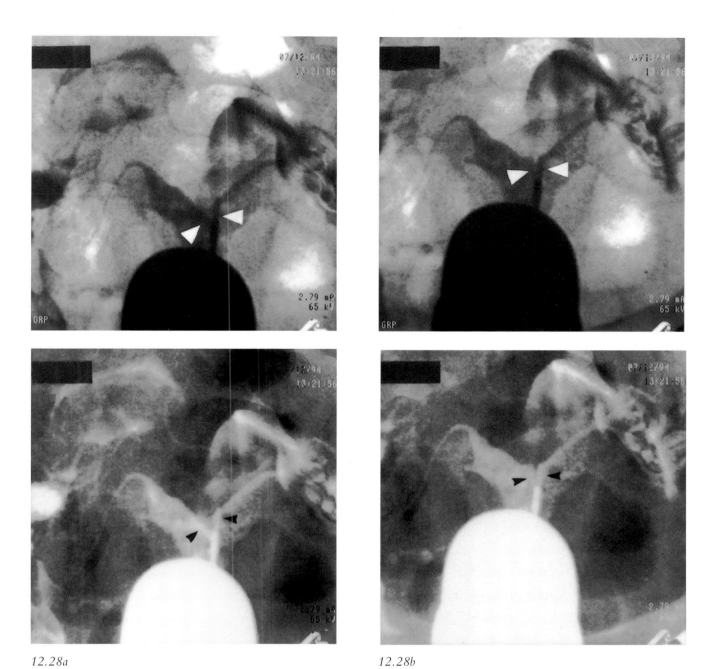

12.28a

12.28b

Figure 12.28: *(a) and (b) Resection of uterine septum with hystero-scopic scissors. The scissors have been passed through the central channel of the cervical cannula and the septum is resected under fluoroscopic guidance. The tip of the scissors (arrowheads) is seen resecting the*

septum (Gleicher et al, 1992a). The procedure can be carried out with minimal discomfort to the patient. This patient had a previous laparoscopy which ruled out a bicornuate uterus.

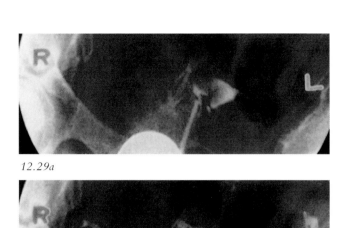

12.29a

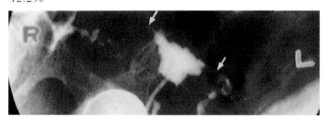

12.29b

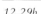

12.29c

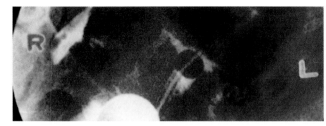

12.29d

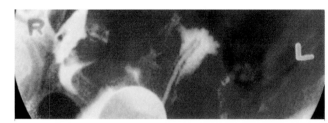

12.29e

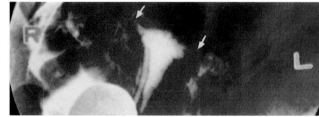

12.29f

Figure 12.29: (a)–(f) *Lysis of intrauterine adhesions. The cervical cannula is advanced into the uterine cavity, where its balloon is distended to lyse the adhesions successfully. This is accomplished with minimal discomfort to the patient, who on occasion is mildly sedated.*

A hysteroscopic scissors can also be passed through the central channel of the cervical cannula to lyse tenacious adhesions (Gleicher et al, 1992a).

REFERENCES

Capitanio GL, Ferrialo A, Croce S, Gazzo R, Anseini P & Cecco L (1991) Transcervical selective salpingography: a diagnostic and therapeutic approach to cases of proximal tubal injection failure. *Fertil Steril* **55**: 1045–1050.

Committee on the Biological Effects of Ionizing Radiation (1980) *The Effect on Populations of Exposure to Low Levels of Ionizing Radiation: Genetic Effects*, pp. 71–134. Washington DC: National Academic Press.

Confino E, Tur-Kaspa I, DeCherney A et al (1990) Transcervical balloon tuboplasty. A multicenter study. *JAMA* **264**: 2079–2082.

Confino E, Tur-Kaspa I & Gleicher N (1992) Sonographic transcervical balloon tuboplasty (TBT). *Hum Reprod* **7**: 1271–1273.

Confino E, Binor Z, Molo MW & Radwanska E (1994) Selective salpingography for the diagnosis and treatment of early tubal pregnancy. *Fertil Steril* **62**: 286–288.

Das K, Nagel TC & Malo JW (1995) Hysteroscopic cannulation for proximal tubal obstruction: a change for the better? *Fertil Steril* **63**: 1009–1015.

Flood JT & Grow DR (1993) Transcervical tubal cannulation: a review. *Obstet Gynecol Surv* **48**: 768–776.

Gleicher N & Pratt D (1994) Transvaginal procedures for infertility. In Behrman SJ, Patton GW Jr & Holtz G (eds) *Progress in Infertility*, 4th edn, pp. 225–248. Boston: Little, Brown.

Gleicher N, Thurmond A, Burry KA & Coulam CB (1992a) Gynecoradiology: a new approach to diagnosis and treatment of tubal disease. *Fertil Steril* **58**: 885–887.

Gleicher N, Parrilli M, Redding L, Pratt D & Karande V (1992b) Standardization of hysterosalpingography and selective salpingography: a valuable adjunct to simple opacification studies. *Fertil Steril* **58**: 1136–1141.

Gleicher N, Parrilli M & Pratt DE (1992c) Hysterosalpingography and selective salpingography in the differential diagnosis of chemical intrauterine versus tubal pregnancy. *Fertil Steril* **57**: 553–558.

Gleicher N, Confino E, Corfman R et al (1993) The multicenter transcervical balloon tuboplasty study: conclusions and comparison to alternative technologies. *Hum Reprod* **8**: 1264–1271.

Hedgepath PL, Thurmond AS, Fry R, Schmidgall JR & Rosch J (1991) Radiographic fallopian tube recanalization: aborted ovarian radiation dose. *Radiology* **180**: 121–122.

ICRP (1991) *1990 Recommendations of the International Commission on Radiological Protection*. Publication 60.

Karande VC, Pratt DE, Rabin DS & Gleicher N (1995a) The limited value of hysterosalpingography in assessing tubal status and fertility potential. *Fertil Steril* **63**: 1167–1171.

Karande VC, Rao R, Pratt DE, Balin M & Gleicher N (1995b) Elevated tubal perfusion pressures during selective salpingography are highly suggestive of endometriosis. *Fertil Steril* **64**: 1070–1073.

Knickerbocker J, Eisermann J, Lopez G et al (1995) Abstract presented at the IXth World Congress on IVF and Alternate Assisted Reproduction, 1995. *J Assist Reprod Genet* **12** (**supplement**).

Martensson O, Nilsson B, Ekelund L, Johansson & Wickman G (1993) Selective salpingography and fluoroscopic transcervical salpingoplasty for diagnosis and treatment of proximal fallopian tube occlusions. *Acta Obstet Gynecol Scand* **72**: 458–464.

Novy MJ, Thurmond AS, Patton P, Uchida BT & Rosch J (1988) Diagnosis of cornual obstruction by transcervical fallopian tube cannulation. *Fertil Steril* **50**: 434–440.

Risquez F & Confino E (1993) Transcervical tubal cannulation, past, present and future. *Fertil Steril* **60**: 211–226.

Risquez F, Forman R, Maleika F, Foulot H, Reidy J & Chapman M (1992) Transcervical cannulation of the fallopian tube for the management of ectopic pregnancy: prospective multicenter study. *Fertil Steril* **58**: 1131–1135.

Rosch J, Thurmond AS, Uchida BT & Sovak M (1988) Selective transcervical fallopian tube catheterization: technique update. *Radiology* **168**: 1–11.

Shuber J (1989) Transcervical sterilization with use of methyl 2-cyanoacrylate and newer delivery system (the FEMCEPT device). *Am J Obstet Gynecol* **160**: 887.

Thurmond A, Rosch J, Patton PE, Burry KA & Novy M (1988) Fluoroscopic transcervical fallopian tube catheterization for diagnosis and treatment of female infertility caused by tubal obstruction. *Radiographics* **8**: 621–639.

Section Two: Appearances and classification of pathology

PART 1

APPEARANCES OF DISORDERS/DISEASES

13 *Infections, atrophy, hyperplasia and polyps of the endometrium*
S de Blok

■ INTRODUCTION

Diagnostic hysteroscopy has been accepted as the most sensitive method for the direct visual evaluation of intrauterine pathology. Hysteroscopic surgical techniques have been developed simultaneously and offer the possibility of endoscopic treatment of intracavitary pathology with less invasive methods, avoiding hysterotomy or hysterectomy in many cases (de Blok and Wamsteker, 1995). In this chapter the imaging of benign diseases of the endometrium with hysteroscopy in comparison with transvaginal ultrasonography, radiology and magnetic resonance imaging (MRI) will be discussed. A practical illustrated guide will be proposed for quick evaluation of structural abnormalities of the endometrium using these techniques.

The endometrial cycle in premenopausal women follows a precisely scheduled series of physiological and morphological events characterized by proliferation, secretory differentiation, degeneration and regeneration of the uterine lining. These events are controlled by estrogen and progesterone and reflect the sensitivity of the hypothalamic–pituitary–ovarian axis. The sensitivity of the endometrium to these hormones remains even after the menopause. Interpretation of pathology of the endometrium with any imaging technique must take this continuous change into account. These changes can be easily illustrated by making transvaginal ultrasound studies of the thickness of the endometrium in the various phases of the cycle (*Figure 13.1*) (see also Chapter 2, *Figure 2.12*).

During hysteroscopy the degree of distension of the uterine cavity influences the appearance of the endometrium, which can be examined most accurately with continuous flow and reduced intrauterine pressure (Wamsteker et al, 1992) (*Figure 13.2*). Thick secretory endometrium may either obscure or suggest intrauterine pathology during transvaginal ultrasonography or hysteroscopy; therefore for detection or exclusion of intrauterine abnormalities these techniques should preferably be scheduled in the first half of the menstrual cycle. With thick secretory endometrium the findings with both techniques must be considered inconclusive, necessitating a repeat procedure after menstruation, which can be either spontaneous or induced by a course of progesterone. MRI, a new diagnostic technique, is a sensitive method of recognizing intracavitary pathology but has the disadvantage of being expensive as a method of routine screening.

The pathogenesis and symptomatology of the different structural abnormalities of the endometrium and the value of diagnostic imaging techniques in these conditions will be discussed separately.

■ ENDOMETRITIS

Inflammation of the endometrium can be distinguished as acute or chronic endometritis.

The cervix is the physiological barrier for microorganisms; except for rare forms of endometritis established by hematogenous implantation or descending infection from the Fallopian tubes, e.g. tuberculosis, most types of endometritis result from an ascending infection via the cervix. The usually impervious cervical barrier is less efficient during menstruation, abortion and delivery and in instrumental interventions such as

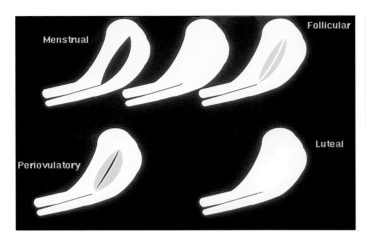

13.1a

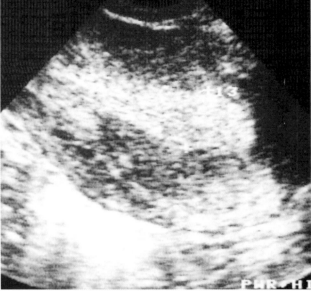

13.1d

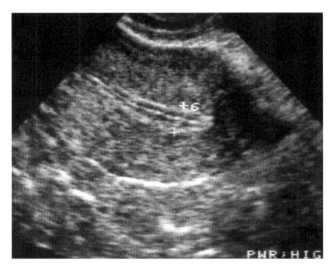

13.1b

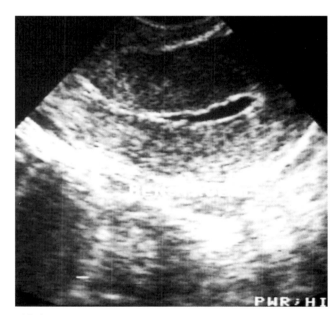

13.1e

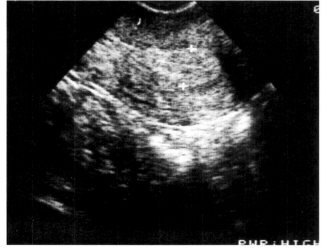

13.1c

Figure 13.1: *Transvaginal ultrasonography. (a) The appearance of the endometrium in the different phases of the endometrial cycle. (b)–(e) Midsagittal section of the uterus showing the endometrium in (b) the proliferative phase, (c) the early secretory phase, (d) the late secretory phase, and (e) menstruation.*

curettage or insertion of an intrauterine contraceptive device, during which the normal vaginal flora can obtain access to the uterine cavity. The bacteriological balance of the vagina can also be disturbed by the use of systemic antibacterial drugs, diabetes or frequent vaginal lavage.

ACUTE ENDOMETRITIS

PATHOGENESIS AND SYMPTOMATOLOGY

In the majority of cases acute endometritis is related to the circumstances mentioned above, which lower the

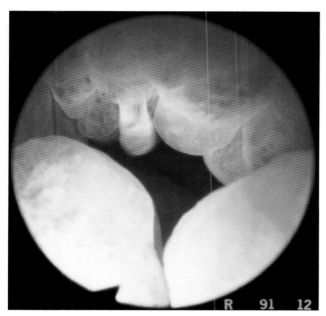

13.2a

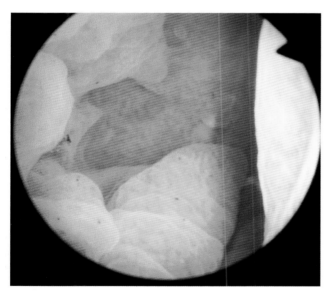

13.2b

Figure 13.2: Hysteroscopy. (a) Secretory endometrium in the isthmic area of the uterine cavity with low pressure continuous flow hysteroscopy. (b) Secretory endometrium showing the thickness corresponding to the ultrasonographic image.

defensive barrier of the cervix, and is usually caused by hemolytic or anaerobic streptococci, staphylococci or organisms related to sexually transmitted disease (STD), such as *Neisseria gonorrhoeae*, *Chlamydia trachomatis* and *Gardnerella* (Bleker et al, 1989). Patients with acute endometritis may present with acute lower abdominal pain, usually after menstruation, delivery or abortion. An increase in temperature (above 38.5°C) will usually be registered and will be accompanied by mucopurulent

vaginal discharge. Urination is rarely painful and defecation is unaffected.

CLINICAL INVESTIGATIONS

The patient will often present with fever and lower abdominal pain. The endocervix and the vagina will contain mucopurulent discharge. Urinary tract infection, pregnancy related disease and appendicitis should be ruled out. The clinical history and tenderness of the uterus and adnexa during bimanual gynecological examination, in combination with elevated leukocyte count, C-reactive protein (CRP) and erythrocyte sedimentation rate (ESR), will provide the diagnosis, especially when supported by microbiological investigation of the cervix.

Transvaginal ultrasonography

This technique will not provide any additional diagnostic clue during the acute phase of endometritis unless the disease is accompanied by hydrosalpinx or pyosalpinx, which give the typical signs of cystic echolucent areas in the adnexal regions.

Diagnostic hysteroscopy

Hysteroscopic examination may aggravate an endometritis, inducing salpingitis by transporting bacteria with the distension medium into the Fallopian tubes, and is contraindicated in the case of suspected acute genital inflammation unless cultures are taken and at least 24 hours of appropriate antibiotic therapy is administered intravenously.

CHRONIC ENDOMETRITIS

PATHOGENESIS AND SYMPTOMATOLOGY

Patients with irregular menstrual bleeding, postmenopausal bleeding, mucopurulent discharge and uterine tenderness may be suffering from chronic endometritis. There may well be a lack of specific symptoms and temperature elevation.

Chronic endometritis can be caused by many types of bacteria and viruses, such as chlamydia, *Neisseria gonorrhoeae*, *Escherichia coli*, staphylococci, streptococci, mycoplasma, *Mycobacterium tuberculosis*, herpes and even cytomegalic inclusion virus, or parasites. The early recognition of STD related cervicitis and endometritis and adequate treatment in the very early phase of clinical symptomatology may prevent many cases of tube related infertility.

Chlamydia trachomatis can be detected in 9% of women during normal routine screening for cervical cancer (Meijer et al, 1989). In many cases of previously suspected infection of the endometrium, chlamydia now seems to play an important role (Mardh et al, 1981). In these cases the diagnosis can be established on clinical history and/or evidence in combination with bacteriological cervical cultures.

CLINICAL INVESTIGATIONS

Inspection of the cervix and vagina may reveal mucopurulent discharge; sampling for bacteriological study and Pap test should be undertaken. On physical examination uterine and sometimes adnexal tenderness will usually be found.

Transvaginal ultrasonography

Imaging of the uterus and adnexa with this method will not provide specific evidence of chronic endometritis. In postmenopausal patients suspected of having this disorder, pyometra or mucoceles may be revealed as echolucent areas within the uterine cavity during ultrasonography (*Figure 13.3*). Endometrial pathology will then be recognized as echodense areas within the echolucent uterine cavity, reflecting irregular thickness of the endometrium.

Diagnostic hysteroscopy

Using microhysteroscopy in cases of chronic endometritis, the first days of proliferation are optimal for recognizing dilated subendometrial vascular architecture. Hysteroscopy should not, however, be considered as a specific diagnostic tool for chronic endometritis.

In postmenopausal patients with mucocele or pyometra the uterine cavity must be evaluated with hysteroscopy to exclude or diagnose endometrial pathology. The external and internal ostia are narrow and sometimes ultrasonography will be needed to reveal the course of the cervical canal in order to prevent perforation during insertion of the hysteroscope. In cases of mucocele the endometrium will be pale pink and

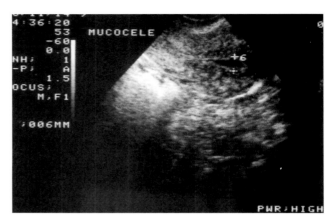

Figure 13.3: Transvaginal ultrasonography. Sagittal section of the uterus of a postmenopausal patient showing occlusion of the cervix and a mucocele.

atrophic and the contents will be clear mucus. No subendometrial vascular injection will be found. Endometrial biopsies will support the diagnosis of atrophy. In cases of pyometra the endometrium is covered with mucopurulent exudate and the subendometrial vasculature is congested.

Chronic endometritis cannot be diagnosed by hysteroscopy alone but must be confirmed by histological examination.

CLINICAL MANAGEMENT

Endocervical cancer and chronic infections must be excluded by cytological and histological investigations. Sometimes occlusions of the cervical canal can be observed with transvaginal ultrasonography, for example in the case of a mucocele (*Figure 13.3*). Using MRI this condition may be recognized and the cervical stroma and glands may also be visualized as a means of revealing or excluding endocervical cancer. The only correct method of gaining access to the uterine cavity in these cases is to use the hysteroscope in order to prevent perforation, as may occur during 'blind' diagnostic curettage. If obstructed, the cervical canal may be opened by using a small diameter diagnostic continuous flow hysteroscope in conjunction with transabdominal ultrasonography, which facilitates the following of the correct route. Flushing with the distension fluid will evacuate purulent collections from the uterine cavity, enabling diagnostic hysteroscopy with tissue sampling for histology to exclude endometrial cancer. The diagnosis 'chronic endometritis' can be established by histological examination, positive cervical cultures and an increased ESR. The condition may be suspected from transvaginal sonographic imaging and hysteroscopy, but other methods, such as culture of cervical secretions and histology, in combination with physical examination are more specific.

▪ ENDOMETRIAL ATROPHY

PATHOGENESIS AND SYMPTOMATOLOGY

The clinical symptom of postmenopausal bleeding in women who are not receiving hormone replacement therapy (HRT) is in many cases based on atrophy of the estrogen sensitive tissue of the vagina, cervix and endometrium. Patients with postmenopausal bleeding based on atrophy may present with brown discharge or true bleeding. Atrophy of the vagina may cause vaginal dryness, coital pain, urinary incontinence and superimposed bacteriological infections.

CLINICAL INVESTIGATIONS

On inspection the vulva and vestibulum are characterized by dryness of the epithelium and cigarette paper-thin pink mucosa. The external orifice of the urethra has a tendency to eversion and is slightly open. On speculum examination the vaginal mucosa also looks very thin and pink, giving a cigarette paper-like appearance. Discharge, if present, may consist of increased vaginal bacteriological flora and old blood remnants. The cervix normally contains no mucus and usually has stiff and narrow external and internal ostia.

The most important clinical diagnoses to be excluded are acute infections and vaginal, cervical and endometrial cancer. Diagnostic hysteroscopy and transvaginal ultrasonography are of utmost importance as minimally invasive techniques for the diagnosis or exclusion of major pathology in these cases, as well as in patients receiving HRT (*Figure 13.4*).

Transvaginal ultrasonography

The endometrium projects as a thin echodense layer with a double thickness, usually less than 4–5 mm in women not using HRT.

Diagnostic hysteroscopy

At diagnostic hysteroscopy both the endocervix and the internal cervical ostium are narrow. The endometrium will present as a pinkish and thin mucosal membrane (*Figures 13.4a* and *13.5*). Sometimes the cornual areas are occluded with filmy adhesions (*Figure 13.6*). Partial

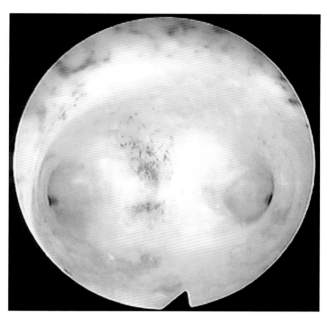

13.4a

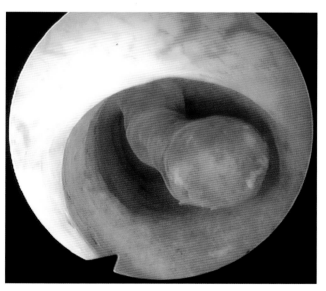

13.4b

Figure 13.4: *(a) Normal uterine cavity and cornual areas with atrophic endometrium. (b) Narrow isthmus with atrophic endometrium and endometrial polyp.*

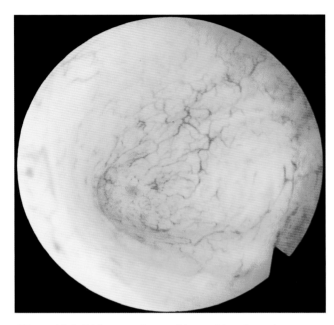

Figure 13.5: Right cornual area with atrophic endometrium.

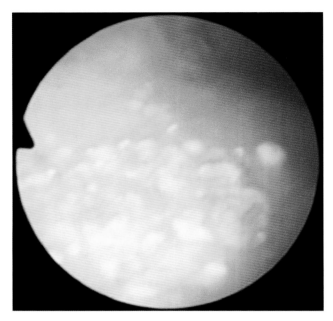

Figure 13.7: Atrophic endometrium with calcifications.

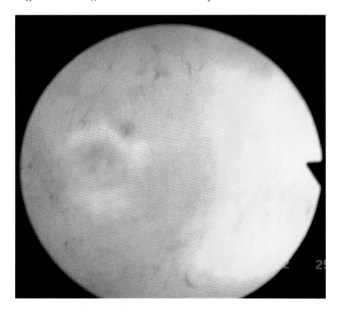

Figure 13.6: Tubal orifice occluded with filmy adhesions.

obliteration may also be present and the tubal orifices may be completely closed. Small cysts and calcifications can sometimes be observed within the thin endometrium (*Figure 13.7*). The vascular architecture shows thin vessels that easily rupture with distension of the uterine cavity which may result in slight bleeding.

INTERPRETATION OF FINDINGS

Endometrial cancer is the most common post-menopausal gynecological malignancy. Histological ex-

amination of the endometrium is essential for diagnosis. The most common technique for tissue sampling is dilatation and curettage under general anesthesia (Grimes, 1982). Other, less invasive techniques for endometrial sampling, such as the Novak technique and the Vabra technique, lack direct visual inspection of the uterine cavity (Grimes, 1982). Diagnostic hysteroscopy has developed into a safe and reliable technique for the diagnosis and treatment of intracavitary pathology (Wamsteker et al, 1992; Wamsteker and de Blok, 1993; de Blok and Wamsteker, 1995). Complete direct visual inspection of the uterine cavity in combination with selective endometrial tissue sampling has proven to be highly accurate in diagnosing intrauterine pathology (Goldrath and Sherman, 1985; Brooks and Serden, 1988; Gimpelson and Rappold, 1988; Loffer, 1989). Comparison of hysteroscopy with dilatation and curettage proved that in 60% of the curettage procedures less than half of the uterine wall was sampled (Stoval et al, 1989). Hysteroscopy with direct visual inspection offers a greater chance of revealing pathology at a far earlier stage of the disease (Stock and Kanbour, 1975).

Although hysteroscopy can be performed on ambulant patients and as an office procedure, transvaginal ultrasonography offers an even less invasive technique. Recent studies with transvaginal ultrasonography report visualization of the endometrial lining in all cases and a sensitivity in diagnosing endometrial pathology of 96–100% at a cut off level of 4–5 mm for the double endometrial layer (Goldstein et al, 1990; Nasri et al, 1990; Osmers et al, 1990; Granberg et al, 1991; Emanuel et al, 1995; Karlsson et al, 1995; Dijkhuizen et al, 1996). The predictive value in a routine clinical setting in excluding endometrial cancer in those patients in which the endometrium was adequately identified with transvaginal ultrasonography was 100% (95% confidence interval 91.4 to 100%) at a cut off level of 5 mm and a predictive value of 90% (95% confidence interval 76.9 to 97.3%) in excluding minor pathology (Dijkman et al, 1996).

CLINICAL MANAGEMENT

For the clinical management of patients presenting with postmenopausal bleeding the following steps are proposed.

The initial investigations consist of a normal gynecological examination with inspection of the vagina and cervix, bacteriological cultures and Pap test, followed by transvaginal ultrasonography. When the endometrium can be visualized properly and the double layer is less than 4 or 5 mm*, expectant management can be proposed. Only when the sonographic findings are inconclusive or indicate an endometrial thickness of 5 mm or more, or when residual bleeding occurs over a period of 3 months, should diagnostic ambulant office hysteroscopy with tissue sampling be considered necessary. The final diagnosis will be established by histological examination.

This management strongly reduces morbidity and may significantly reduce the costs of health care in the diagnostic phase. It is likely that consensus about a safe cut off level of 4 or 5 mm double endometrium thickness will be reached.

▪ ENDOMETRIAL HYPERPLASIA

PATHOGENESIS AND SYMPTOMATOLOGY

Abnormal endometrial proliferations form a morphological continuum ranging from focal glandular crowding through various degrees of hyperplasia and carcinoma. These proliferations are subdivided into noninvasive and invasive forms. The pathogenesis is unknown. Invasive lesions comprise all types of endometrial cancer and are not discussed in this chapter (*Figure 13.8*). Less than 2% of all cases of hyperplasia

without atypia progress to carcinomas, whereas 23% of all cases of hyperplasia with atypia progress to endometrial cancer (Kurman and Norris, 1994). Patients with hyperplasia may present with heavy menstrual bleeding in the perimenopause but hyperplasia can also be found after the menopause. Patients using HRT who have bleeding problems may also have hyperplasia.

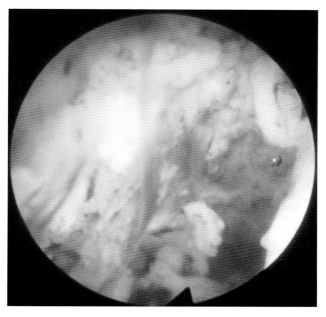

13.8a

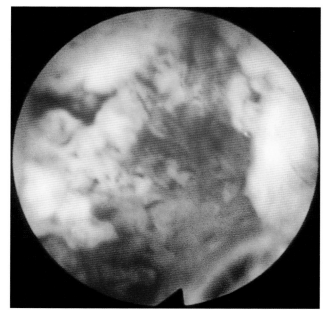

13.8b

Figure 13.8: *(a) and (b) Loss of structural architecture of the epithelium and abnormal growth and branching of vascular architecture in endometrial cancer.*

---

* *Editorial comment* There is no international consensus as to what should be regarded as the cut off level for the endometrial thickness (double layer) for detecting endometrial abnormality at transvaginal ultrasonography.

CLINICAL INVESTIGATIONS

Transvaginal ultrasonography

The endometrium presents as a thick layer containing echolucent and echodense areas, making differentiation from polyps difficult (*Figure 13.9*). The ovaries can be simultaneously studied in order to exclude pathology.

Diagnostic hysteroscopy

The endometrium is usually thick and cystic. The introduction of the hysteroscope must be performed without touching the uterine walls because, in the presence of thick hypervascular endometrium, bleeding will be an immediate result. Continuous flow liquid hysteroscopy has the distinct advantage of distending the uterus and providing for an atraumatic introduction. Sometimes only parts of

the endometrium are hyperplastic, while other parts are normal (*Figure 13.10a,b*). Selective biopsies can be made during hysteroscopy in order to differentiate between pathological and nonpathological areas. With hysteroscopy the histological type of endometrial hyperplasia cannot usually be observed, although the vascular aspect of the tissue can sometimes indicate atypia (*Figure 13.10c*). Polyps can be clearly differentiated from thick hyperplastic endometrium. In premenopausal or perimenopausal

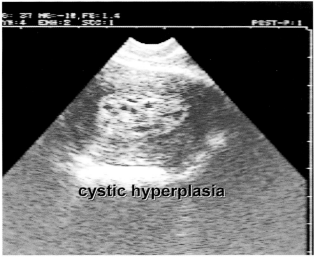

13.9a

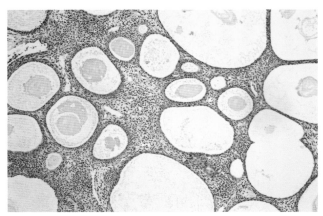

13.9b

Figure 13.9: *(a) Transvaginal ultrasonography. Midsagittal section showing cystic hyperplasia. (b) Histological section of a specimen from the same patient showing simple cystic hyperplasia without atypia (×400).*

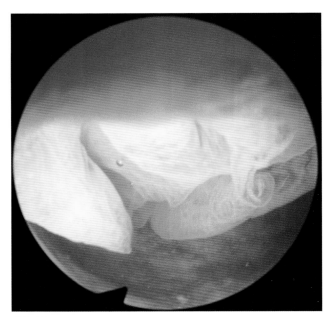

13.10a

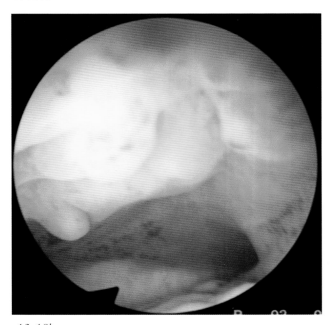

13.10b

Figure 13.10: *(a) and (b) Partial endometrial hyperplasia located at the anterior wall of the uterine cavity.*

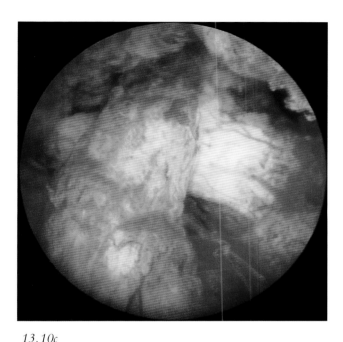

13.10c

Figure 13.10: *(cont.) (c) Massive endometrial hyperplasia with atypical vascular architecture; histology showed atypical adenomatous hyperplasia.*

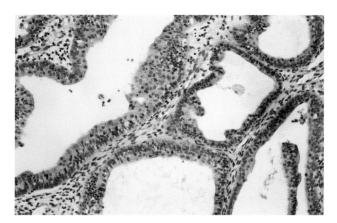

13.11a

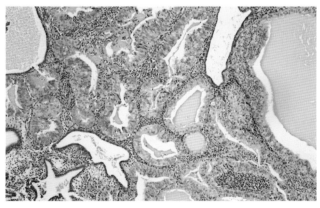

13.11b

Figure 13.11: *(a) Histological section showing simple hyperplasia with atypia (×400). Differentiation cannot be made with ultrasonography. (b) Complex atypical hyperplasia (×400). Differentiation can only be made with histological sections.*

patients the endometrium may be so thick that a reliable hysteroscopy only becomes feasible after a course of progesterone.

INTERPRETATION OF FINDINGS

The differentiation of low grade malignancies, hyperplasia with or without atypia or the late secretory phase cannot be made visually by using the hysteroscope alone, but additionally requires histological examination. The diagnostic differentiation of these conditions depends on their histological distinctions. Histologically, hyperplasia without atypia can be divided into simple and complex types. In simple hyperplasia the glands are cystically dilated (*Figure 13.9b*) and sometimes focally crowded. Complex hyperplasia is characterized by crowded glands with two to four layer epithelial stratification and a mitotic activity of less than 5–10 per ten high power fields.

Hyperplasia with atypia can also be divided into simple and complex types demonstrating cytonuclear atypia (*Figure 13.11* and see *Table 13.2*). Stromal invasion and irregular epithelial lines with back-to-back growth must be considered as signs of endometrial cancer (Kurman and Norris, 1994).

CLINICAL MANAGEMENT

For the clinical management of endometrial hyperplasia, transvaginal sonography and hysteroscopy with tissue sampling for histology are the methods of choice when compared with classic curettage.

The clinical behavior of hyperplasia shows a progression to endometrial cancer, as shown in *Table 13.1* (Kurman et

Table 13.1 *Clinical behavior of endometrial hyperplasia*

Type of hyperplasia	Regression (%)	Persistence (%)	Progression to cancer (%)
Simple	80	19	1
Complex	80	17	3
Simple atypical	69	23	8
Complex atypical	57	14	29

Kurman et al. 1985

al, 1985). This table clearly indicates the risks of hyperplasia progressing to cancer. Since hyperplasia can be diagnosed in both fertile and pre- and postmenopausal women, the clinical management must take into consideration the calculated risk of the possible progression to cancer, the patient's wish to remain fertile or to retain the uterus and her age. Women under the age of 40 with simple atypical hyperplasia without stromal invasion can retain their fertility with conservative treatment with hormonal suppression of progesterone. On the other hand, in those patients with simple atypical hyperplasia with stromal invasion hysterectomy is mandatory. In women over 40 with simple or complex hyperplasia, clinical management of treatment with oral medroxyprogesterone acetate or dilatation and curettage and a control hysteroscopy with histology may be considered.

Nearly 60% of atypical hyperplasia regress but as the likelihood of residual carcinoma in the uterus increases with age, a hysterectomy is advised in women over 50 years of age. Estrogen-producing ovarian tumors should always be excluded. These data may be very important, especially in women receiving HRT who have a withdrawal bleeding once every 3 months. If further diagnostic screening is required, this can be done with transvaginal ultrasonography in combination with office hysteroscopy and tissue sampling in case of abnormal sonographic findings.

CLASSIFICATION

Endometrial hyperplasia is defined as a proliferation of glands of irregular size and shape with an increase in the gland:stroma ratio compared with proliferative endometrium. The process is diffuse but does not always involve the entire endometrium (Kurman and Norris, 1994).

A classification for endometrial hyperplasia, developed by the International Society of Gynecological Pathologits, has been adopted by the World Health Organization (*Table 13.2*) (Scully et al, 1996).

Endometrial hyperplasia is cytologically subdivided into two main categories: hyperplasia without cytological atypia and hyperplasia with cytological atypia (atypical hyperplasia). In both categories the lesions have been further subdivided, depending on the architectural abnormalities, into simple and complex hyperplasia, which refers to the degree of glandular complexity and crowding (Kurman and Norris, 1994).

Table 13.2 *Classification of endometrial hyperplasia*

- Simple hyperplasia
- Complex hyperplasia (adenomatous)
- Simple atypical hyperplasia
- Complex atypical hyperplasia (adenomatous with atypia)

From Kurman RJ & Norris HJ (1994) Endometrial hyperplasia and related cellular changes. In Kurman RJ (ed.) Blaustein's Pathology of the Female Genital Tract, 4th edn, pp 411–417. Copyright Springer-Verlag.

World Health Organization (Scully et al., 1996)

▪ ENDOMETRIAL POLYPS

PATHOGENESIS AND SYMPTOMATOLOGY

Endometrial polyps are benign tumors of the endometrium. They can be pedunculated or sessile. Large polyps can extend down into the cervical canal. The tip of a polyp may sometimes be congested or hemorrhagic as a result of irritation or infarction. In 20% of cases multiple polyps may be observed.

Although polyps can be clinically asymptomatic, patients with endometrial polyps may present before the menopause with irregular nonhormone responding uterine bleeding and in the menopause with bleeding or vaginal discharge symptoms (Burnett, 1964). The role of polyps as a possible cause of infertility is not yet clear.

CLINICAL INVESTIGATIONS

The diagnosis can easily be made with a combination of transvaginal ultrasonography and hysteroscopy (*Figures 13.12* and *13.13*).

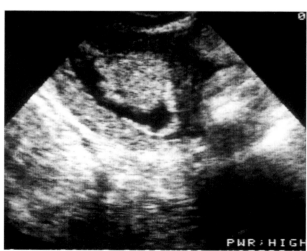

13.12a

Figure 13.12: *(a) Transvaginal ultrasonography. Midsagittal section showing a polyp in a postmenopausal patient.*

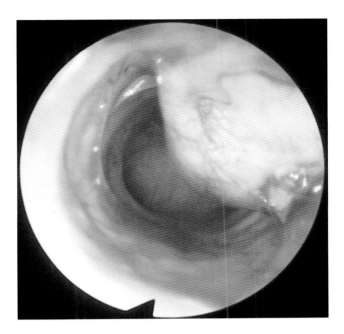

13.12b

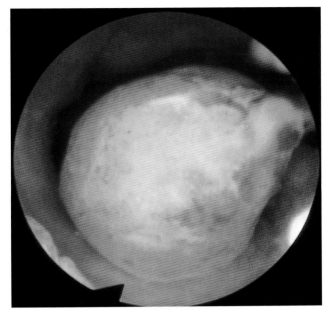

13.13b

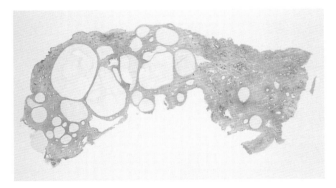

13.12c

Figure 13.12: *(cont.)(b) Hysteroscopic image of the patient shown in Figure 13.12a. (c) Histological section of the complete polyp removed at hysteroscopy (×400).*

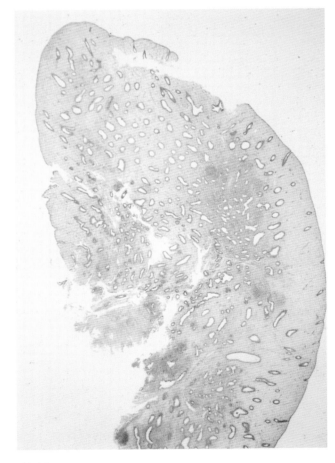

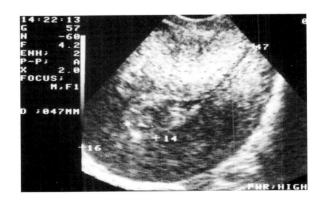

13.13a

13.13c

Figure 13.13: (a)–(f) Examples of polyps seen with transvaginal sonography and hysteroscopy, and comparison with histology.

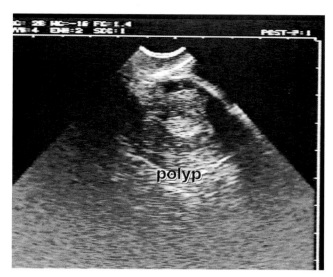

13.13d

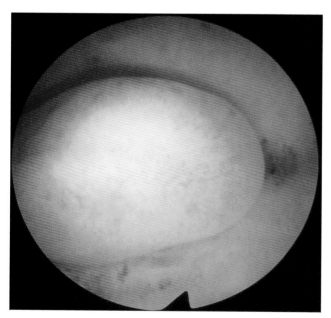

13.13e

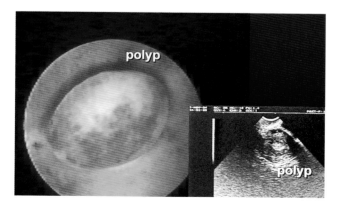

13.13f
Figure 13.13: *continued.*

Transvaginal ultrasonography

Polyps can present as echolucent and echodense areas within the uterine cavity but sometimes differentiation from thick endometrium is difficult. Polyps may even remain undetected unless diagnostic hysteroscopy is performed.

Diagnostic hysteroscopy

Hysteroscopy must be considered the easiest method of detecting even the smallest endometrial polyps. In *Figure 13.14* a very small polyp is shown in the cornual area. Polyps can be differentiated from fibroids by touch

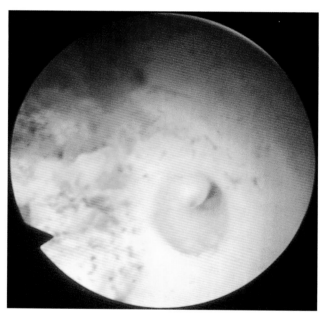

Figure 13.14: *Hysteroscopic image of a cornual polyp obstructing the tubal orifice.*

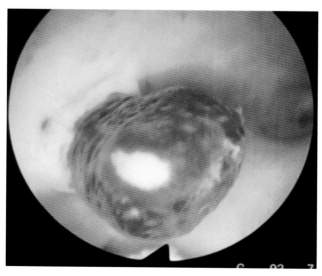

Figure 13.15: *Endometrial polyp with congested surface and bleeding.*

technique using a forceps because they are fragile and usually have a very flexible stalk. Bleeding can be observed on the surface (*Figure 13.15*) and when taking a biopsy the inner structure appears delicate and the glandular tissue is discernible. The main feature that differentiates them from malignancies is the regularity of their vascular and tissue architecture (*Figure 13.16*).

Hysterosalpingography

Occasionally endometrial polyps can be detected at routine hysterosalpingography for investigation of infertility.

During fluoroscopy a polyp will become coated with the contrast medium, producing a sharply defined filling defect, which may be partly or completely obscured by an excess of contrast material (*Figures 13.17* and *13.18*) and may be confused with an air bubble. Inner radiolucent areas may be observed with partial contrast coating of the polyp(s) (*Figure 13.19*).

Magnetic resonance imaging

With T_1-weighted MRI endometrial polyps image with medium signal intensity similar to that of normal endometrium. MRI cannot be considered as a routine diagnostic tool for the detection of endometrial polyps.

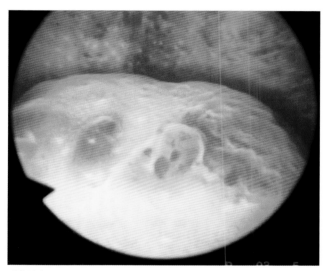

13.16a

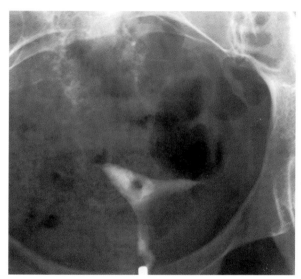

13.17a

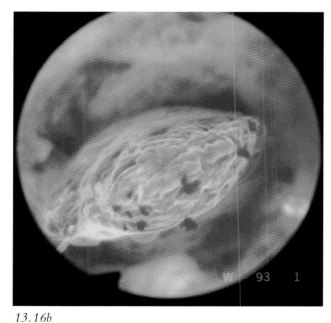

13.16b

Figure 13.16: *(a) and (b) Different surface appearances of benign endometrial polyps.*

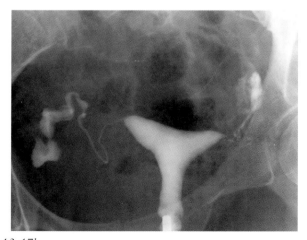

13.17b

Figure 13.17: *Hysterosalpingogram showing (a) a small intracavitary polyp at initial injection of contrast medium; (b) the filling defect has been obscured by an excess of intrauterine contrast medium.*

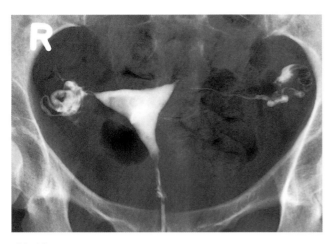

13.18a

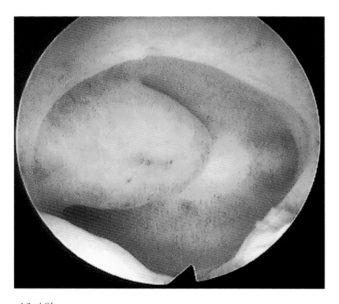

13.18b

Figure 13.18: *(a) Hysterosalpingogram shows a partial filling defect in the right cornual area. (b) Hysteroscopy revealed the filling defect to be an endometrial polyp.*

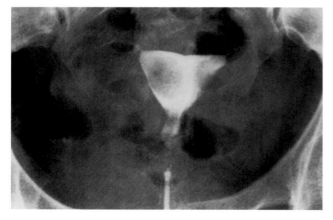

Figure 13.19: *Hysterosalpingogram with partial intracavitary filling defects caused by endometrial polyps.*

INTERPRETATION OF FINDINGS AND CLINICAL MANAGEMENT

The differentiation between a polyp and a fibroid can be made with ultrasonography only if the fibroid contains more echodense connective tissue-like structures. A polyp consists only of endometrial glands, stroma and blood vessels. The differentiation from thick endometrium with transvaginal ultrasonography can be very difficult. In all cases of abnormal bleeding, suspicious transvaginal ultrasound or hysterosalpingographic findings, diagnostic hysteroscopy with tissue sampling for histology is recommended.

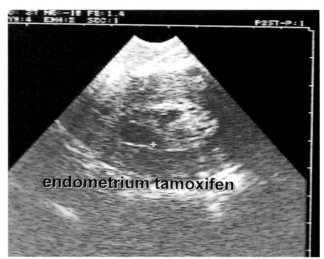

13.20a

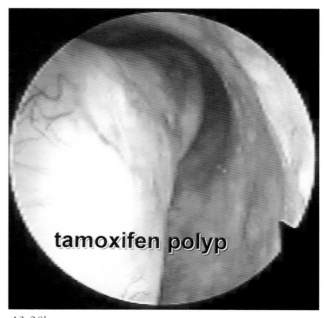

13.20b

Figure 13.20: *(a) Tamoxifen induced changes in the endometrium. (b) Polyp induced by the use of tamoxifen.*

A special group of polyps is formed by those induced by the use of tamoxifen (Berzewsky et al, 1994; Randall and Wallach, 1995). The clinical management of patients using tamoxifen should, nevertheless, be no different from that of those who are counseled for HRT after the menopause. Evaluation with transvaginal ultrasonography and hysteroscopy in case of abnormal findings, is advised (*Figure 13.20*).

REFERENCES

Berzewsky JC, Chalvardjian A & Murray A (1994) Iatrogenic megapolyps in women with breast carcinoma. *Obstet Gynecol* **84**: 727–730.

Bleker OP, Folkertsma K & Dirks-Go SIS (1989) Diagnostic procedures in vaginitis. *Eur J Obstet Gynaecol* **31**: 179–183.

de Blok S & Wamsteker K (1995) Hysteroscopic surgery: possibilities, limitations and future. *Reprod Med Rev* **4**: 101–113.

Brooks P & Serden SP (1988) Hysteroscopic findings after unsuccessful dilatation and curettage for abnormal uterine bleeding. *Am J Obstet Gynecol* **158**: 1354–1357.

Burnett JE (1964) Hysteroscopy controlled curettage for endometrial polyps. *Obstet Gynecol* **24**: 621–625.

Dijkhuizen FPHIJ, Brölmann HAM, Potters AE et al (1996) The accuracy of transvaginal ultrasonography in the diagnosis of endometrial abnormalities. *Obstet Gynecol* **87**: 345–349.

Dijkman AB, de Blok S, Hemrika DJ (1996) The prospective value of transvaginal sonography versus hysteroscopy with tissue sampling in the postmenopause. Submitted for publication *Eur J Obstet Gynaecol* (in press).

Emanuel MH, Verdel MJ, Wamsteker K et al (1995) A prospective comparison of TVS and diagnostic hysteroscopy in the evaluation of patients with abnormal uterine bleeding: clinical implications. *Am J Obstet Gynecol* **172**: 547–552.

Gimpelson RJ & Rappold HO (1988) A comparative study between panoramic hysteroscopy with directed biopsies and dilatation and curettage. *Am J Obstet Gynecol* **154**: 489–492.

Goldrath MH & Sherman AI (1985) Office hysteroscopy and suction curettage: can we eliminate the hospital diagnostic dilatation and curettage? *Am J Obstet Gynecol* **152**: 220–229.

Goldstein SR, Nachiall M, Snyder RJ et al (1990) Endometrial assessment by vaginal ultrasonography before endometrial sampling in patients with postmenopausal bleeding. *Am J Obstet Gynecol* **163**: 119–123.

Granberg S, Wikland M, Karlsson B et al (1991) Endometrial thickness as measured by endovaginal sonography for identifying endometrial abnormality. *Am J Obstet Gynecol* **164**: 47–52.

Grimes DA (1982) Diagnostic dilatation and curettage; a reappraisal. *Am J Obstet Gynecol* **142**: 1–6.

Karlsson B et al (1995) Transvaginal sonography of endometrium in women with postmenopausal bleeding. The Nordic study. *Am J Obstet Gynecol* **172**: 1488–1494.

Kurman RJ & Norris HJ (1994) Endometrial hyperplasia and related cellular changes. In Kurman RJ (ed.) *Blausteins Pathology of the Female Genital Tract*, 4th edn, pp 411–417. Heidelberg: Springer.

Kurman RJ, Kaminski PF & Norris HJ (1985) The behavior of endometrial hyperplasia. A long-term study of 'untreated' hyperplasia in 170 patients. *Cancer* **56**: 403–407.

Loffer FD (1989) Hysteroscopy with selective endometrial sampling compared with D & C for abnormal uterine bleeding: the value of a negative view. *Obstet Gynecol* **73**: 16–20.

Mardh PA, Moeller BR, Ingerselv HJ et al (1981) Endometritis caused by *Chlamydia trachomatis*. *Br J Venereal Dis* **57**: 191–195.

Meijer CJLM, Calame JJ, Windt EJG et al (1989) Prevalence of *Chlamydia trachomatis* infection in a population of asymptomatic women in a screening program for cervical cancer. *Eur J Clin Microbiol Infect Dis* **8**: 127–130.

Nasri MN, Sheperd JH, Setchell ME et al (1990) The role of vaginal scan in measurement of endometrial thickness in postmenopausal women. *Br J Obstet Gynaecol* **98**: 470–475.

Osmers R, Volksen M & Schauer A (1990) Vaginosonography for early detection of endometrial carcinoma? *Lancet* **335**: 1569–1571.

Randall TC & Wallach EE (1995) Tamoxifen: actions, benefits and risks. *Postgrad Obstet Gynecol* **15**: 1–6.

Scully RE, Poulson H & Sobin L (1996) *World Health Organization: Histologic Typing of Tumors of the Female Genital Tract*. Heidelberg: Springer.

Stock RJ & Kanbour A (1975) Pre-hysterectomy curettage. *Obstet Gynecol* **45**: 537–541.

Stoval TG, Solomon SK & Ling FW (1989) Endometrial sampling prior to hysterectomy **7**: 405–409.

Wamsteker K & de Blok S (1993) Diagnostic hysteroscopy: technique and documentation. In Sutton C & Diamond MWB (eds) *Endoscopic Surgery for Gynaecologists*, pp 263–276. London: WB Saunders.

Wamsteker K, de Blok S & Emanuel MH (1992) Instrumentation for transcervical hysteroscopic endosurgery. *Gynaecol Endosc* **1**: 59–67.

14 Adenomyosis
JJ Brosens and NM de Souza

■ INTRODUCTION

Adenomyosis is a disease of the endometrial–myometrial interface. At the cellular level it is characterized by subendometrial smooth muscle hyperplasia and progressive mucosal penetration of the myometrium. The histological criterion for adenomyosis is the presence of ectopic endometrial islets some distance away from the endometrial–myometrial junction. The myoproliferative changes, on the other hand, are often indistinct and difficult to delineate on routine microscopy.

Until recently the diagnosis could only be made with confidence after hysterectomy but new imaging techniques, such as magnetic resonance imaging (MRI) and vaginal sonography, have now made it possible to diagnose adenomyosis in vivo. The MRI and sonographic appearances of adenomyosis are, however, primarily based on the distortion of the normal myometrial architecture due to the smooth muscle hyperplasia, and not on the visualization of ectopic endometrial islets.

New evidence suggests that the myoproliferative changes do not always occur in concert with endometrial penetration of the myometrium; therefore the imaging and pathological findings should be regarded as complementary as they focus on related but potentially disparate features of adenomyosis.

■ PREVALENCE

Adenomyosis is thought to be a disease that mainly affects multiparous women in late reproductive life. Between 70 and 80% of pathologically confirmed cases are indeed found in women in their fourth and fifth decades (Azziz, 1989; Vercellini et al, 1993). Conversely, only 5–25% of cases are reported in patients younger than 39 years, and 5–10% occur in women older than 60 years. Between 80 and 90% of adenomyotic uteri are found in multiparous women. It is important to remember, however, that these data are derived from pathological examination of extirpated uteri and it is therefore not unexpected that the demographic trends in hysterectomy are similar to those mentioned for the prevalence of adenomyosis, namely with a peak incidence in multiparous patients in their late forties. Only one published study can be regarded as free of this bias. In 1931 Lewinski carried out a postmortem study on 54 women with an age range of 20 to more than 70 years old who died from nongynecological causes (Lewinski, 1931). Adenomyosis was found in 29 cases (54%). Reanalyzing the original data of this small study, Vercellini et al (1993) found no difference in the incidence between various age groups.

Selection bias is not the only reason why it has been difficult to determine the true incidence of adenomyosis. Differences in myometrial sampling and the wide range of diagnostic criteria used to define adenomyosis histologically are also important confounding factors. The first point is elegantly illustrated by the experience of Bird and coworkers (1972) who found adenomyosis in 31% of routine histological sections of 200 consecutive hysterectomy specimens; but if six extra blocks of myometrium were examined from six predetermined sites, the incidence rose sharply to 61%. In most series, however, the reported incidence in unselected hysterectomy specimens ranges from 8 to 27%.

The introduction of new imaging techniques in daily practice will not only make a more systematic study possible but is also likely to challenge the concept of adenomyosis as a disease of the older, multiparous woman. For instance, the average age of women with magnetic resonance characteristics of adenomyosis in the limited study by de Souza et al (1995) was only 34.4 years and 10 of 14 patients (71%) were nulliparous.

■ SYMPTOMS AND THEIR RELATION TO PATHOLOGY

MENORRHAGIA

Several clinicopathological studies suggest that symptoms correlate with the depth of endometrial infiltration into the myometrium. Bird and coworkers (1972) reported that superficial penetration of endometrium into the myometrium was a common finding in women who suffered from menorrhagia. Two recent studies appear to confirm this observation: Fraser (1994) and McCausland (1991) reported superficial adenomyosis in 40–60% of women suffering from dysfunctional uterine bleeding.

The existence of superficial adenomyosis as a significant clinicopathological entity remains, however, controversial (Hendrickson and Kempson, 1987). There are several reasons for this. Not only are superficial implants often difficult to distinguish from tangential sectioning of an irregular endometrial–myometrial junction but the presence of additional pelvic pathology, such as uterine fibroids, often provides a more conventional explanation for the symptomatology. But perhaps the main reason for failure to recognize superficial adenomyosis as an important disease entity is a lack of understanding of the causal relationship between superficial implants and dysfunctional uterine bleeding.

MRI studies have demonstrated that extensive distortion of the subendometrial myometrium can be present with minimal or no mucosal penetration into the myometrium (de Souza et al, 1995; Reinhold et al, 1995a). In contrast to the patchy and focal infiltration of endometrial elements, the myoproliferative changes that affect the inner myometrium are diffuse. Although the mechanism of menorrhagia in adenomyosis remains speculative, it may be related to these diffuse smooth muscle changes rather than to the presence of focal and superficial endometrial implants. Incoordinate smooth muscle proliferation in the inner myometrium is likely to compromise the cycle dependent contractions which, in the nongravid uterus, originate exclusively from this layer (de Vries et al, 1990; Martinez-Mir et al, 1990).

During normal menstruation there are antegrade propagated subendometrial contractions from the fundus to the cervix. Some authors have postulated a role for these antegrade contractions in controlling menstrual flow; loss of normal subendometrial motility may thus contribute to excessive menstrual loss (Emge, 1962).

DYSMENORRHEA

Dysmenorrhea appears to be dependent on the presence of mucosal islets deep in the myometrium (Benson and Sneeden, 1958; Nishida, 1991). Nishida (1991) reported that the onset of severe dysmenorrhea requires a depth that exceeds 80% of the total muscle thickness. While superficial lesions are largely unresponsive to sex steroids and unlikely to bleed, deep lesions are characterized by a higher density of implants which partially respond to ovarian sex steroids and which have a hemorrhagic tendency (Benson and Sneeden, 1958; Sandberg and Cohn, 1962). Furthermore, gross hyperplasia of the myometrium is invariably present with extensive and deep adenomyosis. Severe menstrual pain is thus less common than menorrhagia, affecting 20–30% of patients with adenomyosis (Azziz, 1989).

Adenomyotic foci are capable of prostaglandin (PG) synthesis, as demonstrated by the intense immunostaining for cyclooxygenase (the rate limiting enzyme in the PG pathway) in ectopic glandular epithelium (Van Voorhuis et al, 1990). Excessive production of $PGF_{2\alpha}$ can cause uterine spasms and ischemic pain and may explain why the incidence of dysmenorrhea increases with increasing depth and density of mucosal implants in the myometrium. Prostacyclin (PGI_2) production in adenomyotic implants has also been shown to be higher than in eutopic endometrium, myometrium or fibroids, especially during menstruation (Koike et al, 1992). PGI_2 is a potent vasodilator and inhibitor of platelet aggregation, which may contribute to the increased hemorrhagic potential of deep adenomyosis.

INFERTILITY

It is plausible that adenomyosis is a cause of infertility but there is as yet little objective evidence available to substantiate this claim. Using MRI, de Souza and coworkers (1995) reported that 14 of 26 women (53.8%) with infertility and symptoms of menorrhagia or dysmenorrhea had lesions characteristic of adenomyosis. In some cases, smooth muscle hyperplasia around implants in the cornua can cause proximal tubal obstruction and mimic salpingitis isthmica nodosa but reproductive failure in adenomyosis cannot always be explained on mechanical grounds. Although Ota and coworkers (1992) reported that high titers of antiphospholipid autoantibodies are often present in women with adenomyosis, the significance of these autoantibodies in infertility remains unresolved.

On the other hand, in 1962 Sandberg and Cohn identified 27 uteri with adenomyotic implants out of 151 specimens obtained at the time of cesarean hysterectomy, mainly for the purpose of sterilization. This high prevalence (17.9%) in pregnancy appears to contradict the claims that adenomyosis is an important cause of infertility; however, the authors pointed out that the smooth muscle changes which are so characteristically present in the nongravid uterus were absent in these specimens. This observation is in agreement with more recent magnetic resonance findings showing profound changes in the inner myometrium during pregnancy (Barton et al, 1993; Turnbull et al, 1995; Willms et al, 1995).

Controversy also exists around a possible relationship between pelvic endometriosis and adenomyosis. The reported coincidence of both types of heterotopic endometrium at the time of hysterectomy varies from 6 to 20% (Azziz, 1989). More recently, de Souza et al (1995) found that 9 of 14 infertile women with magnetic resonance appearances of adenomyosis also had endometriosis diagnosed at laparoscopy. Although selection bias may account for this high incidence, abnormality of the endometrial–myometrial junction may play a role in the pathogenesis of endometriosis. Salamanca and Beltrán (1995) employed videovaginosonography to study the direction of the inner myometrial contraction waves during menstruation in women with and without endometriosis. Interestingly, retrograde contractions were observed in almost 90% of the patients with endometriosis but in only 5% of the controls. Conversely, antegrade waves, from the fundus to the cervix, were present in 85% of the normal women but absent in all women with endometriosis. If confirmed, then these observations strongly imply that inner myometrial dysfunction commonly present in adenomyosis may result in excessive retrograde menstruation and endometriosis.

'ASYMPTOMATIC' ADENOMYOSIS

Some authors have challenged the concept that adenomyosis is an important clinical entity. Kilkku et al (1984) prospectively interviewed patients undergoing hysterectomy for benign pelvic disease and found no difference in frequency or severity of uterine bleeding, dysmenorrhea or pelvic pain between 28 women with histologically proven adenomyosis and 157 without. They concluded that symptoms attributed to adenomyosis were heterogeneous, nonspecific and probably related to coincidental pathology; however, there was no mention of the number of myometrial blocks examined nor were the criteria for the diagnosis outlined.

In a retrospective review of the clinical notes of 701 cases of adenomyotic uteri, Benson and Sneeden (1958) reported that 16% of the cases were 'incidental'. A prospective study by Lee and coworkers (1984) confirmed this observation and found adenomyosis in 20% of uteri removed for prolapse. This study was, however, designed to correlate preoperative and pathological diagnoses and not to analyze symptomatology. Random diagnostic criteria on histology, small number of myometrial blocks examined, failure to appraise the smooth muscle changes and lack of prospective assessment of the clinical symptoms contribute to the persisting misconception that adenomyosis is a variation of normality.

▪ CLINICAL INVESTIGATIONS

PHYSICAL EXAMINATION

Adenomyosis should be considered in all women suffering from menorrhagia or dysmenorrhea, regardless of their age or the presence of additional pelvic pathology. Historically, repeated bimanual examinations over a period of months, just before and after a menstruation, were recommended. In this way fluctuating changes in contour, size and consistency of the uterus, which typify extensive adenomyosis, could be detected. In 1933, Halban further suggested administration of large doses of estrogen during the second half of the menstrual cycle (Emge, 1962). This not only aggravates menorrhagia

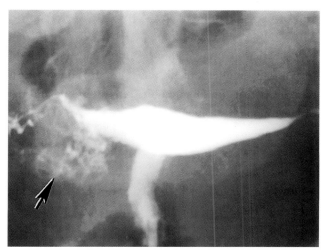

14.1a

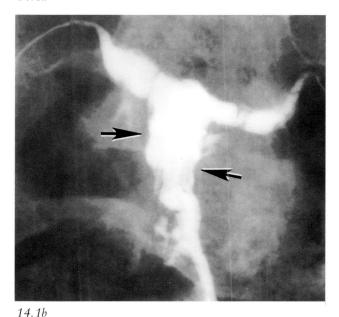

14.1b

Figure 14.1: Hysterosalpingography. (a) Intravasation of contrast medium into the myometrium is seen adjacent to the right uterine wall and right salpinx (arrow). Magnetic resonance imaging of this patient revealed a large adenomyoma (see Figure 14.3b). (b) The uterine cavity is irregular and enlarged. The multiple indentations into the cavity (arrows) proved to be from multiple large fibroids on subsequent magnetic resonance imaging (not shown). No adenomyosis was found.

and intensifies fluctuations in the size of the uterus but also emphasizes the presence of small knob-like nodulations detectable in the outer layer of the myometrium. The use of steroids to exacerbate symptomatology is now obsolete. In practice, there are no pathognomonic signs or symptoms and, even in cases of extensive disease, the reported accuracy of the clinical diagnosis is disappointingly low (Emge, 1962; Gambone et al, 1990).

Table 14.1 *Sonographic features of adenomyosis*

- Asymmetrical uterine enlargement
- Ill defined hypoechoic areas
- Ill defined hyperechoic areas
- Heterogeneous myometrial echotexture
- Small anechoic lakes
- Indistinct endometrial–myometrial border (?)
- Subendometrial halo thickening (?)
- Abnormal inner myometrial contraction waves (?)

(?) The predictive value of these features remains to be determined.

HYSTEROSCOPY AND LAPAROSCOPY

Gross myometrial distortion, which often accompanies extensive adenomyosis, sometimes allows the diagnosis to be made during laparoscopic or hysteroscopic examination. A diffusely enlarged uterus with irregular contours of the serosa or cavity may not only harbor adenomyosis but also multiple small fibroids. Mild and moderate adenomyosis cannot be diagnosed visually. This was clearly demonstrated by McCausland (1991), who found adenomyosis in 33 of 50 women (66%) with menorrhagia and a grossly normal uterine cavity on hysteroscopy.

HYSTEROGRAPHY

Hysterography has been used in the diagnosis of adenomyosis. The most salient diagnostic feature is the demonstration of a spiculated area of contrast intravasation extending perpendicularly from the uterine cavity into the myometrium (*Figure 14.1*). However, the sensitivity of this technique is low: Marshak and Eliasoph (1955) established the diagnosis on hysterography in only 38 of 150 cases with histologically proven adenomyosis.

ULTRASONOGRAPHY

In recent years several studies have appraised the potential role of sonography in the diagnosis of adenomyosis (Fedele et al, 1992; Ascher et al, 1994; Brosens et al, 1995a; Reinhold et al, 1995b). The enhanced resolution of transvaginal ultrasound renders it superior to the abdominal approach. Several sonographic criteria for diffuse adenomyosis have been described (*Table 14.1*). Although adenomyotic uteri tend to be larger, with asymmetrical thickening of the anterior and posterior walls, uterine morphometry alone is insufficient for the diagnosis (Brosens et al, 1995a). The disease is best predicted on the basis of ill defined heterogeneous echotexture within the myometrium (*Figure 14.2*) (Brosens et al, 1995a; Reinhold et al, 1995b). In extensive disease, small anechoic lakes of 1–3 mm diameter are sometimes detected (Fedele et al, 1992). Lakes of this size are at the limit of ultrasonographic resolution and may represent larger cystic implants or, more likely, focal myometrial hemorrhage. Detecting such areas of heterogeneous echogenicity within the myometrium is often complicated by the presence of various artifactual echogenic shadows and compounded by the presence of leiomyomas and vascular calcifications. The diagnosis is therefore best made during the course of the real time examination.

So far, four studies have compared the accuracy of

endovaginal ultrasonography with light microscopy or MRI. The results are summarized in *Table 14.2* and indicate that at present the diagnostic accuracy of this imaging technique remains uncertain. It is important to remember that the sonographic signs are subtle and that the technique is strongly operator dependent. The diagnostic value of color Doppler to assess myometrial perfusion or videovaginosonography to appraise inner myometrial motility patterns remains to be evaluated. It is, however, fair to conclude that endovaginal ultrasound is a useful tool when the clinical suspicion is high.

MAGNETIC RESONANCE IMAGING

Adenomyosis is best demonstrated on T_2-weighted images where the contrast between the low signal inner

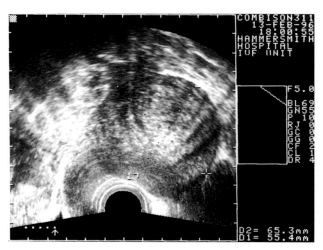

14.2a

Figure 14.2: *(a) Midline sagittal endovaginal ultrasound scan through the uterus. The endometrial stripe is barely visible. The ventral myometrium is grossly enlarged with several ill defined areas of increased echogenicity. Small hypoechoic lakes were seen during real time examination. (b) T_2-weighted (2500/80 msec [TR/TE]) spin echo midline sagittal section through the same uterus demonstrating a large adenomyoma occupying the entire ventral wall (short arrow). The dorsal uterine junctional zone is normal (long arrow).*

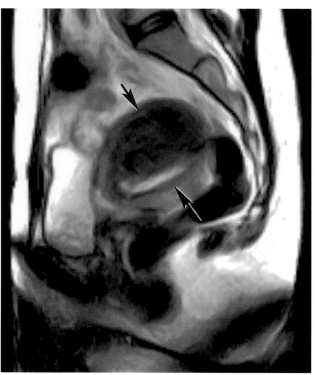

14.2b

Table 14.2 *Specificity, sensitivity and predictive values of endovaginal ultrasonography in the diagnosis of adenomyosis*

	Prevalence (%)	Sensitivity (%)	Specificity (%)	PPV (%)	NPV (%)
Fedele et al (1992)	22/43(51)	80	74	73	81
Ascher et al (1994)	17/20(85)	86	50	90	20
Brosens et al (1995a)	28/56(50)	53	75	86	77
Reinhold et al (1995b)	29/100(29)	86	86	71	94

PPV, positive predictive value; NPV, negative predictive value.

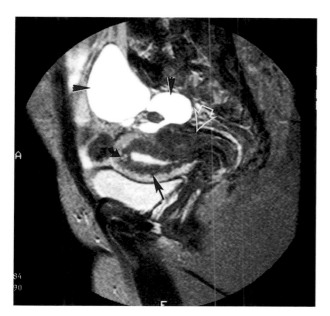

14.3a

Figure 14.3: *(a) Diffuse adenomyosis: T_2-weighted (2500/80 msec [TR/TE]) spin echo midline sagittal section through the uterus showing thickening and irregularity of the low signal band of the junctional zone (black arrow). A focal high signal lesion is seen near the fundus (curved arrow). This may represent cystic adenomyotic implants or focal hemorrhage. An ill defined mixed signal intensity mass occupies the rectovaginal space (white arrow), indicating the presence of extensive rectovaginal endometriosis. Large endometriotic cysts are present on both ovaries (arrowheads). (b) Thirty eight year old nulliparous women suffering from severe menorrhagia and*

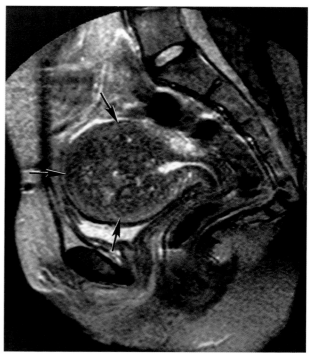

14.3b

dysmenorrhea. T_2-weighted (2500/80 msec [TR/TE]) midline sagittal section through the uterus shows a large mixed signal intensity mass with high signal foci (arrows) indicative of hemorrhage. There is complete loss of myometrial zonal anatomy. Histologically, severe adenomyosis was found, with gross smooth muscle hyperplasia and numerous, often hemorrhagic, implants.

myometrium (junctional zone) and the intermediate signal outer myometrium is maximal. Recognition of this zonal anatomy within the myometrium is essential for detecting the myometrial changes that occur with adenomyosis (Hricak et al, 1983).

On MRI adenomyosis is recognized in a focal and diffuse pattern. In focal adenomyosis there is a localized ill defined mixed signal intensity mass (adenomyoma) within the myometrium (*Figure 14.2b*). In these patients, the junctional zone is often normal in thickness (de Souza et al, 1995). Diffuse adenomyosis, on the other hand, presents with diffuse or irregular thickening of the junctional zone, sometimes with underlying high signal foci (*Figure 14.3*) (Mark et al, 1987; Togashi et al, 1989). Pathologically this has been shown to represent smooth muscle hyperplasia characterized by closely packed smooth muscle fibers that are poorly orientated and less vascular than the smooth muscle of the normal inner myometrium (Togashi et al, 1989). It is the smooth muscle changes that are easily recognized by

MRI, rather than foci of heterotopic glandular epithelium and stroma. These findings seem to support the hypothesis that focal adenomyomas arise from deep Müllerian rests within the myometrium, while diffuse adenomyosis is the result of progressive infiltration of endometrium into the myometrium.

There is no consensus on what constitutes abnormal junctional zone thickening on MRI. Junctional zone widths between 6 and 12 mm have been quoted in the literature as diagnostic for adenomyosis (Mark et al, 1987; Reinhold et al, 1995a). These absolute values for junctional zone widths may not, however, be as meaningful as ratios of junctional zone thickness to the width of the outer myometrium or the cervical stroma. The current confusion has arisen because most studies have attempted to correlate the junctional zone thickness in vivo with the presence or absence of ectopic endometrial islets on histology. These studies are unlikely to be conclusive as there is as yet no consensus on the number of myometrial blocks that should be examined histologically or on the histological definition of superficial adenomyosis. In our experience extensive thickening of the junctional zone can be present with minimal or no penetration of mucosa into the myometrium. Examination of three premenopausal women with severe menorrhagia before hysterectomy revealed junctional zone:outer myometrial ratios of > 1.0 (de Souza et al, 1995). On subsequent pathological examination of eight myometrial blocks there was no evidence of adenomyosis in any of the specimens. We have postulated that the myoproliferative changes may precede the infiltration of mucosa into the myometrium and that the symptoms could be explained on the basis of abnormal smooth muscle proliferation (Brosens et al, 1995b). It may therefore be more meaningful to correlate the junctional zone widths and ratios with an objective assessment of the symptoms.

The use of MRI in the workup for patients with severe menorrhagia or dysmenorrhea has been hampered because of its limited availability and cost. To some extent these factors are determined by the imaging time and at present most MRI studies of the pelvis last for 30 minutes or longer. It may, however, be possible to obtain adequate information with the T_2-weighted sagittal images alone, and improvements in hardware and software are likely to reduce the examination times to the order of a few minutes (Krinsky et al, 1995).

BIOPSY

Myometrial needle biopsies can be taken transabdominally at the time of laparoscopy, or transvaginally under ultrasound guidance. A positive biopsy should provide evidence of ectopic endometrial islets sandwiched between strips of myometrium. Endometrial glands and stroma at the extreme end of the needle core may represent eutopic endometrium and such biopsies should be regarded as negative (*Figure 14.4*).

The sensitivity of random needle biopsies is low and dependent on the number of biopsies and the depth and extent of mucosal infiltration. A recent study using hysterectomy specimens reported that if four 14 Fr needle biopsies were taken at random, one or more would be positive in 70% of uteri with deep adenomyosis (Brosens and Barker, 1995). If only superficial disease was present

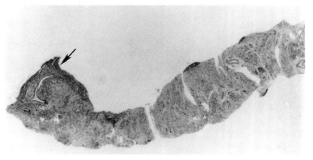

14.4a

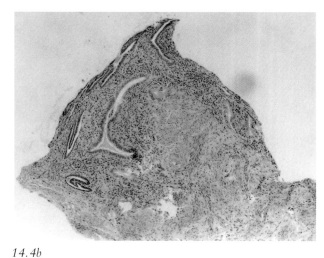

14.4b

Figure 14.4: *(a) and (b) False positive myometrial needle biopsy. The endometrial glands and stroma that are present at the extreme end of this needle core could represent eutopic endometrium. No adenomyosis was found in this uterus. Hematoxylin & eosin; magnification (a) ×30, (b) ×75.*

the sensitivity of this technique dropped to 5%. These findings are similar to a larger study by Popp et al (1993) who took not only needle biopsies immediately after hysterectomy but also at the time of laparoscopy, as well as transvaginally under ultrasound guidance. A single myometrial biopsy picked up only 8–19% of women with adenomyosis. The sensitivity of random needle biopsy is thus too low for clinical practice.

McCausland (1991) advocated hysteroscopic resection of a myometrial strip of the posterior uterine wall for the histological confirmation of the diagnosis. After thorough curettage of the endometrial cavity, a single 1.5–3 cm myometrial biopsy specimen was taken with a 5 mm cutting loop. The myometrial surface of the biopsy was stained with a marking dye and care was taken to avoid tangential sectioning of the specimen. Although it was possible to diagnose adenomyosis, the accuracy of this technique has not yet been compared with conventional histological assessment of hysterectomy specimens. Unlike needle biopsies, it is limited to those women who no longer have a desire to bear children.

■ CONCLUSION

Adenomyosis should no longer be a retrospective diagnosis after hysterectomy. Both endovaginal ultrasonography and MRI are useful tools in the diagnosis but only MRI can at present accurately quantify the extent of the smooth muscle changes associated with the disease. Although these techniques are likely to redefine adenomyosis as primarily a myoproliferative disease of the inner myometrium, more studies are necessary to elucidate the clinical implications of junctional zone hyperplasia.

The role of endoscopic techniques in the diagnosis is limited to cases with extensive disease but even then it may not be possible to differentiate adenomyosis from multiple fibroids. The sensitivity of random multiple myometrial needle biopsies is too low for clinical practice; and even after predetermination of the site of biopsy with ultrasound or MRI a negative biopsy will not exclude the presence of disease. Finally, resection of a myometrial strip at the time of hysteroscopy may be useful for the diagnosis in women who have completed their families. The histological interpretation of these strips will be largely dependent on the criteria used to define superficial adenomyosis.

REFERENCES

Ascher SM, Arnold LL, Patt RH et al (1994) Adenomyosis: prospective comparison of MR imaging and transvaginal sonography. *Radiology* **190**: 803–806.

Azziz R (1989) Adenomyosis: current perspectives. *Obstet Gynecol Clin North Am* **16**: 221–235.

Barton JW, McCarthy SW, Kohorn EI, Scoutt LM & Lange RC (1993) Pelvic MR imaging findings in gestational trophoblastic disease, incomplete abortion and ectopic pregnancy: are they specific? *Radiology* **186**: 163–168.

Benson RC & Sneeden VD (1958) Adenomyosis: a reappraisal of symptomatology. *Am J Obstet Gynecol* **76**: 1044–1061.

Bird CC, McElin TW & Manalo-Estrella P (1972) The elusive adenomyosis of the uterus. *Am J Obstet Gynecol* **112**: 583–593.

Brosens JJ & Barker FG (1995) The role of myometrial needle biopsies in the diagnosis of adenomyosis. *Fertil Steril* **63**: 1347–1349.

Brosens JJ, de Souza NM, Barker FG, Paraschos T & Winston RML (1995a) Endovaginal ultrasonography in the diagnosis of adenomyosis

uteri: identifying the predictive characteristics. *Br J Obstet Gynaecol* **102**: 471–474.

Brosens JJ, de Souza NM & Barker FG (1995b) Uterine junctional zone: function and disease. *Lancet* **356**: 558–560.

de Souza NM, Brosens JJ, Schwieso JE, Paraschos T & Winston RML (1995) The potential value of magnetic resonance imaging in infertility. *Clin Radiol* **50**: 75–79.

de Vries K, Lyons EA, Ballard G, Levi CS & Lindsay DJ (1990) Contractions of the inner third of the myometrium. *Am J Obstet Gynecol* **162**: 679–682.

Emge LA (1962) The elusive adenomyosis. *Am J Obstet Gynecol* **82**: 1541–1562.

Fedele L, Bianchi S, Dorta M et al (1992) Transvaginal ultrasonography in the diagnosis of diffuse adenomyosis. *Fertil Steril* **58**: 94–97.

Fraser IS (1994) Menorrhagia: a pragmatic approach to the understanding of causes and the need for investigations. *Br J Obstet Gynaecol* **101**: 3–7.

Gambone JC, Reiter RC, Lerich JB, Slesinski MJ, Reiter RC & Moore JG (1990) The impact of a quality assurance process on the frequency and confirmation rate of hysterectomy. *Am J Obstet Gynecol* **163**: 545–550.

Hendrickson MR & Kempson RL (1987) Non-neoplastic conditions of the myometrium and uterine serosa. In Fox H (ed.) *Obstetrical and Gynaecological Pathology*, Vol. 1, 3rd edn, pp 405–407. London: Churchill Livingstone.

Hricak H, Alpers C, Crooks LE & Sheldon PE (1983) Magnetic resonance imaging of the female pelvis: initial experience. *Am J Radiol* **141**: 1119–1128.

Kilkku P, Erkolla R & Grönroos M (1984) Nonspecificity of symptoms related to adenomyosis: a prospective comparative survey. *Acta Obstet Gynecol Scand* **62**: 229–231.

Koike H, Egawa H, Ohtsuka T, Yamaguchi M, Ikenoue T & Mori N (1992) Eicosanoids production in endometriosis. *Prostaglandins Leukot Essent Fatty Acids* **45**: 313–317.

Krinsky GA, Rofsky NM, Feinberg DA, Flyer MA & Weinreb JC (1995) Fast MR imaging of the uterus: comparison of four T_2-weighted sequences for diagnosis of adenomyosis and leiomyoma. *Radiology* **197**, SS: 473 (abstract).

Lee NC, Dicker RC, Rubin GL et al (1984) Confirmation of the preoperative diagnosis for hysterectomy. *Am J Obstet Gynecol* **150**: 283–287.

Lewinski H (1931) Beitrag zur Frage der Adenomiosis. *Zentralbl Gynakol* **55**: 2163–2166.

McCausland AM (1991) Hysteroscopic myometrial biopsy: its use in diagnosing adenomyosis and its clinical application. *Am J Obstet Gynecol* **166**: 1619–1628.

Mark SA, Hricak H, Heinrichs LW et al (1987) Adenomyosis and leiomyoma: differential diagnosis with MR imaging. *Am J Radiol* **163**: 527–529.

Marshak RH & Eliasoph J (1955) The roentgen findings in adenomyosis. *Radiology* **64**: 846–851.

Martinez-Mir I, Están L, Morales-Olivas F & Rubio E (1990) Studies of the spontaneous motility and the effect of histamine on isolated myometrial strips of the nonpregnant human uterus: the influence of various uterine abnormalities. *Am J Obstet Gynecol* **163**: 189–195.

Nishida M (1991) Relationship between the onset of dysmenorrhea and histologic findings in adenomyosis. *Am J Obstet Gynecol* **165**: 229–231.

Ota H, Maki M, Shidara Y et al (1992) Effects of danazol at the immunologic level in patients with adenomyosis, with special reference to autoantibodies: a multicenter cooperative study. *Am J Obstet Gynecol* **167**: 481–486.

Popp LW, Schwiedessen JP & Gaetje R (1993) Myometrial biopsy in the diagnosis of adenomyosis uteri. *Am J Obstet Gynecol* **169**: 546–549.

Reinhold C, McCarthy SM, Bret PM et al (1995a) Uterine adenomyosis: prospective comparative analysis of endovaginal US and MR imaging with histopathologic correlation. *Radiology* **197**, SS: 473.

Reinhold C, Atri M, Mehio A, Zakarian R, Aldis AE & Bret PM (1995b) Diffuse uterine adenomyosis: morphologic criteria and diagnostic accuracy of endovaginal sonography. *Radiology* **197**: 609–614.

Salamanca A & Beltrán E (1995) Subendometrial contractility in menstrual phase visualized by transvaginal sonography in patients with endometriosis. *Fertil Steril* **64**: 193–195.

Sandberg EG & Cohn F (1962) Adenomyosis in the gravid uterus at term. *Am J Obstet Gynecol* **84**: 1457–1465.

Togashi K, Ozasa H, Konishi I et al (1989) Enlarged uterus: differentiation between adenomyosis and leiomyoma with MRI. *Radiology* **171**: 531–534.

Turnbull LW, Manton DJ, Horsman A & Killick SR (1995) Magnetic resonance imaging changes in the uterine zonal anatomy during a conception cycle. *Br J Obstet Gynaecol* **102**: 330–331.

Van Voorhuis BJ, Huettner PC, Clark MR & Hill JA (1990) Immunohistochemical localization of prostaglandin H synthase in the female reproductive tract and endometriosis. *Am J Obstet Gynecol* **163**: 57–62.

Vercellini P, Ragni G, Trespidi L, Oldani S, Panazza S & Crosignani PG (1993) Adenomyosis: a déjà vu? *Obstet Gynecol Surv* **12**: 789–794.

Willms AB, Brown ED, Kettritz UI, Kuller JA & Semelka RA (1995) Anatomic changes in the pelvis after uncomplicated vaginal delivery: evaluation with serial MR imaging. *Radiology* **195**: 91–94.

15 *Intrauterine adhesions (synechiae)*
K Wamsteker

■ INTRODUCTION

The occurrence of intrauterine adhesions or synechiae after a curettage was initially recognized by Fritsch in 1894. Asherman reported in 1948 and 1950 on the clinical significance of the syndrome of traumatic intrauterine adhesions with amenorrhea following postpartum and postabortion curettage. Since then intrauterine adhesions generally have been referred to as Asherman's syndrome. Although the incidence of this condition is relatively infrequent, it does have a deleterious effect on fertility. Early recognition and treatment are of utmost importance for optimal anatomical and functional restoration of the uterine cavity. Imaging technology provides the tools for diagnosis and prevention of this condition.

■ CAUSE AND SYMPTOMS

In most cases intrauterine adhesions occur after instrumental intrauterine manipulation related to a pregnancy. In the postpartum or postabortion period the endometrium appears to be much more vulnerable and more susceptible to trauma.

In 1856 reported cases, pregnancy was the predisposing factor in 91%. In 66.7% the related intervention was a postabortion curettage and in 21.5% a postpartum curettage (Schenker and Margalioth, 1982).

The worst cases develop after a postpartum curettage for hemorrhage and/or retained placental tissue (March, 1995). With hysterosalpingography (HSG) after a previous puerperal curettage, Klein and Garcia (1973) observed intrauterine adhesions in 39% of cases. After repeat curettage following evacuation of an incomplete or missed abortion the risk of more extensive adhesion formation is also significantly increased. In such cases a sharp curette is more likely to have been used because of adherence of the tissue.

The incidence of the formation of usually mild adhesions following a primary curettage for incomplete or missed abortion has not yet been adequately studied but it is higher than often suggested and probably occurs in some 5–20% of all cases. The adhesions in such cases are most frequently located in the lower isthmic part of the uterine cavity. Literature reports are inconclusive regarding a difference in frequency of adhesion formation after a curettage for missed abortion or a curettage for incomplete abortion. Adoni et al (1982) found intrauterine adhesions after a missed abortion curettage in 31%, and in only 6% after curettage for incomplete abortion. However, Romer (1994a) did not find a difference in the incidence between those two types of intervention but observed a significantly higher incidence of adhesions in patients with recurrent abortions (48%) than those after a first abortion (19%). In addition, Golan et al (1992) could not identify a significantly higher incidence of intrauterine adhesions after missed abortion curettage. They observed mild adhesions in 16.7% of cases.

After curettage following midtrimester termination of pregnancy, Lurie et al (1991) found intrauterine adhesions in 38.5% of cases, compared with 7.7% in which no curettage had been performed. They therefore recommended that curettage only be performed in cases in which the presence of retained pregnancy products of conception is virtually certain.

Sometimes intrauterine adhesions develop secondary to other intracavitary pathology (*Figure 15.1a*) or an intrauterine device (*Figure 15.1b*). They only occasionally occur after uterine operative procedures like conization, myomectomy of intracavitary myoma(s) and metroplasty, or after diagnostic curettage and/or intrauterine infection. Tuberculous endometritis, however, can cause severe distortion of the uterine cavity with adhesions and amenorrhea.

The most pronounced symptom of moderate and severe adhesions in the uterine cavity is the reduction of the menstrual flow down to hypomenorrhea or amenorrhea, sometimes in combination with cyclic abdominal cramps at the time of the expected menses. In less extensive cases the menstrual flow may be normal without further clinical symptoms.

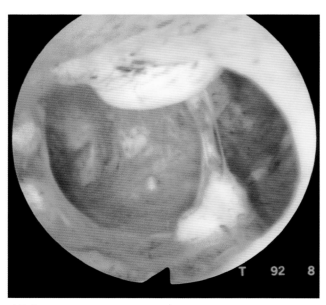

15.1a

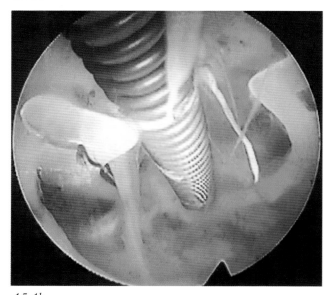

15.1b

Figure 15.1: *(a) Fragile adhesions secondary to intracavitary fibroids. (b) Fundal adhesions partially covering top and arms of intrauterine device.*

In the case of complete obstruction of the lower part of the uterine cavity with normal functioning endometrium in the upper part, a hematometra can occur but is seen only infrequently. Probably some kind of reflex prevents the proliferation and the menstrual shedding of the retained endometrium, which quite often has an inactive aspect at synechiolysis.

Extensive fibrosis and shortage of healthy functioning endometrium resulting from the intrauterine damage and the adhesions can prevent or hamper implantation

and reduce fertility. On pelvic arteriography Polishuk et al (1977) found a decrease of uterine blood flow in patients developing hypomenorrhea or amenorrhea following a pregnancy-related curettage, which may also contribute to the poor reproductive outcome of these women. Pregnancies may end prematurely in an early or late abortion or premature labor. In otherwise successful pregnancies, placenta accreta or increta may complicate separation of the placenta (Jewelewicz et al, 1976).

Any of these symptoms with preceding pregnancy-related intrauterine manipulation should alert the clinician to the possibility of the presence of intrauterine adhesions (March, 1995). The slightest suspicion should result in further diagnostic imaging procedures. The extent of the adhesions and intrauterine fibrosis tend to increase with time and the prognosis for treatment is closely related to these factors and the amount of retained normal endometrium. Blind procedures like sounding, dilatation or dilatation and curettage are contraindicated as they may easily result in the creation of a false route or perforation.

■ CLINICAL INVESTIGATIONS

In cases of hypomenorrhea or amenorrhea with a history of a recent pregnancy-related curettage, intrauterine adhesions should be suspected. Further evidence is the presence of a biphasic basal body temperature pattern and the absence of a withdrawal bleeding following progesterone or estrogen/progesterone provocation.

The most important diagnostic procedures for the disclosure of intrauterine adhesions are hysteroscopy and HSG. Ultrasonography and magnetic resonance imaging so far seem to be only of limited importance.

HYSTEROSALPINGOGRAPHY

Intrauterine adhesions produce irregular filling defects at HSG (*Figure 15.2*). Of great importance is the slow injection of the contrast medium because excessive contrast may obscure the lesions (Hunt and Siegler, 1990). The defects appear as sharply outlined intrauterine structures, which are centrally (*Figure 15.3*) and/or marginally (*Figure 15.4*) located. In more severe cases

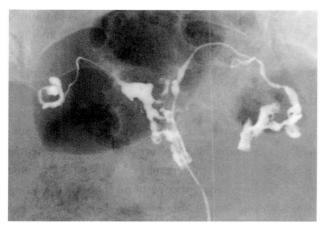

Figure 15.2: A hysterosalpingogram with sharply outlined filling defects in the uterine cavity caused by dense intrauterine adhesions.

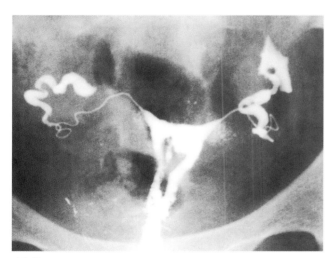

15.3a

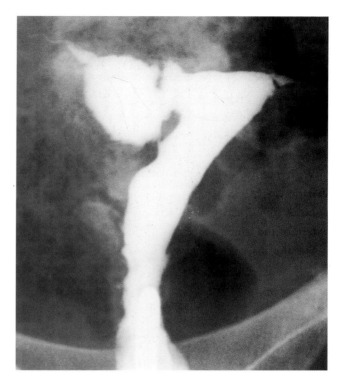

15.4a

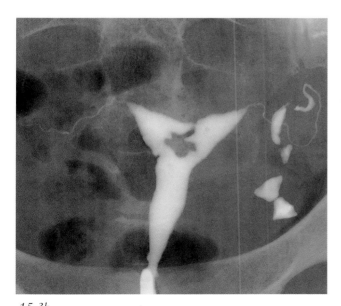

15.3b

Figure 15.3: (a) and (b) Central filling defect due to dense adhesions (grade II).

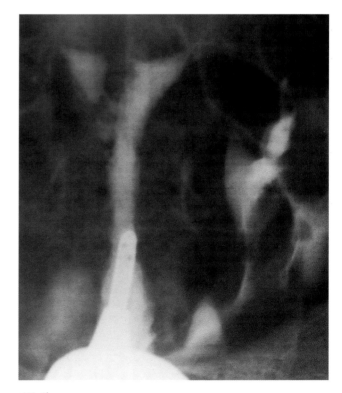

15.4b

Figure 15.4: (a) Intrauterine filling defect due to a marginal adhesion (grade II). (b) Dense marginal adhesions almost completely occluding the right cornual area (grade III).

partial obliteration of the cavity may be observed, its borders may be irregular and either one or both of the tubes may be occluded (*Figure 15.5*). If the covering tissue is defective, vascular intravasation of the contrast medium may occur (*Figure 15.6*). In severe intrauterine adhesions the uterine cavity is completely distorted and narrowed and usually both tubes are occluded (*Figure 15.6b* and *15.7*).

With complete occlusion of the lower part of the uterine cavity HSG will fail to show any intracavitary contrast filling and will provide no information on the extent of the adhesions (*Figure 15.7b*).

For the diagnosis of intrauterine adhesions HSG has

been shown to have a relatively high rate of false positive findings (Raziel et al, 1994; Romer et al, 1994) and hysteroscopic confirmation is always required.

HYSTEROSCOPY

A diagnostic hysteroscopy procedure performed on suspicion of intrauterine adhesions due to clinical symptoms, HSG or ultrasonography should be performed with a diagnostic hysteroscope of no more than 5.5 mm diameter. The uterus must never be sounded, nor should the internal cervical os (ICO) be dilated before hysteroscopic endocervical inspection. In cases of

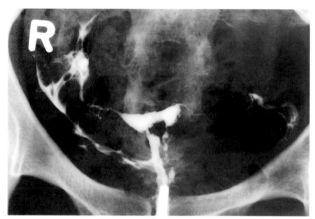

15.5a

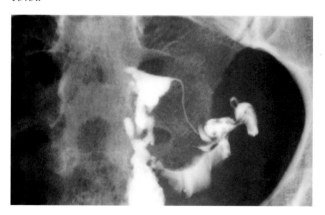

15.5b

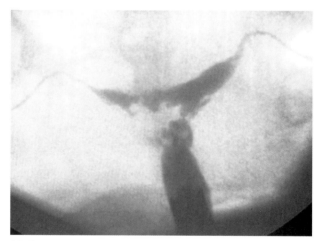

15.5c

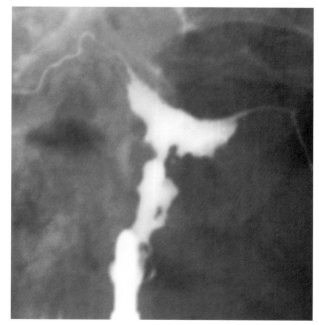

15.5d

Figure 15.5: *(a)–(d) Multiple dense adhesions (grade III) with irregular borders to the uterine cavity; with diagnostic hysteroscopy the fundal areas could not always be evaluated owing to the small openings in the adhesions; hysterosalpingography provides further information on the areas beyond.*

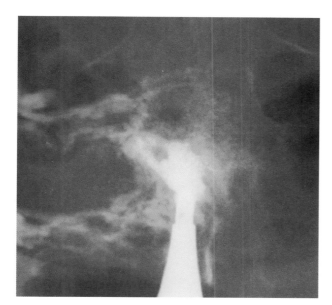

15.6a

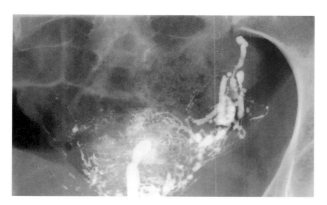

15.6b

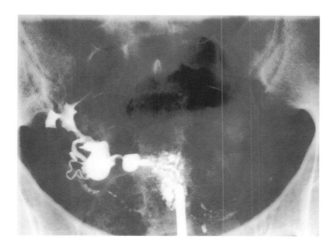

15.6c

Figure 15.6: *(a) Central filling defect in the right cornual area and obliteration of the left cornual area with vascular intravasation due to the defective covering tissue (grade III). (b) and (c) Completely distorted uterine cavities with intravasation (grade IV).*

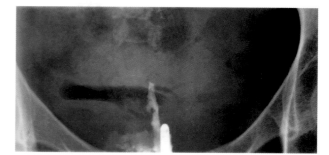

15.7a

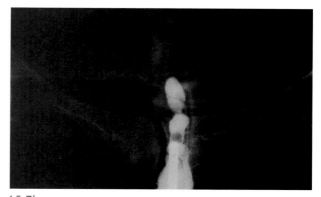

15.7b

Figure 15.7: *(a) Extensive adhesions with narrowed uterine cavity and tubal occlusion (grade IV). (b) Complete occlusion of the upper isthmic area; hysterosalpingography provides no further information on the fundal areas or the Fallopian tubes.*

amenorrhea and complete obstruction this could easily lead to the creation of a false route or even perforation, both of which complicate further therapy.

With carbon dioxide distension it may be difficult to eliminate mucous bubbles from the endocervix before passing the internal os. As the adequate visualization of the endocervix is of vital importance for localizing the ICO or, if present, adhesions in that area, the use of liquid distension media is to be preferred to avoid creating a false route. The hysteroscope must be guided through the endocervix under visual control until the internal os is completely visible or adhesive obstruction is identified. If partial adhesions are present at the ICO region (*Figure 15.8*) it should be carefully ruptured, either with the distension medium or preferably with scissors or forceps, before the hysteroscope is advanced through the internal os (*Figure 15.9*). If the ICO is occluded by membrane-like adhesions, which is seen particularly in patients who develop a secondary amenorrhea following an elective abortion curettage, a gray or faintly blue area may be visible centrally in the white-colored obstructed area (*Figure*

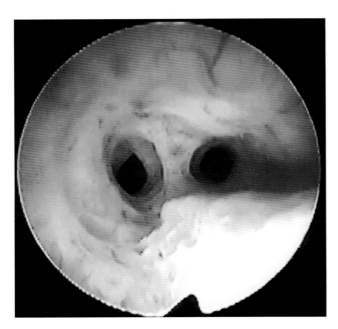

Figure 15.8: Central adhesion with partial obstruction of the internal cervical os.

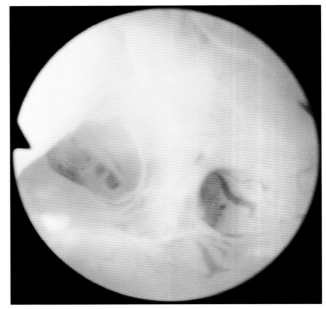

15.10a

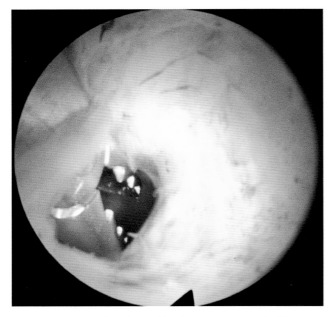

Figure 15.9: *Spreading forceps bluntly rupturing partial adhesions.*

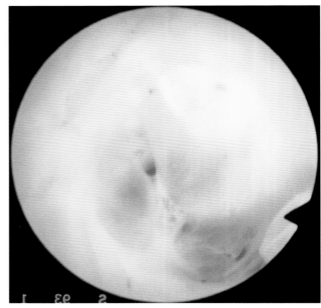

15.10b

Figure 15.10: *(a) and (b) Membrane-like occluding adhesions at the internal cervical os; note the gray areas indicating the thinnest part of the membrane (if no further adhesions exist in the uterine cavity the staging is grade IIa).*

15.10). In the case of dense adhesions and/or complete obstruction the patient must be scheduled for synechiolysis, taking all the necessary precautions.

The two main factors in determining the seriousness of the pathology are the type and extent of the adhesions and the degree of endometrial scarring. In particular, extensive fibrotic scarring of the endometrium (*Figure 15.11*) worsens the prognosis as it significantly reduces the capacity of the endometrium to regenerate.

As a result of the distension of the uterine cavity, intrauterine adhesions appear as strands of tissue representing the artificially stretched adherences between different areas of the uterine cavity. Adhesions may appear in the upper part of the endocervix, at the ICO and elsewhere through the entire uterine cavity. The lower part of the endocervix is usually free of adhesions unless resulting from a previous conization.

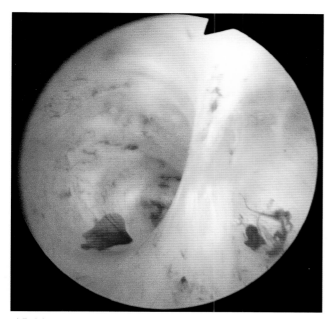

15.11a

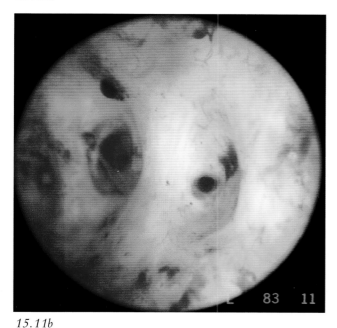

15.11b

Figure 15.11: *(a) and (b) Scarring and fibrosis of the endometrial lining of the uterine cavity.*

Minor adhesions appear as fragile, almost translucent stuctures (*Figure 15.12a,b*) and vascular ingrowth may be visible, indicating organization of the adhesive tissue. With carbon dioxide distension threads of sticky mucus may simulate this type of adhesion (*Figure 15.12c*). More dense adhesions are visible as fibrotic strands, which may be located centrally and/or marginally (*Figure 15.13*). In the case of multiple or transverse

adhesions partial obstruction of the uterine cavity is observed, with one or more small circular holes communicating with the upper part(s) of the uterine cavity (*Figure 15.14*). Sometimes these holes can be mistakenly interpreted as being tubal ostia. Severe adhesions with partial or complete obliteration have a fibrotic

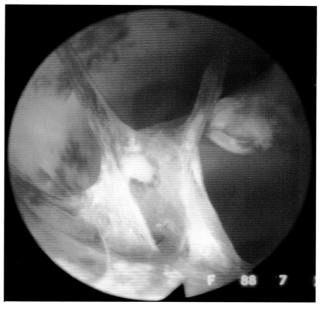

15.12a

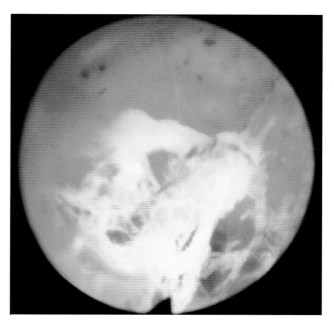

15.12b

Figure 15.12: *(a) Minor fragile adhesions (grade I). (b) Minor adhesions with retained necrotic abortion tissue in the right cornual area (grade I); further organization may lead to occlusion of the right Fallopian tube.*

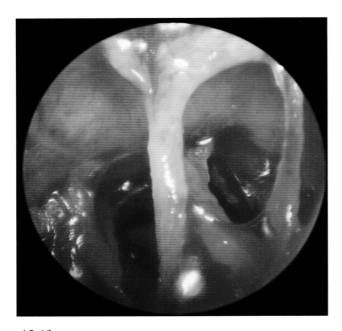

15.12c

Figure 15.12: *(cont.) (c) Endometrium and sticky mucous threads with carbon dioxide distension simulating minor adhesions.*

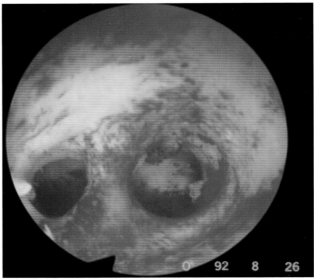

15.13b

appearance (*Figure 15.15*) and the tubal ostia cannot be visualized. The uterine cavity is usually narrowed and shallow (*Figure 15.16a*) which condition also usually results following endometrial ablation (*Figure 15.16b*).

Unless the adhesions are fragile, attempts to rupture them by advancing the hysteroscope sheath should not

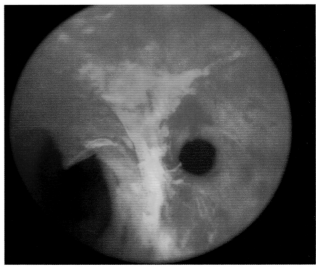

15.13c

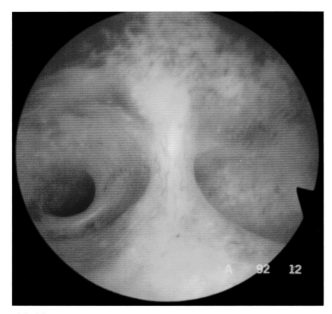

15.13a

Figure 15.13: *Singular dense adhesions (grade II): (a) right cornual area; (b) central, fundal area; (c) and (d) marginal, isthmic area.*

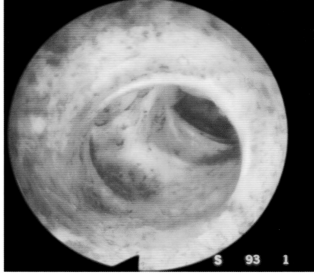

15.13d

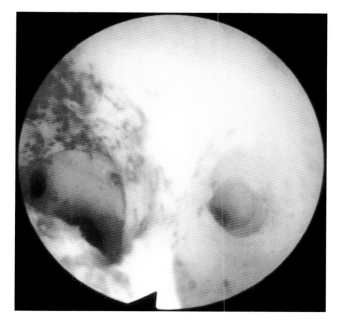

15.14a

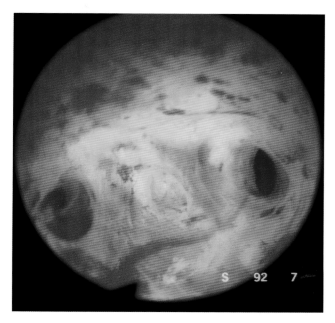

15.15a

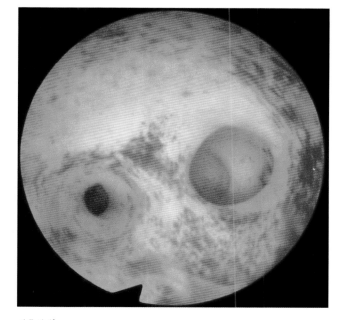

15.14b

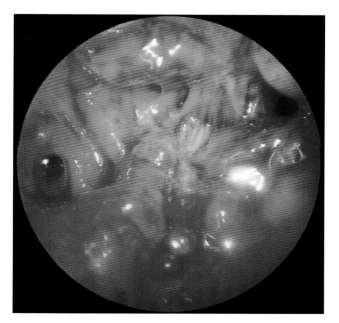

15.15b

Figure 15.14: (a) and (b) Multiple dense adhesions (grade III).

Figure 15.15: (a) and (b) Extensive fibrotic adhesions with partial occlusion of the uterine cavity (grade IV).

be attempted. This can easily lead to a false route or perforation and can further reduce visibility.

ULTRASONOGRAPHY

The benefit of abdominal or transvaginal ultrasonography in the diagnosis of intrauterine adhesions is rather limited. Sometimes the adhered parts of the uterine

wall can appear as asymmetrical dense intrauterine lines (Confino et al, 1985) and irregular endometrial development may also be identified. In the case of a hematometra an anechogenic area filling the uterine cavity may be recognized.

Transvaginal sonography can sometimes be used to demonstrate an area of proliferated endometrium in the upper part of the uterine cavity after estrogenic

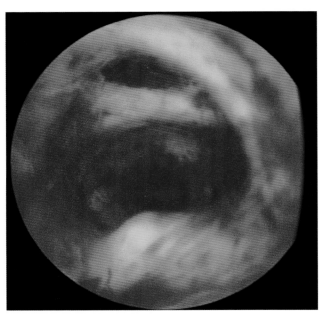

15.16a

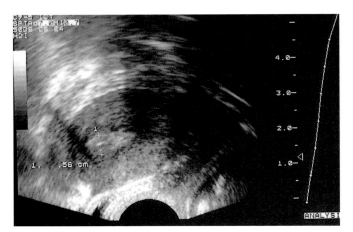

Figure 15.17: Transvaginal sonography in a patient with complete occlusion at hysteroscopy; following preoperative estrogen medication, endometrium with a thickness of 6 mm could be identified in the fundal and cornual areas.

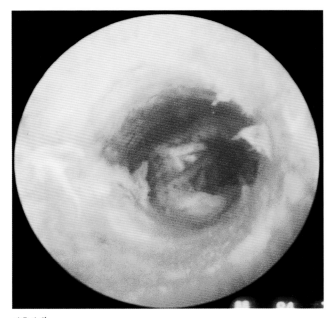

15.16b

Figure 15.16: (a) Rigid and seriously distorted and fibrotic uterine cavity (grade Vb). (b) Narrowed, shallow and fibrotic uterine cavity with obliteration of the cornual areas following endometrial ablation.

stimulation in patients with amenorrhea (*Figure 15.17*). This could indicate that at least part of the uterine cavity is covered by functional endometrium, which facilitates the therapeutic procedure and is of importance for the prognosis of treatment.

Occasionally the presence of intrauterine adhesions may be suspected with ultrasonographic investigation during pregnancy. The adhesions can divide a gesta-tional sac into two communicating compartments and may resemble amniotic bands (Smeele et al, 1989).

Hysterosonography may disclose singular intrauterine adhesions or irregular uterine distension as long as no complete obstruction in the lower part of the uterine cavity exists (Van Roessel et al, 1987).

■ INTERPRETATION OF FINDINGS AND MANAGEMENT

In patients with a history of recurrent abortion, HSG investigation shows intrauterine adhesions in approximately 5% of cases. In only 1% are adhesions found unexpectedly at HSG (Siegler et al, 1990), indicating that the chances of discovering unexpected intrauterine adhesions at routine HSG are small. Usually clinical symptoms or previous interventions lead to further investigation and disclosure of the pathology.

Hysteroscopy is the method of choice for identifying or excluding intrauterine adhesions and should be the first diagnostic step if this kind of pathology is suspected. Adhesions can be localized and assessed and the quality of the endometrium can be observed. Careful inspection of the upper endocervix and the area of the ICO is very important, especially in patients with amenorrhea indicating complete obstruction.

The type and extent of the adhesions in the uterine cavity and the endometrial structure must be examined carefully and, if possible, the cornual areas must be investigated because obstruction of one or both of these areas is important for the classification and the prognosis of treatment.

If more extended adhesions appear to be present in the uterine cavity complete hysteroscopic evaluation will not always be possible (*Figures 15.14* and *15.15*) and HSG is indispensable in determining the extent and assessing the pretreatment classification of the pathology, as well as deciding upon the therapeutic regimen (Valle and Sciarra, 1988; Barbot, 1995). The contrast medium will flow through minor openings in the adhesions through which the hysteroscope cannot pass and will provide further information on the area(s) beyond (*Figure 15.5*). In addition, the accessibility and patency of the Fallopian tubes can be observed.

Although HSG can indicate the presence of intrauterine adhesions and their location, the method is not recommended as the first diagnostic step because false positive results are not uncommon (Raziel et al, 1994; Romer, 1994b). Moreover, minor adhesions could be ruptured by the pressure of the contrast and escape being discovered at all. Although these may be of less clinical importance and may have been treated this way, the true incidence of the occurrence of adhesions will be affected. With hysteroscopy fragile or minor adhesions (*Figure 15.12a,b*) can be identified before they risk being ruptured by the distending medium or the hysteroscope itself.

If suspicion of adhesions arises on clinical symptoms hysteroscopy should be scheduled first, and in the case of extended pathology an HSG must also be performed. If hysteroscopy is not available a hysterosalpingogram can be used as the first diagnostic step. A normal uterine filling pattern at HSG with proper technique excludes major adhesions in the uterine cavity. Minor adhesions of which the clinical significance is unclear can still exist or may have been ruptured. On the other hand, intrauterine defects interpreted as adhesions will not always be confirmed at hysteroscopy, either showing no intrauterine pathology or a different lesion, which necessitates further hysteroscopic investigation.

The place and reliability of hysterosonography in the detection of intrauterine adhesions is as yet unknown.

As intrauterine adhesions have appeared to occur much more frequently after particular pregnancy related interventions, it is worthwhile routinely scheduling a hysteroscopic control examination 6–8 weeks after these procedures (Wamsteker and de Blok, 1993). This will lead to early disclosure of pathology, which facilitates therapy and significantly enhances the results of treatment. The interventions concerned include:

- puerperal curettage for persistent bleeding or retained placental tissue;
- repeat curettage for persistent bleeding or persisting pregnancy products after evacuation of incomplete or missed abortion.

On the other hand hysteroscopy can be also applied during the intervention itself in order to localize the persisting pregnancy products. In such cases the curettage can then be restricted to the region of the uterine cavity affected. A 7 or 8 mm continuous flow operating hysteroscope with low viscosity fluid distension should preferably be used as the ICO is usually dilated and uterine bleeding will be common. Complete removal can be secured by control hysteroscopy after the evacuation of the retained pregnancy tissue. This policy will reduce the damage to areas of the endometrium that are not involved, which in turn reduces the possibility of adhesion formation.

■ CLASSIFICATIONS

In order to be able to assess the pathology, determine the most appropriate therapeutic regimen and to predict and compare the results of treatment, a proper classification of the disease is mandatory.

Several classifications for intrauterine adhesions have been created, two of which are most frequently used. One of these was developed at the Hysteroscopy Training Centre in The Netherlands in 1984 (Wamsteker, 1984) and was adopted by the European Society of Hysteroscopy (ESH), which recently amalgamated with the European Society of Gynecologic Endoscopy (ESGE). The classification was modified in 1993 (Wamsteker and de Blok, 1993) and 1995 and is now in general use in Europe. The second classification was developed by the American Fertility Society (AFS) in 1988 and is currently used in the USA. At present both classifications have been successfully applied.

Other classifications based on hysterographic (Siegler and Kontopoulos, 1981), hysteroscopic (March and

Israel, 1981) or hysteroscopic and histological appearances (Hamou et al, 1983) have been suggested but as these have not received general acceptance they will not be further discussed.

- ▪ *ESH classification*
  The ESH classification (*Table 15.1*) scores the pathology according to the combined HSG and hysteroscopy findings in five different grades, depending on the position and extent of the adhesions, tubal occlusion and the amount of endometrial scarring.
- ▪ *AFS classification*
  With the AFS classification (*Figure 15.18*) the pathology is scored on three different items: extent of involvement of the uterine cavity, type of adhesions and menstrual pattern. Each item has three possibilities and the total score is the sum of the separate scores. The total score divides the patients into three stages: I (mild), II (moderate) and III (severe). The score is calculated for HSG and hysteroscopy separately.

If both classifications are compared, ESH grades I and II relate to AFS stage I, ESH grade III to AFS stage II, and ESH grades IV and V to AFS stage III.

For clinical management it is important to realize that the treatment of severe intrauterine adhesions is generally considered to be the most difficult type of hysteroscopic surgery and should only be performed in centers equipped for these procedures and by surgeons with wide experience in transcervical endosurgery. Adhesions ESH grades I or II (AFS stage I) can usually be treated by all experienced hysteroscopists. In cases classified as ESH grade III, IV or V (AFS stage II or III) the therapeutic regimen generally requires laparoscopic and/or hysterographic control during synechiolysis (Lancet and Mass, 1981) and extensive experience with hysteroscopic endosurgery.

Table 15.1 *European Society of Hysteroscopy classification of intrauterine adhesions*

Grade	Extent of intrauterine adhesions*
I	Thin or fragile adhesions (*Figure 15.12a, b*)
	− easily ruptured by hysteroscope sheath alone
	− cornual areas normal
II	Singular dense adhesion (*Figures 15.3, 15.4a* and *15.13*)
	− connecting separate areas of the uterine cavity
	− visualization of both tubal ostia possible
	− cannot be ruptured by hysteroscope sheath alone
IIa	Occluding adhesions only in the region of the internal cervical os (*Figure 15.10*)†
	− upper uterine cavity normal
III	Multiple dense adhesions (*Figures 15.2, 15.4b, 15.5, 15.6a* and *15.14*)
	− connecting separate areas of the uterine cavity
	− unilateral obliteration of ostial areas of the tubes
IV	Extensive dense adhesions with (partial) occlusion of the uterine cavity (*Figures 15.6b,c, 15.7* and *15.15*)
	− both tubal ostial areas (partially) occluded
Va	Extensive endometrial scarring and fibrosis (*Figure 15.11*) in combination with grade I or grade II adhesions
	− with amenorrhea or pronounced hypomenorrhea
Vb	Extensive endometrial scarring and fibrosis (*Figure 15.11*) in combination with grade III or grade IV adhesions (*Figure 15.16*)†
	− with amenorrhea

* *From findings at hysteroscopy and hysterography.*
† *Only to be classified during hysteroscopic treatment.*
Wamsteker K, Hysteroscopy Training Centre NL, 1984/1993/1995
Spaarne Hospital, Haarlem, The Netherlands.

AFS Classification of Intrauterine Adhesions

Patient's Name _____ Date _____ Chart# _____

Age _____ G _____ P _____ Sp Ab _____ VTP _____ Ectopic _____ Infertile Yes _____ No _____

Other Significant History (i.e. surgery, infection, etc.) _____

_____

HSG _____ Sonography _____ Photography _____ Laparoscopy _____ Laparotomy _____

Extent of Cavity involved	<1/3	1/3 – 2/3	>2/3
	1	2	4
Type of Adhesions	Filmy	Filmy & Dense	Dense
	1	2	4
Menstrual Pattern	Normal	Hypomenorrhea	Amenorrhea
	0	2	4

Prognostic Classification   HSG*   Hysteroscopy   **Additional Findings:** _____
                                 Score   Score

_____

Stage I   (Mild)   1–4 _____ _____   _____

Stage II   (Moderate) 5–8 _____ _____   _____

Stage III   (Severe)   9–12 _____ _____   _____

*All adhesions should be considered dense

DRAWING

Treatment (Surgical Procedures): _____

_____

_____

HSG Findings

Prognosis for Conception & Subsequent Viable Infant*

_____ Excellent   (> 75%)

_____ Good   (50 – 75%)

_____ Fair   (25 – 50%)

_____ Poor   (< 25%)

* Physician's judgement based upon tubal patency.

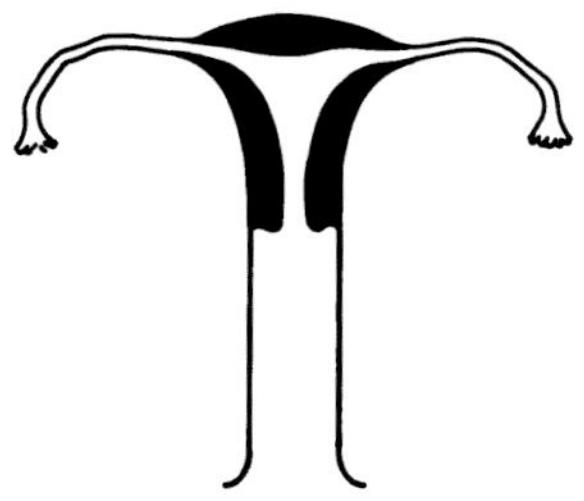

Hysteroscopy Findings

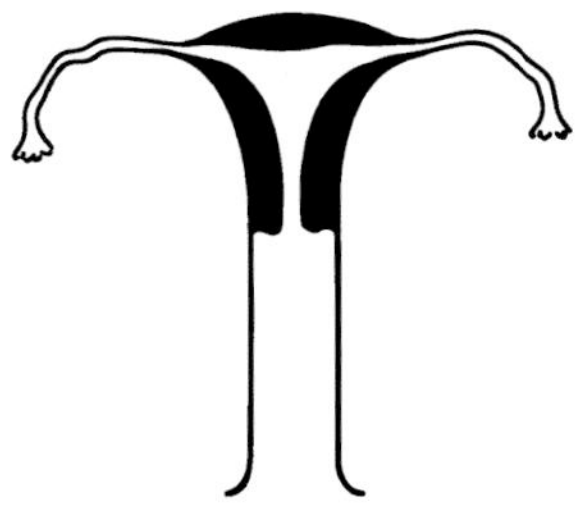

Recommended Followup Treatment: _____

_____

_____

*Figure 15.18:The American Fertility Society classification of intrauterine adhesions. From The American Fertility Society (1988) The American Fertility Society classifications of adnexal adhesions, distal tube occlusion, tubal occlusion secondary to tubal ligation, tubal pregnancies, Müllerian anomalies and intrauterine adhesions. Fertil Steril **49**: 944–955. Reproduced with permission of the publisher, the American Society for Reproductive Medicine (formerly The American Fertility Society).*

REFERENCES

Adoni AS, Palti Z, Milwidsky A et al (1982) The incidence of intrauterine adhesions following spontaneous abortion. *Int J Fertil* **27**: 117.

American Fertility Society (1988) The American Fertility Society classifications of adnexal adhesions, distal tubal occlusion, tubal occlusion secondary to tubal ligation, tubal pregnancies, Müllerian anomalies and intrauterine adhesions. *Fertil Steril* **49**: 944–955.

Asherman JG (1948) Amenorrhoea traumatica (atretica). *J Obstet Gynaecol Br Empire* **55**: 23–30.

Asherman JG (1950) Traumatic intrauterine adhesions. *J Obstet Gynaecol Br Empire* **57**: 892–896.

Barbot J (1995) Hysteroscopy and hysterography. *Obstet Gynecol Clin North Am* **22**: 591–603.

Confino E, Friberg J, Giglia RV & Gleicher N (1985) Sonographic imaging of intrauterine adhesions. *Obstet Gynecol* **66**: 596–598.

Fritsch H (1894) Ein Fall von volligen Schwund der Gebärmutterhöhle nach Auskratzung. *Zentralbl Gynäk* **18**: 1337.

Golan A, Schneider D, Avrech O et al (1992) Hysteroscopic findings after missed abortion. *Fertil Steril* **58**: 508–510.

Hamou J, Salat-Baroux J & Siegler AM (1983) Diagnosis and treatment of intrauterine adhesions by microhysteroscopy. *Fertil Steril* **39**: 321–326.

Hunt RB & Siegler AM (1990) *Hysterosalpingography: Techniques and Interpretation*. Chicago: Year Book Medical.

Jewelewicz R, Khalaf S, Neuwirth RS & Vande Wiele RL (1976) Obstetric complications after treatment of intrauterine synechiae (Asherman's syndrome). *Obstet Gynecol* **47**: 701.

Klein SM & Garcia CR (1973) Asherman's syndrome: a critique and current review. *Fertil Steril* **24**: 722–735.

Lancet M & Mass N (1981) Concomitant hysteroscopy and hysterography in Asherman's syndrome. *Int J Fertil* **26**: 267–272.

Lurie S, Appelman Z & Katz Z (1991) Curettage after midtrimester termination of pregnancy: is it necessary? *J Reprod Med Obstet Gynecol* **36**: 786–788.

March CM (1995) Intrauterine adhesions. *Obstet Gynecol Clin North Am* **22**: 491–505.

March CM & Israel R (1981) Gestational outcome following hysteroscopic lysis of adhesions. *Fertil Steril* **36**: 455.

Polishuk WZ, Siew FP, Gordon R & Lebenshart P (1977) Vascular changes in traumatic amenorrhea and hypomenorrhea. *Int J Fertil* **22**: 189–192.

Raziel A, Arieli S, Bukovsky I et al (1994) Investigation of the uterine cavity in recurrent aborters. *Fertil Steril* **62**: 1080–1082.

Romer T (1994a) Post-abortion hysteroscopy: a method for early diagnosis of congenital and acquired intrauterine causes of abortion. *Eur J Obstet Gynecol Reprod Biol* **57**: 171–173.

Romer T (1994b) Intrauterine adhesionen: Ätiologie, Diagnostik, Therapie und Präventionsmöglichkeiten. *Zentralbl Gynakol* **116**: 311–317.

Romer T, Bojahr B & Lober R (1994) Hysteroskopie versus Hysterosalpingographie in der Sterilitäts- und Infertilitätsdiagnostik. *Zentralbl Gynakol* **116**: 24–27.

Schenker JG & Margalioth EJ (1982) Intrauterine adhesions: an updated appraisal. *Fertil Steril* **37**: 593.

Siegler AM & Kontopoulos VG (1981) Lysis of intrauterine adhesions under hysteroscopic control. *J Reprod Med* **26**: 372–374.

Siegler AM, Valle RF, Lindemann HJ et al (1990) *Therapeutic Hysteroscopy: Indications and Techniques*. St Louis: CV Mosby.

Smeele B, Wamsteker K, Sarstadt T & Exalto N (1989) Ultrasonic appearance of Asherman's syndrome in the third trimester of pregnancy. *J Clin Ultrasound* **17**: 602–606.

Valle RF & Sciarra JJ (1988) Intrauterine adhesions: hysteroscopic diagnosis, classification, treatment, and reproductive outcome. *Am J Obstet Gynecol* **158**: 1459–1470.

Van Roessel J, Wamsteker K & Exalto N (1987) Sonographic investigation of the uterus during artificial uterine cavity distension. *J Clin Ultrasound* **15**: 439.

Wamsteker K (1984) Hysteroscopy in Asherman's syndrome. In Siegler AM and Lindemann HJ (eds) *Hysteroscopy Principles and Practice*, pp 198–203. Philadelphia: JB Lippincott.

Wamsteker K & de Blok S (1993) Diagnostic hysteroscopy: technique and documentation. In Sutton S & Diamond MP (eds) *Endoscopic Surgery for Gynaecologists*, pp 263–276. London: WB Saunders.

16 Uterine leiomyomas
MH Emanuel and K Wamsteker

■ INTRODUCTION

Leiomyomas, myomas or fibroids are the most common benign neoplasms of the uterus. They are said to occur in nearly one-quarter of women over the age of 35 and are likely to be present in an occult fashion even more. Although myomas are also found in younger women, it is largely a disease of women in their fourth and fifth decades. Myomas do not occur normally prepubertally or after menopause, so their growth during these periods would point towards a malignancy. The development of myomas varies from initial growth and size stabilization to rapid growth of multiple tumors.

Myomas have been found to possess estrogen and progesterone receptors in greater concentration than the surrounding myometrium. Their size and growth are more endocrine dependent than normal myometrium. They are usually multifocal and although their etiology is uncertain it seems clear that leiomyomas arise from a single neoplastic parent cell derived from the smooth muscle element of the myometrium. Cytogenetical leiomyomas show clonal cell lines of which 50% are abnormal. Some correlation was found between cytogenetical and histological abnormalities (Meloni et al, 1992). Although estrogen may help to explain the growth of leiomyomas, factors responsible for the initial neoplastic transformation are unknown and may involve an as yet undetermined genetic predisposition. Furthermore, varying estrogen levels do not explain differences in the rate of growth of myomas, which may also depend upon genetically determined tendencies or upon differences in blood supply to the tumors.

The tumors are composed of smooth muscle and connective tissue in whorled configurations and are nourished by a vascular supply from encircling uterine tissue, constituting a pseudocapsular layer. The retraction of the surrounding myometrium causes the tumors to project somewhat above the surface, enabling ready resection or enucleation from the uterine wall after opening of the pseudocapsule. Histological changes associated with degeneration include hyalinization, liquefaction, calcification and hemorrhage.

Strictly speaking, leiomyomas can arise in many different organs containing smooth muscle. They can also develop in other Müllerian tissues, such as the round and broad ligaments, in the cervix and in the vagina. This chapter will concentrate on the uterine variety.

■ SYMPTOMS

The leiomyomas may either be asymptomatic, detected by bimanual pelvic examination or routine ultrasonography, or be related to significant symptomatology (in 20–50% of cases). The pathology effected by leiomyomas can be divided into that causing uterine symptoms and that resulting in anatomical distortion which, in turn, affects other organ systems. The severity of symptoms experienced by a patient will depend on the number, size and location of the tumors. The common subdivision of the tumors is into the subserous, the interstitial or intramural, and the submucous varieties, according to whether the growth is located just beneath the serosa, within the uterine muscular wall or just beneath the mucosa, respectively (*Figure 16.1*).

The subserous tumors may present as knobby excrescences or as masses that have developed distinct pedicles, the so-called pedunculated myomas. Not infrequently, lateral growths may extend outward between the folds of the broad ligament. Such intraligamentary tumors, when large, may burrow far outward and form retroperitoneal masses.

The intramural growths, when small, may cause no change in the contour of the uterus. When larger, they produce an enlargement of the organ, giving it a hilly or

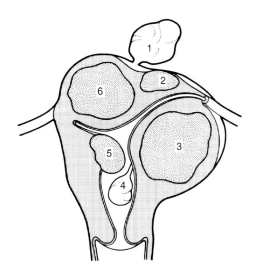

Figure 16.1: Different types/subdivisions of myoma: 1, penduncu-lated subserous; 2, subserous; 3, intramural; 4, pendunculated sub-mucous (type 0); 5, sessile submucous (type I); 6, intramural, distorting part of the Fallopian tube.

nodular contour. In the majority of such cases, more-over, some of the intramural tumors become subserous or submucous as they increase in size.

Although the submucous tumors constitute the least common group numerically (estimated at between 5 and 10%), they are perhaps the most important clinically, and may be considered a rather specific group. The preva-lence is probably underestimated because of diagnostic difficulties. Whereas other myomas attain large size with frequently no symptomatology, even a small tumor in a submucous location may impinge on the blood vessels of the endometrium and produce bleeding. As they grow in size they bring about a dome-like protrusion into the uterine cavity, with impingement on the opposite wall and marked distortion and enlargement of the cavity.

In a 4 year observational study of 1202 hysteroscopies for abnormal uterine bleeding a prevalence of 14.7% (95% confidence interval 12.1 to 17.6) was found for the presence of submucous myomas in an unselected group of patients referred by general practitioners (Emanuel et al, 1995a).

Abnormal bleeding, characterized as specifically menor-rhagia or metrorrhagia, with or without dysmenorrhea, is often due to submucous or large intramural myomas. Direct pressure effects on the endometrium, congestion

and dilatation of the subjacent endometrial venous plexuses, enlargement of the endometrial surface area or impaired contractility of the myometrium are all feasible etiologic explanations but all remain unsubstantiated.

Reproductive capacity can be impaired by increased fetal loss, premature labor and possible infertility because of cavity or tubal distortion. Other suggestions are the impaired transport of sperm due to interference with rhythmic uterine contractions by leiomyomas, the increased distance sperm may have to travel in a distorted uterine cavity, or endometrial changes, such as atrophy or ulceration associated with submucous myomas, as pos-sible causes for improper nidation. Since leiomyomas typically arise later in reproductive life, the trend towards delaying pregnancy may increase their prevalence among women who wish to conceive and also contribute to the incidence of leiomyomas in a population with fertility problems.

Large subserosal and intramural leiomyomas can com-press nerves, vessels or adjacent organs, causing pain, heaviness and urinary or bowel difficulties. Pedunculated submucous myomas can protrude into the cervix and vagina, accompanied by pain, discharge, infection or bleed-ing. Even uterine inversion has been reported as a rare complication of submucous leiomyoma. During preg-nancy leiomyomas can grow very fast and ischemic changes can lead to painful degeneration due to swelling of the myomatous tissue. Sarcomatous degeneration is uncommon and sometimes unexpected as clinically reli-able indicators can be lacking, except growth before puberty, after menopause or despite gonadotropin releasing hormone (GnRH) analogue medication. In the literature the incidence of leiomyosarcomas varies from 0.17% to 0.49% (Montague et al, 1965; Novak and Woodruff, 1979; Liebsohn et al, 1990; Emanuel et al, 1992). The true inci-dence is extremely difficult to calculate because the basis for these figures is neither well defined nor comparable. One should realize the bias of not taking into considera-tion the high incidence of asymptomatic myomas in most populations. Furthermore, conflicting opinions as to the precise histological features necessary to justify the diagno-sis of leiomyosarcoma still exist (Novak and Woodruff, 1979; Clement et al, 1992).

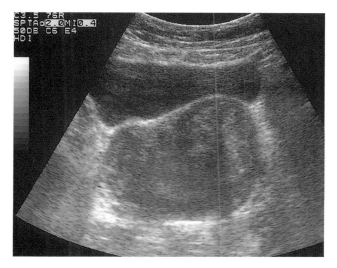

Figure 16.2: Transabdominal sonogram of a large solitary intramural myoma.

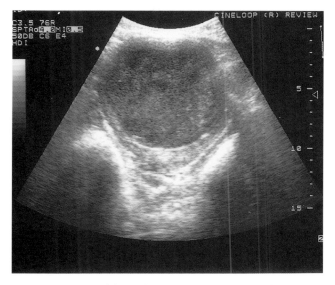

Figure 16.3: Transabdominal sonogram of a pedunculated subserous myoma that may simulate an adnexal mass separate from the uterus.

■ CLINICAL INVESTIGATIONS

TRANSABDOMINAL ULTRASONOGRAPHY

The ultrasonographic diagnosis of uterine myomas is generally accepted as accurate. The use of transabdominal ultrasonography (TAS) is widely reported for the evaluation and sizing of uterine enlargements. In particular, in the follow up of conservative medical treatment it is often the technique of choice for assessing shrinkage of the volume of the uterus or the myoma. However, due to the

heterogeneous echogeneity of myomas precise details of measurements and localization can be difficult and smaller myomas may even remain unnoticed. The most reliable and useful information will be obtained in cases of massive uterine enlargement or large, solitary, intramural or subserous myomas (*Figures 16.2* and *16.3*). Different forms of degeneration like liquefaction, hemorrhage and calcification can cause areas that are anechoic, hypoechoic and hyperechoic respectively.

Disadvantages of the technique are its limitations in obese patients and the need for the patient to have a full bladder, with its associated discomfort.

TRANSVAGINAL ULTRASONOGRAPHY

The acceptance of the use of transvaginal ultrasonography (TVS) for the depiction of abnormal endometrium and intracavitary pathology is growing. Transvaginal probes are generally of high frequency (5–7.5 MHz), giving excellent resolution despite high magnifications; however, the high frequency results in less penetration and a shorter effective field of vision. One must define the target organ by 'palpation' with the probe because the panoramic view one may be accustomed to with TAS is not available. This actually is the most important practical disadvantage of TVS.

The gold standard control in most studies describing the diagnostic value of TVS has been histological examination of specimens obtained by dilatation and curettage (D&C) or blind endometrial biopsy (Osmers et al, 1990). As D&C appeared to be unreliable in excluding intracavitary pathology, particularly submucous myomas (Burnett, 1964; Beazley, 1972; Stock and Kanbour, 1975; Brooks and Serden, 1988; Gimpelson and Rappold, 1988), studies were performed to assess the diagnostic value of TVS in patients with abnormal uterine bleeding, with diagnostic hysteroscopy and histology as the gold standard. These studies show good predictive values of a normal sonogram in excluding intracavitary pathology (Fedele et al, 1991; Emanuel et al, 1995b).

The abnormal or inconclusive sonogram reveals an important limitation of the technique as it is not always possible to differentiate between a submucous myoma and an endometrial polyp (*Figure 16.4*). In addition, in the secretory phase of the menstrual cycle small intracavitary

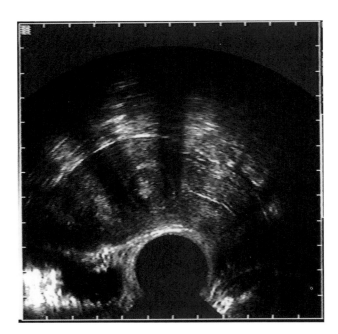

Figure 16.4: Transvaginal sonogram showing a submucous myoma.

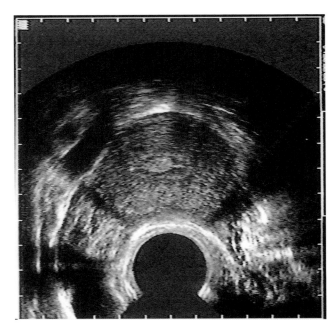

Figure 16.6: Transvaginal sonogram showing a transverse plane of proliferative hypoechoic endometrium with a small intracavitary structure clearly visible.

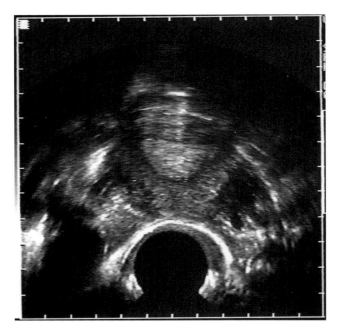

Figure 16.5: Transvaginal sonogram showing a transverse plane of secretory hyperechoic endometrium in which a polyp can be easily missed.

pathology can be missed in the hyperechoic endometrium, particularly when it is located centrally in the cavity (*Figure 16.5*). If the endometrium is very thick and hyperechoic it is therefore advisable to repeat the procedure in the proliferative phase of the cycle after menstruation (*Figure 16.6*).

Although the presence of submucous myomas is often suggested by the patient's clinical history, it has become apparent that bimanual pelvic examination should be combined with TVS because these tumors are generally missed at physical examination.

ULTRASONOHYSTEROGRAPHY

A promising new development for the detection of intracavitary pathology is ultrasonohysterography (Parsons and Lense, 1993; Goldstein, 1994; Dubinsky et al, 1995). Fluid instillation or uterine cavity distension improves the ultrasonographic image. It was first tested with TAS, controlled with hysteroscopy (van Roessel et al, 1987). This extension of TVS, combined with diagnostic hysteroscopy, could be very helpful with mapping or classifying submucous myomas (*Figure 16.7*). The classification of submucous myomas according to their intramural extension is discussed more extensively later in the chapter.

The use of ultrasonographic contrast instilled in the uterus in testing tubal patency has recently been described. Its role in mapping myomas is as yet unclear.

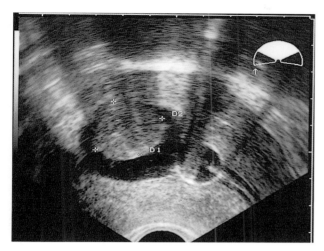

Figure 16.7: *Transvaginal sonogram with fluid instillation showing the balloon catheter and a filling defect of the uterine cavity caused by a type I submucous myoma.*

TRANSVAGINAL (COLOR) DOPPLER

This technique can be used for assessing the physiological and pathological characteristics of the uterine artery as well as myoma vascularization. Color flow imaging facilitates the visualization of vascularization (*Figure 16.8*) and increases the reproducibility of the Doppler measurements. Blood flow impedance is reflected by the resistance index (RI) and the pulsatility index (PI). Kurjak et al (1992) found lower resistance indices and pulsatility indices in both uterine arteries of 101 patients with palpable myomas. This means that the arterial resistance is decreased and therefore the total arterial blood flow in these myomatous uteri is increased. The waveform analysis of myoma vessels was characterized by lower resistance indices in the case of necrosis and secondary degenerative and inflammatory changes within the myoma.

LAPAROSCOPY

Diagnostic laparoscopy has a particularly useful role in the clarification of the nature of pelvic masses for which other techniques are not conclusive. In the case of a myomatous uterus the enlargement can be observed and classified. The most common laparoscopic findings in cases of uterine enlargement are intramural and sessile or pedunculated subserous myomas (*Figure 16.9a–c*). Occasionally myomas originating from different Müllerian

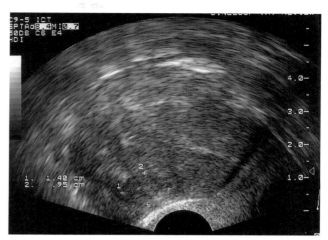

16.8a

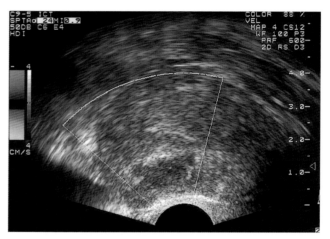

16.8b

Figure 16.8: *(a) Transvaginal sonogram showing a small intramural myoma with indistinct margins. (b) Color flow imaging facilitates the visualization of the myoma by revealing its vascularization.*

structures can be detected (*Figure 16.9d*). If discovered in infertile patients during diagnostic laparoscopy and tubal testing with methylene blue, attention should be paid to the site, volume and number of myomas and their relation to the intramural part of the tubes. If there is a regularly shaped, diffuse, enlarged uterus, the surface should be carefully examined because a reddish and whitish spotted appearance may suggest adenomyosis.

HYSTEROSCOPY

The development of new techniques and methods for diagnostic hysteroscopy and hysteroscopic surgery has altered the management of women with abnormal uterine bleeding due to benign intrauterine pathology.

With the use of continuous flow hysteroscopy differ-

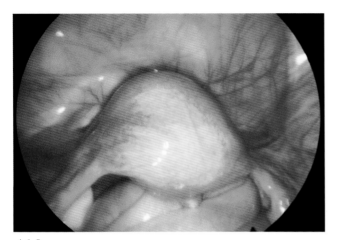

16.9a

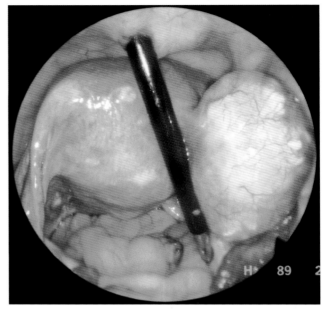

16.9c

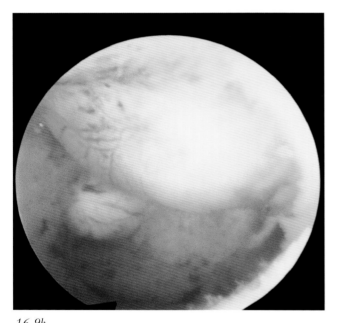

16.9b

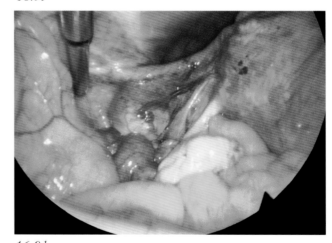

16.9d

Figure 16.9: *(a) Laparoscopic image of an intramural myoma with more or less subserous extension of the anterior surface. (b) Hysteroscopic image of the same intramural myoma showing submucous extension from the anterior wall. (c) Laparoscopic image of a calcified subserous myoma. The abdominal sonogram was suggestive of a dermoid cyst. (d) Laparoscopic image of a myoma originating from the left uterine round ligament.*

ent degrees of uterine distension can be chosen, enabling a better observation of the vascular structure of lesions and the recognition of specific patterns. Submucous myomas typically appear as dense, white intracavitary tumors with a superficial complex network of stretched and dilated blood vessels covered by thin and compressed endometrium (*Figure 16.10*). The submucous myoma may even break through the mucosa (*Figure 16.11*). Evidence of recent hemorrhage can be seen in the form of adherent blood clots or subepithelial hematomas. The sinus-like vessels are often very vulnerable and rupture easily if touched. This appearance contrasts with most

endometrial polyps, which usually consist of soft tissue with a surface that looks like normal endometrium (*Figure 16.12*). The vascular architecture of endometrial polyps shows much smaller and more uniform vessels, although irregular, spiral-like coiling and kinking vessels may be accompanied by atypia of the epithelium. The endometrial vasculature, even in areas relatively remote from submucous myomas, can also demonstrate distorted vessels with an atrophic endometrial appearance, probably due to compression. In the case of active bleeding, continuous flow hysteroscopy with low viscosity liquid distension is preferred. Submucous myomas can be

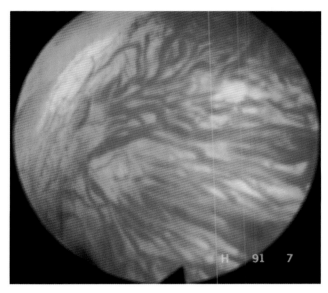

Figure 16.10: Submucous myoma with networks of stretched, thin walled, dilated vessels covering an almost absent endometrium.

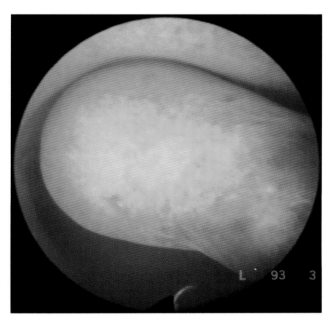

Figure 16.12: Endometrial polyp covered with more or less normal endometrium.

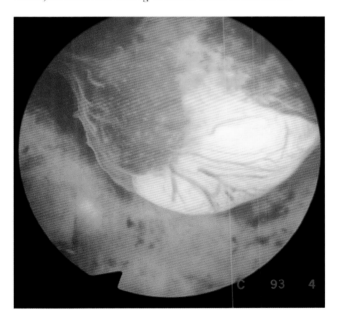

Figure 16.11: Submucous myoma breaking through endometrial layer.

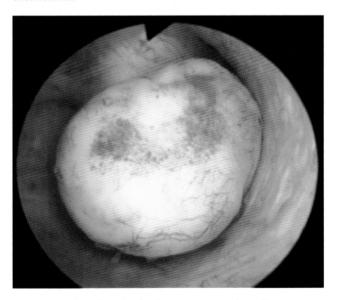

Figure 16.13: Pedunculated submucous myoma (type 0).

pedunculated (*Figure 16.13*) or sessile (*Figures 16.14 and 16.15*), and single or multiple (*Figure 16.16*). Criteria for categorization of submucous myomas are further discussed in the section on classification.

MAGNETIC RESONANCE IMAGING AND COMPUTED TOMOGRAPHY

Although computed tomography (CT) affords complete delineation of the pelvis and abdomen in superb anatomical detail, magnetic resonance imaging (MRI) is often advocated as a better alternative. MRI shares with ultrasonography a number of advantages over CT, the most important of which is the ability to image the uterus in various planes as well as the absence of the use of ionizing radiation. In addition, MRI generates images with greater inherent tissue contrast than that of CT (*Figure 16.17*), in which, in those cases where attenuation difference between normal and myomatous tissue is minimal, one may have to rely on contour deformity and size alone.

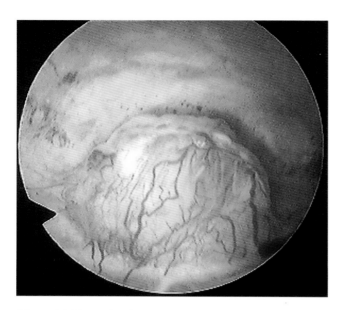

Figure 16.14: Sessile submucous myoma (type I).

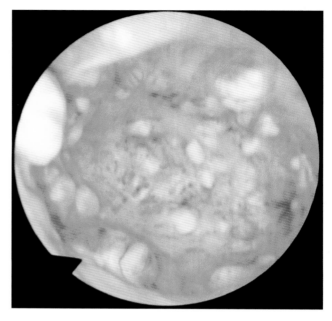

Figure 16.16: Hysteroscopic view of numerous submucous myomas.

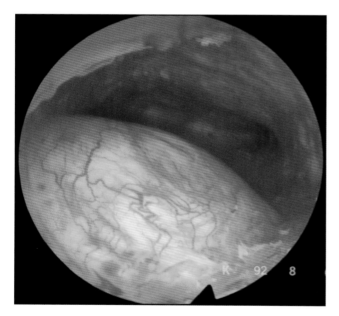

Figure 16.15: Sessile submucous myoma (type II).

HYSTEROSALPINGOGRAPHY

In many centers hysterosalpingography (HSG) is used as a primary invasive procedure in the investigation of infertility and may occasionally disclose an intrauterine filling defect caused by a submucous myoma. In cases of known or suspected uterine myomas, HSG can also provide additional information on the degree of cavity distorsion by submucous and/or intramural myomas and on tubal patency, particularly in cases where the tumors are

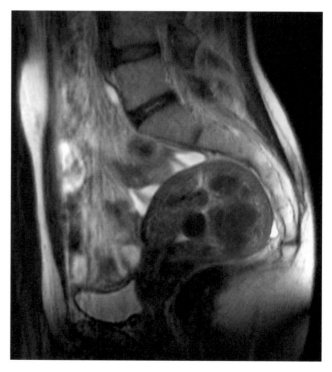

Figure 16.17: Magnetic resonance image of a large bulky myomatous uterus.

encroaching on the tubal cornua (*Figures 16.18* and *16.19*).

The use of HSG in the diagnostic evaluation of patients with known or suspected myomas without fertility problems is not common because of the limited information on size and site of the myomas that it provides.

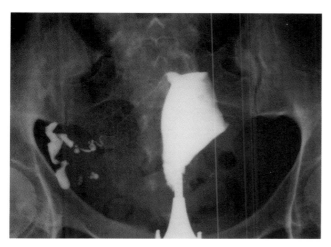

Figure 16.18: Hysterosalpingogram showing cavity distorsion of the left tubal cornu and tubal impatency caused by a submucous and/or intramural myoma.

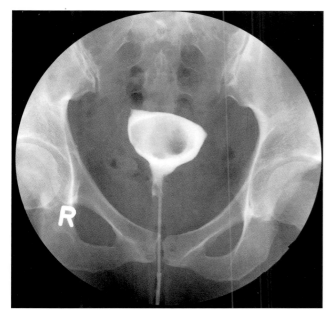

Figure 16.19: Hysterosalpingogram showing a centrally located submucous myoma causing a filling defect of the uterine cavity.

■ INTERPRETATION OF FINDINGS AND CLINICAL MANAGEMENT

Before signs and symptoms can be attributed to uterine myomas the diagnosis has to be established, after bimanual pelvic examination, by imaging or endoscopic techniques in many cases. The only type of myoma that is detected without any of these techniques is the cervically expelled submucous myoma (*Figure 16.20*).

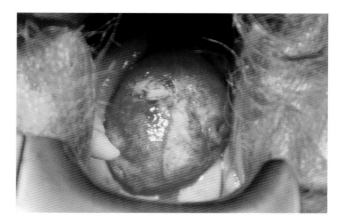

Figure 16.20: Cervically expelled large submucous myoma.

In the case of an *enlarged* uterus TAS alone may be insufficient and often needs to be combined with other imaging techniques. TAS provides little information about submucous myomas. They are missed quite often, particularly when the myoma is small and the patient obese. Sometimes the variety of ultrasonographic appearances and presentations of myomas creates difficulty in interpretation, even leading to diagnostic pitfalls. Pedunculated subserous myomas, especially if they are on a narrow stalk, may simulate adnexal masses that are separate from the uterus. A laterally bulging intramural or subserous myoma can create a more or less symmetric bilobed uterine appearance like a bicornuate uterus. Different forms of degeneration of myomas can mimic predominantly cystic or multiseptate adnexal masses when located at the periphery of the uterus, or even an abnormal intrauterine gestational sac when located centrally. Various ultrasonographic patterns of calcified myomas may contribute to misdiagnosis as ovarian tumors, such as dermoid cysts. Awareness of these potential problems may be helpful in further management. In such cases laparoscopy is indispensable and often conclusive.

The differential diagnosis in patients with uterine enlargement can be very difficult if no myomas are readily identified whichever technique is used. Adenomyosis can cause uterine enlargement and may be misconstrued as intramural myomas. MRI may have a role in the clarification of the nature of pelvic masses for which ultrasonography is unsatisfactory and laparoscopy inconclusive. The number of studies that show the advantages of MRI over the more conventional techniques in imaging uterine myomas is still very limited (Dudiak et al, 1988; Zawin, 1990). Moreover, poorer clinical availability and higher costs restrict the routine use of MRI in patients with uterine myomas, in whom alternative techniques are satisfactory. Some authors claim MRI to be the only noninvasive technique that can diagnose adenomyosis (McCarthy, 1990); others demonstrate the diagnostic value of TVS as well (Fedele et al, 1992; Brosens et al, 1995).

In patients with more or less *normal sized* uteri and abnormal uterine bleeding, submucous myomas and endometrial polyps often appear not to have been diagnosed during D & C. With failure of hormonal treatment, this lack of diagnosis could eventually result in hysterectomy because of persisting 'dysfunctional' bleeding. TVS could be introduced as the routine first step procedure to exclude intracavitary pathology in the evaluation of patients with abnormal uterine bleeding from an unenlarged uterus. The place of diagnostic hysteroscopy, combined with histology, will be that of gold standard after an abnormal or inconclusive sonogram, or in the case of persistent complaints in spite of a normal sonogram. Using this approach, the number of invasive diagnostic procedures could be reduced by approximately 50% without missing intracavitary pathology of any importance.

Treatment options for uterine myomas vary greatly and depend on several factors. These factors can be subjective, like complaints, desire for fertility, expectations or wishes, such as the use of hormonal replacement therapy, or more objective, like the age of the patient, myoma volume, growth, location, number or uterine distortion. Whatever the treatment options are, the topographical distribution of myomas within the uterus is the cornerstone for making decisions about their management. This mapping of myomas is a very challenging part of diagnostic imaging and endoscopy in gynecology. Most of the techniques are not antagonistic but complementary to one another. After weighing the pros and cons, a decision will be made concerning the therapeutic options: expectant treatment by observation, conservative treatment by medication (particularly GnRH analogues), myomectomy, either transcervical or transabdominal, or radical treatment by hysterectomy. The number of randomized controlled trials demonstrating the justification for these different treatment options is limited.

Many small, asymptomatic, intramural or subserous myomas are initially detected during ultrasonography or laparoscopy, particularly when carried out for the investigation of subfertility or, less commonly, in women undergoing sterilization. Given the high prevalence of myomas in women of reproductive age, it is not surprising to find that a significant proportion of women attempting to conceive are affected. Should we pay much attention to these more or less coincidental findings? The relation between myomas and infertility is unclear and it is still unknown whether myomas are really the cause for subfertility or merely a chance association. It has, however, been accepted that myomas occluding the intramural part of both tubes or severely distorting the uterine cavity may cause subfertility.

When the indications for myomectomy are subfertility, occasional pain, pressure or growth of the myomas, laparoscopy is mandatory in the preoperative assessment. Location, number and volume are the main factors determining whether the myomectomy will be by laparotomy or by laparoscopy. In these cases hysteroscopy should be performed as well to exclude undetected submucous myomas.

As a consequence of its limited field of view, TVS will be less informative the larger the uterus. The role of this technique in the preoperative workup preceding myomectomy is therefore restricted to the mapping of submucous myomas in unenlarged uteri. The efficacy of transcervical resection of myomas is related more to the degree of intramural extension of submucous myomas than to their size or number (Wamsteker et al, 1993). This intramural extension can be assessed in most cases by combining TVS and diagnostic hysteroscopy in a thorough preoperative assessment.

▪ CLASSIFICATION

Techniques for hysteroscopic surgery enable the selective resection of submucous myomas, which necessitates the development of criteria for preoperative assessment to determine the possibilities for hysteroscopic surgery and to compare the results of treatment. Hysteroscopic assessment includes the determination of nature, size, number, location and degree of intramural extension of the tumors.

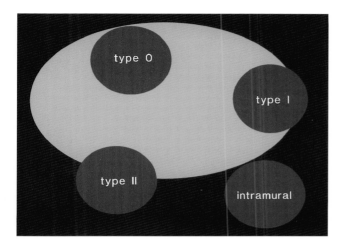

Figure 16.21:The ESH classification of the submucous myomas.

Table 16.1 *European Society of Hysteroscopy classification of submucous myomas*

Type	Extent of submucous myomas
0	Pedunculated submucous myomas without intramural extension
I	Sessile submucous myomas with intramural extension of less than 50%
II	Myomas with intramural extension of 50% or more

From Wamsteker and de Blok (1993).

Two different classifications of submucous myomas have been developed.The one at present most frequently used was developed at the Hysteroscopy Training Centre in The Netherlands and was adopted by the European Society of Hysteroscopy (ESH) in 1990 (Wamsteker and de Blok, 1993) (*Table 16.1; Figure 16.21*). Pedunculated submucous myomas without intramural extension are classified as type 0 myomas (*Figure 16.13*); if the submucous myoma is sessile and the intramural part constitutes less than 50%, the myoma is classified as type I (*Figure 16.14*); with an intramural extension of equal to or more than 50% the myoma is classified as type II (*Figure 16.15*). The degree of intramural extension can be assessed by observation of the angle of the myoma with the normal endometrium at the attachment to the uterine wall. Careful inspection with varying degrees of uterine distension is necessary because the endometrium may smooth away the actual angle (*Figure 16.22*), and with a lower intrauterine pressure the myoma is expelled further into the uterine cavity. Some patients have

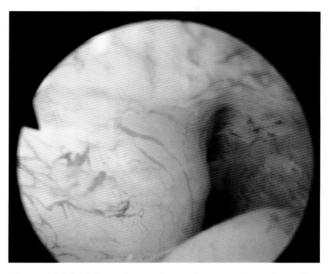

Figure 16.22: Endometrium at the attachment to the uterine wall, smoothing away the actual angle of the myoma with the normal myometrium.

Table 16.2 *Classification of submucous myomas according to Donnez et al (1993)*

Class	Extent of submucous myomas
1	Submucous myomas with greatest diameter inside the uterine cavity
2	Submucous myomas with greatest diameter inside the uterine wall
3	Multiple (>2) submucous myomas (submucous and intramural myomas diagnosed by hysterosalpingography and ultrasonography)

numerous submucous myomas that cannot all be described in detail.

The type 0 and type I myomas are the most suitable varieties for transcervical resection. Depending on the amount of intramural extension, concomitant laparoscopic control during resection of type I myomas may be necessary in some cases. Endoresection of type II myomas requires much more experience, poses an increased risk of excessive intravasation of the distension fluid and more often necessitates multiple procedures to obtain complete removal of the myoma(s) (Wamsteker et al, 1993). Laparoscopic control is mandatory in these cases.

A second classification was developed by Donnez et al (1993) by the review of hysterosalpingographic data (*Table 16.2*).

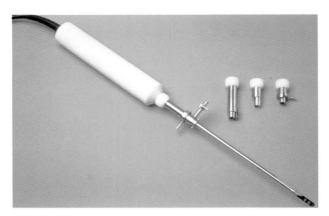

Figure 16.23: The Kretz® intracavitary probe with a 7.5 and 10 MHz transducer for intravesical scanning (Kretztechnik Aktiengesellschaft, Zipf, Austria).

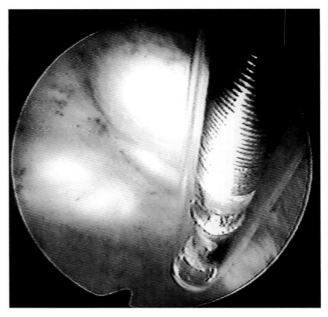

Figure 16.25: The transducer placed against the attachment of the submucous myoma to the uterine wall (Aloka Co. Ltd, Mitaka-shi, Tokyo, Japan).

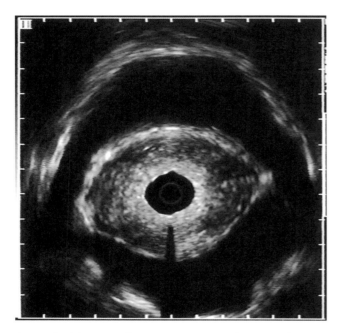

Figure 16.24: A normal intrauterine sonogram (transverse plane).

■ FUTURE DEVELOPMENTS

For specific clinical questions the techniques available have been expanded with recent developments. We need more informative methods for assessing the degree of intramural extension of submucous myomas under circumstances comparable with transcervical resection, in other words during cavitary distension. One of the new developments that could be useful is *intrauterine ultrasonography*. Kretz® (Kretztechnik Aktiengesellschaft, Zipf, Austria) developed an intracavitary probe with a 7.5 and 10 MHz transducer for use with uterine disten-

sion (*Figures 16.23* and *16.24*). An alternative, more recent technique is the use of 192 cm long and very thin (6 and 8 Fr) rotating transducers of 10, 15 and 20 MHz, made by Aloka® (Aloka Co. Ltd, Mitaka-shi, Tokyo, Japan), which are introduced through the working channel of a continuous flow hysteroscope. The transducer can be placed against the attachment of the submucous myoma to the uterine wall (*Figure 16.25*). Careful inspection with varying degrees of uterine distension is possible with the visualization of the intramural part (*Figure 16.26*). These methods may become valuable for the more accurate preoperative assessment of the intramural extent of submucous myomas in the future.

Three-dimensional ultrasonography equipment is gradually becoming available to clinicians. In gynecology the anatomical view of the uterus can be optimized with a transverse section through the whole uterus from fundus to cervix, an image that cannot be obtained from conventional two-dimensional imaging (*Figure 16.27*). Theoretically three-dimensional volume measurements of the uterus or single myomas should be more accurate. This potential advantage can be helpful for more objective observation of growth or shrinkage of the uterus during expectant or medical management of myomas.

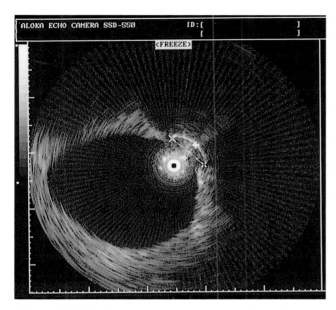

Figure 16.26: The intrauterine sonogram corresponding to Figure 16.25, showing a small submucous myoma, with almost no intramural extension, that could not be assessed hysteroscopically.

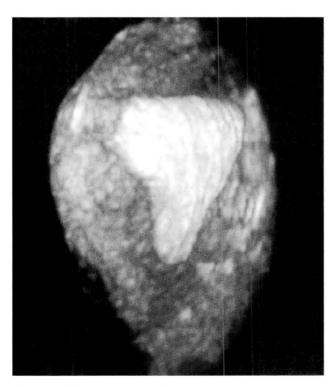

Figure 16.27: A normal three-dimensional transvaginal sonogram (7.5 MHz, Combison 530®, Kretztechnik Aktiengesellschaft, Zipf, Austria). From Steiner H, Staudach A, Spitzer D, Graf AH & Wienerroither H (1993) 3D-sonography provides new aspects in obstetrical and gynecological ultrasound. Geburtshilfe Frauenheilkd **53**: 779–782. Reproduced with permission of Georg Thieme Verlag, Stuttgart.

■ CONCLUSION

Diagnosis and treatment of uterine myomas in modern gynecology is impossible without taking account of the results of continuously improving diagnostic imaging and endoscopic techniques. Nowadays more and more patients therefore have the opportunity of choosing not to have their myomatous uterus removed but to have strongly individualized conservative treatment with preservation of the uterus. This is beneficial for the wellbeing of women in general, and for health care systems in terms of lower costs. Follow up studies are necessary to demonstrate whether these benefits will last in the long term.

REFERENCES

Beazley JM (1972) Dysfunctional uterine haemorrhage. *Br J Hosp Med* **7**: 573–578.

Brooks PG & Serden SP (1988) Hysteroscopic findings after unsuccessful dilatation and curettage for abnormal uterine bleeding. *Am J Obstet Gynecol* **158**: 1354–1357.

Brosens JJ, de Souza NM, Barker FG, Paraschos T & Winston RM (1995) Endovaginal ultrasonography in the diagnosis of adenomyosis uteri: identifying the predictive characteristics. *Br J Obstet Gynaecol* **102**: 471–474.

Burnett JE (1964) Hysteroscopy-controlled curettage for endometrial polyps. *Obstet Gynecol* **24**: 621–625.

Clement PB & Scully RE (1992) Pathology of uterine sarcomas. In Copplesone M, Monaghan J, Morrow CP & Tattersall MHN (eds) *Copplesone Gynaecologic Oncology*, 2nd edn, pp 827–840. Edinburgh: Churchill Livingstone.

Donnez J, Nisolle M, Grandjean P, Gillerot S & Clerckx F (1993) The place of GnRH agonists in the treatment of endometriosis and fibroids by advanced endoscopic techniques. *Br J Obstet Gynaecol* **13**: 69–71.

Dubinsky TJ, Parvey R, Gormaz G, Curtis M & Maklad N (1995) Transvaginal hysterosonography: comparison with biopsy in the evaluation of postmenopausal bleeding. *J Ultrasound Med* **14**: 887–893.

Dudiak CM, Turner DA, Patel SK, Archie JT, Silver B & Norusis M (1988) Uterine leiomyomas in the infertile patient: preoperative localization with MR imaging versus US and hysterosalpingography. *Radiology* **167**: 627–630.

Emanuel MH, Wamsteker K, Eastham WN & Kroeks MVAM (1992) Leiomyosarcoma or cellular leiomyoma diagnosed after hysteroscopical transcervical resection of a presumed leiomyoma. *Gynaecol Endosc* **1**: 161–164.

Emanuel MH, Verdel MJC, Stas H, Wamsteker K & Lammes FB (1995a) An audit of true prevalence of intra-uterine pathology: the hysteroscopical findings controlled for patient selection in 1202 patients with abnormal uterine bleeding. *Gynaecol Endosc* **4**: 237–241.

Emanuel MH, Verdel MJC, Wamsteker K & Lammes FB (1995b) A prospective comparison of transvaginal ultrasonography and diagnostic hysteroscopy in the evaluation of patients with abnormal uterine bleeding: clinical implications. *Am J Obstet Gynecol* **172**: 547–552.

Fedele L, Bianchi S, Dorta M, Brioschi D, Zanotti F & Vercellini P (1991) Transvaginal ultrasonography versus hysteroscopy in the diagnosis of uterine submucous myomas. *Obstet Gynecol* **77**: 745–748.

Fedele L, Bianchi S, Dorta M, Zanotti F, Brioschi D & Carinelli S (1992) Transvaginal ultrasonography in the differential diagnosis of adenomyoma versus leiomyoma. *Am J Obstet Gynecol* **167**: 603–606.

Gimpelson RJ & Rappold HO (1988) A comparative study between panoramic hysteroscopy with directed biopsies and dilatation and curettage. A review of 276 cases. *Am J Obstet Gynecol* **158**: 489–492.

Goldstein SR (1994) The use of ultrasonohysterography for triage of perimenopausal patients with unexplained uterine bleeding. *Am J Obstet Gynecol* **170**: 565–570.

Kurjak A, Kupesic-Urek S & Miric D (1992) The assessment of benign uterine tumor vascularization by transvaginal color Doppler. *Ultrasound Med Biol* **18**: 645–649.

Liebsohn S, d'Ablaing G, Mishell DR & Schlaerth JB (1990) Leiomyosarcoma in a series of hysterectomies performed for presumed uterine leiomyomas. *Am J Obstet Gynecol* **162**: 968–976.

McCarthy S (1990) Magnetic resonance imaging in the evaluation of infertile women. *Magn Reson Q* **6**: 239–249.

Meloni AM, Surti U, Contento AM, Davare J & Sandberg AA (1992) Uterine leiomyomas: cytogenetic and histologic profile. *Obstet Gynecol* **80**: 209–217.

Montague AC, Swartz DP & Woodruff JD (1965) Sarcoma arising in a leiomyoma of the uterus. *Am J Obstet Gynecol* **92**: 421–427.

Novak ER & Woodruff JD (eds) (1979) Sarcoma and allied lesions of the uterus. In *Novak's Gynecological and Obstetric Pathology*, 8th edn, pp 291–305. Philadelphia: WB Saunders.

Osmers R, Völksen M & Schauer A (1990) Vaginosonography for early detection of endometrial carcinoma? *Lancet* **335**: 1569–1571.

Parsons AK & Lense JJ (1993) Sonohysterography for endometrial abnormalities: preliminary results. *J Clin Ultrasound* **21**: 87–95.

Stock RJ & Kanbour A (1975) Prehysterectomy curettage. *Obstet Gynecol* **45**: 537–541.

van Roessel J, Wamsteker K & Exalto N (1987) Sonographic investigation of the uterus during artificial uterine cavity distension. *J Clin Ultrasound* **15**: 439–450.

Wamsteker K & de Blok S (1993) Diagnostic hysteroscopy: technique and documentation. In Sutton C & Diamond MP (eds) *Endoscopic Surgery for Gynaecologists*, pp 263–276. London: WB Saunders.

Wamsteker K, Emanuel MH & de Kruif JH (1993) Transcervical hysteroscopic resection of submucous fibroids for abnormal uterine bleeding: results regarding the degree of intramural extension. *Obstet Gynecol* **82**: 736–740.

Zawin M, McCarthy S, Scoutt LM & Comite F (1990) High-field MRI and US evaluation of the pelvis in women with leiomyomas. *Magn Reson Imaging* **8**: 371–376.

17 *Endometrial cancer and uterine sarcoma*
D Timmerman and I Vergote

ENDOMETRIAL CANCER

■ SYMPTOMS AND THEIR RELATIONSHIP TO PATHOLOGY

In many Western countries endometrial cancer is the most common gynecological malignancy. Survival is generally good because most cases present at an early stage with abnormal vaginal bleeding. Ninety percent of patients with endometrial cancer are postmenopausal (Pettersson, 1991). Endometrial cancer is found in 10–15% of women with postmenopausal bleeding. Other causes of postmenopausal bleeding include exogenous estrogens (30%), atrophic endometritis or vaginitis (30%), endometrial or cervical polyps (10%), endometrial hyperplasia (5%) and other diseases, such as uterine sarcoma, trauma and cervical cancer (10%) (Hacker, 1994). Probably about 5% of endometrial cancers are found in patients without any vaginal bleeding (Carter and Twiggs, 1993). Occasionally, a pyometra or endometrial cells on a Papanicolaou smear in asymptomatic postmenopausal women are the first signs of endometrial cancer. The risk of endometrial cancer is strongly related to the exposure to unopposed estrogens. Estrogen replacement therapy, obesity and estrogen-secreting tumors are considered as risk factors, whereas oral contraceptives, progesterone therapy and early menopause exert a risk reduction (La Vecchia et al, 1984; Lesko et al, 1985; Parazzini et al, 1991, 1995).

■ CLINICAL INVESTIGATIONS

DETECTION OF ENDOMETRIAL CANCER IN PATIENTS WITH POSTMENOPAUSAL BLEEDING

Despite a false negative rate of 2–6% (Granberg et al, 1991), the histopathological diagnosis obtained at *curettage* is used as the gold standard for distinguishing between benign and malignant endometrium. Several methods have been developed to reduce the need for curettage. *Aspiration methods* have never been able to decrease significantly the number of curettages performed in women with postmenopausal bleeding. Using *transvaginal sonography* (TVS) a thin hyporeflective endometrial line can be seen in postmenopausal patients. Atrophic endometrium is characterized by a maximal total endometrial thickness of less than 5 mm (Nasri et al, 1991; Varner et al, 1991; Karlsson et al, 1993). The false negative rate of TVS for the detection of pathology is similar to other existing techniques, such as dilatation and curretage (D&C), and in the best hands TVS is a very reliable tool for excluding endometrial cancer (Granberg et al, 1991; Karlsson et al, 1995; Dijkhuizen et al, 1996). It may therefore be possible to reduce the number of operative procedures by about 50% if patients with postmenopausal bleeding and an endometrial thickness of more than 4 mm were to be referred for diagnostic hysteroscopy or D&C; however, in less experienced hands a surprisingly high rate of endometrial cancer has been reported among patients with postmenopausal bleeding associated with an endometrial thickness of less than 5 mm (15/212) (Dørum et al, 1993; Schramm et al, 1995; Seelbach–Göbel et al, 1995). Although many recent papers (*Table 17.1*) advise that curettage be limited to patients with postmenopausal bleeding associated with an endometrial thickness of ≥ 5 mm at ultrasonography, we recommend that an office endometrial sampling be performed in

Table 17.1 *Prevalence of endometrial cancer in patients with postmenopausal bleeding in relation to (double layer) endometrial thickness (ET) at transvaginal sonography*

Reference	ET < 5 mm	ET ≥ 5 mm	Mean ET in endometrial cancer (mm)
Nasri and Coast (1989)	0/37	7/63	24.4 (11.5–38)
Goldstein et al (1990)	0/11	1/19	NR
Osmers et al (1990)	0/46	13/57	NR
Bourne et al (1991)*	0/NR	17/NR	20 (6–41)
Ghirardini et al (1991)	0/30	5/8	NR
Granberg et al (1991)	0/150	18/55	18.2 (9–35)
Nasri et al (1991)	0/51	6/42	22.2 (8–38)
Smith et al (1991)	0/22	4/23	18.2 (14–22)
Dørum et al (1993)	3/54	12/45	20 (2–30)
Karlsson et al (1993)*	0/≤57	15/≥48	NR (5–NR)
Kurjak et al (1993)*	0/NR	35/NR	NR
Dhont and Beghin (1994)	0/34	12/48	NR
Sladkevicius et al (1994)*	0/NR	23/NR	24 (7–56)
Emanuel et al (1995)*	0/NR	7/NR	14.3 (9–20)
Karlsson et al (1995)	0/518	114/620	21.2 (5–68)
Malinova and Pehlivanov (1995)*	0/≤35	57/≥83	18.4 (7–40)
Schramm et al (1995)	10/74	19/121	11 (0–20)
Seelbach-Göbel et al (1995)	2/86	37/146	23.6 (NR)
Van den Bosch et al (1995)*	0/NR	6NR	22.5 (13–35)
Total	15/1113	248/1247	

* *Not included for statistical analysis (insufficient data).*

NR, not recorded.

Overall prevalence of endometrial carcinoma: 11.1%.

TVS (5 mm cut off): sensitivity 94.3%; specificity 52.4%; positive predictive value 19.9%; negative predictive value 98.6%; accuracy 57.0%.

patients presenting with postmenopausal bleeding and with an endometrial thickness of less than 5 mm*. From the meta-analysis (*Table 17.1*) of reported studies we can conclude that endometrial cancer will be found in 11% of patients presenting with postmenopausal bleeding. If the subsequent TVS reveals an endometrial thickness of 5 mm or more, this figure rises to 20%. With an endometrial thickness of less than 5 mm, the risk for endometrial cancer in patients with postmenopausal bleeding is only 1.4%.

The initial reports on the use of *color Doppler sonography* were promising (Hata et al, 1989; Bourne et al, 1991; Mercé et al, 1991) but more recent reports suggest that the contribution of a Doppler examination to the differential diagnosis in women with postmenopausal bleeding is very limited (Carter et al, 1994; Sladkevicius et al, 1994).

Using a negative contrast agent (e.g. normal saline), *sonohysterography* has the potential to improve the diagnostic performance of transvaginal sonography (Bourne et al, 1994; Gaucherand et al, 1995). It can be used as a secondary test in patients with a thickened endometrial line at TVS, to distinguish between intracavitary polyps or fibroids and endometrial thickening (hyperplasia or carcinoma) (Parsons and Lense, 1993; Cohen et al, 1994; Goldstein, 1994). This may allow appropriate preoperative triage for operative hysteroscopy.

Three-dimensional ultrasonography can still be considered as an experimental technique for the evaluation of endometrial pathology.

Endometrial cancer shows a variety of appearances at *diagnostic hysteroscopy*. It can appear as polypoid tumors, usually with atypical vascular architecture, such as tortuosity

* *Editorial comment* There is no international consensus for what should be regarded as the cut off level for the endometrial thickness (double layer) for detecting endometrial abnormality at transvaginal ultrasonography.

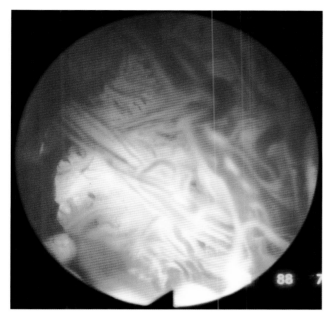

17.1a

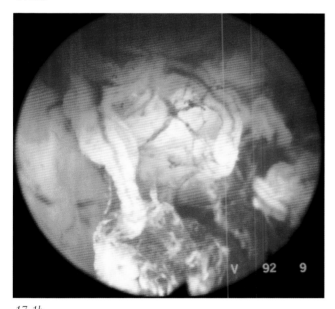

17.1b

Figure 17.1: (a) Hysteroscopic appearance of well differentiated adeno-carcinoma of the endometrium; note the abnormal vascular architecture and the papillary structures predominantly consisting of dilated blood vessels. (b) Hysteroscopic appearance of well differentiated papillary adenocarcinoma of the endometrium; note the irregular white papillary structures and the atypical vascular architecture with caliber changes; on the left side normal smooth atrophic endometrium can be observed.

and caliber changes. Sometimes typical papillary proliferations can be observed in well differentiated tumors (*Figure 17.1*). More extended endometrial malignancies appear as broadly based irregular, raw and polypous masses covering a major part of the uterine cavity. Necrotic, fragile and easily bleeding tissue may be observed. Usually the extension of

the tumor into the endocervix can be clearly determined, which enables a preoperative differentiation between stage I and stage II cases. Although endometrial malignancy generally will be suspected by experienced hysteroscopists from the macroscopic appearance, histological diagnosis of tissue specimens obtained by directed biopsies or curettage is always mandatory to confirm the diagnosis.

Hysteroscopy was found to be superior to curettage in 276 women with abnormal bleeding in making an accurate diagnosis of pathological conditions in the uterine cavity (Gimpelson and Rappold, 1988). In 45 women with postmenopausal bleeding hysteroscopy had a higher specificity but a lower sensitivity for the detection of endometrial pathology compared with TVS (Cacciatore et al, 1994). In this study, hysteroscopy failed to detect two out of four endometrial cancers. Other studies, however, have indicated that hysteroscopy may increase the chance of early detection of small endometrial cancers and facilitates the determination of location, size and extent of the neoplasia and/or its precursors (see Chapters 3 and 13). Some authors suggest that hysteroscopy with biopsy is superior to curettage for evaluation of endometrial pathology and should be preferred for further evaluation in case of abnormal or inconclusive sonographic findings (Emanuel et al, 1995; Dijkhuizen et al, 1996) (see also Chapter 2).

Finally the debate as to whether hysteroscopy (or sonohysterography) can worsen the prognosis of endometrial cancer by retrograde seeding of malignant cells has not yet ended (Romano et al, 1992) (see also Chapter 3).

Magnetic resonance imaging (MRI) is not useful in the detection of endometrial carcinoma. The signal intensity of endometrial carcinoma is often similar to normal high intensity endometrium on T_2-weighted images (Popovich and Hricak, 1994).

The algorithm in *Figure 17.2* summarizes the investigations in postmenopausal patients presenting with bleeding or with an enlarged uterus.

STAGING OF ENDOMETRIAL CANCER

The classical staging procedures in endometrial cancer are physical examination and chest X-ray.

Transabdominal sonography (TAS) is considered to be unreliable for staging of endometrial cancer (Requard et

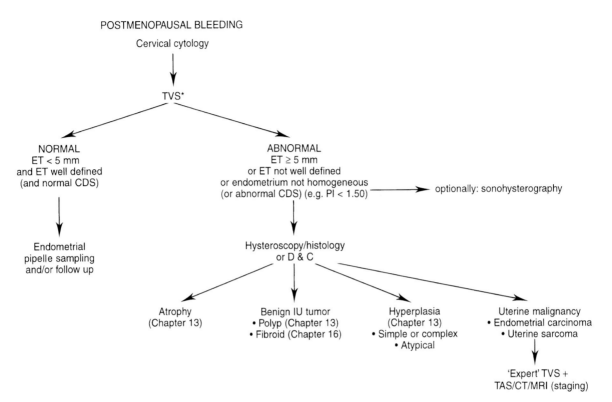

Figure 17.2: Investigations for the detection of endometrial cancer in postmenopausal patients. CDS, Color Doppler sonography; CT, computed tomography; D&C, dilatation and curettage; ET, endometrial thickness; IU, intrauterine; MRI, magnetic resonance imaging; PI, pulsatility index; TAS, transabdominal sonography; TVS, transvaginal sonography. * *In cases with enlarged uterus TAS should be added. (*Editorial Comment: *Note that there is no international consensus for what should be regarded as the cut off level for the endometrial thickness (double layer) for detecting endometrial abnormality at transvaginal ultrasonography.)*

al, 1981), whereas TVS can be helpful in predicting the depth of myometrial invasion (Karlsson et al, 1992; Artner et al, 1994; Prömpeler et al, 1994). The low cost and absence of ionizing radiation are the obvious advantages of this technique. The disadvantages include operator and machine dependency and the limited depth of visualization, which prevents proper evaluation of the pelvic lymph nodes.

Diagnostic hysteroscopy with directed biopsies can be applied for determination of the extension of the tumor into the endocervix, assisting in the pretreatment staging between stage I and stage II cases (see also Clinical Investigations).

Computed tomography (CT) is similar to MRI in that it can offer a complete delineation of the pelvis and the abdomen and it has an ability to detect involved lymph nodes. On the other hand, it is an expensive examination that utilizes ionizing radiation. In our opinion, however, CT of the abdomen could be performed to exclude metastases in the upper abdomen or in

retroperitoneal lymph nodes. Even if TVS suggests little or no myometrial invasion (stage Ia or Ib), a lymphadenectomy should be performed if CT shows pathological lymph nodes.

MRI combines an absence of ionizing radiation with images of greater inherent tissue contrast than CT images. Additionally, it makes imaging in various planes possible. Contrast enhanced images are highly accurate for staging of endometrial cancer (depth of myometrial invasion, extension into the cervix and detection of extrauterine disease) (Popovich and Hricak, 1994). It is, however, not better than CT for detecting pathological lymph nodes. The main disadvantage is that MRI is a very expensive technique.

Cystoscopy can be useful for staging patients with endometrial cancer if extension of the disease into the bladder is suspected.

A recent retrospective study of *preoperative colonoscopy* in 212 gynecological oncology patients found 17 cases of colonic polyps, five cases of synchronous colon cancer and two cases of cancer metastatic to the colon. The authors concluded that colon screening is not needed in the asymptomatic patient under 50 years of age but a full colonoscopy during the preoperative investigations in patients aged 70 or over seems to be appropriate (Saltzman et al, 1995).

SCREENING FOR ENDOMETRIAL CANCER

Screening for endometrial cancer in asymptomatic women has become technically feasible by the introduction of *high resolution TVS* and *office endometrial sampling techniques (Figure 17.3).*

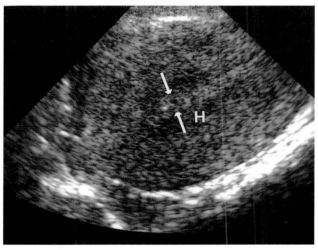

17.3a

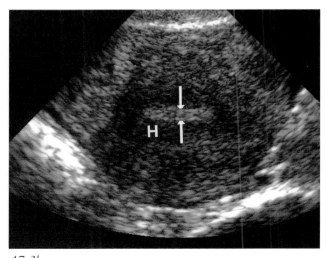

17.3b

Figure 17.3: *Transvaginal sonographic image of a normal and thin endometrial line (between arrows) surrounded by an intact myometrial halo (H). (a) Longitudinal view. (b) Transverse view.*

TVS with color flow imaging and blood flow analysis might improve the accuracy of endometrial thickness measurements alone. More prospective studies in this area are required.

Currently it is not indicated that all postmenopausal women should be regularly screened with TVS or other techniques (e.g. pipelle de Cornier). The final answer to the most important question of whether screening for the presence of endometrial pathology really does benefit the patient can only be offered by very large randomized trials, but given the low incidence of the disease and the fact that it seems to present early, screening is unlikely to be of value. In the mean time it seems to make sense to use TVS to screen postmenopausal patients at *high risk* for endometrial carcinoma. These would include women with a personal or familial history of several epithelial cancers (e.g. breast, ovary, endometrium).

In cases of thickened or otherwise abnormal endometrium or inconclusive sonographic findings further investigation is indicated. Office endometrium sampling (e.g. pipelle de Cornier) could be the first step to exclude endometrial cancer (Silver et al, 1991; Fothergill et al, 1992; Goldschmit et al, 1993; Van den Bosch et al, 1995); however, diagnostic hysteroscopy with tissue sampling or D&C should be performed in case of doubt.

A special group of patients at risk consists of postmenopausal breast cancer patients treated with *tamoxifen*. It has been extensively shown that these patients are more likely to develop endometrial polyps, hyperplasia and endometrial cancer (Hardell, 1988; Neven et al, 1989; Corley et al, 1992; Kedar et al, 1994; Timmerman and Vergote, 1996). After treatment with tamoxifen the endometrial appearance at TVS typically changes from a postmenopausal, atrophic (1–2 mm) endometrium into a characteristic endometrial pattern: it thickens and becomes hyperechogenic, with or without the presence of cysts. The junctional area is irregular and not clearly defined. In most of these cases hysteroscopy shows only an apparent atrophic endometrium with many cysts (*Figure 17.4*). The histological findings are most often consistent with an atrophic endometrium (Perrot et al, 1994). Some authors suggest the routine use of hysteroscopy as a screening method in postmenopausal

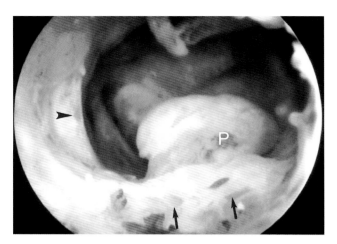

Figure 17.4: *Hysteroscopic image of the endometrial cavity of the postmenopausal patient with breast cancer treated with tamoxifen. There is a polyp (P) on the posterior wall. Note the presence of thin and friable endometrium (arrows) and microcysts (arrowhead). Courtesy of the Department of Obstetrics and Gynecology, Algemene kliniek St-Jan, Brussels 1000.*

breast cancer patients treated with tamoxifen (Neven et al, 1994). On the other hand some large polyps might prove difficult to detect at hysteroscopy but can easily be detected by sonohysterography (Bourne et al, 1994). Again, larger studies need to be awaited to know whether screening for endometrial pathology is indicated for patients treated with tamoxifen and, if so, what screening protocol should be used.

■ INTERPRETATION OF FINDINGS

CHARACTERISTICS

ULTRASONOGRAPHY *(Figures 17.5 and 17.6)*

General appearance of endometrial cancer (Carter and Twiggs, 1993; Kurjak et al, 1993)

- Thickened endometrium (hyperechoic (45%) or mixed echogenic (45%) or hypoechogenic (10%).
- Uterus enlarged and distended.
- Absence of a central echodense line.
- Structure of endometrium is not homogeneous
- Irregular margins of the uterine cavity.
- Ascites may be found.
- Presence of significant intrauterine fluid (variable importance in different studies).

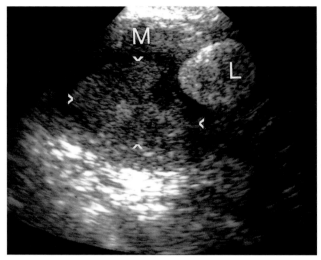

17.5a

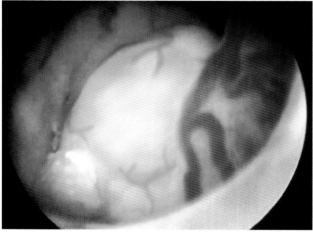

17.5b

Figure 17.5: *(a) Transvaginal sonographic appearance of a well differentiated endometrial adenocarcinoma, stage Ib (between arrows). Note the presence of a well circumscribed hyperreflective intramural (M) leiomyoma (L). In the posterior wall the myometrial halo has disappeared as a result of tumor invasion. (b) Hysteroscopic view of another endometrial adenocarcinoma. Typically a pronounced neovascularization is present. Courtesy of the Department of Obstetrics and Gynecology, Algemene kliniek St-Jan, Brussels 1000.*

Assistance in staging of endometrial cancer (Cacciatore et al, 1989; Karlsson et al, 1992)

Stage Ia: absence of myometrial invasion. No endometrial echoes or an intact halo surrounding the endometrial echoes. Stage Ic: myometrial invasion > 50%. Diameter of total endometrial echo is more than 50% of the diameter of the anteroposterior uterine distance in the longitudinal plane or in the transverse plane.

Stage II: tumor extension to the cervix. No clear demarcation of the endometrial echo towards the cervical canal.

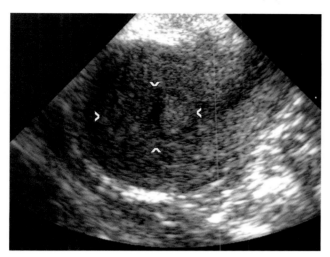

17.6a

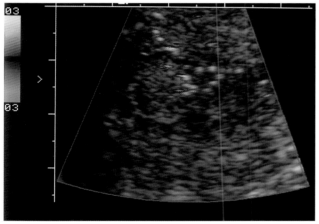

17.6b

Figure 17.6: *Endometrial clear cell adenocarcinoma (between arrowheads) in a 47 year old patient with menometrorrhagia for 5 months. Although the invasion was limited to the inner half of the myometrium and the cervix was free of disease, two lymph nodes in the obturator fossa were invaded by the tumor (stage IIIc). (a) Transvaginal sonographic image (longitudinal view). (b) Transvaginal color Doppler image. The tumor contained multiple small blood vessels (red).*

MRI (Popovich and Hricak, 1994)

Assistance in staging of endometrial cancer

Stage Ia: without myometrial invasion (junctional zone preserved).

Stage Ib: with myometrial invasion (disruption of the junctional zone and tumor limited to inner half of myometrium).

Stage Ic: with myometrial invasion (tumor extension into the outer half).

Stage II: with tumor extension into the cervix.

Stage III and IV: with extrauterine disease.

DIAGNOSTIC PITFALLS

The problems affecting the accuracy of ultrasonography include polypoid growths of endometrial cancer and the presence of adenomyosis and myomas deforming the uterine shape and volume.

In symptomatic women if it is not possible to measure the endometrial thickness with TVS, then an invasive procedure (hysteroscopy and/or D&C) is indicated.

Over one third of premenopausal patients with endometrial cancer present with heavy but regular periods.

Postmenopausal breast cancer patients treated with tamoxifen can display a variety of abnormal endometrial images.

Pitfalls and artifacts in color Doppler ultrasound are beyond the scope of this chapter and have been described elsewhere (Zalud and Kurjak 1994).

DIFFERENTIAL DIAGNOSIS (AT ULTRASONOGRAPHY)

It should be noted that abnormal ultrasonographic findings always warrant further investigation leading to a histopathological diagnosis (*Figure 17.2*).

ENDOMETRIAL HYPERPLASIA

- Highly reflective, thick endometrium.
- Often homogeneous structure of endometrium, sometimes loose with echo-free areas.
- Intact halo surrounding endometrium.
- Sonomorphological differentiation of different forms of hyperplasia or endometrial cancer is not possible.

TREATMENT WITH TAMOXIFEN OR HORMONE REPLACEMENT THERAPY

- Very thick endometrium with or without the presence of cysts. If polyps are suspected sonohysterography may be used.

ENDOMETRIAL POLYPS

- Easily visualized with sonohysterography (or three-dimensional ultrasonography) (*Figure 17.7*).

ENDOMETRITIS

- Presence of intrauterine free fluid also possible.
- Clinical presentation.

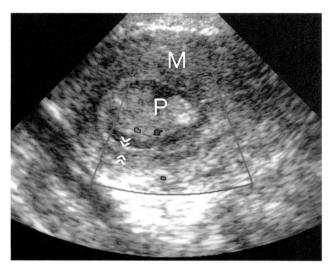

17.7a

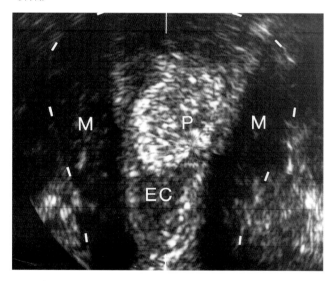

17.7b

Figure 17.7: *Endometrial polyp (2.1 × 1.0 cm) in a 35 year old nulligravid patient. (a) Transvaginal sonographic image of the polyp (P) surrounded by some intracavitary blood. The endometrium (between double arrowheads) measured only 2 mm (single layer). (b) Reconstructed image of the endometrial cavity (EC) and the same polyp (P) in the absence of intracavitary blood (three-dimensional ultrasound, Kretztechnik Aktiengesellschaft, Zipf, Austria). Dotted lines indicate the outline of the myometrium.*

UTERINE SARCOMA

Mixed Müllerian tumor or endometrial stromal sarcoma (*Figure 17.8*).

- Thickened hyperechoic endometrium.
- Enlarged uterus.
- No intact halo surrounding endometrium.
- Polypoid endometrial tumor.

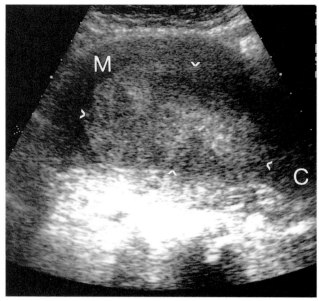

17.8a

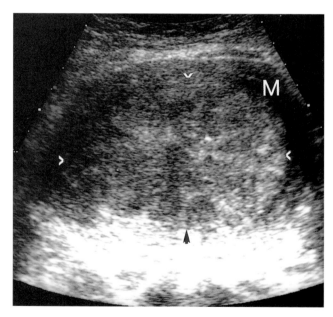

17.8b

Figure 17.8: *(a)–(e) Images of a large uterine carcinosarcoma.*

ADENOMYOSIS

- Asymmetrical uterine enlargement.
- Distorted endometrial and myometrial echo texture (Brosens et al, 1995).
- Occasionally small cystic areas.
- Usually there are no outer feeding arteries around the adenomyomatous lesion without distinct contour (Hirai et al, 1995).
- MRI is highly accurate in the detection and characterization of both focal

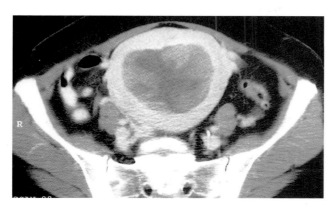

17.8c

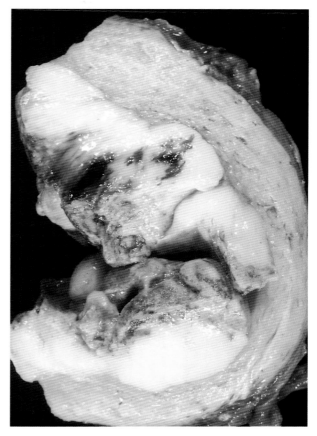

17.8e

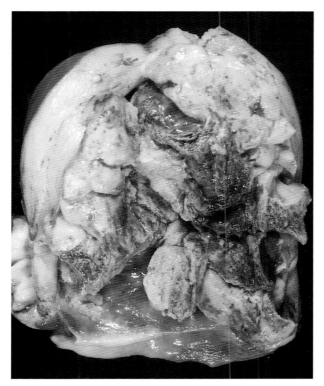

17.8d

Figure 17.8: *(cont.)Images of a large uterine carcinosarcoma (stage I mixed Müllerian tumor) in a 58 year old patient. The invasion was limited to the inner half of the myometrium (M) and the cervix (C) was free of disease. (a) Transabdominal ultrasonography revealed a large (9.9 × 9.2 × 6.6 cm) oval-shaped intrauterine mass with hyper- and hyporeflective areas (between arrowheads). Longitudinal view. (b) Transverse view. (c) CT image of this large intrauterine mass after contrast injection. (d) Surgical specimen of the uterus with a polypoid mass protruding into the uterine cavity. (e) There was limited myometrial invasion. Note the green necrotic areas.*

and diffuse adenomyosis (Togashi et al, 1989). Diffuse adenomyosis is suspected when the myometrial zonal anatomy is distorted by a diffuse and irregular thickening of the junctional zone. Focal adenomyosis appears as mixed signal intensity lesions with ill defined margins (Mark et al, 1987).

HYDATIDIFORM MOLE

Unusual in this age group.

- Typical 'grape-like' vesicles, usually only present in second trimester.
- In the first trimester the sonographic picture is not specific. The enlarged uterus contains an echogenic oval mass within a gestational sac, or it may appear as a heterogeneous mass within an enlarged uterus (DeBaz and Lewis, 1995).

- Color Doppler sonography seems to be useful in these patients. An association between pulsatility index, beta human chorionic gonadotropin (ß-hCG) and prognosis has been reported (Carter et al, 1993).
- CT or MRI findings are helpful (DeBaz and Lewis, 1995).

MISSED ABORTION

Unusual in this age group.

- Large hyperechoic mass filling the uterine cavity.

SENSITIVITY AND SPECIFICITY OF DIAGNOSTIC TECHNIQUES

See *Table 17.2.*

Table 17.2 *Sensitivity and specificity of diagnostic techniques – endometrial cancer*

Technique	Sensitivity (%)	Specificity (%)	Accuracy (%)	References
Curettage	94–98	±100	—	Granberg et al (1991)
Screening with TVS	94	52	57	*Table 17.1*
Deep myometrial invasion				
with TVS	79	100	87	Karlsson et al (1992)
	93	71	81	Prömpeler et al (1994)
	80	77	78	Cagnazzo et al (1992)
with MRI	87	78	83	Cagnazzo et al (1992)
	—	—	85	Hricak et al (1991)
	88	85	86	Sironi et al (1992)

■ CLASSIFICATION AND ITS USE IN CLINICAL MANAGEMENT

For details of the current classification, see Chapter 29.

UTERINE SARCOMA

■ SYMPTOMS AND THEIR RELATIONSHIP TO PATHOLOGY

Uterine sarcoma is a rare tumor, accounting for only 2–6% of malignant tumors of the corpus uteri (Olah and Kingston, 1994). In a retrospective analysis of 318 cases of uterine sarcoma, one sarcoma was found for every 11 endometrial adenocarcinomas (Olah et al, 1991). The age at presentation ranged from 24 to 95 years (mean 60.5 years). Mixed Müllerian tumors tend to occur predominantly in postmenopausal patients, whereas endometrial stromal sarcomas and leiomyosarcomas usually present in younger women. Abnormal vaginal bleeding is a presenting symptom in 76% of cases. *Tables 17.3* and *17.4* list the presenting symptoms and signs.

Multiple possible risk factors for uterine sarcomas have been suggested by several authors (Zaloudek and Norris, 1981; Olah et al, 1991; Schwartz et al, 1993; Olah and Kingston, 1994); they include nulliparity or low parity (not for leiomyosarcoma), previous breast cancer (leiomyosarcoma), previous pelvic irradiation (for mixed Müllerian tumors), previous endocervical or endometrial 'polyps' (for adenosarcoma and adenofibroma) and obesity, diabetes and hypertension (only for carcinosarcoma).

Table 17.3 *Presenting symptoms in uterine sarcoma*

Symptom	%
Postmenopausal bleeding (especially in MMT and ESS)	49
Abdominal pain	27
Abdominal distension	20
Menstrual irregularity	15
Menorrhagia	12
Urinary symptoms (e.g. dysuria, frequency)	11
Weight loss	5.5
Bowel symptoms	5.5
Infertility	1

*ESS, Endometrial stromal sarcomas; MMT, mixed Müllerian tumors.
Adapted from Olah et al (1991).*

Table 17.4 *Presenting signs in uterine sarcoma*

Sign	%
Enlarged uterus	78
Mass/polyp visible on speculum examination (especially in MMT and ESS)	18
Parametrial involvement (sometimes rubbery parametrial induration)	12
Pelvic mass (other than uterus)	8.5
Lymphadenopathy	3
Ascites	2.5
Hepatomegaly	1.5

*ESS, Endometrial stromal sarcomas; MMT, mixed Müllerian tumors.
Adapted from Olah et al (1991) and Olah and Kingston (1994).*

■ CLINICAL INVESTIGATIONS

Since uterine sarcoma is a rare tumor, the various imaging techniques in this malignancy have only been described in case reports and small series. It is therefore difficult to compare the accuracy of the different techniques.

A negative result with the *cervical Papanicolaou smear* does not give any information. A positive result can only be obtained if the sarcoma is endometrial, polypoid and friable, and even then cytological interpretation is difficult (Bennani et al, 1995).

Diagnostically *curettage* is a good tool for endometrial stromal sarcoma and mixed Müllerian tumors (positive in 50–70% of women with carcinosarcoma). Curettage is not reliable in diagnosing leiomyosarcoma (Olah and Kingston, 1994). Overall, curettage or biopsies from intravaginal masses were diagnostic in 20–60 % of cases (Bennani et al, 1995), whereas experience with *hysteroscopy* and *hysterosalpingography* is limited.

TAS cannot differentiate between leiomyosarcoma and a benign leiomyoma (which is 800 times more common) (Hata et al, 1990).

The images obtained with *TVS* are also nonspecific. In a review of 20 patients with uterine leiomyosarcoma, the tumor presented as the largest or the only uterine mass in 19 patients (95%) (Schwartz et al, 1993); it has therefore been suggested that the largest myoma should be monitored closely during conservative management of a uterus containing leiomyomas. Mixed Müllerian tumors and endometrial stromal sarcomas were associated with a heterogeneous pattern with high intensity and hypoechoic areas scattered in the myometrium in five cases out of seven. In the remaining two cases the sonographic picture was indistinguishable from that of leiomyomas. The depth of invasion was correctly predicted in five cases and there was a slight overestimation of the invasion in two cases (Cacciatore et al, 1989). In a clinicopathological study of 25 cases of uterine adenosarcoma the only morphological feature that correlated with the aggressive behavior of this tumor was deep myometrial invasion (Zaloudek and Norris, 1981).

The experience with *color Doppler sonography* in uterine sarcoma is too limited to draw any conclusion. The presence of irregular, thin, randomly dispersed vessels with low impedance (resistance index (RI) 0.32–0.42) as well as low velocity (peak systolic velocity 9–27 cm/s) of the intra- and peritumoral blood flow was found in eight uterine sarcomas (Kurjak and Shalan, 1994). On the contrary, Hata and colleagues did find a normal impedance (RI 0.77) and a high velocity (peak systolic velocity 124 cm/s) in a case of uterine leiomyosarcoma (Hata et al, 1990). Another report described the presence of a

low impedance (RI 0.286) in a high grade endometrial stromal sarcoma compared with an RI of 0.523 in a low grade endometrial stromal sarcoma (Tepper et al, 1994). We found rather low impedance vessels (RI 0.55; pulsatility index 0.88) and a rather high velocity (29 cm/s) in a large uterine carcinosarcoma (mixed Müllerian tumor) (*Figure 17.8*). These values are commonly encountered in large uterine leiomyomas. This seems to limit the possibilities for differential diagnosis between a sarcoma and a leiomyoma, based on color Doppler sonography.

CT findings in 118 patients with leiomyosarcoma were reviewed by McLeod and colleagues. The series included 19 uterine leiomyosarcomas. The CT appearance was not specific, but a large mass with central necrosis or liquefaction was a frequent finding. Calcification was not observed (McLeod et al, 1984).

MRI was more accurate than CT in delineating the extent and tissue characteristics in a case of uterine leiomyosarcoma (Janus et al, 1989). Malignant degeneration should be considered on magnetic resonance images of any degenerated leiomyoma showing an irregular contour (Pattani et al, 1995).

We can conclude that there are no pathognomonic features for detecting a sarcoma with an imaging technique. The ultimate diagnosis will always be based on histopathological examination of resected specimens.

■ INTERPRETATION OF FINDINGS

CHARACTERISTICS

ULTRASONOGRAPHY

Leiomyosarcoma

- Large size (usually 5–18 cm).
- Broad based and pedunculated and have no preferential uterine location.
- Ninety five percent of cases limited to one mass (Schwartz et al, 1993).
- Enlarged uterus with an inhomogeneous and bizarre internal echo pattern at transabdominal sonography (Hata et al, 1990).
- Mixed high echogenic part and a poor echogenic part surrounded by a thinned myometrium (Hata et al, 1990).

Mixed Müllerian tumor or endometrial stromal sarcoma

See differential diagnosis in endometrial cancer, p. 206.

MRI

Leiomyosarcoma

- Tumor with heterogeneous areas consistent with debris and hemorrhage within the lesion. Absence of calcification.
- 'Degenerated leiomyoma' with an irregular contour (Pattani et al, 1995).

Mixed Müllerian tumor

- Massive invasive endocervical and/or intracavitary mass without unique magnetic resonance signal intensity characteristics; may simulate invasive endometrial carcinoma. Mildly inhomogeneous, low intensity mass on T_1-weighted images, heterogeneous appearance on T_2-weighted images (Worthington et al, 1986).

DIAGNOSTIC PITFALLS

Curettage, endometrial sampling or hysteroscopy are not reliable for the diagnosis of leiomyosarcoma. The histopathology will only be positive in patients with submucosal leiomyosarcomas (Schwartz et al, 1993).

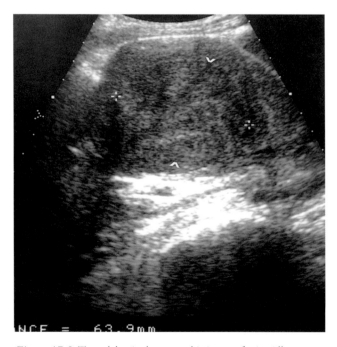

Figure 17.9: Transabdominal sonographic image of a 'rapidly growing tumor' (between calipers) (6.4 × 5.0 cm) in a 34 year old patient. Five months later the tumor measured 9.5 × 7.5 cm. Only after hysterectomy could the presence of a sarcoma be completely excluded. The tumor consisted of a benign submucous leiomyoma with degenerated areas.

In cases of carcinosarcoma curettage will be diagnostically helpful in only 50–70% of patients (Olah and Kingston, 1994).

The various imaging techniques are nonspecific so that in uterine masses managed conservatively close follow up should be arranged to detect rapid growth of a possible uterine sarcoma (*Figure 17.9*).

DIFFERENTIAL DIAGNOSIS

ENDOMETRIAL CANCER

See p. 204.

LEIOMYOMAS

- Concentric round masses with distinct margins (size varying usually between microscopic and 5 cm).
- False capsule of compressed myometrium with peripheral flow on color Doppler sonography.
- Sharply defined, homogeneous masses of decreased signal intensity on routine MRI.
- Can undergo degeneration (cystic, hyaline, fatty myxomatous or mucinous). On T_2-weighted MRI, degenerated leiomyomas have a variable appearance.

SENSITIVITY AND SPECIFICITY OF DIAGNOSTIC TECHNIQUES

- Curettage: sensitivity 20–60%; specificity ?; accuracy? (Bennani et al, 1995).

The reported series are too small to obtain reliable figures for the other diagnostic techniques.

■ CLASSIFICATION AND ITS USE IN CLINICAL MANAGEMENT

Mixed Müllerian tumors and endometrial stromal sarcomas arise within the endometrial cavity, whereas leiomyosarcomas arise within the myometrium. Patients with mixed Müllerian tumors present with more advanced disease than those with either leiomyosarcomas or endometrial stromal sarcomas (Olah et al, 1991).

No staging system for uterine sarcoma has been proposed by the International Federation of Gynecology and Obstetrics (FIGO) but customarily the FIGO staging for endometrial adenocarcinoma has been adopted for these tumors (Quinn et al, 1992):

Stage I: sarcoma confined to uterus.

Stage II: sarcoma involving corpus and cervix.

Stage II: sarcoma spread beyond uterus, not outside the pelvis.

Stage IV: sarcoma spread beyond uterus, outside the pelvis or into bladder/rectum.

REFERENCES

Artner A, Bösze P & Gonda G (1994) The value of ultrasound in preoperative assessment of the myometrial and cervical invasion in endometrial carcinoma. *Gynecol Oncol* **54**: 147–151.

Bennani O, Himmi A, Laghzaomi M et al (1995) Les sarcomes de l'uterus: à propos de 25 cas. *Rev Fr Gynécol Obstet* **90**: 12–16.

Bourne TH, Campbell S, Steer CV et al (1991) Detection of endometrial cancer by transvaginal ultrasonography with color flow imaging and blood flow analysis: a preliminary report. *Gynecol Oncol* **40**: 253–259.

Bourne TH, Lawton F, Leather A et al (1994) Use of intracavity saline instillation and transvaginal ultrasonography to detect tamoxifen-associated endometrial polyps. *Ultrasound Obstet Gynecol* **4**: 73–75.

Brosens JJ, de Souza NM, Barker FG et al (1995) Endovaginal ultrasonography in the diagnosis of adenomyosis uteri: identifying the predictive characteristics. *Br J Obstet Gynaecol* **102**: 471–474.

Cacciatore B, Lehtovirta P, Wahlström J et al (1989) Ultrasound findings in uterine mixed Müllerian sarcomas and endometrial stromal sarcomas. *Gynecol Oncol* **35**: 290–293.

Cacciatore B, Ramsay T, Lehtovirta P et al (1994) Transvaginal sonography and hysteroscopy in postmenopausal bleeding. *Acta Obstet Gynecol Scand* **73**: 413–416.

Cagnazzo G, D'Addario V, Martinelli G et al (1992) Depth of myometrial invasion in endometrial cancer: preoperative assessment by transvaginal ultrasonography and magnetic resonance imaging. *Ultrasound Obstet Gynecol* **2**: 40–43.

Carter J, Fowler J, Carlson J et al (1993) Transvaginal color flow Doppler sonography in the assessment of gestational trophoblastic disease. *J Ultrasound Med* **12**: 595–599.

Carter JR & Twiggs LB (1993) The role of transvaginal sonography in gynecologic oncology. In Studd J (ed.) *Progress in Obstetrics and Gynaecology*, vol. **10**, pp 341–357. London: Churchill Livingstone.

Carter JR, Lan M & Saltzman AK (1994) Gray scale and color flow Doppler characterisation of uterine tumors. *J Ultrasound Med* **13**: 835–840.

Cohen JR, Luxman D, Sagi J et al (1994) Sonohysterography for distinguishing endometrial thickening from endometrial polyps in postmenopausal bleeding. *Ultrasound Obstet Gynecol* **4**: 227–230.

Corley D, Rowe J, Curtis MT et al (1992) Postmenopausal bleeding from unusual endometrial polyps in women on chronic tamoxifen therapy. *Obstet Gynecol* **79**: 111–116.

DeBaz BP & Lewis TJ (1995) Imaging of gestational trophoblastic disease. *Semin Oncol* **22**: 130–141.

Dhont M & Beghin C (1994) Endometriumcarcinoom. Epidemiologie, etiologie en screening. *Tijdschr Geneesk* **50**: 1560–1566.

Dijkhuizen FPHLJ, Brölmann HAM, Potters AE et al (1996) The accuracy of transvaginal ultrasonography in the diagnosis of endometrial abnormalities. *Obstet Gynecol* **87**: 345–349.

Dørum A, Kristensen GB, Langebrekke A et al (1993) Evaluation of endometrial thickness measured by endovaginal ultrasound in women with postmenopausal bleeding. *Acta Obstet Gynecol Scand* **72**: 116–119.

Emanuel MH, Verdel MJ, Wamsteker K et al (1995) A prospective comparison of TVS and diagnostic hysteroscopy in the evaluation of patients with abnormal uterine bleeding: clinical implications. *Am J Obstet Gynecol* **172**: 547–552.

Fothergill DJ, Brown VA, Hill AS et al (1992) Histological sampling of the endometrium: a comparison between formal curettage and the pipelle sampler. *Br J Obstet Gynaecol* **99**: 779–780.

Gaucherand, Piacenza JM, Salle B et al (1995) Sonohysterography of the uterine cavity: preliminary investigations. *J Clin Ultrasound* **23**: 339–348.

Ghirardini G, Montanari R & Gualerzi C (1991) Vaginosonography in primary prevention of endometrial oncological pathology. *Clin Exp Obstet Gynecol* **18**: 149–151.

Gimpelson RJ & Rappold HO (1988) A comparative study between hysteroscopy with directed biopsies and dilatation and curettage. *Am J Obstet Gynecol* **158**: 489–492.

Goldschmit R, Katz Z, Blickstein I et al (1993) The accuracy of endometrial pipelle sampling with and without sonographic measurement of endometrial thickness. *Obstet Gynecol* **82**: 727–730.

Goldstein SR (1994) Use of ultrasonohysterography for triage of perimenopausal patients with unexplained uterine bleeding. *Am J Obstet Gynecol* **170**: 565–570.

Goldstein SR, Nachtigall M, Snyder JR et al (1990) Endometrial assessment by vaginal ultrasonography before endometrial sampling in patients with postmenopausal bleeding. *Am J Obstet Gynecol* **163**: 119–123.

Granberg S, Wikland M, Karlsson B et al (1991) Endometrial thickness as measured by endovaginal ultrasonography for indentifying endometrial abnormality. *Am J Obstet Gynecol* **164**: 47–52.

Hacker NF (1994) Uterine cancer. In Berek JS & Hacker NF (eds) *Practical Gynecologic Oncology*, 2nd edn, pp 285–326. Baltimore: Williams and Wilkins.

Hardell L (1988) Tamoxifen as a risk factor for carcinoma of the corpus uteri. *Lancet* **ii**: 563.

Hata T, Hata K, Senoh D et al (1989) Doppler ultrasound assessment of tumor vascularity in gynecologic disorders. *J Ultrasound Med* **8**: 309–314.

Hata K, Hata T, Makihara K et al (1990) Sonographic findings of uterine leiomyosarcoma. *Gynecol Obstet Invest* **30**: 242–245.

Hirai M, Shibata K, Sagai H et al (1995) Transvaginal pulsed and color Doppler sonography for the evaluation of adenomyosis. *J Ultrasound Med* **14**: 529–532.

Hricak H, Rubinstein L, Gherman G et al (1991) MR imaging evaluation of endometrial carcinoma: results of an NCI cooperative study. *Radiology* **179**: 829–832.

Janus C, White M, Dottino P et al (1989) Uterine leiomyosarcoma: magnetic resonance imaging. *Gynecol Oncol* **32**: 79–81.

Karlsson B, Norström A, Granberg S et al (1992) The use of endovaginal ultrasound to diagnose invasion of endometrial carcinoma. *Ultrasound Obstet Gynecol* **2**: 35–39.

Karlsson B, Gransberg S, Wikland M et al (1993) Endovaginal scanning of the endometrium compared to cytology and histology in women with postmenopausal bleeding. *Gynecol Oncol* **50**: 173–178.

Karlsson B, Granberg S, Wikland M et al (1995) Transvaginal sonography of the endometrium in postmenopausal women to identify endometrial abnormality: a Nordic multi-center study. *Am J Obstet Gynecol* **172**: 1488–1494.

Kedar RP, Bourne TH, Powles TJ et al (1994) Effects of tamoxifen on uterus and ovaries of postmenopausal women in a randomised breast cancer prevention trial. *Lancet* **343**: 1318–1321.

Kurjak A & Shalan H (1994) Malignant uterine tumors. In Kurjak A (ed.) *An Atlas of Transvaginal Color Doppler,* 2nd rev. edn, pp 265–277. London: Parthenon.

Kurjak A, Shalan H, Sosic A et al (1993) Endometrial carcinoma in postmenopausal women: evaluation by transvaginal color Doppler sonography. *Am J Obstet Gynecol* **169**: 1597–1603.

La Vecchia C, Franceschi S, Decarli A et al (1984) Risk factors for endometrial cancer at different ages. *J Natl Cancer Inst* **73**: 667–671.

Lesko SM, Rosenberg L, Kaufman DW et al (1985) Cigarette smoking and the risk of endometrial cancer. *N Engl J Med* **313**: 593–596.

McLeod AJ, Zornoza J & Shirkhoda A (1984) Leiomyosarcoma: computed Tomographic findings. *Radiology* **152**: 133–136.

Malinova M & Pehlivanov B (1995) Transvaginal sonography and endometrial thickness in patients with postmenopausal uterine bleeding. *Eur J Obstet Gynaecol* **58**: 161–165.

Mark AS, Hricak H, Heinrichs LW et al (1987) Adenomyosis and leiomyoma: differential diagnosis with MR imaging. *Radiology* **163**: 527–529.

Mercé LT, Garcia GL & de la Fuente F (1991) Doppler ultrasound assessment of endometrial pathology. *Acta Obstet Gynecol Scand* **70**: 525–530.

Nasri MN & Coast GJ (1989) Correlation of ultrasound findings and endometrial histopathology in postmenopausal women. *Br J Obstet Gynaecol* **96**: 1333–1338.

Nasri MN, Shepherd JH, Setchell ME et al (1991) The role of vaginal scan in measurement of endometrial thickness in postmenopausal women. *Br J Obstet Gynaecol* **98**: 470–475.

Neven P, De Muylder X, Van Belle Y et al (1989) Tamoxifen and the uterus and endometrium. *Lancet* **i**: 375.

Neven P, De Muylder X, Van Belle Y et al (1994) Tamoxifen and the uterus. *BMJ* **309**: 1313–1314.

Olah KS and Kingston RE (1994) Uterine sarcoma. In Studd J (ed.) *Progress in Obstetrics and Gynaecology,* vol. 11, pp 427–449. London: Churchill Livingstone.

Olah KS, Gee H, Blunt S et al (1991) Retrospective analysis of 318 cases of uterine sarcoma. *Eur J Cancer* **27**: 1095–1099.

Osmers R, Völksen M & Schauer A (1990) Vaginosonography for early detection of endometrial carcinoma? *Lancet* **335**: 1569–1571.

Parazzini F, La Vecchia C, Bocciolone L et al (1991) The epidemiology of endometrial cancer: review. *Gynecol Oncol* **41**: 1–16.

Parazzini F, La Vecchia C, Negri E et al (1995) Smoking and risk of endometrial cancer: results from an Italian case–control study. *Gynecol Oncol* **56**: 195–199.

Parsons A & Lense JJ (1993) Sonohysterography for endometrial abnormalities: preliminary results. *J Clin Ultrasound* **21**: 87–95.

Pattani SJ, Kier R, Deal R et al (1995) MRI of uterine leiomyosarcoma. *Magn Reson Imaging* **13**: 331–333.

Perrot N, Guyot B, Antoine M & Uzan S (1994) The effects of tamoxifen on the endometrium. *Ultrasound Obstet Gynecol* **4**: 83–84.

Pettersson F (1991) Annual report on the results of treatment in gynecological cancer. *Int J Gynaecol Obstet* **21**: 132–237.

Popovich MJ & Hricak H (1994) The role of MRI in the evaluation of gynecologic disease. In Callen PW (ed.) *Ultrasonography in Obstetrics and Gynecology,* 3rd edn, pp 660–688. Philadelphia: WB Saunders.

Prömpeler HJ, Madjar H, du Bois A et al (1994) Transvaginal sonography of myometrial invasion depth in endometrial cancer. *Acta Obstet Gynecol Scand* **73**: 343–346.

Quinn MA, Anderson MC & Coulter CAE (1992) Malignant disease of the uterus. In Shaw R, Soutter P & Stanton S (eds) *Gynaecology*, pp 533–546. London: Churchill Livingstone.

Requard CK, Wicks JD & Mettler FA (1981) Ultrasonography in the staging of endometrial carcinoma. *Radiology* **140**: 781–785.

Romano S, Shimoni Y, Muraler D et al (1992) Retrograde seeding of endometrial carcinoma during hysteroscopy. *Gynecol Oncol* **44**: 116–118.

Saltzman AK, Carter JR, Fowler JM et al (1995) The utility of preoperative screening colonoscopy in gynecologic oncology. *Gynecol Oncol* **56**: 181–186.

Schramm Th, Kürzl R, Schweighart C et al (1995) Endometriumkarzinom und Vaginalsonographie: Untersuchungen zur diagnostischen Validität. *Geburtshilfe Frauenheilkd* **55**: 65–72.

Schwartz LB, Diamond MP & Schwarz PE (1993) Leiomyosarcomas: clinical presentation. *Am J Obstet Gynecol* **168**: 180–183.

Seelbach-Göbel B, Rempen A & Kristen P (1995) Transvaginaler Ultraschall am Endometrium in der Postmenopause. *Geburtshilfe Frauenheilkd* **55**: 59–64.

Silver MM, Miles P & Rosa C (1991) Comparison of Novak and Pipelle endometrial biopsy instruments. *Obstet Gynecol* **78**: 828–830.

Sironi S, Taccagni G, Garancini P et al (1992) Myometrial invasion by endometrial carcinoma: assessment by MR imaging. *AJR* **158**: 565–569.

Sladkevicius P, Valentin L & Marsal K (1994) Endometrial thickness and Doppler velocimetry of the uterine arteries as discriminators of endometrial status in women with postmenopausal bleeding: a comparative study. *Am J Obstet Gynecol* **171**: 722–728.

Smith P, Bakos O, Heimer G et al (1991) Transvaginal ultrasound for identifying endometrial abnormality. *Acta Obstet Gynecol Scand* **70**: 591–594.

Tepper R, Altaras M, Goldberger S et al (1994) Color Doppler ultrasonographic findings in low and high grade endometrial stromal sarcomas. *J Ultrasound Med* **13**: 817–819

Timmerman D & Vergote I (1996) Clincial images in medicine: tamoxifen-induced endometrial polyp. *N Engl J Med* (in press).

Togashi K, Ozasa H, Konishi I et al (1989) Enlarged uterus: differentiation between adenomyosis and leiomyoma with MR imaging. *Radiology* **171**: 531–534.

Van den Bosch T, Vandendael A, Van Schoubroeck D et al (1995) Combining vaginal ultrasonography and office endometrial sampling in the diagnosis of endometrial disease in post-menopausal women. *Obstet Gynecol* **85**: 349–352.

Varner RE, Sparks JM, Cameron CD, Roberts LL & Soong SJ (1991) Transvaginal sonography of the endometrium in postmenopausal women. *Obstet Gynecol* **78**: 195–199.

Worthington JL, Balfe DM, Lee JKT et al (1986) Uterine neoplasms: MR imaging. *Radiology* **159**: 725–730.

Zaloudek CJ & Norris HJ (1981) Adenofibroma and adenosarcoma of the uterus: a clinicopathologic study of 35 cases. *Cancer* **48**: 354–366.

Zalud I & Kurjak A (1994) Pitfalls and artifacts in Doppler ultrasound. In Kurjak A (ed.) *An Atlas of Transvaginal Color Doppler,* 2nd rev. edn, pp 353–358. London: Parthenon.

18 *Acute and chronic pelvic inflammatory disease*
LTGM Geerts and HJ Odendaal

■ INTRODUCTION

'Pelvic inflammatory disease' (PID) refers to a whole range of upper genital tract infections of varying sites and severity (Stacey et al, 1991). For the purpose of this chapter, the term PID will be used for the clinical syndrome attributed to the ascending spread of microorganisms from the vagina and cervix to the endometrium, Fallopian tubes and/or continguous structures (Weström, 1983). To decrease the high worldwide morbidity and mortality due to the acute disease process as well as the frequently occurring long-term sequelae of PID, prevention and early diagnosis accompanied by appropriate treatment is a prerequisite.

■ SYMPTOMS AND THEIR RELATION TO PATHOLOGY

The signs and symptoms of acute PID (APID) are extremely variable and differ drastically between causative organisms (Jacobson and Weström, 1969). They do not correlate with the severity of PID and are not specific for the tissues or the disease process involved (Kahn et al, 1991).

Lower abdominal pain is the main complaint but it is unclear whether it is caused predominantly by cervicitis, endometritis or salpingitis (Jacobson and Weström, 1969). The presence of a purulent vaginal discharge is a strong predictor of APID because microorganisms spread from a lower genital tract infection (Hadgu et al, 1986). Damage to the tubal mucosa causes diapedesis of granulocytes, increased blood flow and vascular permeability in the damaged area and accumulation of pus within the tubal lumen. The tubes become edematous and distended and are often covered by a fibrinous exudate or adhesions with the surrounding peritoneum. Peritonitis, with rebound tenderness, is caused by leakage of pus, either contained within the pouch of Douglas or disseminated in the peritoneal cavity. Agglutination of fimbriae leads to occlusion of the tubal ostia and formation of a pyosalpinx. Ovarian involvement is often limited to perioophoritis and adhesion to the tubal serosa forming a tubo-ovarian complex. In more severe infection, involvement of the ovarian stroma leads to disappearance of ovarian and tubal configuration and formation of a tubo-ovarian abscess. These adnexal changes are often detected as adnexal or cervical excitation tenderness or a palpable adnexal mass. Associated perihepatitis causes adhesions between liver surface and diaphragm, with pain and tenderness in the right hypochondrium. Abnormal vaginal bleeding is caused by the usually accompanying endometritis (Paavonen et al, 1985). Systemic symptoms of infection include fever, rigors, anorexia, nausea, vomiting and general malaise. Symptoms of urinary tract infection or proctitis are often present.

In chronic PID, clinical features are related to persistent low grade infection, recurrent episodes of PID or long-term sequelae (Berland et al, 1982). Permanent bridging of mucosal folds leads to impaired tubal function and ectopic pregnancies or infertility. Adnexal masses (hydrosalpinx or remnants of a tubo-ovarian abscess), adhesions, inflammatory cysts and fibrosis may persist and distort normal anatomy, causing chronic pelvic pain, dysmenorrhea or dyspareunia. Reactive sacroiliitis may lead to chronic lumbosacral pain (Mozas et al, 1994).

■ CLINICAL INVESTIGATIONS

ULTRASONOGRAPHY

CHARACTERISTICS AND PATHOLOGICAL APPEARANCES

The early stage of APID is likely to produce no sonographic abnormalities. In the majority of patients with APID however, especially with more severe disease,

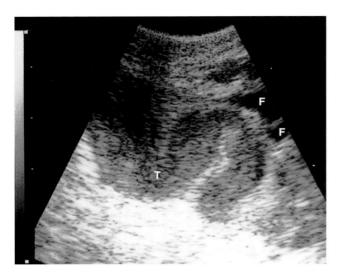

Figure 18.1: A pyosalpinx appears on transvaginal sonography as a tubular structure filled with echogenic fluid and displaying a distinctly folded configuration. Note the free fluid (F) to the right of the tube (T).

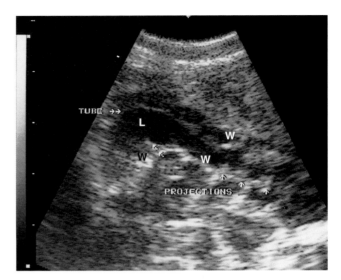

Figure 18.3: This image illustrates the classic characteristics of a pyosalpinx on transvaginal sonography: a tubular appearance, a fluid-filled lumen (L), an echogenic wall (W) and linear projections protruding into the lumen (representing mucosal folds)(↑).

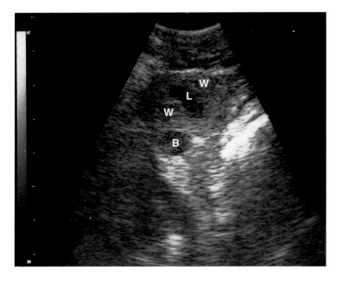

Figure 18.2: A transverse section of a pyosalpinx on transvaginal sonography clearly shows the fluid-filled lumen (L) surrounded by a thick, more echogenic wall (W). B, transverse section of iliac vessel.

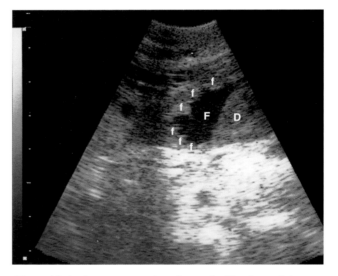

Figure 18.4: A transverse section of a grossly dilated pyosalpinx on transvaginal sonography demonstrates the typical appearance of tubal mucosal folds (f). A clear fluid (F)–debris (D) level is visible with echogenic material collecting in the most dependent part of the patient (to the right of the image).

transvaginal sonography (TVS) will show some abnormality (Spirtos et al, 1982; Patten et al, 1990).

Uterine signs (see Figure 18.10).

Uterine inflammation in APID is often not visible on ultrasonography (Patten et al, 1990). The uterus may appear enlarged and display poorly margined borders (the 'indefinite uterus' sign) due to edema or the contiguity of the uterine image with the surrounding purulent fluid (the 'silhouette' sign). Hypoechogenicity of the myometrium is

often but not consistently recognized (Berland et al, 1982). The endometrial line can be indistinct or totally absent, although prominent central uterine echoes or fluid in the cavity have been described (Bulas et al, 1992).

Tubal signs (Figures 18.1–18.5)

Hyperemia of the tubes cannot be visualized on ultrasonography (Golden et al, 1987). Pyosalpinges usually have a tubular shape and sometimes a folded configura-

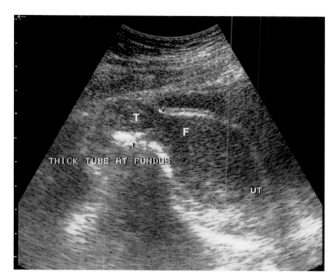

Figure 18.5: *This transvaginal sonogram shows the origin of the thickened tube (T) from the uterine fundus (F). Note the indistinct appearance of the uterus (UT).*

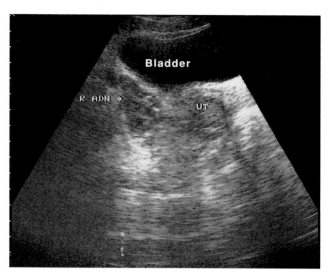

18.7a

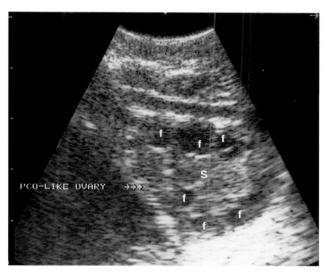

Figure 18.6: *Transvaginal sonography demonstrates the typical polycystic appearance of the ovary. Multiple small follicles (f) are located peripherally to increased ovarian stroma (S). Note the indistinct contours of the ovary.*

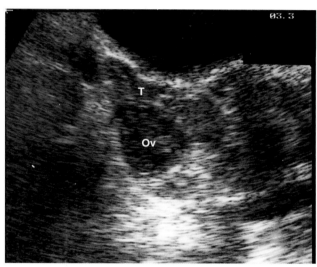

18.7b

Figure 18.7: *(a) The adnexal image obtained with abdominal sonography shows an enlarged adnexa (R ADN) to the right of the uterus (UT). Ovary and tube cannot easily be separated due to lack of definition. (b) The image obtained by transvaginal sonography in the same patient allows clear recognition of an ovary (Ov) adjacent to the tube (T), confirming the presence of a tubo-ovarian complex and excluding the diagnosis of a tubo-ovarian abscess.*

tion. They can be differentiated from loops of bowel and vessels by the absence of flow or peristalsis (Tessler et al, 1989). Occasionally the origin from the uterine cornu can be visualized. The wall is well defined and echogenic and can contain linear echoes (mucosal folds) protruding in the lumen.

Ovarian signs *(Figures 18.6 and 18.7)*

Periovarian inflammation may manifest itself as ovarian enlargement, ill defined contours, periovarian fluid or a solid mass due to multiple adhesions (Patten et al, 1990). Although proven adhesions often cause no abnormalities on ultrasonography, 'adnexal adherence' is diagnosed when no definite distance can be identified between the adnexa and the uterine wall (Kirkpatrick et al, 1979; Golden et al, 1987). Polycystic-like ovaries are probably caused by inflammatory exudate and edema in the vascular pole and prevention of normal follicular growth by a thickened capsule (Cacciatore et al, 1992). In a tubo-ovarian complex, ovarian and tubal definition is lost and

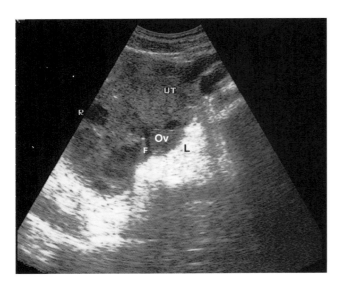

Figure 18.8: *A transverse transvaginal sonogram depicts the uterus (UT) without a clear endometrial line, a normal left (L) ovary (Ov) posterior to the uterus and separated by a small fluid collection (F) from a complex mass involving the right adnexa (R).*

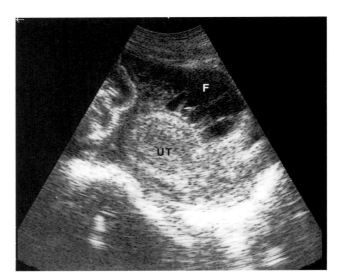

Figure 18.10: *A sagittal transvaginal sonogram of the pelvis demonstrates the uterus (UT) with indistinct contours and absence of a normal endometrial line. A large collection of free fluid (F) anterior to the uterus contains multiple loculations and internal echoes.*

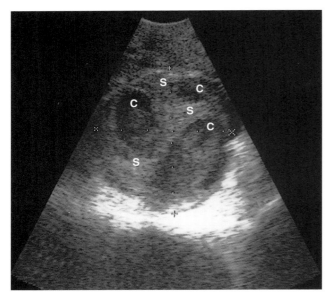

Figure 18.9: *A detailed image of Figure 18.8 shows a right tubo-ovarian abscess, displayed as a well defined complex adnexal mass with several cystic areas (C) filled with echogenic fluid and interspersed with more solid appearing echodense areas (S). Tubal and ovarian anatomy cannot be recognized.*

the thickened fluid-filled tube is fixed to the ovary (Lande et al, 1988).

Tubo-ovarian abscess (*Figures 18.8–18.9*)

A tubo-ovarian abscess can appear as a totally anechoic mass with well defined, sharp, smooth walls. More frequently it appears as a mass with variable echogenicity,

irregular contours, septations and occasionally a gas–fluid or debris–fluid level (Gagliardi et al, 1988). Acoustic enhancement and ringdown can often be demonstrated. Tubal or ovarian anatomy cannot be recognized and adjacent structures are distorted, sometimes rendering the ultrasound image uninterpretable (Berland et al, 1982; Lande et al, 1988). With Doppler ultrasonography measurable low resistance flow has been demonstrated at the margins of tubo-ovarian abscesses. Resistance is lowest in the acute phase and correlates inversely with disease severity. With progressive healing resistance increases and flow becomes undetectable.

Free fluid (*Figure 18.10*)

Free fluid is often present in the pouch of Douglas (Patten et al, 1990). An irregular wall, loculations and internal echoes make an infectious origin of the fluid more likely (Berland et al, 1982). The Fitz-Hugh–Curtis syndrome has been demonstrated ultrasonographically in a patient with ascites (Van Dongen, 1993).

Chronic PID

In chronic PID, adhesions may present on ultrasonography as a complex pattern of pelvic fluid collections or masses due to fixation of bowel or omentum (Berland et al, 1982). The uterus has usually regained its sharp borders and normal echogenicity. The tube can still be thick walled and enlarged as a result of chronic interstitial salpingitis. A hydrosalpinx may present as a tubular structure, but more often as a large unilocular cyst with sharp smooth walls, clear fluid and sometimes a visible fluid-filled tail at the junction with the uterus. After healing, tubo-ovarian abscesses become echo-free fluid collections with sharply defined, thin walls. Inflammatory peritoneal cysts present as large, clear, multiloculated, thin walled cysts adherent to the tubes. In chronic PID, low resistance flow remains demonstrable around tubo-ovarian abscesses (Tinkanen and Kujansuu, 1993).

DIFFERENTIAL DIAGNOSIS

The ultrasonographic findings of APID are not pathognomonic and should be interepreted within the clinical context.

A prominent central uterine echo can represent a decidual reaction in an ectopic pregnancy and poorly marginated uterine borders also occur in endometriosis, ovarian malignancy or leiomyomas (Berland et al, 1982). An inflamed appendix can be confused with salpingitis (Terry and Forrest, 1989). Complex adnexal masses can represent ectopic pregnancies, endometriomas, leiomyomas, abscesses of nongenital origin, ovarian neoplasms or cysts with hemorrhage, rupture or torsion. Sterile fluid collections like lymphoceles, urinomas, seromas, hematomas, a dilated distal ureter or even fluid-filled loops of bowel can all mimic tubo-ovarian abscesses (Berland et al, 1982). Free fluid in the pouch of Douglas can occur with normal ovulation or menstruation, as well as with ectopic pregnancy, cyst rupture, ascites or malignancy. Low resistance flow on Doppler is also present in malignancy, ectopic pregnancy or even a normal corpus luteum (Schiller and Grant, 1992).

DIAGNOSTIC PITFALLS

False negative ultrasound findings, even of obvious lesions, are often due to the limited field of view, poor acoustic accessibility or technical difficulties. When a lesion is small or inflammation mild or diffuse, the diagnosis can be missed (Patten et al, 1990). False positive findings are usually caused by the misinterpretation of adhesions or loops of bowel. A mass should not be diagnosed unless it is easily reproducible (Lawson and Albarelli, 1977). One must be cautious not to overinterpret subtle subjective findings.

SENSITIVITY AND SPECIFICITY

In assessing the accuracy of ultrasonography in the diagnosis of PID, a clear distinction has to be made between transvaginal (TVS) and transabdominal scanning (TAS). Although TAS allows easier orientation and visualization of a much wider area, TVS gives significantly better information about the origin and internal architecture of pelvic masses (Leibman et al, 1988; Mendelson et al, 1988; Fleischer et al, 1989) and has better interobserver agreement on the severity of APID (Bulas et al, 1992).

It should also be acknowledged that it is not clear to which diagnostic gold standard the accuracy of ultrasonography should be compared. The value of laparoscopy in this regard has recently been questioned (Sellors et al, 1991).

The characteristic appearance of a dilated tube on TVS makes the technique a good tool for accurate diagnosis (Tessler et al, 1989). Sensitivity is in the range of 85–93%, specificity and positive predictive values approach 100%, the negative predictive value for APID is around 95% and the overall accuracy 93% (Patten et al, 1990; Cacciatore et al, 1992). Signs of periovarian inflammation have a sensitivity of 90% and an overall accuracy of 91% (Patten et al, 1990). In a small study, polycystic-like ovaries had a sensitivity of 100%, specificity of 71%, positive predictive value of 54% and negative predictive value of 91% (Cacciatore et al, 1992), but these results await confirmation. The presence of free fluid in the pouch of Douglas is not very accurate (sensitivity of 77%, specificity of 79% (Cacciatore et al, 1992)) nor are the signs of uterine inflammation (sensitivity only 25% (Patten et al, 1990)). In retrospective studies on intra-abdominal abscesses, the sensitivity (60–100%), specificity (78–93%) and accuracy (87–96%) of ultrasonography vary depending on abscess localization and patient selection (Dobrin et al, 1986; Gagliardi et al, 1988). In a prospective study on TAS in intra-abdominal abscesses the general sensitivity fell to 43–48% for a specificity of 90% (McNeil et al, 1981). No large prospective series with specific data on pelvic abscesses or the use of TVS are available. Some studies found no significant difference in sensitivity and specificity between pelvic and other abdominal abscesses, while others report discrepant results in the pelvis (Taylor et al, 1978; Jasinsky et al, 1987).

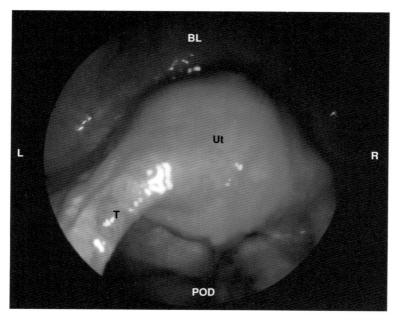

Figure 18.11: Laparoscopy demonstrates hyperemia and edema of the uterus (Ut) and the proximal left tube (T) in a patient with mild acute pelvic inflammatory disease. BL, bladder; POD, pouch of Douglas; L, left; R, right.

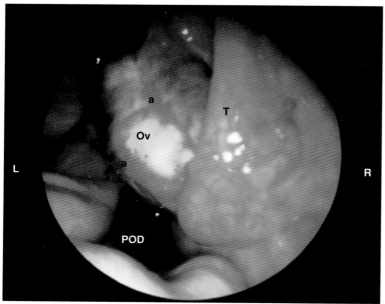

Figure 18.12: On laparoscopy, the distal end of the right tube (T) appears red and swollen. The right ovary (Ov) is covered by a sticky exudate and fresh adhesions (a). A serosanguineous purulent exudate is present in the pouch of Douglas (POD). L, left; R, right.

The specificity of ultrasonography can be increased by performing serial examinations showing typical changes with time (Golden et al, 1987; Cacciatore et al, 1992). The accuracy can also be improved by incorporating ultrasound-guided aspiration of fluid collections, by administering water enemas or by abdominal palpation during real time ultrasonography (Berland et al, 1982).

The role of ultrasonography in chronic PID is limited to the documentation of sequelae.

LAPAROSCOPY

CHARACTERISTICS AND PATHOLOGICAL APPEARANCES *(Figures 18.11–18.16)*

Laparoscopy has revolutionized current thinking on the etiology and pathogenesis of PID (Landers and Sweet, 1985). Pronounced hyperemia and edema of the tubal wall are usually accepted as minimum criteria for the diagnosis of APID (Jacobson, 1964). Very often a sticky or fibrinous exudate can be demonstrated on the tubal surface and surrounding structures, as well as oozing of

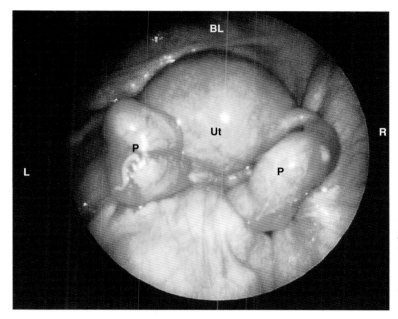

*Figure 18.13: In more severe pelvic infection, bilateral pyosalpinges (P) are seen on laparoscopy, with both tubes adhering to the posterior aspect of the uterus (Ut). BL, bladder; L, left; R, right. Reprinted with permission from Soper DE (1991) Diagnosis and laparoscopic grading of acute salpingitis. Am J Obstet Gynecol **164 (5/2)**: 1370–1376.*

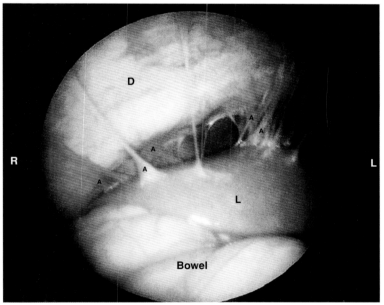

*Figure 18.14: A laparoscopic image of the Fitz-Hugh–Curtis syndrome, with extensive adhesions between liver surface (L) and diaphragm (D). R, right; L, left. Reprinted with permission from Soper DE (1991) Diagnosis and laparoscopic grading of acute salpingitis. Am J Obstet Gynecol **164 (5/2)**: 1370–1376.*

pus from the tubal ostia and free pus in the pouch of Douglas. With more severe APID, the free moveability of the tubes is lost due to fresh adhesions. A pyosalpinx can often be seen after occlusion of the fimbrial stoma. Sometimes no portion of the ovary can be recognized within the inflammatory conglomeration. Perihepatic violin string adhesions can be seen in perihepatitis (Jacobson, 1964).

In chronic PID, dilated tubes, blocked ostia, widespread adhesions, fibrosis and residual masses can be visualized.

DIFFERENTIAL DIAGNOSIS

One of the main advantages of laparoscopy is that it can exclude other pathology in patients who are clinically suspected of having APID (Jacobson, 1980). When visualization of the pelvis and the whole length of the tube is satisfactory, interpretation of the laparoscopic features is straightforward. It can, however, be difficult to distinguish very mild salpingitis from normal, or to determine whether the observed pathology is due to acute or past and inactive PID (Stacey et al, 1991). With only slight uterine hyperemia the presence of a normal pregnancy has to be considered (Jacobson, 1964). The appendix

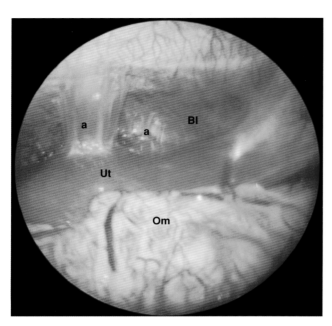

Figure 18.15: In a patient with severe pelvic infection, the pelvis could not be completely visualized by laparoscopy owing to extensive adhesions (a) between the uterus (Ut), bladder (Bl) and omentum (Om).

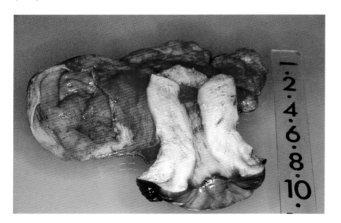

Figure 18.16: A hysterectomy specimen of a patient with a tubo-ovarian abscess illustrates the presence of an abscess wall and the absence of any recognizable tubal or ovarian structures.

and the upper abdomen should always be visualized to exclude any other primary focus of infection (Spirtos et al, 1987).

The structural changes of chronic PID can be confused with adhesions due to other intraperitoneal inflammation or endometriosis.

DIAGNOSTIC PITFALLS

False positive diagnoses can occur when signs are very mild and the hyperemia can be attributed to the carbon dioxide pneumoperitoneum or the phase in the men-

strual cycle (Sellors et al, 1991). It has been demonstrated by fimbrial histology that false positive diagnoses are also caused by a considerable expectation bias from managing gynecologists (Sellors et al, 1991). Early disease with limited inflammation can easily be missed on laparoscopy as the outside of the tube can still look normal while endometritis, parametritis and endosalpingitis are already present (Jacobson and Weström, 1969; Paavonen et al, 1985).

SENSITIVITY AND SPECIFICITY

Routine laparoscopy as the gold standard for PID diagnosis has never been validated (Jacobson and Weström, 1969). In some patients, the procedure fails due to inappropriate visualization of the pelvis. The incidence of false positive and negative diagnoses with laparoscopy (Soper, 1991b) is presently unknown and its accuracy may be markedly lower than generally accepted. When compared with pathologically proven salpingitis, laparoscopy had a sensitivity of only 50%, a specificity of 80%, a positive predictive value of 55% and a negative predictive value of 77% (Sellors et al, 1991). Exactly the same histopathological confirmation rate was observed in patients with tubal hyperemia and edema, either with or without tubal exudate (Sellors et al, 1991). The incorporation of a tubal exudate in the minimum criteria for APID decreases the number of false positive diagnoses, but will lower sensitivity. All these observations indicate that the diagnostic gold standard for PID should be reviewed (Kahn et al, 1991).

The accuracy of laparoscopy may be increased by combining it with endometrial biopsy, cotton tip intratubal swabs, nontraumatic tubal cytobrushes, fimbrial minibiopsies or endosalpingoscopy (Sellors et al, 1991; Cianci et al, 1994). Results on these techniques are still awaited.

COMPUTED TOMOGRAPHY

CHARACTERISTICS AND PATHOLOGICAL APPEARANCES (*Figure 18.17*)

In contrast to plain X-rays, computed tomography (CT) gives more direct evidence of PID. In the absence of a discrete abscess or hydrosalpinx, however, CT images are not specific and definition of the pelvic structures is usually

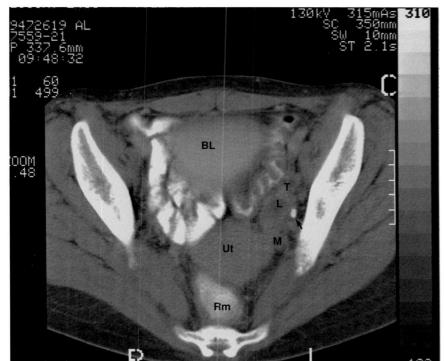

Figure 18.17: Computed tomography with contrast in a patient with a suspected pelvic abscess confirmed the presence of a tubular structure (T) in the left adnexa with low attenuation values in the center (L), without rim enhancement. It also illustrates the thickening of the mesosalpinx (M), the loss of definition of the uterine borders (Ut) and anterolateral displacement of the left ureter (arrow). Rm, rectum. Courtesy of Dr N Smuts, Department of Radiology, Tygerberg Hospital, University of Stellenbosch.

poor because of permeation of the fat planes by the inflammatory process (Raskin, 1980). CT can demonstrate endometrial thickening, fluid in the endometrial cavity or loss of definition of the uterine border. At times a pyosalpinx can be recognized due to its tubular shape (Wilbur et al, 1992). Tubo-ovarian abscesses have a widely varied appearance on CT but often present as well defined masses with low attenuation values in the center, not enhancing with intravenous contrast except for the rim (Callen, 1979; Koehler and Moss, 1980). They can also be multinodular, contain internal septations or form a more diffuse mass with ill defined borders of increased density (Koehler and Moss, 1980). Gas bubbles, although the most specific sign of abscess formation, are unusual in tubo-ovarian abscess (Wilbur et al, 1992). Anterior displacement and thickening of the ipsilateral mesosalpinx around the mass is highly suggestive of an adnexal origin (Wilbur et al, 1992). CT can detect adhesions around a pelvic mass by the obliteration of normally occurring fat, the presence of fuzzy uterine borders, angularly shaped intestines or irregularly thickened walls of bladder, bowel or peritoneum (Ozasa et al, 1986; Ellis et al, 1991). Thickening of the uterosacral ligaments as well as increased density of the presacral and perirectal fat is due to edema. Infiltration of perirectal fat can cause luminal narrowing of the rec-

tosigmoid and indistinct margins between bowel and internal genitalia. Ureter compression and hydronephrosis can accompany a tubo-ovarian abscess and can be demonstrated after intravenous contrast injection. Inflammatory para-aortic lymph nodes and loculated fluid collection in the pouch of Douglas may be visualized (Langer and Dinsmore, 1992).

DIFFERENTIAL DIAGNOSIS

CT cannot differentiate tubo-ovarian abscesses from noninfected inflammatory masses. Hematomas, tumors, seromas, endometriomas, thick walled cysts or loops of bowel can all mimic such abscesses (Callen, 1979; Koehler and Moss, 1980). Pelvic abscesses of nongenital origin can also be confused with tubo-ovarian abscesses (Langer and Dinsmore, 1992).

DIAGNOSTIC PITFALLS

Due to lack of perivisceral fat, CT can be inaccurate in very thin patients (Raskin, 1980). Nonopacified bowel can be misinterpreted as a mass, abscess or phlegmon (Gagliardi et al, 1988). Artifacts can be created by metal clips, bone and gas (Raskin, 1980; Gagliardi et al, 1988). An abscess wall can be invisible on CT early in the inflammatory process or when the fluid content is highly cellular (Callen, 1979). Lesions are often missed when they simulate bowel, are diffuse or drain spontaneously (Baldwin and Wraight, 1990).

SENSITIVITY AND SPECIFICITY

CT has excellent anatomical resolution in the pelvis because of the clear outlining of the solid organs by extraperitoneal fat and the intravenous, oral and rectal administration of contrast media (Langer and Dinsmore, 1992). CT is very accurate in the detection of intra-abdominal abscesses. Retrospective studies reported sensitivities of 78–100%, specificities of 85–100% and overall accuracies of 90–100% (Korobkin et al, 1978; Koehler and Moss, 1980; Moir and Robins, 1982; Parikh et al, 1982; Gagliardi et al, 1988). Results are, however, area dependent (Jasinsky et al, 1987) and influenced by prior knowledge of results of other tests. In a prospective study on CT as a first line test for the detection of intra-abdominal abscesses, sensitivity fell below 60% for a specificity of 90% (McNeil et al, 1981). Scanty information is available on the accuracy of CT for the diagnosis of tubo-ovarian abscesses (Landers and Sweet, 1985). For pelvic abscesses a sensitivity of 93% and an accuracy of 86% have been reported (Dobrin et al, 1986; Jasinsky et al, 1987). CT can accurately predict adhesions around tubo-ovarian abscesses but results are somewhat poorer for adhesions with other structures than the uterus (sensitivity 75 versus 100%, specificity 77 versus 91%, accuracy 76 versus 95%) (Ozasa et al, 1986).

The accuracy of CT can be increased by using CT guided fluid aspiration to differentiate between infected and noninfected fluid.

MAGNETIC RESONANCE IMAGING

Magnetic resonance imaging (MRI) has a superb soft tissue resolution allowing a good differentiation of pelvic organs from surrounding tissues (Bryan et al, 1984). The normal pelvic images are now well known and MRI demonstrates soft tissue changes like edema and inflammation particularly well (Brown et al, 1986). There is not yet vast experience with MRI changes in PID. Thickening of the tubal wall or mucosal folds is not evident on MRI and normal ovaries cannot usually be identified (Jain and Jeffrey, 1994). Tubo-

ovarian abscesses display relatively low signal intensity indicating long T_1 values and may contain a fluid level (Bryan et al, 1984). MRI is inadequate for diagnosing fibrosis or adhesions (Mitchell, 1992) and cannot make tissue specific diagnoses (Bryan et al, 1984). Currently, there are no data available on the accuracy of MRI in the evaluation of PID.

RADIONUCLIDE INFECTION IMAGING (SCINTIGRAPHY)

CHARACTERISTICS AND PATHOLOGICAL APPEARANCES (*Figure 18.18*)

Radionuclide studies are very rarely used in patients with PID. In contrast with other imaging modalities, scintigraphy depicts organ function rather than morphology. Inflammatory lesions are characterized on scintigrams by focal increased uptake of activity (Gagliardi et al, 1988). Radionuclide scanning highlights regions of suspected abnormality but cannot localize lesions precisely enough for therapeutic use without confirmation with higher resolution methods (Gagliardi et al, 1988). Different radiopharmaceuticals are available. Leukocytes labeled either with ^{111}In or ^{99m}Tc-hexamethylpropyleneamineoxime (HMPAO) are currently most widely used for acute infections, while ^{67}Ga appears to be the better agent for localizing more chronic infections. Other agents include radiolabeled nonspecific polyclonal IgG or, currently less widely available, monoclonal antibodies and chemotactic peptides. Although these agents seem promising, their use is still predominantly experimental (Datz, 1994).

DIFFERENTIAL DIAGNOSIS

The above mentioned radiopharmaceuticals are not only localized in infectious lesions but also accumulate in sterile, noninfective inflammation, as in certain neoplasms, inflammatory bowel disease, tissue damage or infarction (Seabold et al, 1984; Gagliardi et al, 1988; Baldwin and Wraight, 1990). Venous thrombosis can cause increased uptake due to clumped leukocytes or labeled red blood cells and platelets (Baldwin and Wraight, 1990).

DIAGNOSTIC PITFALLS

Techniques based on leukocyte labeling give false negative results when leukocytes fail to accumulate at the site

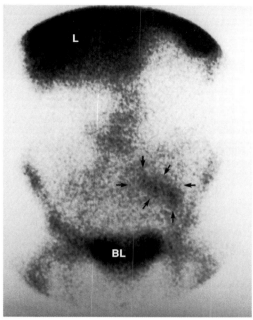

18.18a

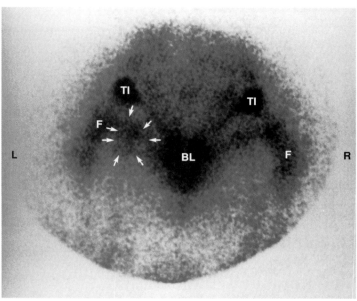

18.18b

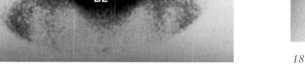

Figure 18.18: *(a) Anterior view and (b) tail-on-collimator view of a* ^{99m}*Tc-HMPAO labeled leukocyte scan (4 hours after injection), in a patient with suspected postabortal pelvic infection and an equivocal fluid collection on ultrasonography, confirmed abnormal leukocyte*

accumulation (arrows) in the vicinity of the parametrium on the left side. BL, bladder; L, liver; S, spleen; F, femur; TI, tuber ischiadicum. Courtesy of the Department of Nuclear Medicine, Tygerberg Hospital, University of Stellenbosch.

of infection. Although this could be the case with chronic abscesses lacking a significant inflammatory response and surrounded by a thick capsule, this has not been consistently found (Knochel et al, 1980; Datz, 1993). Antibiotic treatment has also been considered a possible reason for false negative results because of reduced leukocyte chemotaxis (Knochel et al, 1980); however, this phenomenon seems not to be important at normal therapeutic doses (Datz, 1993). Hyperalimentation, hyperglycemia and hemodialysis as well as leukopenia or immunosuppression can also alter leukocyte chemotaxis (Knochel et al, 1980; Seabold et al, 1984). Inflammation with round cell response due to fungi, *Mycobacterium tuberculosis* and other opportunistic organisms can be missed with labeled leukocytes, but not with leukocyte independent techniques like ^{67}Ga or labeled nonspecific polyclonal IgG (Datz, 1993). Another diagnostic pitfall is normal excretion of activity in the bowel on ^{99m}Tc-HMPAO leukocyte studies, as this may be misinterpreted as abscesses. When this agent is used, it is extremely important to obtain early images (30–90 minutes) as bowel activity is not seen before 2 hours.

Small lesions in or near areas of normal background uptake can easily be missed (Baldwin and Wraight, 1990).

SENSITIVITY AND SPECIFICITY

None of the radionuclide techniques has been well studied for the diagnosis of tubo-ovarian abscesses as such, and the diagnostic accuracy has only been evaluated for intra-abdominal abscesses in general. ^{111}In labeled leukocyte scans had a sensitivity of 84–100%, a specificity of 91–95% and an overall accuracy of 87% (Seabold et al, 1984; Baldwin and Wraight, 1990) for the detection of intra-abdominal abscesses. In retrospective studies, ^{67}Ga scans had sensitivities of 73–96%, specificities of 65–81% and accuracies of 78% (Moir and Robins, 1982; Dobrin et al, 1986) for diagnosing intra-abdominal abscesses, but in a prospective study on ^{67}Ga scans as a first line test the sensitivity was only 57–59% (McNeil et al, 1981). ^{111}In or ^{99m}Tc labeled polyclonal IgG had a sensitivity of 91–100% and a specificity of 100% for focal infection, including chronic and nonbacterial infections (Rubin et al, 1989).

One of the advantages of scintigraphy is the diagnosis of a septic focus outside the abdomen in a significant

Table 18.1 *Clinical diagnostic criteria for acute pelvic inflammatory disease*

Hager*	Soper†
Major criteria (must all be present)	
Abdominal tenderness	Adnexal tenderness
Cervical motion tenderness	Signs of LGTI
Adnexal tenderness	
Minor criteria (one or more must be present)	
GND on endocervical Gram's stain	Endometritis on biopsy
Temperature (> 38°C)	Temperature > 38°C
Leukocytosis (> 10 000)	Leukocytosis
Purulent fluid POD	Elevated CRP/ESR
Pelvic complex (PV/US)	Chlamydia or GC positive

LGTI, lower genital tract infection; GND, Gram-negative diplococci; ESR, erythrocyte sedimentation rate; CRP, C-reactive protein; GC, Neisseria gonorrhoeae; POD, pouch of Douglas; PV, per vaginam examination; US, ultrasonography.

* *Reprinted with permission from The American College of Obstetricians and Gynecologists and modified from Hager WD et al (1983) Criteria for diagnosis and grading of salpingitis.* Obstet Gynecol **61**: 113–114.

† *Modified with permission from Soper DE (1991) Diagnosis and laparoscopic grading of acute salpingitis.* Am J Obstet Gynecol **164 (5/2)**: 1370–1376.

number of patients because unlike other imaging modalities, the whole body can be scanned without increasing the radiation burden (Seabold et al, 1984).

■ CLASSIFICATION AND ITS USE IN CLINICAL PRACTICE

The diagnosis of PID has been plagued by a lack of accuracy and standardization. In order to make data from different reports comparable, standardized criteria are necessary.

The clinical diagnostic criteria, as formulated by Hager (Hager et al, 1983) and endorsed by the Infectious Disease Society for Obstetrics and Gynecology, are widely accepted but have not been validated. Recent literature suggests that the presence of a lower genital tract infection should receive more emphasis, as opposed to abdominal pain or tenderness, supporting new criteria as proposed by Soper (Soper, 1991a) (*Table 18.1*).

Pronounced hyperemia of the tubal surface, edema of the tubal wall and a sticky exudate on the tubal surface and from the fimbriated ends when patent are still widely accepted as the minimum criteria for the laparoscopic diagnosis of APID (Jacobson and Weström, 1969).

From a prognostic point of view, it is important to determine the severity of disease (Chaparro et al, 1978; Bernstine et al, 1987); moreover, this may have therapeutic implications (Hager, 1983; Monif, 1983). A clinical and laparoscopic grading system was suggested by Hager (Hager et al, 1983) but their relationship has not been determined (*Table 18.2*).

■ DISCUSSION

Acute salpingitis should be suspected in every woman with lower abdominal discomfort. Clinical diagnosis of APID has repeatedly been shown to be unreliable (Hadgu et al, 1986; Jacobson and Weström, 1969; Kahn et al, 1991; Sellors et al, 1991) but it is often not feasible to confirm the diagnosis routinely by laparoscopy, especially in developing countries lacking the necessary facilities (Pastorek, 1989; Stacey et al, 1991). Alternative cost effective diagnostic approaches are thus needed, using simple and noninvasive methods first (Soper, 1991a).

A combination of clinical features and laboratory investigations was used in mixed mathematical models to indicate in which patients laparoscopy would be mandatory and in which the diagnosis would be satisfactorily certain to warrant no further testing. Selec-

Table 18.2 *Grading of acute pelvic inflammatory disease*

Grade	Clinical examination	Laparoscopy
Mild	Uncomplicated: limited to tubes/ovaries, ± pelvic peritonitis	Erythema, edema, no spontaneous purulent exudate, tubes freely moveable
Moderate	Complicated: inflammatory mass or abscess of tubes/ovaries, ± pelvic peritonitis	Gross purulent material, more marked erythema and edema, tubes may not be freely moveable and fimbria stoma not patent
Severe	Spread to structures beyond pelvis, i.e. ruptured tubo-ovarian abscess	Pyosalpinx/inflammatory complex; abscess

Reprinted with permission of The American College of Obstetricians and Gynecologists and modified from Hager WD et al (1983) Criteria for diagnosis and grading of salpingitis. Obstet Gynecol **61**: 113–114.

tive use of laparoscopy in this limited and systematic manner can achieve maximal sensitivity at less cost and operative morbidity than routine laparoscopy (Hadgu et al, 1986).

Other authors feel that the diagnostic aggressiveness should be dictated by the severity of the disease (Kahn et al, 1991). To minimize underdiagnosis of mild PID, a certain degree of overdiagnosis would be acceptable (Weström, 1983). Signs, symptoms and simple laboratory tests would be sufficient for the diagnostic workup and these patients should be treated empirically and followed up to exclude alternative diagnoses. In the seriously ill patient, however, high diagnostic accuracy is mandatory, allowing appropriate management of serious competing diagnoses. This necessitates the simultaneous presence of several clinical indicators and the selective incorporation of more elaborate tests (Kahn et al, 1991).

Despite its limitations, pelvic ultrasonography is often used as a single, first line imaging investigation in APID because of the many advantages (safety, cost, availability, portability, speed and repeatability) (Moir and Robins, 1982; Langer and Dinsmore, 1992). Its major role is detecting complications, localizing abscesses and determining their response to treatment or their amenability to drainage (Berland et al, 1982). Since TVS diagnoses many clinically unsuspected masses (Golden et al, 1989), more liberal or even routine use of ultrasonography in PID may be of benefit (Berland et al, 1982).

Laparoscopy should be used whenever the diagnosis is uncertain, the patient is severely ill, treatment fails, symptoms recur or when the patient is particularly worried about her fertility (Kahn et al, 1991; Soper 1991b).

Apart from exclusion of other pathology, it gives the opportunity to take appropriate samples for culture or histology and allows intervention by draining abscesses or pyosalpinges (Landers and Sweet, 1985; Teisala et al, 1990). Negative laparoscopies should probably be complemented by appropriate sampling for culture or histology (Sellors, 1991; Soper, 1991a).

Imaging studies other than ultrasonography presently have no significant role in PID and are almost never necessary. CT can be used as an adjunct when sonographic results are equivocal or even as a primary investigation when ultrasonography is expected to be unsatisfactory (Knochel et al, 1980; Landers and Sweet, 1985; Jasinsky et al, 1987). Due to its cost, irradiation, immobility and the fact that CT is not always readily available, the routine use of CT as a first line test cannot be supported. Although MRI could become directly competitive with CT as far as image quality is concerned, its value in PID will remain limited. Radionuclide scanning should be reserved for patients without localizing signs, who are not critially ill, who had recent surgery or in whom sonographic assessment is not diagnostic (Moir and Robins, 1982; Seabold et al, 1984; Gagliardi et al, 1988). Potentially life threatening disease requires accurate diagnosis and benefits from the use of multiple imaging modalities because of their complementary features (Korobkin et al, 1978). The sequence of the examinations should be dictated by the clinical circumstances (Knochel et al, 1980; Gagliardi et al, 1988; Baldwin and Wraight, 1990). In patients with a suspected ruptured tubo-ovarian abscess, emergency laparotomy is indicated and valuable time should not be lost by imaging studies.

REFERENCES

Baldwin JE & Wraight EP (1990) [111]Indium labelled leucocyte scintigraphy in occult infection: a comparison with ultrasound and computed tomography. *Clin Radiol* **42**: 199–202.

Berland LL, Lawson TL, Foley WD & Albarelli JN (1982) Ultrasound evaluations of pelvic infections. *Radiol Clin North Am* **20**: 367–381.

Bernstine R, Kennedy WR & Waldron J (1987) Acute pelvic inflammatory disease: a clinical follow-up. *Int J Fertil Menopausal Stud* **32**: 229–232.

Brown CEL, Lowe TW, Cunningham FG & Weinreb JC (1986) Puerperal pelvic thrombophlebitis: impact on diagnosis and treatment using X-ray computed tomography and magnetic resonance imaging. *Obstet Gynecol* **68**: 789–794.

Bryan PJ, Butler HE & LiPuma JP (1984) Magnetic resonance imaging of the pelvis. *Radiol Clin North Am* **22**: 897–915.

Bulas DI, Ahlstrom PA, Sivit CJ, Nussbaum Blask AR & O'Donnell RM (1992) Pelvic inflammatory disease in the adolescent: comparison of transabdominal and transvaginal sonographic evaluation. *Radiology* **183**: 435–439.

Cacciatore B, Leminen A, Ingman-Friberg S, Ylöstalo P & Paavonen J (1992) Transvaginal sonographic findings in ambulatory patients with suspected pelvic inflammatory disease. *Obstet Gynecol* **80**: 912–916.

Callen PW (1979) Computed tomographic evaluation of abdominal and pelvic abscesses. *Radiology* **131**: 171–175.

Chaparro MV, Ghosh S, Nashed A & Poliak A (1978) Laparoscopy for the confirmation and prognostic evaluation of pelvic inflammatory disease. *Int J Gynaecol Obstet* **15**: 307–309.

Cianci A, Furneri PM, Tempera G, Nicoletti G, Roccasalva L & Palumbo G (1994) Laparoscopy diagnosis of chlamydial salpingitis by using a tubal cytobrush. *Fertil Steril* **61**: 181–184.

Datz FL (1993) The current status of radionuclide infection imaging. *Nucl Med Annu* 47–76.

Datz FL (1994) Letter from the Guest Editor. *Semin Nucl Med* **2**: 89–91.

Dobrin PB, Heer Gully P, Greenlee HB et al (1986) Radiologic diagnosis of an intra-abdominal abscess. *Arch Surg* **121**: 41–46.

Ellis JH, Francis IR, Rhodes M, Kane NM & Fechner K (1991) CT findings in tuboovarian abscess. *J Comput Assist Tomogr* **15**: 589–592.

Fleischer AC, Gordon AN & Entman SS (1989) Transabdominal and transvaginal sonography of pelvic masses. *Ultrasound Med Biol* **15**: 529–533.

Gagliardi PD, Hoffer PB & Rosenfield ST (1988) Correlative imaging in abdominal infection: an algorithmic approach using nuclear medicine, ultrasound, and computed tomography. *Semin Nucl Med* **4**: 320–334.

Golden N, Cohen H, Gennari G & Neuhoff S (1987) The use of pelvic ultrasonography in the evaluation of adolescents with pelvic inflammatory disease. *Am J Dis Child* **141**: 1235–1238.

Golden N, Neuhoff S & Cohen H (1989) Pelvic inflammatory disease in adolescents. *J Pediatr* **114**: 138–143.

Hadgu A, Weström L, Brooks CA, Reynolds GH & Thompson SE (1986) Predicting acute pelvic inflammatory disease: a multivariate analysis. *Am J Obstet Gynecol* **155**: 954–960.

Hager WD (1983) Follow-up of patients with tubo-ovarian abscess(es) in association with salpingitis. *Obstet Gynecol* **61**: 680–684.

Hager WD, Eschenbach DA, Spence MR & Sweet RL (1983) Criteria for diagnosis and grading of salpingitis. *Obstet Gynecol* **61**: 113–114.

Jacobson L (1964) Laparoscopy in the diagnosis of acute salpingitis. *Acta Obstet Gynecol Scand* **43**: 160–174.

Jacobson L (1980) Differential diagnosis of acute pelvic inflammatory disease. *Am J Obstet Gynecol* **138**: 1006–1011.

Jacobson L & Weström L (1969) Objectivized diagnosis of acute pelvic inflammatory disease. *Am J Obstet Gynecol* **105**: 1088–1098.

Jain KA & Jeffrey RB (1994) Evaluation of pelvic masses with magnetic resonance imaging and ultrasonography. *J Ultrasound Med* **13**: 845–853.

Jasinsky RW, Glazer GM, Francis IR & Harkness RL (1987) CT and ultrasound in abscess detection at specific anatomic sites: a study of 198 patients. *Comput Med Imaging Graph* **11**: 41–47.

Kahn JG, Walker CK, Washington AE, Landers DV & Sweet RL (1991) Diagnosing pelvic inflammatory disease. A comprehensive analysis and considerations for developing a new model. *JAMA* **266**: 2594–2604.

Kirkpatrick RH, Nikrui N, Wittenberg J, Hann L & Ferrucci JT (1979) Gray scale ultrasound in adnexal thickening: correlation with laparoscopy. *J Clin Ultrasound* **7**: 115–118.

Knochel JQ, Koehler PR, Lee TG & Welch DM (1980) Diagnosis of abdominal abscesses with computer tomography, ultrasound, and ^{111}In leukocyte scans. *Radiology* **137**: 425–432.

Koehler PR & Moss AA (1980) Diagnosis of intra-abdominal and pelvic abscesses by computerized tomography. *JAMA* **244**: 49–52.

Korobkin M, Callen PW, Filly RA, Hoffer PB, Shimshak RR & Kressel HY (1978) Comparison of computed tomography, ultrasonography, and gallium-67 scanning in the evaluation of suspected abdominal abscess. *Radiology* **129**: 89–93.

Lande IM, Hil MC, Cosco FE & Kator NN (1988) Adnexal and cul-de-sac abnormalities: transvaginal sonography. *Radiology* **166**: 325–332.

Landers DV & Sweet RL (1985) Current trends in the diagnosis and treatment of tuboovarian abscess. *Am J Obstet Gynecol* **151**: 1098–1110.

Langer JE & Dinsmore BJ (1992) Computed tomographic evaluation of benign and inflammatory disorders of the female pelvis. *Radiol Clin North Am* **30**: 831–842.

Lawson TL & Albarelli JN (1977) Diagnosis of gynecologic pelvic masses by gray scale ultrasonography: analysis of specificity and accuracy. *AJR* **128**: 1003–1006.

Leibman AJ, Kruse B & McSweeney MB (1988) Transvaginal sonography: comparison with transabdominal sonography in the diagnosis of pelvic masses. *AJR* **151**: 89–92.

McNeil BJ, Sanders R, Alderson PO et al (1981) A prospective study of computed tomography, ultrasound, and gallium imaging in patients with fever. *Radiology* **139**: 647–653.

Mendelson EB, Bohm-Velez M, Joseph N & Neiman HL (1988) Gynecologic imaging: comparison of transabdominal and transvaginal sonography. *Radiology* **166**: 321–324.

Mitchell DG (1992) Benign disease of the uterus and ovaries. Applications of magnetic resonance imaging. *Radiol Clin North Am* **30**: 777–787.

Moir C & Robins RE (1982) Role of ultrasonography, gallium scanning, and computed tomography in the diagnosis of intraabdominal abscess. *Am J Surg* **143**: 582–585.

Monif GRG (1983) The staging of acute salpingitis and its therapeutic ramifications. *J Reprod Med* **28**: 712–715.

Mozas J, Castilla JA, Alarcón JL, López JM, Garcia JL & Herruzo AJ (1994) Reactive sacroiliitis as late sequela after severe pelvic inflammatory disease verified by laparoscopy or laparotomy. *Acta Obstet Gynecol Scand* **73**: 324–327.

Ozasa H, Noda Y, Mori T, Togashi K & Nakano Y (1986) Diagnostic capability of ultrasound versus CT for clinically suspected ovarian mass with emphasis on detection of adhesions. *Gynecol Oncol* **25**: 311–318.

Paavonen J, Aine R, Teisala K et al (1985) Comparison of endometrial biopsy and peritoneal fluid cytologic testing with laparoscopy in the diagnosis of acute pelvic inflammatory disease. *Am J Obstet Gynecol* **151**: 645–650.

Parikh SJ, Peters JC & Kihm RH (1982) Abdominal and pelvic abscesses: computed tomography diagnosis. *Comput Med Imaging Graph* **6**: 99–108.

Pastorek II JG (1989) Pelvic inflammatory disease and tubo-ovarian abscess. *Obstet Gynecol Clin North Am* **16**: 347–361.

Patten RM, Vincent LM, Wolner-Hanssen P & Thorpe E (1990) Pelvic inflammatory disease. Endovaginal sonography with laparoscopic correlation. *J Ultrasound Med* **9**: 681–689.

Raskin MM (1980) Combination of CT and ultrasound in the retroperitoneum and pelvis examination. *Crit Rev Diagn Imaging* **13**: 173–228.

Rubin RH, Fisherman AJ, Callahan RJ et al (1989) ^{111}In-labeled nonspecific immunoglobulin scanning in the detection of focal infection. *N Engl J Med* **321**: 935–940.

Schiller VL & Grant EG (1992) Doppler ultrasonography of the pelvis. *Radiol Clin North Am* **30**: 735–742.

Seabold JE, Wilson DG, Lieberman LM & Boyd CM (1984) Unsuspected extra-abdominal sites of infection: scintigraphic detection with indium-111-labeled leukocytes. *Radiology* **151**: 213–217.

Sellors J, Mahony J, Goldsmith C et al (1991) The accuracy of clinical findings and laparoscopy in pelvic inflammatory disease. *Am J Obstet Gynecol* **164**: 113–120.

Soper DE (1991a) Diagnosis and laparoscopic grading of acute salpingitis. *Am J Obstet Gynecol* **164**: 1370–1376.

Soper DE (1991b) Surgical considerations in the diagnosis and treatment of pelvic inflammatory disease. *Surg Clin North Am* **71**: 947–962.

Spirtos NJ, Bernstine RL, Crawford WL & Fayle J (1982) Sonography in acute pelvic inflammatory disease. *J Reprod Med* **27**: 312–320.

Spirtos NM, Eisenkop SM, Spirtos TW, Poliakin RI & Hibbard LT (1987) Laparoscopy: a diagnostic aid in cases of suspected appendicitis. *Am J Obstet Gynecol* **156**: 90–94.

Stacey CM, Barton SE & Singer A (1991) Pelvic inflammatory disease. *Prog Obstet Gynecol* **9**: 259–271.

Taylor KJW, Wasson JFMcI, De Graaff C, Rosenfield AT & Andriole VT (1978) Accuracy of grey-scale ultrasound diagnosis of abdominal and pelvic abscesses in 220 patients. *Lancet* **i**: 83–84.

Teisala K, Heinonen PK & Punnonen R (1990) Laparoscopic diagnosis and treatment of acute pyosalpinx. *J Reprod Med* **35**: 19–21.

Terry J & Forrest T (1989) Sonographic demonstration of salpingitis. Potential confusion with appendicitis. *J Ultrasound Med* **8**: 39–41.

Tessler FN, Perrella RR, Fleischer AC & Grant EG (1989) Endovaginal sonographic diagnosis of dilated Fallopian tubes. *AJR* **153**: 523–525.

Tinkanen H & Kujansuu E (1993) Doppler ultrasound findings in tubo-ovarian infectious complex. *J Clin Ultrasound* **21**: 175–178.

Van Dongen PW (1993) Diagnosis of Fitz-Hugh–Curtis syndrome by ultrasound. *Eur J Obstet Gynecol Reprod Biol* **50**: 159–162.

Weström L (1983) Clinical manifestations and diagnosis of pelvic inflammatory disease. *J Reprod Med* **28**: 703–708.

Wilbur AC, Aizenstein RI & Napp TE (1992) CT findings in tuboovarian abscess. *AJR* **158**: 575–579.

19 *Endometriosis*
I Brosens

■ INTRODUCTION

Endometriosis, a disease affecting many women during their reproductive life, is classically defined by the presence of glands and stroma outside the uterine cavity. Progress in pelvic endoscopy has led to an increased recognition of endometriosis, but at the same time it has become questionable whether the mere presence of what is defined by histology as endometriosis can be equated per se with the presence of disease. Its presence in symptomatic women can therefore be a finding that is not necessarily the cause of the symptom. This chapter describes, illustrates and discusses the symptoms and their relationship to the pathology, the clinical appearances, the investigational techniques and finally the problems of staging.

Historically three distinctive types of endometriotic lesions have been described. For obvious reasons the initial description of the disease was focused on severe lesions that were palpable by pelvic examination and apparently represented lesions which today are described as deep nodular endometriosis (*Figure 19.1*). The comprehensive work by T. S. Cullen (1920) recognized the disease as a complex affecting the uterus and different pelvic structures, particularly the ligaments and septa and having the histological characteristics of 'a matrix of non-striped muscle and fibrous tissue . . . and scattered throughout this matrix or groundwork an isolated gland or group of glands lying in direct contact with the muscle but usually in characteristic stroma' (Benagiano and Brosens, 1991).

Interest in the hemorrhagic cysts of the ovary was started by W. W. Russel in 1899, when he described a case of a woman of premenopausal age who had 'the right ovary enveloped in adhesions of the posterior face of the broad ligament' and on microscopic examination showed, to his astonishment, 'areas which were an exact prototype of normal uterine mucous membrane'. It took more than

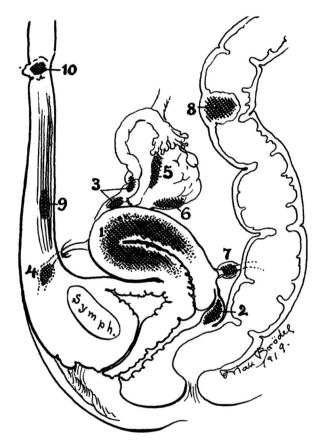

Figure 19.1: Diagram prepared by Cullen (1920) showing the sites of nodular endometriosis or adenomyosis externa in the pelvic supportive structures and wall of the pelvic organs. Reproduced with permission from Cullen TS (1920) The distribution of adenoma containing uterine mucosa. Arch Surg 1: 215–283. Copyright 1920, American Medical Association.

20 years before the endometrial tissue was recognized as a cause of the hemorrhagic cyst by Sampson (1921), and the cyst was later called endometrioma (*Figure 19.2*).

Sampson (1927) is considered as the discoverer of endometriosis because he observed similarity between the peritoneal implants and eutopic endometrium and formulated the hypothesis that peritoneal endometriosis originates by a mechanism of menstrual regurgitation and implantation. Sampson's theory so much impressed the scientific community that the disease is now uniformly

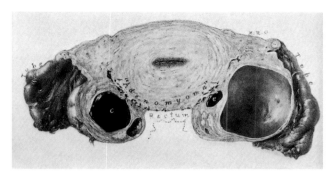

Figure 19.2: Sampson's illustration of the ovarian endometrial cyst. Note the adhesions between the anterior side of the ovary and the posterior side of the uterus and the stigma central in the adhesions which was described by Sampson as the site of perforation but represents the site of inversion of the ovarian cortex. Reproduced with permission from Sampson JA (1921) Perforating hemorrhagic (chocolate) cysts of the ovary. Arch Surg 3: 245–323. Copyright 1921, American Medical Association.

defined as the presence of glands and stroma outside the uterine cavity, although the associated changes such as bleeding, smooth muscle cell hyperplasia, chronic inflammatory reaction and adhesions to a large extent determine the progression and clinical significance of the disease.

■ SYMPTOMS AND THEIR RELATIONSHIP TO PATHOLOGY

PELVIC PAIN

Although chronic pelvic pain, dysmenorrhea, deep dyspareunia and infertility are considered to be the main symptoms of pelvic endometriosis, many women are completely asymptomatic.

A recent large prospective study (Mahmood et al, 1991) has shown that women with endometriosis experience *dysmenorrhea* more frequently than women with sequelae of pelvic infection or laparoscopically normal pelvis; however, the same study demonstrated that 32% of women with endometriosis did not have dysmenorrhea.

Deep dyspareunia and *chronic pelvic pain* affect respectively one in three and one in two women with endometriosis (Mahmood et al, 1991; Fedele et al, 1992). There has been a surprising lack of correlation between the stage of the disease as determined by revised Ameri-

can Fertility Society (r-AFS) classification and the prevalence and severity of symptoms (Fedele et al, 1992). Pain in endometriosis has been related to adhesions in restricted mobility of the organs, but treatment regimens have often produced relief of pain without affecting the adhesion score. Sites of focal tenderness on examination are associated strongly with the presence of disease on the uterosacral ligaments and cul-de-sac and are associated significantly with deeper and larger volumes of implants (Koninckx et al, 1991). The deep nodular implants, particularly in the rectovaginal septum, frequently have the histological characteristics of adenomyosis (Brosens, 1994).

It should be remembered that chronic pelvic pain in women is of complex origin and can be effected by a variety of physical causes. In addition, the psychological status of the woman can influence the perception of pain and it is difficult to know in individual cases whether the psychological disturbance precedes or aggravates the pain or is the result of the chronic exposure to it. On the other hand, pain due to other causes may be incorrectly attributed to endometriosis and gynecologists must remain aware of these possibilities.

INFERTILITY

Despite the fact that endometriosis is the most frequently made diagnosis in infertile couples, it has never been proven that the implants themselves are the cause of infertility. The treatment of endometriosis in infertility remains one of the most controversial issues in gynecology. Until a causal relationship can be established it remains just as plausible that infertility causes endometriosis as it does that endometriosis causes infertility.

The relationship between endometriosis and infertility has been examined by the prevalence of the disease in both fertile and infertile couples. The incidence of endometriosis in the female partner of infertile couples undergoing laparoscopy is currently estimated to range from 20 to 50%, while the incidence of endometriosis in the general population of women of reproductive age is between 2 and 22% (Moen and Muus, 1991). This has led many clinicians to consider the endometriosis implants to be responsible in some way for the concurrent infertility, despite the absence of a defined mechanism; however, these data can only serve to support the notion of an association but not a causal relationship.

A second approach to determine if a causal relationship exists has been the correlation between the amount of endometriosis and some degree of infertility. While this approach has worked well in oncology, this has not been the case with endometriosis associated infertility. The various staging systems for endometriosis have not taken into account cell volume and activity of the implants and are mixed with factors such as size of endometriotic cyst (or hematoma) and extent of pelvic adhesions, without data to suggest this is justified. In addition, factors such as age or duration of infertility have not been adequately accounted for in considering the fertility prognosis. For the moment endometriosis associated infertility can be best divided into infertility in women with peritoneal implants alone and infertility in women with factors in the form of adhesive disease compromising the tubo-ovarian relationship or the ovarian function.

▪ CLINICAL INVESTIGATIONS

PERITONEAL ENDOMETRIOSIS

Although peritoneal endometriosis can be observed at laparotomy, it is only since the introduction of laparoscopy that peritoneal endometriosis has been accurately described. Peritoneal endometriosis can present multiple appearances, and lesions have been described using a variation of colorful terminology (*Table 19.1*). Suspected or atypical lesions, especially if they do not have the characteristics of subtle or classical lesions, should be biopsied because they can be confused with other possibly malignant lesions of the peritoneum (*Table 19.2*).

Visible peritoneal implants have been described and classified as red, black and white lesions or a combination of these lesions. The color reflects the degree of vascularization, hemorrhage, hemopigmentation and fibrosis.

The *pink or red lesion* includes papular and vesicular structures and is characterized by a well developed vascularization or microhemorrhage (*Figure 19.3*). The peritoneal surroundings also display increased vascularization or hemorrhage (flame-like lesion) without fibro-

Table 19.1 *Terminology used to describe peritoneal endometriosis*
- Powder burn, puckered black lesion
- Vascularized glandular papule
- Vesicular lesions
    serous, surrounded by marked vascularization
    red hemorrhagic
- Red, flame-like
- Petechial peritoneum
- Hypervascularized area
- Discolored area
    yellow-brown
    blue
    white
- White scarring
- Peritoneal defects
- Cribriform peritoneum
- Subovarian adhesions

Table 19.2 *Nonendometriotic peritoneal lesions*
- Hemangioma
- Epithelial inclusions
- Foreign body reaction to oil-based contrast medium, talc, old suture
- Inflammatory cystic inclusions
- Psammoma body reaction
- Adrenal rest
- Walthard rest
- Ovarian cancer
- Splenosis
- Endosalpingiosis
- Ectopic pregnancy
- Secondary trophoblast implantation

sis. The implants are covered by normal mesothelium. The papular type is formed by cystic dilatation of an endometrial gland while the vesicular type frequently has a polypoidal structure (*Figure 19.4*). Both types are considered as an active endometriosis and are seen more frequently in young women (Redwine, 1987).

The *black lesion* is the classical, puckered blue-black or so-called gunshot lesion (*Figure 19.5*). Microscopic examination shows that the lesion contains not only glands and stroma but also a variable amount of fibrosis, pigmentation and inflammatory cell reaction. The hormonal response of this lesion is variable and has been related to the extent of fibrosis and decrease of vascularization (Nisolle et al, 1993).

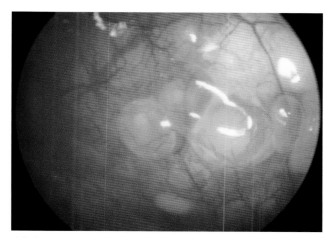

19.3a

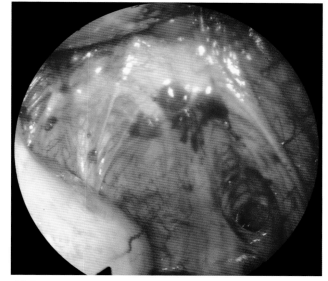

19.3c

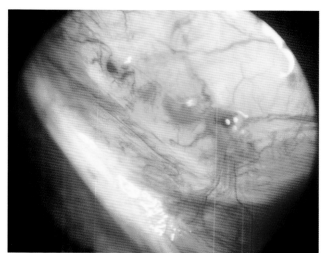

19.3b

Figure 19.3: *Early peritoneal endometriosis. (a) Papular lesion. Note the fine vascularization on the papule. Bleeding has not occurred and there is absence of fibrosis. (b) Serohemorrhagic lesion. Note the early hemorrhage and the absence of fibrosis. (c) Red vesicular lesions and peritoneal fibrosis and retraction. (d) A well vascularized endometrial polyp is seen inside the vesicle.*

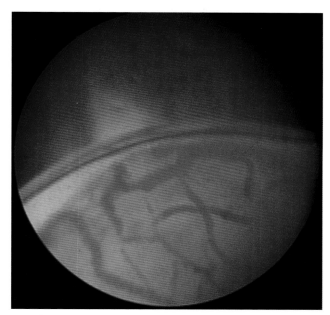

19.3d

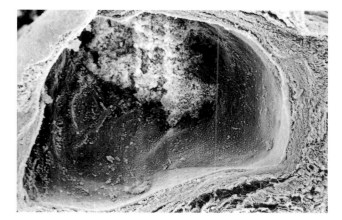

19.4a

Figure 19.4: *(a) Scanning electron microscopy shows that the papule represents a distended gland with secretory products (×150).*

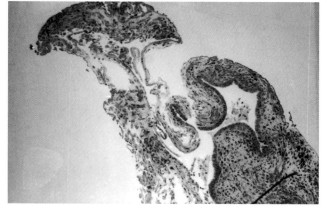

19.4b

(b) Polypoidal structure emerging from a distended glandular structure in a vesicular lesion (×235).

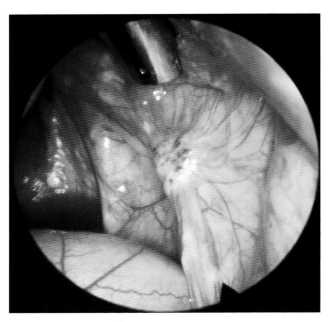

Figure 19.5: Classical blue-black puckered lesion of peritoneal endometriosis.

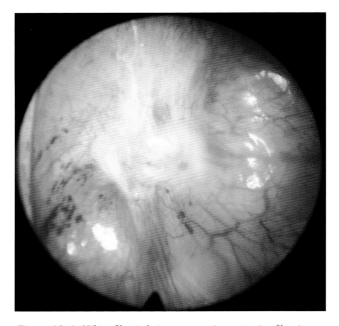

Figure 19.6: White fibrotic lesion representing extensive fibrosis; however, the presence of some active endometriotic cells cannot be excluded.

The *white lesion* reveals microscopically fibrous tissue with some inactive glandular tissue and scanty or no stroma and vascularization (*Figure 19.6*). Sequential observations have shown that peritoneal implants, and in particular the red lesions, can appear and disappear spontaneously on the peritoneal surface (Wiegerinck et al, 1993). When related to age, the red lesions precede the

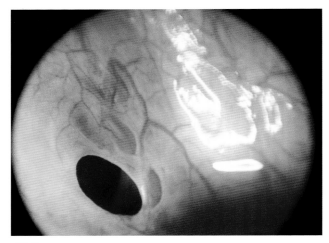

19.7a

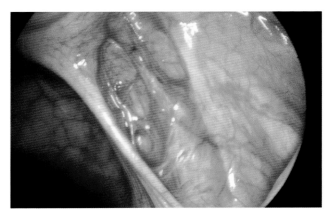

19.7b

Figure 19.7: Peritoneal defects. (a) Open peritoneal defect: in this case an endometrial implant with the full histological characteristics of superficial endometrium was identified inside the defect. (b) The defect has been peritonealized. A small pigmented endometriotic implant is seen.

others and with time their presence decreases, being replaced by black and ultimately white lesions (Redwine, 1987). Peritoneal endometriosis is frequently found to be associated with peritoneal defects (*Figure 19.7*) and adhesions (*Figure 19.8*).

Microscopic endometriosis was first described in scanning electron microscopy studies of the peritoneum as an area where the mesothelium is replaced by endometrial surface epithelium (Vasquez et al, 1984). This lesion has been identified as occurring in normal-looking peritoneum (Murphy et al, 1986). The origin of this lesion is not clear but can be explained by the rupture of a vesicular implant leaving glandular surface covering the peritoneal surface. Transition of peritoneal mesothelium into endometrial surface epithelium has not been documented. Nonvisible

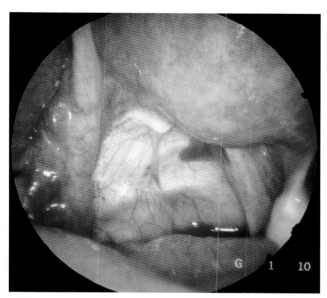

19.8a

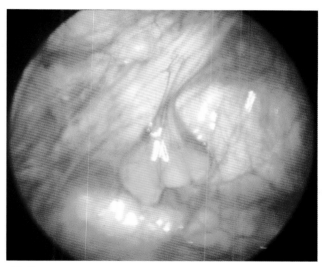

19.8b

Figure 19.8: *Peritoneal adhesions of questionable origin. (a) Filmy adhesions in the pouch of Douglas: such lesions can also represent sequelae of chronic pelvic inflammatory disease. (b) Vesicular lesion: note the absence of vascularization. Such vesicles are likely to be of inflammatory rather than endometriotic origin.*

implants, such as foci of glands and stroma underlying normal-looking peritoneum, were described in biopsies of normal-looking sacrouterine ligaments in 6% of the patients with endometriosis (Nisolle et al, 1990).

OVARIAN ENDOMETRIOMA

The term 'chocolate cyst' was applied by Sampson (1921) to describe the endometrial cyst of the ovary. The term is, however, purely descriptive and can be mis-

leading if only the chocolate colored contents of the cyst are noted, as hemorrhagic functional cysts can have the same content. Careful histological studies using step serial sections of ovaries with in situ endometriomas have demonstrated that in 93% of cases the wall of the endometrioma is formed by ovarian cortex and that the endometrioma is an extraovarian pseudocyst (Hughesdon, 1957). The frontal surface of the ovary is the most frequent site where the folding-in process has occurred and the stigma of inversion can be identified. Using the technique of ovarian cystoscopy the site of retraction and inversion can be identified in situ (Brosens et al, 1994). Inside, the ovarian cortex can be recognized in the early stage by its pearl-white appearance but with time the wall becomes more and more pigmented and changes from white to yellow and brown-black. The endometrial implants are seen as red, vascularized or hemorrhagic foci scattered over the ovarian cortex and connected by an extensive network of superficial vascularization. At the site of invagination small foci of superficial endometrial mucosa, including surface epithelium, glands and stroma, can be found, while in other areas the cortex is covered by not more than surface epithelium, with or without stroma. The terminology of deep endometriosis for the ovarian endometrioma is misleading. First, the type of implant is not more than surface epithelium or functional superficial endometrium; second, most endometriomas are structurally extraovarian pseudocysts; and third, there is no histological proof that the endometrial tissue is invading ovarian stroma (Hughesdon, 1957).

SONOGRAPHY

Endometriomas present different sonographic patterns, such as purely cystic, cystic with few septations or minimal debris, complex combinations of cystic and solid elements and largely solid (Athey and Diment, 1989; Fried et al, 1993). The sensitivity, specificity and accuracy of ultrasonographic diagnosis are reported as 84, 90 and 88% respectively (Mais et al, 1993). Due to the nonspecificity of the ultrasound examination the mass has to be differentiated from other ovarian cysts and occasionally from a cystadenoma or tubo-ovarian abscess. The technique is, however, useful for identifying the presence and location of endometriomas and may also be helpful in following the size of the cyst in response to therapy. Aspiration of the cyst under ultrasound can reveal the chocolate content but a similar chocolate colored hemorrhagic content may be found in some follicle hematomas, lutein cysts or even in cystadenomas.

MAGNETIC RESONANCE IMAGING

Sonography continues to be the initial modality of choice for evaluating adnexal masses, but magnetic resonance imaging (MRI) is increasingly used for problem solving when further characterization is needed. MRI has a higher accuracy than ultrasonography and appears to be the most accurate method of differentiating an endometrioma from other gynecological masses (Togashi et al, 1991). The hemorrhagic cyst can be accurately distinguished from the nonhemorrhagic cyst by MRI. The blood elements of a chronic stage hematoma exhibit hyperintense signal on both T_1- and T_2-weighted images and the thick viscous content is likely to explain the shading of the signal intensity of the fluid. The signal intensity typical of acute hematomas (intermediate intensity on T_1-weighted masses) and subacute hematomas (hyperintensity with a distinct central area of hypointensity on T_1-weighted images) allows differentiation from chronic bleeding in the endometrial cyst (Sugimura et al, 1992, 1993). In addition, MRI can reflect some specific features of an endometrioma, such as the typical localization and the adhesions between the endometrioma and the uterus or parametrium (*Figure 19.9*). The multilocularity or the presence of two or more hyperintense cysts communicating with each other or adhering to each other or to neighboring organs can be visualized. On the basis of the data of Togashi et al (1991) the overall diagnostic sensitivity, specificity and accuracy for MRI diagnosis of endometrial cysts were 90, 98 and 96% respectively. Given the 96% accuracy, MRI was proposed as an acceptable diagnostic test on which clinical decisions can be based.

LAPAROSCOPY

The laparoscopic features of a typical endometrioma include:

- ovarian cysts no more than 12 cm in diameter;

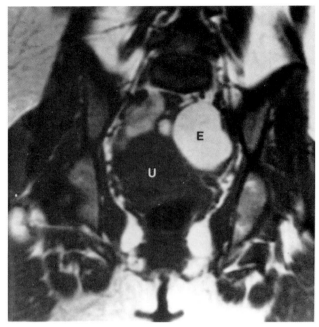

19.9a

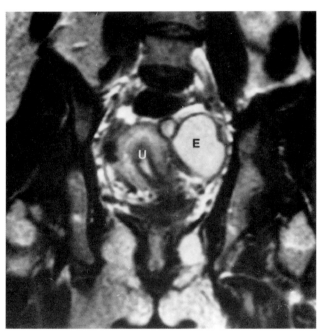

19.9b

Figure 19.9: *Endometrioma. Coronal T_1-weighted (a) and T_2-weighted (b) images. On the T_1-weighted image, the endometrioma (E) is of high signal intensity consistent with hemorrhage. The endometrioma demonstrates multilocularity and an indistinct interface with the adjacent uterus (U). From Popovich and Hricak (1994), courtesy of Professor H Hricak.*

- adhesions to the pelvic side wall and/or the posterior broad ligament;
- 'powder burns' and minute red or blue spots with adjacent puckering on the surface;
- tarry, thick, chocolate colored fluid content (*Figure 19.10*).

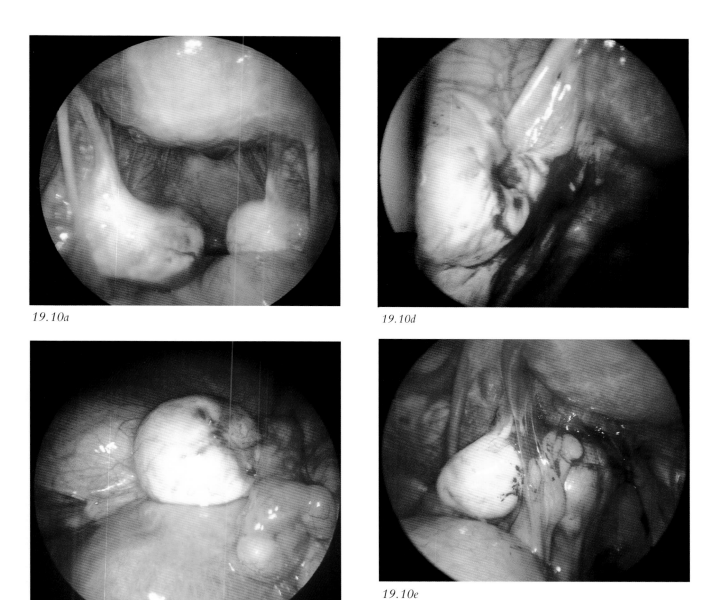

19.10a

19.10b

19.10d

19.10e

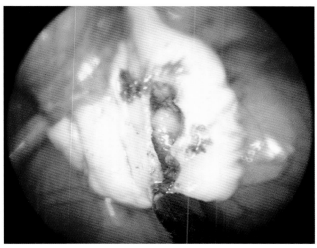

19.10c

Figure 19.10: *Ovarian endometrioma. (a) At laparoscopy the typical features are not usually seen as the endometrioma is located on the anterior side of the ovary. (b) The ovary has been rotated and the typical features of the endometrioma are exposed: anterior location, hemorrhagic and pigmented lesions in the center of the retraction. (c) After opening the pseudocyst the inverted ovarian cortex is exposed. (d) Adhesions at the hilus of the ovary between the ovarian cortex and the peritoneum with a hemorrhagic endometrial implant in the center. Note the depression of the ovarian cortex. (e) Ovarian endometrioma with extensive adhesions on the anterior side of the ovary.*

Table 19.3 *Diagnosis of ovarian endometrioma*

Technique	Sensitivity (%)	Specificity (%)	Accuracy (%)
Sonography	84	90	88
MRI	90	98	96
Visual inspection	97	95	96

The visual diagnosis of a typical endometrioma remains the most accurate method for detecting and diagnosing the endometrioma and has a sensitivity, specificity and accuracy of 97, 95 and 96% respectively (Vercellini et al, 1990) (*Table 19.3*).

In the absence of typical features a deep cyst or a cyst obscured by dense adhesions can be detected by aspiration of chocolate content (Candiani et al, 1990), but there is a need for histological confirmation. The diagnosis of an endometrioma should not be based on inspection of the aspirate alone. Cytology of the aspirate does not, as in most ovarian cysts, contribute to the diagnosis because of the poor yield of cells. CA-125 and steroid hormone assays of the cyst fluid have been suggested as being helpful in the differential diagnosis between an endometrioma and a functional cyst (Koninckx et al, 1992).

OVARIAN CYSTOSCOPY AND BIOPSY

Biopsy is essential for the detection of malignancy or atypia (Barbieri, 1992); however, random biopsies frequently fail to yield representative endometrial tissue. Ovarian cystoscopy has recently been proposed as a useful additional technique for the identification of the internal features of the endometrioma and the localization of implants for biopsy (Brosens and Puttemans, 1989; Brosens et al, 1994). The typical features of the wall of the endometrioma cyst are the capsule retraction, the presence of hemorrhagic foci at the site where on the outside retraction and adhesions are seen, and the network of superficial vascularization between the filmy superficial red implants (*Figure 19.11a–c*). In early endometriomas the color of the wall appears pearl-white, like normal ovarian cortex, and the red, hemorrhagic foci are easily dislodged from the surface by

manipulation. At histology the red foci are frequently found to be typical superficial endometrial tissue (*Figure 19.11d*) (Martin and Berry, 1990). At the site of retraction small foci of full thickness endometrial mucosa can be found, while at a distance only surface epithelium with or without stroma is found, suggesting a progressive outgrowth of endometrial tissue over the inverted cortex from the site of invagination. Biopsies from the pearl-white surface confirm the presence of cortex with or without primordial follicles, while pigmented and dark areas represent progressive fibrosis infiltrated with hemosiderin-loaded macrophages. Luteinized follicles in the inverted cortex are also seen as red areas, but in contrast to the endometrial implants they are located in the wall and are not detachable. Microbiopsies of 1–2 mm in size obtained under ovarioscopic guidance produce more representative endometriosis tissue than large, randomly taken biopsies or resected specimens (Brosens et al, 1994). The ovarioscopic technique allows identification of the characteristics of an endometrioma, particularly in cases where the laparoscopic inspection fails to reveal typical features. Recurrent chocolate cysts after previous surgery for endometriosis have been found to be functional hemorrhagic cysts in 73% of cases. Follicular and serous cysts are characterized by a smooth undulating or flat surface with a fine, retinal network of vascularization (*Figure 19.12a*). Lutein cysts present a uniform, granular and yellow appearance with discrete vascularization (*Figure 19.12b*).

NODULAR ENDOMETRIOSIS

True deep endometriosis is a nodular lesion. Histologically, it is characterized by dense tissue composed of fibrous and smooth muscle cells with islands or strands of glands and stroma. It is not surprising that, on descriptive grounds, the lesion had been called adenomyosis externa. Although the terminology was discarded after Sampson's 1921 publication, there are several reasons for reappraising the terminology for this specific type of implant.

Deep nodular endometriosis occurs particularly in the supportive structures of the pelvis, such as the uterosacral ligament, the retrocervical area, the rectovaginal and uterovesical septa. The major component of the nodular

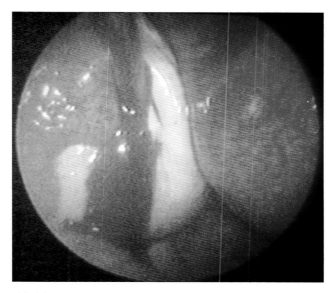

19.11a

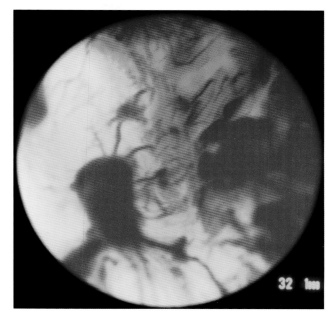

19.11c

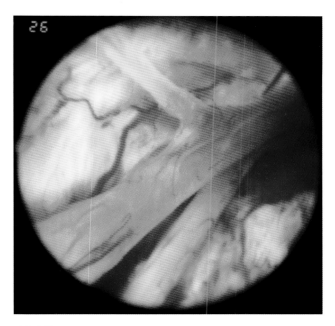

19.11b

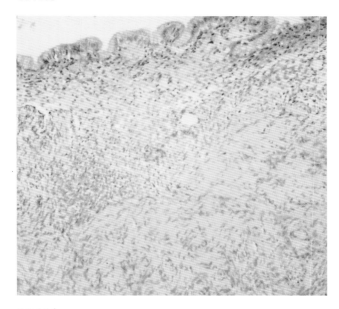

19.11d

Figure 19.11*: Ovarioscopy. (a) The endometrioma is distended and flushed by saline. (b) Identification of the site of retraction. (c) The red lesion with a prominent vascularization is very suggestive of* endometriotic implants and is the preferred site for biopsy. (d) Biopsy of the red implant shows superficial endometrium proliferating on ovarian cortex (×235).

lesion is not endometrial but fibromuscular tissue with sparse, finger-like extensions of glandular and stromal tissue. Small cysts filled with blood are seen in or around the nodule. In addition, with the well known resistance to current hormonal therapy, the lesion is morphologically and functionally similar to advanced adenomyosis of the uterus. This type of myoproliferative lesion was found in 25 and 91% of nodular lesions of the uterosacral ligament and rectovaginal septum respectively (Brosens, 1994).

A specific disadvantage of laparoscopy is that the two-dimensional view and the absence of palpation make it difficult to evaluate the size and depth of the nodule. A small retraction of the peritoneum may be the only visible lesion (*Figure 19.13*).

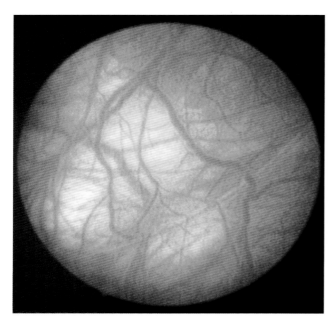

19.12a

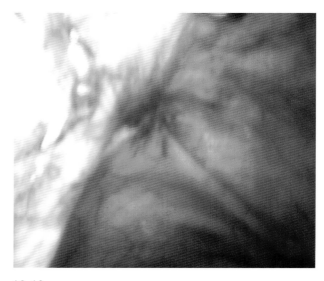

19.13a

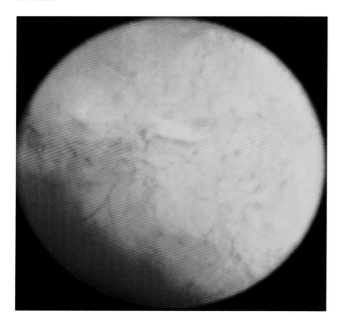

19.12b

Figure 19.12: Ovarioscopy of cysts with hemorrhagic content. (a) Serous cyst with retinal network of vascularization and a smooth surface. (b) Lutein cyst shows a yellow granular wall and a fine regular vascularization.

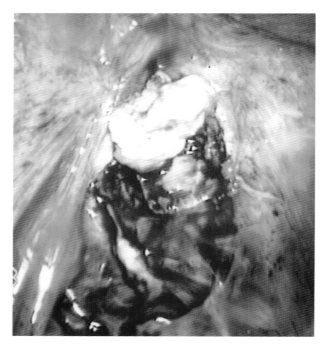

19.13b

Figure 19.13: Deep nodular endometriosis. (a) Only a small area of retraction is seen on the peritoneal surface. (b) A deep nodule is excised at this site.

▪ CLASSIFICATION

As accurate laparoscopic diagnosis requires optimal visualization, the prerequisites for accurate laparoscopic staging of endometriosis are very similar to those for laparoscopic surgery of endometriosis (Canis et al, 1992b, 1993). As usual, patients should be informed of a possible laparotomy. A bowel preparation should be administered on the day before surgery, facilitating the laparoscopic procedure and minimizing the consequences of a bowel injury.

The technique for laparoscopic exploration in gynecology has been described in Chapter 4. In cases of endometriosis special attention should be given to the following additional procedures.

1. To diagnose ovarian endometriomas a complete inspection of the ovarian surface is necessary, particularly the hilus of the ovary. This may require a complete ovariolysis. Ovariolysis should be performed slowly and carefully following the plane of cleavage between ovarian capsule and adherent peritoneum to avoid entering the peritoneum and risking unnecessary damage to the ureter and ovarian hilus vessels.

2. Enlarged ovaries and star-like ovarian scars are routinely punctured looking for small endometriomas (Candiani et al, 1990); however, the chocolate aspirate is not a pathognomonic sign of an endometrial cyst and can represent a lutein cyst.

3. The posterior cul-de-sac and the rectum are assessed using, when necessary, peroperative vaginal examination and/or vaginal and rectal probes (Reich et al, 1991).

4. If an ovarian endometrioma has been ruptured or punctured, the pelvis should be copiously irrigated and washed; the internal cyst wall is then inspected and a biopsy is taken from the red areas or other representative or suspected tissues in order to rule out malignancy and to differentiate endometriomas from functional or neoplastic chocolate cysts (Martin and Berry, 1990).

5. Finally, the upper abdomen is carefully inspected for bowel or appendicular endometriosis.

Expertise in operative laparoscopy is a prerequisite for accurate staging of patients with severe disease. Similarly, awareness of the various appearances of peritoneal and ovarian endometriotic implants is required. Martin et al (1989) clearly demonstrated that the recognition of subtle lesions increases with the surgeon's expertise. In their study, the rate of patients diagnosed with subtle lesions increased from 15% in 1986 to 65% in 1988, whereas the rate of patients with typical lesions rose only from 43 to 60%.

It was not until 1973 that the first classification based specifically on surgical inspection was designed to correlate with the postoperative pregnancy rate. This scheme is known as the Acosta classification (Acosta et al, 1973). Although it allowed a more exact staging of actual lesions it had its drawbacks – for example, lack of discrimination between unilateral and bilateral adnexal lesions and absence of deep subperitoneal lesions such as rectovaginal endometriosis. In view of the need for a widely accepted system, The American Fertility Society (AFS) published (in 1979) its first official classification, designed for use in connection with laparotomy or laparoscopy and based on the attribution of a score varying with the location and extent of lesions. A series of obvious defects became apparent in the AFS scoring

method and in 1985 the society published the revised AFS (r-AFS) classification of endometriosis in which the stage or degree of disease is based on a weighted point system (see *Table 29.2* and Chapter 29). This new scheme included improvements such as a two-dimensional and a three-dimensional assessment, a high score for dense adhesions enclosing the fimbriae and for complete posterior cul-de-sac obliteration, and the points attributed to a solitary adnexa are multiplied by two.

One of the criticisms often levelled at the r-AFS classification is that the scores for the subgroups can be added to give a global score of severity, whereas the involvement of the peritoneum, the ovary or the rectovaginal septum are different entities; therefore the score for endometriosis of the peritoneum, ovary and supporting pelvic tissues should be kept separately. Indeed, the score should be considered within each structure, as there can be no alleviation of severity by changes occurring in the opposite direction. Second, the visual classification of peritoneal endometriosis should also be complemented by a classification to include aspects of activity and healing. Third, the staging should take into account the presence or absence of regular menstruation. Some modifications have been proposed for the classification of endometriosis (Brosens et al, 1993).

PERITONEAL ENDOMETRIOSIS

A simple morphological classification can be added to the current r-AFS staging, including those lesions which have been confirmed histologically (Jansen and Russell, 1986; Stripling et al, 1988; Martin et al, 1989):

- Red lesion: a flame-like lesion, or a hemorrhagic vesicle or a vascularized or papular lesion.
- Black lesion: a puckered, blue-black lesion.
- White lesion: scarred tissue with or without some pigmentation.
- Atypical lesion: other lesions can be included under this heading if they are histologically proven.

For clinical purposes the number of implants can be counted; for research work they can be mapped on a peritoneal diagram and evaluated by their number or diameter.

Table 19.4 *Pelvic pain symptoms score.* (Adapted from Biberoglu and Behrman, 1981.)

Dysmenorrhea

0	= Absent	No discomfort/amenorrhea
1	= Mild	Some loss of work efficiency
2	= Moderate	In bed for part of one day
3	= Severe	In bed for one or more days

Dyspareunia

0	= Absent	No discomfort
1	= Mild	Tolerated discomfort
2	= Moderate	Intercourse painful to the point of interruption
3	= Severe	Avoids intercourse because of pain

Not applicable if not sexually active.

Pelvic pain

0	= Absent	No discomfort
1	= Mild	Occasional pelvic discomfort (i.e. any time during the cycle)
2	= Moderate	Noticeable discomfort for most of the cycle
3	= Severe	Pain persisting during the cycle, or pain requiring strong analgesics

The scores for each of the three symptoms must be added to obtain the total pelvic symptoms score.

Physical findings

Pelvic tenderness

Absent	No tenderness
Mild	Minimal tenderness on palpation
Moderate	Extensive tenderness on palpation
Severe	Unable to palpate because of tenderness

Pelvic induration

Absent	No induration
Mild	Uterus freely mobile, induration of the cul-de-sac
Moderate	Thickened and indurated adnexa and cul-de-sac, restricted uterine mobility
Severe	Nodular adnexa and cul-de-sac, frozen uterus

DEEP ENDOMETRIOSIS

This should include lesions visible on the peritoneal surface which are estimated to extend 1 cm or more below the peritoneal surface; they should be properly indicated on the peritoneal diagram. As the depth has been correlated with pain, it is recommended that a nodular lesion be scored by its estimated diameter (e.g. 1–2 cm, 2–3 cm, more than 3 cm) (Cornillie et al, 1990). It is important to distinguish rectovaginal from peritoneal endometriosis because they do not always coexist. Lesions should be biopsied for histological characterization (Nieminen, 1962; Brosens, 1994). In cul-de-sac obliteration adhesiolysis may be indicated for the location and diagnosis of the presence of true nodular lesions.

OVARIAN ENDOMETRIOSIS

Superficial ovarian endometriosis should be distinguished from cystic ovarian endometriosis. In addition, it is important always to examine the posterior ovarian surface; therefore, in the presence of adhesions it is essential to perform adhesiolysis and liberate the ovary for full inspection.

SUPERFICIAL LESIONS

Superficial lesions should be identified as red, black or white, using the same criteria as for peritoneal endometriosis. The scoring can also be expressed in 'number' or 'size' of implants on one or both ovaries.

ENDOMETRIOTIC CYST

It is rare to find an endometrioma without other evidence of endometriosis on the ovary. To detect an endometriotic cyst it may be helpful to use needle aspiration for the presence of the typical dark, chocolate cyst fluid; however, the wall of all hemorrhagic cysts should be fully inspected and biopsies should be obtained. Inspection is performed after opening the cyst or by ovarioscopy and can differentiate between those with red, vascularized foci on a white or yellow pigmented surface (red cysts) and those with a dark, pigmented and fibrotic wall (black cysts). Biopsies representative of endometriosis are most likely to be obtained from the red lesions. This distinction is suggested as the red cysts can be treated conservatively by adhesiolysis, eversion and coagulation while the black cysts may require excision (Brosens et al, 1996).

ADHESIONS

Only adhesions involving the Fallopian tube and ovary are of real relevance in terms of restoration of fertility. Other adhesions could therefore be excluded from a scoring aimed at predicting future fertility potential. Adhesions involving the Fallopian tube and ovary should be scored separately. In addition, only those tubal adhesions involving the ampullary portion are of relevance. They should perhaps be divided into categories, such as one third or two thirds, or complete occlusion/fixity of the ampullary portion of the tube. None the less, these other adhesions may be relevant in long-term management and/or in evaluating pain (particularly when there is fixation to other organs, such as the uterus in marked retroversion or the bowel being kinked and fixed).

The distinction between filmy and dense adhesions should be maintained in the new classification because this may indicate the likelihood of performing surgical division of the adhesions. The operability of ovarian endometriomas depends more on the degree and type of adhesions than on the size of the cystic structure (Canis et al, 1992a, 1992b).

PELVIC PAIN

The following steps are recommended to improve classification of this symptom:

1. Indicate other possible etiologies of lower abdominal pain (orthostatic, digestive, urinary); undertake investigations of possible contributing factors of pelvic pain (infertility, infection, depression, sexual abuse).
2. Describe the sites and use a scoring system for dysmenorrhea, dyspareunia and pelvic pain such as the one proposed in *Table 19.4*.

REFERENCES

Acosta AA, Buttram VC, Besch PK, Malinak LR, Franklin RR & Vanderheyden JD (1973) A proposed classification of pelvic endometriosis. *Obstet Gynecol* **42**: 19–23.

American Fertility Society (1985) Revised American Fertility Society classification of endometriosis. *Fertil Steril* 43: 351–352.

Athey PA & Diment DD (1989) The spectrum of sonographic findings in endometriomas. *J Ultrasound Med* **8**: 487–491.

Barbieri RL (1992) Visual diagnosis of endometriosis – reliability? *Fertil Steril* **58**: 221–222 (letter).

Benagiano G & Brosens I (1991) The history of endometriosis: identifying the disease. *Hum Reprod* **7**: 963–968.

Biberoglu KO & Behrman SJ (1981) Dosage aspects of danazol therapy in endometriosis: short-term and long-term effectiveness. *Am J Obstet Gynecol* **139**: 645–654.

Brosens IA (1994) New principles in the management of endometriosis. *Acta Obstet Gynecol Scand* **159**: 18–21.

Brosens IA & Puttemans PJ (1989) Double-optic laparoscopy. Salpingoscopy, ovarian cystoscopy and endo-ovarian surgery with the argon laser. *Baillière's Clin Obstet Gynaecol* 3: 595–608.

Brosens IA, Donnez J & Benagiano G (1993) Improving the classification of endometriosis. *Hum Reprod* **8**: 1792–1795.

Brosens IA, Puttemans PJ & Deprest J (1994) The endoscopic localization of endometrial implants in the ovarian chocolate cyst. *Fertil Steril* **65**: 1034–1038.

Brosens IA, Van Ballaer P, Puttemans P & Deprest J (1996) Reconstruction of the ovary containing large endometriomas by an extraovarian endosurgical technique. *Fertil Steril* **66**: 517–521.

Candiani GB, Vercellini P & Fedele L (1990) Laparoscopic ovarian puncture for correct staging of endometriosis. *Fertil Steril* **53**: 994–997.

Canis M, Mage G, Wattiez A, Chapron C, Pouly JL & Bassil S (1992a) Second-look laparoscopy after laparoscopic cystectomy of large ovarian endometriomas. *Fertil Steril* **58**: 617–619.

Canis M, Pouly JL, Wattiez A, Manhes H, Mage G & Bruhat MA (1992b) Incidence of bilateral adnexal disease in severe endometriosis (revised American Fertility Society (AFS), stage IV): should a stage V be included in the AFS classification? *Fertil Steril* **57**: 691–692.

Canis M, Bouquet de Jolinières J, Wattiez A et al (1993) Classification of endometriosis. *Baillière's Clin Obstet Gynaecol* **7**: 758–772.

Cornillie F, Oosterlynck D, Lauwereyns JM & Koninckx PR (1990) Deeply infiltrating pelvic endometriosis: histology and clinical significance. *Fertil Steril* **53**: 978–983.

Cullen TS (1920) The distribution of adenomyoma containing uterine mucosa. *Arch Surg* **1**: 215–283.

Fedele L, Bianchi S, Bocciolone L et al (1992) Pain symptoms associated with endometriosis. *Obstet Gynecol* **79**: 767–769.

Fried AM, Rhodes RA & Morehouse IR (1993) Endometrioma: analysis and sonographic classification of 51 documented cases. *South Med J* **86**: 297–301.

Hughesdon PE (1957) The structure of endometrial cysts of the ovary. *J Obstet Gynaecol Br Empire* **44**: 481–487.

Jansen RPS & Russell P (1986) Non-pigmented endometriosis: clinical laparoscopic and pathologic definition. *Am J Obstet Gynecol* **155**: 1154–1159.

Koninckx PR, Meuleman C, Demeyere S, Lesaffre E & Cornillie FJ (1991) Suggestive evidence that pelvic endometriosis is a progressive disease, whereas deeply infiltrating endometriosis is associated with pelvic pain. *Fertil Steril* **55**: 759–765.

Koninckx PR, Muyldermans M, Moerman P, Meuleman C, Deprest J & Cornillie F (1992) CA 125 concentrations in ovarian 'chocolate' cyst fluid can differentiate an endometriotic cyst from a cystic corpus luteum. *Hum Reprod* **7**: 1314–1317.

Mahmood TA, Templeton AA, Thomson L & Fraser C (1991) Menstrual symptoms in women with pelvic endometriosis. *Br J Obstet Gynaecol* **98**: 558–563.

Mais V, Guerriero S, Ajossa S, Angiolucci M, Paoletti AM & Melis GB (1993) The efficiency of transvaginal ultrasonography in the diagnosis of endometrioma. *Fertil Steril* **60**: 776–780.

Martin DC & Berry JD (1990) Histology of chocolate cysts. *J Gynecol Surg* **6**: 43–46.

Martin DC, Hubert GD, Vander Zwaag R & El-Zeky F (1989) Laparoscopic appearances of peritoneal endometriosis. *Fertil Steril* **51**: 63–67.

Moen MH & Muus KM (1991) Endometriosis in pregnant and non-pregnant women at tubal sterilization. *Hum Reprod* **6**: 699–702.

Murphy A, Green W, Bobbie D et al (1986) Unsuspected endometriosis documented by scanning electron microscopy in visually normal peritoneum. *Fertil Steril* **46**: 522–524.

Nieminen U (1962) Studies on the vascular pattern of ectopic endometrium with special reference to cyclic changes. *Acta Obstet Gynecol Scand* **41 (suppl 3)**: 1–81.

Nisolle M, Paindaveine B, Bourdon A et al (1990) Histologic study of peritoneal endometriosis in infertile women. *Fertil Steril* **53**: 984–988.

Nisolle M, Casanas-Roux F, Anaf V, Mine JM & Donnez J (1993) Morphometric study of the stromal vascularization in peritoneal endometriosis. *Fertil Steril* **59**: 681–684.

Popovich MJ & Hricak H (1994) The role of magnetic resonance imaging in the evaluation of gynecologic disease. In Callen PW (ed.) *Ultrasonography in Obstetrics and Gynecology*, 3rd edn, p 677. Philadelphia: Saunders.

Redwine DB (1987) The distribution of endometriosis in the pelvis by age groups and fertility. *Fertil Steril* **47**: 173–175.

Reich H, McGlynn F & Salvat J (1991) Laparoscopic treatment of cul de sac obliteration secondary to retrocervical deep endometriosis. *J Reprod Med* **36**: 516–522.

Russel WW (1899) Aberrant portions of the Müllerian duct found in an ovary. *Johns Hopkins Hosp Bull* **10**: 8–10.

Sampson JA (1921) Perforating hemorrhagic (chocolate) cysts of the ovary. *Arch Surg* **3**: 245–323.

Sampson JA (1927) Peritoneal endometriosis due to the menstrual dissemination of endometrial tissue into the peritoneal cavity. *Am J Obstet Gynecol* **14**: 422–469.

Stripling MC, Martin DC, Chatman DL, Vander Zwaag R & Poston WM (1988) Subtle appearances of endometriosis. *Fertil Steril* **49**: 427–431.

Sugimura K, Takemori M, Sugiura M, Okizuka H, Kono M & Ishida T (1992) The value of magnetic resonance relaxation time in staging ovarian endometrial cysts. *Br J Radiol* **65**: 502–506.

Sugimura K, Okizuka H, Imaoka I et al (1993) Pelvic endometriosis: detection and diagnosis with chemical shift MR imaging. *Radiology* **188**: 435–438.

Togashi K, Nishimura K, Kimura I et al (1991) Endometrial cysts: diagnosis with MR imaging. *Radiology* **180**: 73–78.

Vasquez G, Cornillie F & Brosens IA (1984) Peritoneal endometriosis: scanning electron microscopy and histology of minimal pelvic endometriotic lesion. *Fertil Steril* **42**: 696–703.

Vercellini P, Vendola N, Bocciolone L, Rognoni M, Carinelli S & Candiani G (1990) Reliability of the visual diagnosis of ovarian endometriosis. *Fertil Steril* **53**: 1198–1200.

Wiegerinck MAHM, Van Dop PA & Brosens IA (1993) The staging of peritoneal endometriosis by the type of active lesion in addition to the revised American Fertility Society classification. *Fertil Steril* **3**: 461–464.

20 *Anovulation: a therapeutically oriented diagnosis*
B Lunenfeld, E Lunenfeld and SL Tan

■ INTRODUCTION

The field of reproductive medicine has witnessed major technological advances in the area of imaging since the mid-1980s. Certainly, a major contribution to imaging has been in the field of ultrasonography. Pelvic ultrasonography as a diagnostic tool for gynecologists and reproductive endocrinologists has enjoyed an impressive and sustained growth in its short (two decades) existence. Integral to this progression has been the continuous development of new instruments with improved resolution, smaller scan units, the introduction of endovaginal probes and the increased number of skilled ultrasonographers. This progressive expansion of the field of gynecological ultrasonography has allowed the incorporation of this technology into routine clinical practice. The introduction of transvaginal ultrasonography has greatly enhanced the use of sonography in the diagnosis and management of infertility.

■ SONOGRAPHIC EXPLORATIONS AND INTERPRETATION

The main advantage of the transvaginal approach is that pictures of the ovaries and uterus are generally larger and clearer (*Figures 20.1* and *20.2*) than those produced by abdominal sonography, so that measurements taken are much more accurate (*Figures 20.3* and *20.4*). This is because the ovaries and uterus are closer to the vaginally placed ultrasound transducer, allowing the use of higher ultrasound frequencies, and artifactual echoes caused by multiple reflections from intervening tissues are minimized. Moreover, the patient does not need to have a full bladder and therefore it is much more convenient (Tan et al, 1992a). Ultrasonography has become an integral part of the primary evaluation and management

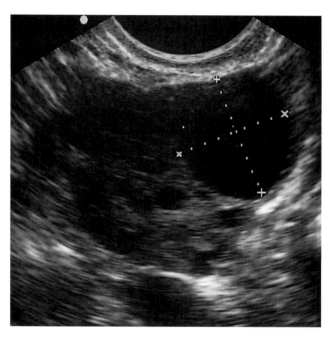

Figure 20.1: *An ovary with a dominant follicle as seen on transvaginal ultrasonography.*

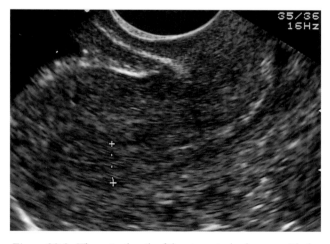

Figure 20.2: *The entire length of the uterus is clearly seen, with the endometrium visible along the axis of the uterus.*

of female infertility and for the detection of possible complications during ovarian stimulation. While it cannot totally replace laparoscopy, which allows direct visualization of pelvic structures, or hysterosalpingography (HSG), which has been traditionally used to detect tubal

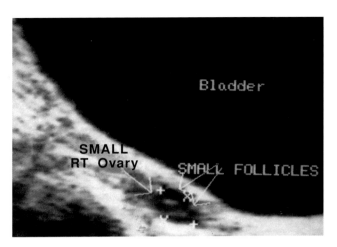

Figure 20.3: *The ovary as seen on transabdominal ultrasonography. Note that the ovary appears much smaller than it does on transvaginal ultrasound scan. It is important that the patient has a full bladder for transabdominal ultrasonography of the ovaries and uterus.*

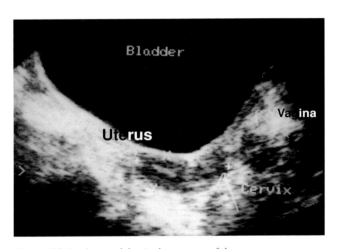

Figure 20.4: *A transabdominal sonogram of the uterus.*

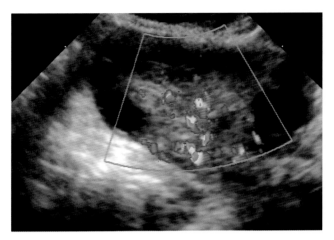

Figure 20.5: *A polycystic ovary with increased blood flow in the ovarian stroma.*

diseases, its uses are continually expanding. For example, with regard to the evaluation of tubal patency, several studies have shown that the use of hysterosalpingo contrast sonography (HyCoSy) with echo enhancing agents such as Echovist® (SHU 454; Schering AG, Germany) may allow diagnosis of tubal blockage to be reliably made (Campbell et al, 1994). Occasionally, transvaginal ultrasound may also diagnose the presence of hydrosalpinges (Tan et al, 1992a). Because it is a noninvasive and relatively convenient procedure for the patient, ultrasonography is of primary importance in obtaining valuable information in the clinical decision making process of several conditions.

More recently, the introduction of transvaginal color Doppler ultrasonography (see Chapter 12) has further

expanded the horizons of sonography in infertility. It may help in the diagnosis of polycystic ovarian syndrome by demonstrating increased blood flow in the ovarian stroma in the early follicular phase (*Figure 20.5*) (Zaidi et al, 1995a) and luteinized unruptured follicle syndrome (Zaidi et al, 1995b). Transvaginal color Doppler ultrasonography is an accurate investigative tool (Steer et al, 1995); using this technique, impedance to uterine artery blood flow has been found to be significantly different in women with different causes of infertility as compared with that in women of normal fertility (Steer et al, 1994).

Thus, even at the onset of an 'infertility workup' ultrasonography can direct the reproductive endocrinologist or reproductive gynecologist to continue investigations either towards mechanical infertility or towards functional infertility, or towards both. If mechanical infertility has been suspected by the ultrasound procedure, it must be confirmed by HSG or laparoscopy, as appropriate according to the information obtained by sonography, as a second step in the investigation of infertile patients.

In the management of infertility, sonographic procedures can confirm ovarian response to various pharmacological regimens for induction of ovulation and can guide the treating physician to increase or decrease doses of ovulation inducing agents, or withhold therapy if excessive stimulation is obtained in order to avoid the occurrence of ovarian hyperstimulation syndrome. If sonographic assessment of follicular growth is combined

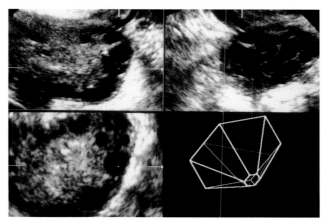

20.6a

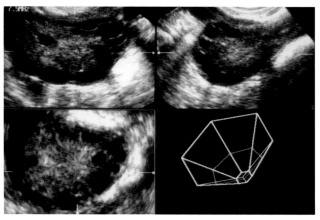

20.6c

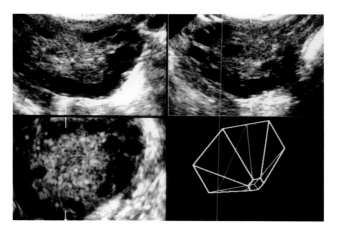

20.6b

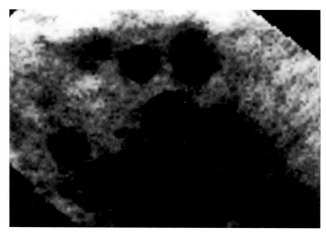

20.6d

Figure 20.6: *(a)–(c) A polycystic ovary visualized in three planes using a three-dimensional ultrasound scan machine.*

(d) A three-dimensional reconstruction of the ovary.

with blood flow measurements of the intraovarian arteries it may permit early recognition of poor response due to poor ovarian neovascularization (Zaidi et al, 1996). In induction of ovulation for anovulatory infertility, ultrasonography should be performed before starting ovarian stimulation, and if an ovarian cyst is noted at the beginning of the cycle, we would normally advise that treatment be delayed until a subsequent cycle when the cyst has disappeared. In the context of assisted reproduction, however, because these cysts will be aspirated at the time of oocyte collection, the same advice does not necessarily apply. A number of studies have suggested that, with respect to in vitro fertilization (IVF), there is no significant difference in the total number of follicles developed, oocytes retrieved and fertilized or in the final outcome between patients who have aspiration of the cysts compared with those where the cysts have been left alone (Rizk et al, 1990).

■ INTERPRETATION OF FINDINGS

Transvaginal sonography gives an excellent opportunity for the study of the normal physiology of the ovarian and endometrial cycle and permits the detection of both major and minor abnormalities in follicular and endometrial development. The selection and dynamic development of follicles can be observed. With the introduction of vaginal sonography and color Doppler imaging, the possibilities have opened for the study of human ovaries and uterus in both physiological and pathological conditions; however, conventional transvaginal sonography has limitations in imaging pelvic structures as it is restricted to only two dimensions. Recently, three-dimensional ultrasound machines have been developed, which will probably increase the precision of imaging pelvic structures (Kyei-Mensah et al, 1996a, 1996b) *(Figure 20.6)*.

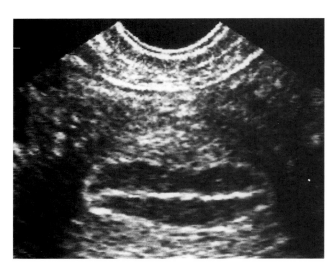

Figure 20.7: *The endometrial lining shows a triple line appearance consistent with a receptive endometrium.*

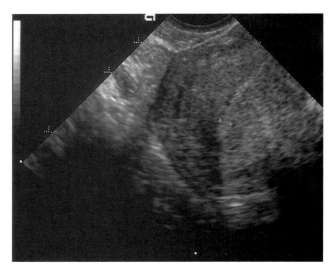

Figure 20.8: *Note the thin endometrium in the early follicular phase, as seen on the baseline ultrasound scan, consistent with an unstimulated endometrium.*

THE OVARIAN AND UTERINE CYCLE

Traditionally, ultrasonography is used to give us information regarding the number and size of follicles, while simultaneous estrogen measurement permits the assessment of the functional capacity or integrity of the growing follicles. However, the possibility of measuring the endometrial thickness (*Figure 20.2*) and texture (*Figure 20.7*) (Adams et al, 1988), together with measurements of blood flow to the uterus and the ovary, may reduce the need for frequent estrogen measurements and permit the patient to be her 'own personal specific bioassay'.

The bioendocrine assessment of endometrial response to estrogens initially and later to progesterone are important elements for understanding the diagnosis and management of infertility. An unstimulated endometrium appears as a thin echogenic line suggestive of a hypoestrogenic state (*Figure 20.8*). As a result of gradual follicular maturation in the follicular phase there is a progressive increase in endometrial thickness. Often the presence of endometrial stromal edema results in the appearance of a clear echo-free space surrounding the periphery of the echogenic endometrial line, producing the so-called triple line appearance (*Figure 20.7*). This picture is normally seen together with at least one dominant follicle with an average diameter greater than 18 mm. In the immediate post-ovulatory period, due to a sudden fall in estrogen con-

centration following follicular rupture, there is regression of stromal edema. This results in the echo-free space surrounding the echogenic endometrial line losing its echo-free nature and the development of fine dispersed echoes within the space.

INDUCTION OF OVULATION AND SUPEROVULATION

Thus the integration of ultrasonography in the management of infertility could increase the precision of the diagnostic workup of the infertile patient to help elucidate the cause of infertility, and reduce the cost of induction of ovulation and superovulation regimens by avoiding the need for frequent estrogen assays. It also increases convenience to the patient. The ultrasonic assessment of spontaneous follicle growth can be easily monitored. It has been shown that the intraobserver and interobserver variation of ultrasound assessment of ovarian follicle diameter is very small, with one study reporting an intraobserver standard variation of 0.6 mm and interobserver standard deviation of 1.2 mm (Eissa et al, 1985), even though the abdominal approach was used to measure follicular diameters in this study.

In superovulated cycles, however, greater care has to be taken to measure the diameters of the follicles because the reliability of standard ultrasound techniques of follicular measurements is influenced by the shape and numbers of

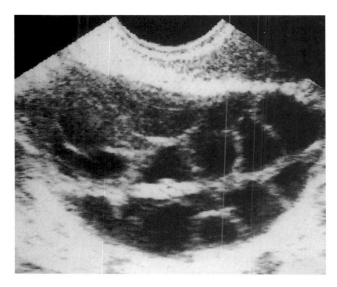

Figure 20.9: An ovary with multiple follicles developing as a result of ovarian stimulation. The shapes of the follicles are distorted because of compression by adjacent follicles.

the follicles. There may be technical difficulty in measuring the diameters of the follicle when its shape is distorted because of compression by adjacent follicles (*Figure 20.9*). Penzias et al (1994) showed that mean follicular diameter accurately predicted volume in round and polygonal follicles, but not in those that were ellipsoid. It is therefore imperative that there be a standardized approach to measuring the three diameters of the follicle when conventional ultrasound scanning is performed in the presence of multiple follicles. In this connection, the recent introduction of three-dimensional (3-D) ultrasound scanning is a major advance. This is because 3-D measurement is not affected by follicular shape as the changing contours are outlined serially to obtain specific volume measurements (*Figure 20.10*). In a recent study it has been shown that the volume of large follicles in IVF cycles is more accurately determined by 3-D ultrasound than by calculations from three follicular diameters obtained using conventional two-dimensional ultrasound (Kyei-Mensah et al, 1996a).

We have alluded to the usefulness of a baseline ultrasound scan before commencing ovarian stimulation for assisted reproduction. A major reason for this scan is to determine if the patient has polycystic ovaries (*Figure 20.11*) (Adams et al, 1985), a finding which has significant impact on prognostic outcome. In a recent study in which a group of patients with polycystic ovaries

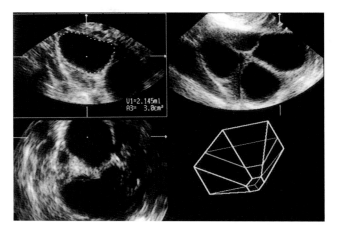

20.10a

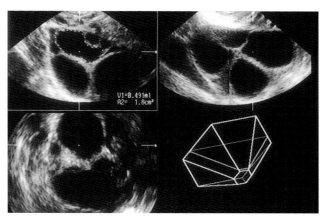

20.10b

Figure 20.10: (a) and (b) Measuring the volume of a follicle by outlining the changing contours serially.

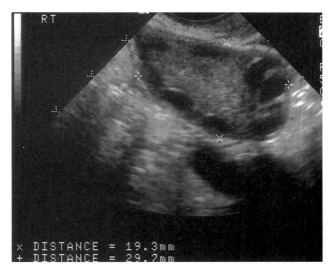

Figure 20.11: The polycystic ovary is typically enlarged with multiple small cysts seen around its periphery, with increased echogenic stroma.

diagnosed on pretreatment ultrasound scan were compared with control patients who had normal ovaries and who were matched for age, cause of infertility and ovarian stimulation regimen, all of whom were undergoing superovulation for IVF, it was found that patients with polycystic ovaries, as compared with controls, required significantly less human menopausal gonadotropin to stimulate their ovaries, but produced significantly higher serum estradiol levels on the day of human chorionic gonadotropin (hCG) administration, and more oocytes, but lower fertilization rates (MacDougall et al, 1993). Importantly, 10.5% of the patients with polycystic ovaries developed moderate or severe ovarian hyperstimulation syndrome, compared with none of the controls (MacDougall et al, 1993). Another reason would be to exclude the presence of uterine fibromyomas, which may distort the endometrial lining. The use of color Doppler ultrasound allows the position of the myoma in relation to the endometrium to be clearly established (*Figure 20.12*).

More recently, there have been studies to determine if measurement of intraovarian blood flow in the early follicular phase is related to subsequent ovarian responsiveness in IVF treatment (Zaidi et al, 1996). This is particularly useful because the ability to predict ovarian response is important. If an inadequate dose of gonadotropins is used there may be a relatively poor response, which reduces the number of oocytes retrieved. On the other hand, if an excessive dose is used, ovarian hyperstimulation syndrome, which is the most dangerous complication of IVF treatment, may occur.

Although measurement of the baseline follicle stimulating hormone (FSH) level may be useful in predicting some cases of poor response, the majority of patients have normal FSH levels and, to date, there is no reliable method for predicting ovarian response in these patients. A recent study correlated the velocity of blood flow in the ovarian stroma measured before ovarian stimulation was commenced with subsequent ovarian response (Zaidi et al, 1996). The results showed that there was a significant positive independent relationship between the maximum ovarian stromal blood flow velocity at the baseline ultrasound scan and the subsequent ovarian response. There was no relationship between resistance to blood flow in the ovarian stroma and follicular response, implying that the results reflect varying degrees of intraovarian perfusion in the stromal vessels at the baseline ultrasound scan. The reason for these observations may be because women with greater ovarian stromal blood flow have increased intraovarian perfusion so that, in response to the same dosage of gonadotropins, a relatively greater amount of gonadotropin is delivered to the granulosa–thecal cell complex, which leads to a greater number of follicles being produced. It has been previously reported that women with polycystic ovaries have significantly greater maximum ovarian stromal blood flow velocity (*Figure 20.5*) and this may be the reason why patients with polycystic ovaries tend to respond excessively to the administration of gonadotropins (Zaidi et al, 1995).

Sonography can aid recognition of imminent ovulation. The reasons for precise timing of this process include:

■ optimizing the harvesting of ova for assisted reproductive technology (ART) programs;

■ scheduling insemination with husband or donor sperm;

■ deciding whether to withhold ovulation induction with hCG or perform follicular reduction before or after the administration of hCG to avoid the development ovarian hyperstimulation syndrome.

Severe ovarian hyperstimulation syndrome, although occurring only in 0.5–2% of ovulation induction cases, is a major complication, which if not recognized and promptly treated can progress to massive ovarian enlargement, multiple luteal and hemorrhagic cysts, ascites, pleural effusion, hypovolemia, renal failure and possible death. Ovarian

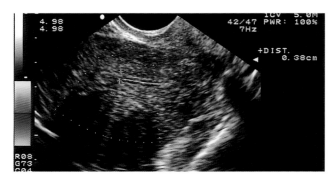

Figure 20.12: *A uterine fibroid in the posterior wall of the uterus. Note that the margin of the fibroid is outlined by the color Doppler ultrasound and can be seen not to impinge on the endometrial lining.*

sonography may allow determination and classification of hyperstimulation syndrome according to ovarian size. We have shown that follicular phase scanning demonstrating multiple intermediate follicles associated with high serum estradiol concentrations is predictive of the occurrence of luteal phase ovarian hyperstimulation syndrome.

Ultrasonography can suggest that ovulation has occurred and it can identify, at a very early stage, the ovarian hyperstimulation syndrome, which may help avert a medical complication. Furthermore, ultrasonography in the luteal phase may depict the beginning of luteal cyst formation, detect the beginning of ascites and allow the estimation of the volume of peritoneal fluid, permitting the physician an early diagnosis and prompt intervention. In patients with severe ascites and respiratory compromise, ultrasonic needle-guided paracentesis plays a major role in the treatment of ovarian hyperstimulation syndrome. Sonography also reduces the risk of accidental puncturing of the vulnerable ovary during paracentesis.

In ART procedures the laparoscopic approach for oocyte recovery was initially popular because gynecologists were familiar with the procedure; however, it is invasive and requires general anesthesia. Nowadays ultrasound directed follicular aspiration (*Figure 20.13*) has more or less replaced laparoscopy worldwide as the technique of choice for ovum collection. It has made ART an ambulatory procedure. It has greatly simplified IVF and allows the concept that patients should be encouraged to attempt several IVF treatment cycles because the cumulative pregnancy rate would be much higher (Tan et al, 1992b, 1994a, 1994b). Ultrasound directed follicular aspiration does not require general anesthesia or full operating theatre facilities and is simpler, faster and requires fewer staff compared with the laparoscopic approach. It can be performed even if extensive pelvic adhesions are present, and it has effectively converted ART into an ambulatory technique (Hussein et al, 1992; Tan et al, 1992c).

For the patient, IVF with ultrasound is therefore a much simpler procedure than gamete intrafallopian transfer (GIFT) and possibly future improvements in ultrasound technology may permit placing of the embryo precisely in the desired part of the uterus or tube under ultrasound guidance or transfer of ova and sperm or zygotes into the Fallopian tube.

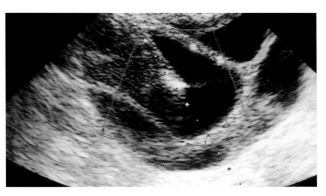

20.13a

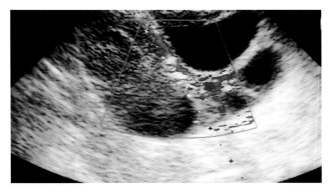

20.13b

Figure 20.13: *An ultrasound directed follicular aspiration. (a) The needle is clearly seen within the follicle. (b) The follicle has been totally emptied.*

■ CLASSIFICATION OF ANOVULATION

Whether or not a mechanical problem is suspected, it is useful to schedule the 'presumed ovulatory' female for a cycle evaluation. This would include sonographic assessment of follicular and endometrial growth and development, determination of the cervical score, a postcoital test in the preovulatory period and determination of the midluteal serum progesterone levels. These tests will indicate the presence or absence of cervical problems or problems associated with the deposition of sperm and assess follicular development, ovulation and endometrial development.

During the last three decades a variety of effective ovulation inducing agents have been developed. According to their mode of action each category of these therapeutic agents will be useful only in a specific situation. Therefore, in order to use these drugs effectively in anovulatory patients, the etiological diagnosis has first to be established. For the purpose of general organization, the female is classified in one of the following ways:

- having presumed ovulatory cycles;
- being amenorrheic;
- having presumed anovulatory cycles which may be regular or irregular;
- being amenorrheic or having anovulatory cycles associated with clinical signs of androgenization.

HYPERPROLACTINEMIA

In about 20% of cases of anovulation, elevated prolactin levels associated with disturbances in luteinizing hormone releasing hormone (LHRH) pulsatility are expressed by an unpredictable variety of cycle disturbances, ranging from luteal phase defects to amenorrhea. Sonographic procedures will help to assess the degree of lack of follicular and endometrial development. It is useful to measure prolactin levels in all patients with anovulation. If elevated on repetitive assays, and iatrogenic causes have been excluded, an elevated thyroid stimulating hormone (TSH) level may uncover a subclinical hypothyroidism. In primary hypothyroidism the administration of thyroxine usually normalizes prolactin levels and restores ovulatory cycles. A space occupying lesion in the hypothalamic–pituitary region may be diagnosed by appropriate imaging techniques. The diagnosis of a space occupying lesion is less important for deciding when to employ medical therapy and when to choose the surgical approach.

Modern imaging techniques may be combined with endocrine assessment to arrive at a therapeutically rendered classification of anovulatory infertility. Bevan et al (1987) correlated the serum prolactin concentration with histological diagnosis in a series of 128 patients with sella enlargement who were referred for the diagnosis of a presumed pituitary adenoma. A pituitary prolactin concentration of more than 8000 iu/l was always due to a prolactinoma, while all three patients with stalk defect and none of the patients with a large prolactinoma had a prolactin concentration less than 3000 iu/l. These results suggest that a pituitary tumor with hyperprolactinemia less than 3000 iu/l should be regarded as a nonfunctional tumor and treated surgically (Soule and

Jacobs, 1995). Conversely, if the prolactin concentration is greater than 8000 iu/l, the lesion is likely to be a true prolactinoma and should respond to dopamine agonist therapy with a reduction in tumor volume. Patients with prolactin concentration in the 3000–8000 iu/l range may reasonably be given a trial of dopamine agonist therapy. The strategy for managing patients with prolactinoma who are about to embark on pregnancy has undergone a major modification in recent years. The 50–70% enlargement of the normal pituitary during pregnancy poses little threat to the patient harboring a microprolactinoma (Soule and Jacobs, 1995). There is only a 1.6% risk of significant symptomatic enlargement of a microprolactinoma during pregnancy in patients not previously treated with bromocriptine (Molitch, 1992).

In a patient with microprolactinoma, bromocriptine should therefore be advocated to induce ovulation and allow conception. At the other end of the spectrum, the approach to the management of a macroprolactinoma in a patient desiring pregnancy is a little more contentious.

Advocates of prophylactic debulking surgery have overestimated the overall risk of macroprolactinomic expansion during pregnancy, while failing to appreciate adequately the prophylactic efficacy of adequate pretreatment with dopamine agonists in causing tumor shrinkage to within the confines of the sella turcica (Tan et al, 1986). It is reasonable to recommend primary therapy with bromocriptine in patients with macroprolactinoma seeking pregnancy, initially while using varying methods of contraception. Once follow up with pituitary imaging has documented regression of the tumor within the confines of the sella, contraception is discontinued and bromocriptine withdrawn once pregnancy is confirmed. If significant suprasellar extension remains after 3 months of treatment with bromocriptine, then another dopamine agonist may be tried. Alternatively, selective pituitary adenectomy may be undertaken. Should headache and impairment of visual field develop during pregnancy, the pituitary should be examined promptly by magnetic resonance imaging and bromocriptine reinstituted if significant tumor extension is evident. Once the patient has resumed spontaneous menstrual cycles, ultrasound monitoring will help follow restoration of normal follicular and endometrial development.

HYPOTHALAMIC DYSFUNCTION WITH NORMAL PROLACTIN AND ANDROGEN LEVELS

Failure to ovulate in the nonandrogenized normoprolactinemic woman secondary to chronic hypothalamic dysfunction is a frequent cause of menstrual dysfunction. Patients in this category also present with a variety of symptoms that may range from luteal phase defects to amenorrhea. This form of amenorrhea usually responds to a progesterone challenge with vaginal bleeding. Stress, alterations in body weight and excessive athletic activity can result in chronic hypothalamic anovulation. If change in lifestyle does not restore ovulation, clomiphene citrate is the first line therapy. Only in patients who fail to ovulate with doses of up to 100–150 mg/day for 5 days should gonadotropin therapy or pulsaltile LHRH administration be initiated.

If the patient ovulates in response to clomiphene citrate but does not conceive after six cycles of treatment, gonadotropin therapy may be contemplated. In this instance the aim would be a degree of superovulation in the expectation that if the patient develops a few follicles, the chance of one of the oocytes fertilizing and implanting would be increased; however, this approach would be associated with an increased risk of multiple pregnancy. If gonadotropin treatment is used, serial ultrasound scanning will help determine the number of follicles that grow, as well as the sizes of the follicles. hCG is given when a mean diameter of the largest follicle reaches about 18 mm.

PREMATURE LUTEINIZATION

A specific category of anovulation is premature luteinization. This entity is frequently unrecognized, or misdiagnosed as unexplained infertility, luteal phase defect, or luteinized unruptured follicle syndrome. This situation will occur if an untimely luteinizing hormone (LH) surge occurs in response to rising estrogen at a time when the follicle is still immature. It can only be diagnosed if an LH peak is detected in the presence of immature follicles as seen by ultrasonography. It can be speculated that the etiology of this entity is an exaggerated sensitivity of the pituitary in response to rising estrogen levels. This assumption may explain the failure

of clomiphene citrate, human menopausal gonadotropin (hMG) or FSH in restoring ovulation in these cases. All these agents cause multiple follicular development, with exaggerated estrogen response; thus a premature LH peak is even more likely. In these cases the only rational therapy is to abolish the estrogen evoked positive feedback mechanism. This can be effectively accomplished by the use of a potent LHRH agonist. Thus the treatment of choice for anovulation due to recurrent premature luteinization is a triphasic therapeutic approach. LHRH agonist is administered until the positive feedback is abolished (2–4 weeks); thereafter FSH is given in conjunction with the agonist until at least one follicle reaches maturation as judged by ultrasonography and measurement of estrogen levels. hCG is then administered to induce ovulation.

HYPOTHALAMIC–PITUITARY INSUFFICIENCY

The etiology of amenorrhea in women who fail to have withdrawal vaginal bleeding following progesterone challenge may be due to target unresponsiveness or hypothalamic–pituitary insufficiency. Bleeding following cyclic estrogen and progesterone administration, together with ultrasound assessment, will eliminate the diagnosis of uterine causes, such as congenital abnormalities, or severe uterine adhesions, such as in Asherman's syndrome. The presence of a thin endometrium (less than 5 mm) will support the diagnosis of estrogen deficiency. A low or normal FSH and LH concentration will rule out ovarian failure and point to pituitary insufficiency. All cases with pituitary insufficiency will benefit from hMG/hCG therapy.

HYPOTHALAMIC–PITUITARY DYSFUNCTION ASSOCIATED WITH HYPERANDROGENISM

The androgenized anovulatory patient usually presents with a past or present history of acne, seborrhea and hirsutism, which may or may not be associated with obesity. Investigation must be oriented towards both the source and quantity of excessive androgens. Proper evaluation of the source of elevated androgen synthesis, either from the ovaries, the adrenal cortex or both, is necessary for choosing the correct treatment in order to restore ovulation. In an androgenized patient with normal or elevated serum testosterone concentration but in the presence of a normal dehydroepiandrosterone sulfate level, polycystic ovaries can be suspected. An elevated LH:FSH ratio (usually greater than 3) is a characteristic biochemical feature of this diagnostic entity. High resolution ultrasound imaging of the pelvis permits confirmation of this diagnosis (Adams et al, 1985). In severe cases, the typical distribution of peripheral cysts of average diameter of 4–6 mm and an echodense central stroma can be observed (*Figure 20.11*). This corresponds well with the macroscopic appearance of the cut surface of the polycystic ovary. In patients with polycystic ovary syndrome chronic increased LH secretion will continuously stimulate the proliferation of stromal and thecal cells and increase intraovarian and intrafollicular androgens. Intrafollicular androgens are associated with follicular atresia, probably as a result of inhibition of both FSH and LH receptors. This mechanism fits well with the hormonal pattern and morphological appearance described above. The chronic elevated LH secretion may, however, have manifold etiologies. It may be initiated through increased androstenedione/testosterone production from either ovarian or adrenal source. Its peripheral conversion to estrone/estradiol (mainly by adipose tissue) will enhance LH secretion. The relationship of obesity with polycystic ovary syndrome is unequivocal and its impact on the clinical expression of the syndrome is most important; however, a hypothalamic–pituitary disorder as an originator of this syndrome cannot be excluded. The first line treatment of polycystic ovary syndrome, regardless of its etiology, is clomiphene citrate. This will increase gonadotropin secretion, and in some women will allow the selection, growth and maturation of a follicle. In some instances it will cause many follicles to grow and result in hyperstimulation. In cases with an inappropriate response to clomiphene citrate, gonadotropin therapy, preferably using a purified FSH preparation, should be used in order to attempt to override the FSH:LH imbalance. In cases where both of these types of therapy have failed, a more rational approach may be indicated.

Chronic administration of gonadotropin releasing hormone (GnRH) agonists has been shown to be effective in downregulating pituitary gonadotropin secretion (Porter et al, 1984; Fleming et al, 1985). Fleming and Coutts (1990) successfully used GnRH agonists in con-

junction with gonadotropins in patients with polycystic ovary syndrome who had previously failed to conceive with exogenous gonadotropin therapy alone. We (Insler et al, 1989; Insler and Lunenfeld, 1990) have shown that during LHRH agonist therapy gonadotropin secretion diminishes and the FSH:LH imbalance is corrected within 3–4 weeks. When this stage has been accomplished, treatment with FSH is initiated.

This short review is not meant to give an exhaustive overview on this impressive and promising technique but it expresses our thoughts of how to integrate imaging techniques into the endocrine workup and management of the infertile woman.

REFERENCES

Adams J, Polson DW, Abdulwahid N et al (1985) Multifollicular ovaries: clinical and endocrine features in response to pulsatile gonadotropin releasing hormone. *Lancet* **ii**: 1375–1378.

Adams J, Tan SL, Wheeler M, Morris D, Jacobs HS & Franks S (1988) Uterine growth in the follicular phase of spontaneous ovulatory cycles and during LHRH induced cycles in women with normal or polycystic ovaries. *Fertil Steril* **49**: 52–55.

Bevan GS, Burke CW, Esirim M & Adams CBT (1987) Misinterpretation of prolactin levels leading to management errors in patients with sella enlargement. *Am J Med* **82**: 29–32.

Campbell S, Bourne TH, Tan SL & Collins WP (1994) Hysterosalpingo contrast sonography (HyCoSy): future role within the investigation of infertility in Europe. *Ultrasound Obstet Gynecol* **4**: 245–253.

Eissa M, Hudson K, Docker M, Sawers R & Newton J (1985) Ultrasound follicular diameter measurement: an assessment of interobserver and intra-observer variation. *Fertil Steril* **44**: 751–754.

Fleming R & Coutts JRT (1990) The use of exogenous gonadotropins and GnRH-analogues for ovulation induction in PCO syndrome. *Res Clin Forums* **11**: 77–85.

Fleming R, Haxton MJ & Hamilton R (1985) Successful treatment of infertile women with oligomenorrhea using a combination of an LHRH agonist and exogenous gonadotropins. *Br J Obstet Gynaecol* **92**: 369–373.

Hussein EL, Balen A & Tan SL (1992) A prospective study comparing the outcome of oocytes retrieved in the aspirate with those retrieved in the flush during transvaginal ultrasound directed oocyte recovery for in vitro fertilisation. *Br J Obstet Gynaecol* **99**: 841–844.

Insler V & Lunenfeld B (1990) Polycystic ovarian disease: a challenge and controversy. *Gynecol Endocrinol* **4**: 51–69.

Insler V, Potashnik G, Lunenfeld E, Meizner I & Levy J (1989) The combined suppression/stimulation therapy in IVF-ET programmes: expectations and facts. *Gynecol Endocrinol* **4** (Suppl): 47–51.

Kyei-Mensah A, Zaidi J, Pitroff R, Shaker A, Campbell S & Tan SL (1996a) Transvaginal 3-dimensional ultrasound: accuracy of follicular volume measurements. *Fertil Steril* **65**: 377–381.

Kyei-Mensah A, Maconochie N, Zaidi J, Pitroff R, Campbell S & Tan SL (1996b) Intra- and inter-observer variation in 3-dimensional measurements of the ovarian stromal and endometrial volumes. *Fertil Steril* (in press).

MacDougall MJ, Tan SL, Balen A & Jacobs SH (1993) A controlled study comparing patients with and without polycystic ovaries undergoing in vitro fertilization. *Hum Reprod* **8**: 233–237.

Molitch ME (1992) Pathologic hyperprolactinemia. *Endocrinol Metab Clin North Am* **21**: 877–901.

Penzias AS, Emmi AM, Dubey AK, Layman LC, Dejourney AH & Reindollar RH (1994) Ultrasound prediction of follicle volume: is the mean diameter reflective? *Fertil Steril* **62**: 1274–1276.

Porter RN, Smith W, Craft IL, Abdulwahid NA & Jacobs HS (1984) Induction of ovulation for IVF using buserelin and gonadotropins. *Lancet* **ii**: 1284–1285.

Rizk B, Tan SL, Kingsland C, Steer C, Mason BA & Campbell S (1990) Ovarian cyst aspiration and outcome of in-vitro fertilisation. *Fertil Steril* **54**: 661–664.

Soule SG & Jacobs HS (1995) Prolactinoma: present day management. *Br J Obstet Gynaecol* **102**: 117–181.

Steer C, Tan SL, Mason BA & Campbell S (1994) Mid luteal phase vaginal color Doppler assessment of uterine artery impedance in a subfertile population. *Fertil Steril* **61**: 53–58.

Steer C, Williams J, Zaidi J, Campbell S & Tan SL (1995) Intraobserver, inter-observer, inter-ultrasound transducer and inter-cycle variation in colour Doppler assessment of uterine artery impedance. *Hum Reprod* **10**: 479–481.

Tan SL & Jacobs HS (1986) Management of prolactinomas. *Br J Obstet Gynaecol* **93**: 1025–1029.

Tan SL, Steer C & Campbell S (1992a) Ultrasound and infertility. In Brinsden P & Rainsbury P (eds) *Bourn Hall Textbook of IVF*, pp 127–138. London: Parthenon.

Tan SL, Royston P, Campbell S et al (1992b) Cumulative conception in live birth rates after in vitro fertilisation. *Lancet* **339**: 1390–1394.

Tan SL, Waterstone J, Wren M & Parsons J (1992c) A prospective randomized study comparing aspiration only with aspiration flushing for transvaginal ultrasound directed oocyte recovery. *Fertil Steril* **58**: 356–360.

Tan SL, Doyle P, Manconochie N et al (1994a) Pregnancy and live birth rates after IVF by life-table analysis in women with, and without, previous IVF pregnancies: a study of 8000 cycles undertaken at one center. *Am J Obstet Gynecol* **170**: 34–40.

Tan SL, Maconochie N, Doyle P et al (1994b) Cumulative conception in live birth rates after in vitro fertilization with, and without, the long, short and ultrashort regimens of the luteinizing hormone releasing hormone agonist buserelin. *Am J Obstet Gynecol* **171**: 513–520.

Zaidi J, Campbell S, Pitroff R, Shaker A, Jacobs HS & Tan SL (1995a) Ovarian stromal blood flow in women with polycystic ovaries: a possible new marker for diagnosis. *Hum Reprod* **10**: 1992–1996.

Zaidi J, Jurkovic D, Campbell S, Collins W, McGregor A & Tan SL (1995b) Luteinized unruptured follicle: morphology, endocrine function and blood flow changes during the menstrual cycle. *Hum Reprod* **10**: 44–49.

Zaidi J, Barber J, Kyei-Mensah A, Bekir J, Campbell S & Tan SL (1996) Relationship of ovarian stromal blood flow at the baseline ultrasound scan to subsequent follicular response in an IVF program. *Obstet Gynecol* **88**: 1–6.

21 *Benign and malignant adnexal masses*
D Querleu, M Cosson and J Decocq

■ INTRODUCTION

A number of imaging techniques that improve the preoperative diagnosis of the adnexal mass have been described. This concept, initially limited to the clinical palpation of a pelvic mass lateral to the uterus, has now evolved and has been extended to the finding of an enlarged or cystic ovary at ultrasonographic examination. As a matter of fact, the evaluation of pelvic mass is nowadays based as much on imaging techniques as it is on clinical grounds. The goal of evaluation of the adnexal mass is to manage the patient with a minimum of surgical trauma and a maximum of oncological safety. In some cases, simple observation or transvaginal cyst aspiration will be recommended, while in others referral for surgery by a gynecologic oncologist is required. Generally, between these two extremes, the patient may be confidently managed by a laparoscopic approach. The goal of the preoperative workup, including imaging techniques and direct laparoscopic visualization, is to classify patients into one of these three groups.

Both clinical examination and imaging techniques, especially when interpreted by inexperienced observers, may lead to a false positive diagnosis of adnexal mass, organic cyst or cancer. As far as cancer is concerned, the contradictory goals of improving sensitivity or specificity may lead to two drawbacks: overdiagnosis of cancer means unnecessary surgery; underdiagnosis may impair the patient's chances of cure. Even a test with a 100% sensitivity and a 98% specificity would yield 50 false positives for every single case of cancer identified (Westhoff and Randall, 1991). In this regard, the concept of 'suspicious' adnexal mass remains imprecise, depending on the cut off level chosen to discriminate benign from malignant masses.

The differential diagnosis is wide and varied. It includes both benign neoplastic (uterine and ligamentous myomas, parovarian cyst, tubal carcinoma) and nonneoplastic (pregnancy, abscess, hydrosalpinx) gynecological conditions, in addition to pathologies or incidental findings affecting the bowel (stool in colon, tumors of the bowel, diverticular or appendiceal abscess, Crohn's disease), urinary tract (full bladder, pelvic kidney) or other systems (retroperitoneal tumors, anterior sacral meningocele).

The structure of the ovary and its anatomical location in the peritoneal cavity require the assessment of both its internal structure by noninvasive techniques and its external appearance by invasive techniques. As a consequence, laparoscopic examination, more adapted to diagnostic procedures than laparotomy, has become the most efficient tool for completing the diagnosis of the adnexal mass, and must be considered as an imaging technique.

The gold standard is ultimately the pathological examination of an operative specimen. However, the assessment of the accuracy of a diagnosis may differ according to the pathological endpoint, depending on the inclusion of tumors of low malignant potential in cancer cases. The development of laparoscopic surgery, including specific instrumentation and skills required to avoid spillage of tumor cells into the peritoneal cavity or the abdominal wall, has led to the concept of simultaneous diagnosis and surgical therapy of the adnexal mass. In most cases, laparoscopic cystectomy (in younger women) or salpingo-oophorectomy (in menopausal women) ensures proper diagnosis and definitive cure of the adnexal mass, provided it is benign.

The ultimate goals of imaging techniques may be summarized thus:

- screening for ovarian disease;
- selection of patients for laparoscopic surgery, whether the mass has been identified clinically or by ultrasound screening;
- exclusion of malignancy.

■ SYMPTOMS AND THEIR RELATIONSHIP TO PATHOLOGY

A vast majority of adnexal masses, whether benign or malignant, are asymptomatic or revealed by coincidental symptoms related to the pelvic area or abdomen, thus leading to the performance of a clinical and/or ultrasound examination of the pelvis. As enlargement occurs, compression of the surrounding structures may produce urinary frequency, constipation, pelvic discomfort and pain of various degrees. Masses exceeding 12–15 cm in diameter rise out of the pelvis, and abdominal enlargement occurs. In the case of malignant tumors, abdominal pain and swelling due to tumor growth or ascites are the two most common complaints. Occasionally, severe pain may create a surgical emergency.

The clinical palpation of the ovary in postmenopausal patients, in whom the so-called 'postmenopausal palpable ovary syndrome' has been defined, is definitely unreliable, with an accuracy as low as 10% (Cohen and Jennings, 1994). This generally accepted finding has for years been an incentive for the development of screening techniques, including imaging and biological techniques. Solid, bilateral, fixed masses and masses with ascites are more likely to be malignant, but none of these features is pathognomonic of cancer. Even though Schutter et al (1994) found a surprisingly high accuracy of clinical examination in differentiating benign from malignant adnexal masses, the generally accepted relative inaccuracy of clinical examination in the differential diagnosis of cancer, endometriosis and benign adnexal cyst warrants the use of imaging techniques.

■ CLINICAL INVESTIGATIONS

TRANSABDOMINAL ULTRASONOGRAPHY

Early attempts at assessment of the internal structure of adnexal masses using B-mode ultrasonography have been overtaken by the development of two-dimensional ultrasound imaging, improved by the gray scale and real time technologies. Transabdominal sonography (TAS) is still useful for the screening of the abdominal and pelvic cavities, the diagnosis of abdominal adnexal masses and the detection of ascites.

Owing to the relatively poor resolution associated with the use of lower frequency diagnostic ultrasound, the accuracy of TAS in the presurgical diagnosis of ovarian masses is, however, less than ideal (Benacerraf et al, 1991), missing a significant number of ovarian cancers.

TAS has also been assessed in screening programs (Campbell et al, 1989). The criterion used was the estimated ovarian volume, computed after measurement of the maximum transverse, anteroposterior and longitudinal diameters of both ovaries. Although they apparently missed no case of ovarian cancer in their study of 5479 self referred women, Campbell et al observed a false positive rate of 2.3%. The odds that a positive result on screening indicated the presence of an ovarian cancer were only 1 in 67.

TRANSVAGINAL ULTRASONOGRAPHY

The use of endovaginal probes of higher frequency (6.5 to 7.5 MHz) has improved dramatically the discrimination of pelvic structures, and particularly of the inner structure of ovarian masses. Using transvaginal ultrasonography (TVS), Granberg et al (1989) concluded that a unilocular cyst measuring less than 10 cm in diameter without papillary formation had an extremely low chance of being malignant, regardless of the age of the patient. Many other authors, however, have chosen a cut off value of 5 cm to exclude cancer in anechogenic cysts.

The criteria for the assessment of adnexal masses became more reliable and reproducible, and were refined in scores. Finkler et al, in 1988, designed a scoring system using a multiparameter analysis of ultrasound reports. Sassone et al, in 1991, published a scoring system for TVS achieving an 83% specificity and a 100% sensitivity. This score was later modified in the same institution (Lerner et al, 1994), using a computer based linear regression analysis. These authors found, using the new scoring system with a cut off level of 3, a 77% specificity and a 97% sensitivity, which is not superior to the accuracy obtained in the first version of the score with arbitrarily selected point value assignments. DePriest et al (1993a) combined tumor volume, wall structure and septal structure. In a study of 121 sonograms of patients presenting with ovarian masses, they found that 80 ovarian tumors with a score of less than 5 were benign. Using the same score in a screening program setting, they screened three ovarian cancers in 3220 asymptomatic postmenopausal women, at the cost of 41 surgical explorations including 21 serous cystadenomas (DePriest et al, 1993b). None of these patients had elevated serum CA-125 or evidence of an ovarian tumor at clinical examination.

Botta and Zarcone (1995) compared the diagnostic accuracy of the Sassone and DePriest scoring systems. They found, using a cut off value of 9 in Sassone's score and of 5 in DePriest's score, a high number of false positive results and a considerable overlap in the scores of benign and malignant tumors. The two systems showed similar diagnostic value, with an 89% sensitivity for both systems, and similar specifities (73% for the Sassone scoring system, 70% for the DePriest scoring system). The conclusion was that the addition of ovarian volume to the list of criteria does not improve the accuracy of scoring systems.

DOPPLER FLOW IMAGING

The evaluation of adnexal lesions by color Doppler sonography has been under investigation. Reports on the accuracy of Doppler flow imaging in discriminating benign from malignant ovarian lesions are conflicting. Some groups are enthusiastic (Fleischer et al, 1993; Kurjak et al, 1993), while others state that it adds little information to TVS (Schneider et al, 1993; Bromley et al, 1994; Valentin et al, 1994). These discrepancies can be accounted for by lack of universal criteria and by differences in sensitivity between scanners. Some investigators use pulsatility index, others resistance index. The cut off value is not standardized, ranging from 0.4 to 0.8 for the resistance index, and from 0.65 to 1.25 for the pulsatility index, and this obviously influences the specificity and sensitivity. Each scanner has its own accuracy in terms of sensitivity and flow determination. Operator dependence is also a variable. The use of a single flow parameter is thus not applicable for distinguishing between benign and malignant masses because of the overlapping of index values and the lack of universally applicable criteria. It can only be stated that most benign cysts lack detectable blood flow, and that the resistance index tends to be lower in malignant masses.

The morphological appearance of tumor vascularity is a potential tool for discriminating between benign and malignant masses. Malignancies tend to exhibit neovascularity in the center, or septum, or papillary projections with a diffuse dispersed vascular arrangement, whereas benign masses are associated with peripheral or pericystic vascularity (Kurjak et al, 1993). These findings must be included in a multiparameter description of the suspicious adnexal mass, and may be of clinical importance; however, Doppler flow imaging should be used as a secondary technique after primary screening or evaluation by conventional TVS.

ABDOMINAL RADIOGRAPHY

A plain film of the abdomen and pelvis may help to identify dermoid cysts from three radiographic features: calcifications due to tooth or bone formation; radiolucent areas due to the lipidic cyst contents; and radiodensity circumscribing the cyst. All these features may also be detected by ultrasonography.

Many other benign or malignant tumors may be associated with radiographically visible calcifications. Psammocarcinomas may be detected by the presence of multiple pelvic and abdominal calcifications.

COMPUTED TOMOGRAPHY

Computed tomography (CT) used to be the preferred imaging technique for the assessment or monitoring of ovarian cancer because it offers excellent visualization of ascites and of subclinical implants; however, owing to the lack of resolution of fine architectural detail, characteristic nodules of less than 1–2 cm may be missed, and the technique has limited value in the diagnosis of early ovarian cancer. It may be used to detect mature cystic teratomas, characterized by the low density of their dermoid fluid contents.

MAGNETIC RESONANCE IMAGING

Magnetic resonance imaging (MRI) can differentiate endometriosis, mature cystic teratomas and malignant tumors. Using a 1.5 T system and T_1- and T_2-weighted images, Hata et al (1992) obtained a 97% specificity in 68 ovarian neoplasms, which was higher than that of ultrasonography, Doppler flow imaging and CA-125 studies; however, the sensitivity was only 67%, lower than that of TVS and Doppler flow imaging. Because of its cost, the use of MRI is limited to the gathering of additional information on certain equivocal adnexal lesions.

RADIOIMMUNOSCINTIGRAPHY

This technique, using radiolabeled monoclonal antibodies, is currently under investigation. The sensitivity and specificity of current techniques using antibodies to OC 125 or TAG 72 are as yet lower than those obtained using less costly techniques.

LAPAROSCOPY

Adnexal masses are one of the most controversial indications for laparoscopic surgery. The problem lies between the overtreatment, by laparotomy, of benign masses, and the undertreatment, by laparoscopy, of ovarian cancers. To avoid the discovery of unsuspected ovarian cancer during a laparoscopy performed by surgeons not qualified in gynecologic oncology, all adnexal masses must be investigated preoperatively. Only patients with CA-125 levels below 35 iu/ml (see discussion on tumor markers below) and benign ultrasound patterns should undergo laparoscopy in nonspecialized settings. Most solid masses, excluding mature teratomas, should not be managed laparoscopically.

Laparoscopic surgery is, in this context, a satisfactory diagnostic tool for early ovarian malignancy, with a false negative rate of less than 1% in experienced hands (Nezhat et al, 1992; Canis et al, 1994). Nezhat et al

found four false negatives in a series of 1011 laparoscopies. Canis et al. did not miss a single case of ovarian cancer in a series of 819 masses, including seven cancers and 12 low malignant potential tumors, but falsely diagnosed cancer in 27 patients (*Table 21.1*). Translated into a diagnostic performance measurement, the diagnostic value of laparoscopy is 100% sensitivity and 97% specificity; however, the positive predictive value is only 42% is this series, owing to the high level of precautions taken to exclude laparoscopic management of ovarian cancer. On the other hand, false positive cancer diagnosis is not uncommon in the preoperative workup of adnexal masses. Screening for ovarian cancers may lead to a number of unnecessary laparotomies, impairing the cost efficiency of the screening program. Diagnostic laparoscopy is an ideal tool for the assessment of ovarian tumors if an invasive technique is required to ensure definitive diagnosis and appropriate therapy.

Of interest in the French series (Canis et al, 1994) is that 11.5% of ovarian cysts diagnosed as functional are in fact benign organic cysts. As a consequence, simple aspiration, fenestration or biopsy is inadequate in a significant number of apparently functional cysts. The conclusion is that the entire cystic wall must be removed in all cases. On the other hand, only 5% of apparently organic cysts were functional and were overtreated by surgery in these series.

Laparoscopy provides visual access and a magnified view of the pelvis and peritoneal cavity. It is particularly valuable for looking into difficult areas, including the pouch of Douglas and the subdiaphragmatic area. Biopsies and material for cytology may be obtained with minimal surgical trauma. The occurrence of complications arising from diagnostic or surgical laparoscopy must, however, not be neglected (Querleu et al, 1993). Laparoscopic surgery may lead to spillage of tumor cells,

Table 21.1 *Accuracy of laparoscopic diagnosis of adnexal masses*

	Pathology			
Laparoscopic diagnosis	*Functional*	*Benign*	*Borderline*	*Cancer*
Functional	<u>115</u>	15	0	0
Benign	32	<u>611</u>	0	0
Suspicious or malignant	2	25	<u>12</u>	<u>7</u>

The numbers underlined indicate diagnostic concordance.
Reprinted with permission from The American College of Obstetricians and Gynecologists from Canis M et al (1994) Laparoscopic diagnosis of adnexal cystic masses: a 12-year experience with long-term followup. Obstet Gynecol **83**: 707.

aggravating the prognosis if there is a delay between diagnosis and definitive therapy (Maiman et al, 1991; Blanc et al, 1994). If some part of the tumor is removed without special precautions being taken, tumoral grafts to the abdominal wall are to be anticipated. Radical surgery must be carried out as soon as possible after laparoscopic diagnosis, and ideally at the time of primary surgery. As a consequence, the laparoscopic surgeon must be aware of the macroscopic features of ovarian cancer.

The visual findings suggesting malignancy are papillary or solid growth on the external surface of the ovary and suspicion of metastatic peritoneal implants. Even if the ovarian and peritoneal surfaces are normal, a diagnosis of cancer cannot be totally excluded. We advise aspiration and lavage of the cyst with a minimum of spillage. The internal surface of the cyst is then inspected in search of papillary growth. If papillary growth is found on either surface of the cyst, the simple cystectomy procedure must be aborted.

Abdominal exploration requires observation of every aspect of the abdominal cavity, the entire surface of the parietal peritoneum and the surfaces of the intraperitoneal organs. A magnified view is obtained when the tip of the endoscope is placed close to the peritoneum. The normal peritoneum shows a fine microvascular network and a transparent smooth surface. Papillary growth, thickening of the peritoneum, whitish areas or enlarged capillaries suggest the presence of malignancy. The pattern of the involved peritoneum is quite similar to the colposcopic view of a malignant tumor of the cervix. In fact, the magnified laparoscopic view of the peritoneum is superior to standard inspection at the time of conventional surgery. Biopsies are taken with the help of two instruments: the suspect area is grasped with a forceps, and removed with scissors. We do not advise the use of standard biopsy forceps. They are traumatic and remove only small specimens. Material for peritoneal cytological examination must be obtained. Lymph node assessment is also mandatory in some cases.

The pelvis is first thoroughly inspected. The patient is placed in a slight (10°) Trendelenburg position. The entire surface of the ovaries is examined. Ovarian masses are carefully manipulated to avoid rupture and subsequent spillage, but their external surface must be thoroughly inspected. The peritoneal surface of the uterus, broad ligaments and anterior and posterior cul-de-sac is inspected.

The exploration of the upper abdomen follows, mainly in cases of obvious ovarian malignancy. The operating table is placed in a 10° Trendelenburg position and tilted to the left. The video monitor is placed at the head of the operating table and the surgeon either stands to the side of the patient or between her legs. The abdominal cavity is thoroughly explored, including the surface of the diaphragm, the liver, the omentum, the mesentery, the colon, the appendix and the small bowel. Every loop of the small bowel must be carefully moved and sequentially inspected, from the ileocecal junction up to the duodenojejunal junction.

The operation ends by ensuring that hemostasis is complete and undertaking copious lavage of the peritoneal cavity. The ancillary incisions are also washed to avoid tumor grafting, especially in the case of peritoneal disease.

When an unsuspected ovarian cancer is found, biopsies of the ovarian surface may be of help, but frozen sections may be difficult to interpret. Four choices are possible, depending upon the availability of a trained gynecologic oncologist, the level of training of the surgeon in advanced operative laparoscopy and the degree of informed consent given by the patient.

1. The first option is to perform, with a gynecologic oncologist, a laparotomy with comprehensive staging and radical surgery of the ovarian carcinoma.

2. The second option is to take biopsies, without rupturing the cystic portion of the tumor, and to await the results of permanent sections before definitive therapy or referral of the patient.

3. The third option is to perform, laparoscopically or by laparotomy, a salpingo-oophorectomy for definitive pathological examination of the entire ovary.

4. The fourth option is limited to the rare surgeon trained in gynecological oncology and at the same time skilled in laparoscopic surgery, and involves, after frozen section examination, performance of definitive laparoscopic surgery for ovarian carcinoma, which includes total hysterectomy and bilateral salpingo-oophorectomy (or unilateral salpingo-oophorectomy in selected cases), pelvic and para-aortic node sampling, and abdominal staging.

▪ APPEARANCES

Figures 21.1–21.13 illustrate the appearance of various adnexal masses.

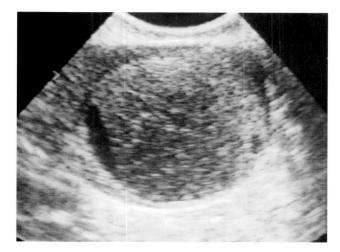

21.1a

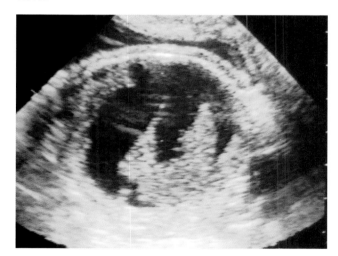

21.1b

Figure 21.1: *(a) and (b) Hemorrhagic corpus luteum. Transvaginal sonography shows a diffuse irregular echogenicity.*

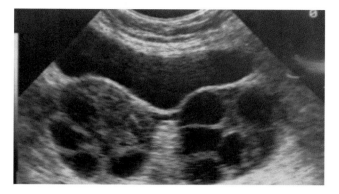

Figure 21.2: *Functional cysts after ovarian stimulation. Enlarged ovary with multiple cystic structures.*

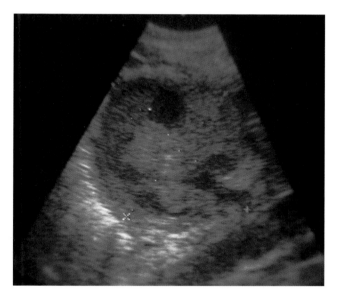

21.3a

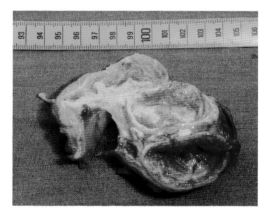

21.3b

Figure 21.3: *Pyosalpinx. (a) Multilocular tumor with solid areas. (b) Pathological specimen.*

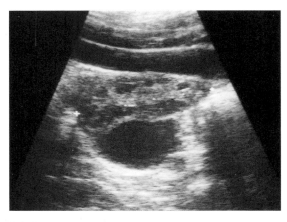

21.4a

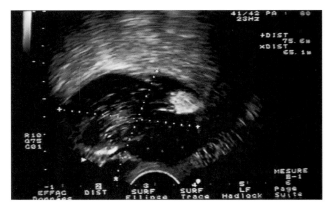

21.5b

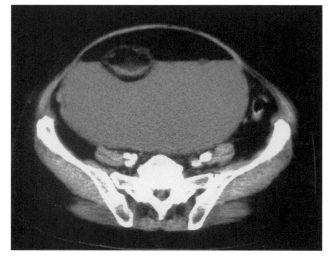

21.4b

Figure 21.4: *(a) and (b) Parauterine cyst. Solitary thin walled, anechoic cyst.*

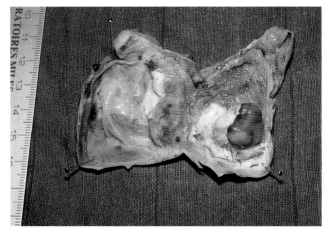

21.5c

Figure 21.5: *Benign ovarian teratoma. (a) Computed tomographic image, characterized by the low density of the dermoid fluid content. (b) Transvaginal sonography. The tumor is complex with irregular solid parts. Echogenicity is higher than that of clear fluid, but much lower than that of a solid tumor. (c) Pathological specimen.*

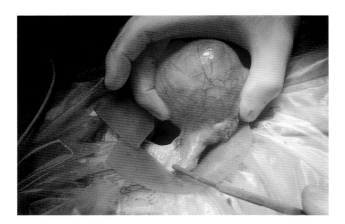

21.5a

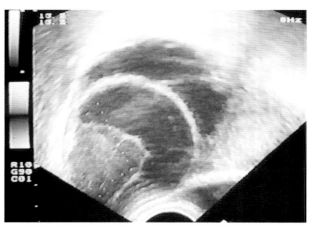

21.6a

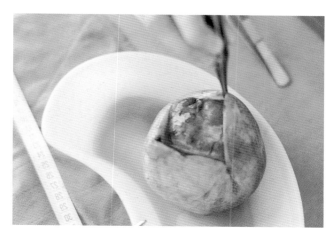

21.6b

Figure 21.6: *(a) Mucinous benign ovarian cyst. Multilocular, thin walled and with echogenic cystic content. (b) Ovoid mass with a smooth capsule, usually translucent.*

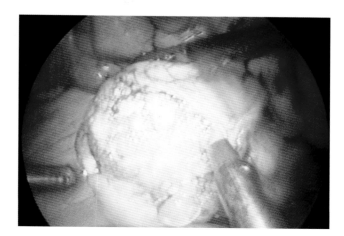

Figure 21.8: *Laparoscopy: fibroma of the ovary.*

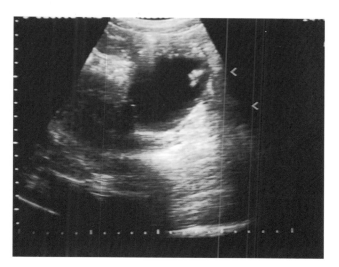

21.7a

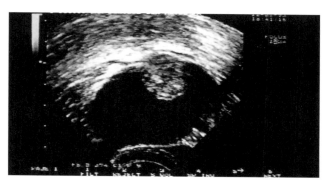

21.9a

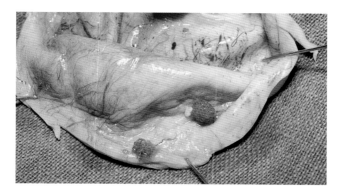

21.7b

Figure 21.7: *Cystadenoma. (a) Thin walled cyst with papillary formation. (b) Pathological specimen.*

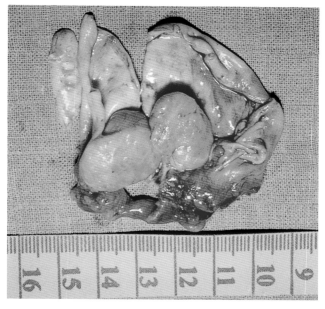

21.9b

Figure 21.9: *Thecoma of the ovary. (a) Unusual presentation as a unique papillary formation in a unilocular cyst. (b) Pathological specimen.*

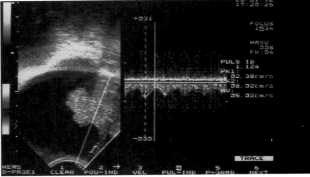

21.10a

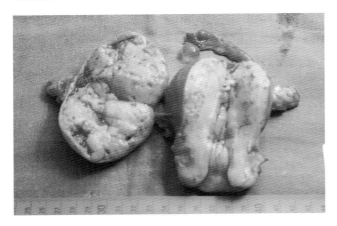

21.10b

Figure 21.10: *(a) Granulosa cell tumor. (b) Pathological specimen.*

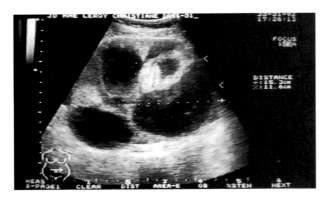

Figure 21.11: *Borderline tumor: multilocular mass with thick septa and echogenic area. These tumors are very difficult to distinguish from invasive ovarian cancer.*

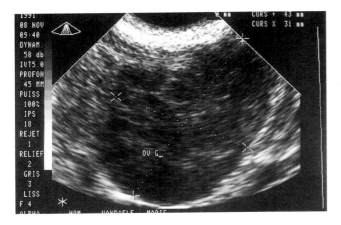

21.12a

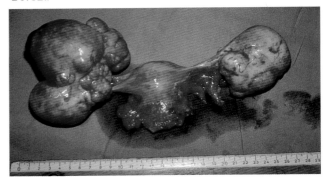

21.12b

Figure 21.12: *Malignant ovarian tumor. (a) Papillary formations in the inside of the tumor with highly suspicious neovascularization. (b) Pathological specimen.*

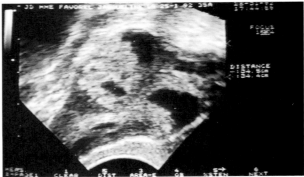

21.13a

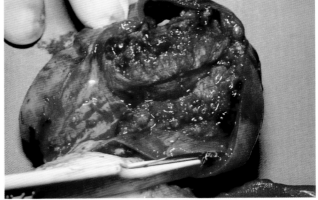

21.13b

Figure 21.13: *(a) Secondary adenocarcinoma of the ovary in a case of endometrial cancer. (b) Multilocular tumor with solid areas.*

■ INTERPRETATION OF FINDINGS

UNEXPECTED CANCER

Mismanagement, spillage or delay in diagnosis or therapy of an ovarian cancer are of utmost clinical importance. Some potentially curable patients with stage I tumors may present with stage III tumors after unnecessary delay or chronic abdominal spillage of tumor contents. In four large series in the literature (Hulka et al, 1992; Nezhat et al, 1992; Blanc et al, 1994; Canis et al, 1994), the incidence of malignancy in patients presenting with a non-suspicious adnexal mass was between 0.3 and 2.9%. A recent survey of gynecological oncologists in the United States found 42 tumors, including 12 ovarian cancers, managed laparoscopically. Most patients did not have proper staging and surgical management for weeks after laparoscopy. A similar survey was conducted in France (Blanc et al, 1994). Sixty borderline and 18 invasive tumors were managed laparoscopically in a combined series of 5307 ovarian cysts; 26 of them were true false negatives, with a benign preoperative workup, but 52 tumors could have been identified preoperatively with at least one positive test at clinical examination, ultrasound or CA-125 level. Fifty nine percent of tumors were not suspected laparoscopically, including 6 of 18 invasive cancers. As there is evidence that rupture of tumor is not detrimental to the patient provided it is followed by immediate surgical management, peritoneal lavage and adequate adjuvant therapy (Berek, 1995), it is logical to affirm that laparoscopy of itself is not the cause for mismanagement of cancer. The cause of mismanagement in both the American and the French studies was primarily the surgeon's poor understanding of the macroscopic features of ovarian cancer and lack of knowledge of the management of ovarian carcinomas. However, even an experienced surgeon, operating by laparoscopy or laparotomy after a careful preoperative workup, may be confronted with a pathological diagnosis of ovarian borderline or invasive tumor. The lesson is that all ovarian cysts, whether managed laparoscopically or by open surgery, should be sent for pathological examination. In case of unsuspected ovarian tumor, a gynecological oncologist must be consulted without any delay.

NATURAL HISTORY OF OVARIAN CANCER

Small clear cysts may be found in menopausal women enrolled in screening programs. The malignant potential of asymptomatic, apparently benign cysts is in question owing to our lack of understanding of the early stages of ovarian carcinogenesis. In early ovarian cancers, benign serous epithelial lining may be found adjacent to borderline or malignant epithelium. Although it is generally accepted (Curtin, 1994) that small anechogenic cysts are benign, Luxman et al (1991) found two malignant tumors in 33 patients with a 'simple cyst' smaller than 5 cm detected by abdominal ultrasonography. On the other hand, no cancer was diagnosed in a series of 32 simple ovarian cysts in postmenopausal women managed conservatively and followed for up to 9 years (Kroon and Andolf, 1995). Furthermore, up to 14.8% prevalence of simple adnexal cysts has been found in a population of 149 women aged 50 or older (Wolf et al, 1991). Of 22 patients in these series, 20 had cysts of 3 cm or less. It would not make sense to propose surgery to all these patients.

ASPIRATION OF SIMPLE CYSTS

Fine-needle aspiration of simple cysts, whether performed under laparoscopic or ultrasound guidance, has been advocated as it involves a lack of immediate morbidity; however, it is unlikely to improve dramatically the level of care in the diagnosis and management of adnexal masses. The diagnostic value of cytological examination is poor, with sensitivity as low as 26% in one series (Moran et al, 1993). Aspiration of a malignant cyst involves a risk of dissemination (Trimbos and Hacker, 1993) if the definitive surgical therapy is delayed for weeks, corresponding to the time necessary to detect recurrence of an apparently simple cyst with negative cytology. The failure rate, combining failure to empty the cyst and recurrence, ranges from 8 to 67% (mean 20%) in a review of five series of the literature (Trimbos and Hacker, 1993). For all these reasons, fine-needle aspiration, while improving the specificity from 97.3% for ultrasound alone to 99.5% when ultrasound and aspiration are combined, does not improve significantly the results of a screening program (Schincaglia et al, 1994).

However, determination of CA-125 and estradiol level in the cystic fluid may help to differentiate functional cysts, in which hormonal levels are high and CA-125 levels are low, from organic cysts, in which hormonal levels are low and CA-125 levels are high (Audra et al, 1991).

FUNCTIONAL CYSTS

Functional cysts may occur in premenopausal women and even during the early menopause. Functional cysts usually present as anechogenic structures less than 8 cm in diameter, but they may be septated, or contain blood. Hemorrhagic functional cysts show either diffuse echogenicity, and may mimic endometriosis, or endocystic echogenic clots resembling papillary projections. Functional cysts may be associated with increased vascularity. Low impedance blood flow is common in premenopausal ovaries in relation to ovulation and corpus luteum formation; however, no vascularity is found in the central area, even in echogenic structures.

As a consequence, not only anechogenic cysts in younger women may be functional: the probability of a functional cyst may be raised in the case of an echogenic cyst or in early menopausal women. A majority of patients with an ovarian abnormality should be reassessed at an interval to allow for spontaneous resolution, which may take up to several months; however, it seems important to avoid unnecessary delay in operative investigation and to propose surgery if the cyst persists for longer than 3 months. The popular prescription of a combination oral contraceptive pill to hasten the involution of functional cysts is useless (Steinkampf et al, 1990). Immediate surgery is required only:

- in the case of a clinically significant dermoid cyst;
- in masses measuring over 10 cm;
- in highly suspicious masses.

▪ CLASSIFICATION AND ITS USE IN CLINICAL MANAGEMENT

ARE MORE PREOPERATIVE INVESTIGATIONS WORTHWHILE?

The use of imaging techniques is usually limited to TVS with or without Doppler flow imaging. Ultrasonography is generally accepted as a noninvasive and relatively reliable method; however, the diagnostic accuracy of ultrasonography alone does not yield a satisfactory preoperative discrimination of benign and malignant masses. Many investigators have tried to combine ultrasonography with other techniques to improve the preoperative diagnosis of adnexal masses.

There has been considerable interest in tumor marker determination in the diagnosis of the adnexal mass and in the screening of ovarian cancer; however, no tumor marker is unique to ovarian cancer. CA-125 has been shown to combine the highest sensitivity and specificity for ovarian cancer (Malkasian et al, 1988), with a generally accepted cut off level of 35 iu/ml. Human chorionic gonadotropin, α-fetoprotein and lactate dehydrogenase levels may be of help in the case of a solid tumor in younger patients, as they can be elevated in germ cell tumors. CA-125 levels are, however, elevated in only approximately half of patients with stage I ovarian cancer and are falsely elevated in many benign conditions – in nonovarian cancer, endometriosis and during the menstrual cycle and pregnancy. It is therefore more accurate in menopausal patients. In all patients, CA-125 findings should be viewed with caution, as they may cloud the differential diagnosis of ovarian masses.

As CA-125 level is not suitable as a test on its own, it is combined with ultrasonography, which improves the overall accuracy. The combination of abdominal ultrasound and CA-125 >35 iu/ml has a 78% sensitivity and an 82% specificity (Maggino et al, 1994). Jacobs et al (1990) have designed a 'risk of malignancy index' computed as the product of CA-125 level, menopausal status (premenopausal patients were scored 1, postmenopausal patients were scored 3) and ultrasound score. Ultrasound reports were scored 1 point for each of the following characteristics: multilocular cyst, evidence of solid areas, evidence of metastases, presence of ascites, bilateral lesions. Ultrasonography alone, using a cut off level of 2, provided a 71% sensitivity and an 83% specificity. The risk of malignancy index, using a cut off level of 200 chosen after receiver operator characteristics (ROC) curve investigation, improved the diagnostic accuracy of ultrasound alone and of CA-125 alone, reaching an 85% sensitivity and a

Table 21.2 *Criteria for a preoperative classification of ovarian masses*

1 *Probably benign* if *all* the following criteria are observed:

TVS: size less than 5 cm, nonechogenic or dermoid content, up to three thin (< 3 mm) septa

DFI: no vascularization or peripheral vascularization, high resistance

CA-125: < 35 iu/ml

2 *Equivocal* if *one* of the following criteria is observed:

TVS: solid homogeneous content, more than three or thick septa

CA-125: 35 to 65 iu/ml

3 *Probably malignant* if *one* of the following criteria is observed:

TVS: endocystic vegetation, thick and irregular septa, ascites

DFI: central vascularization, low resistance

CA-125: >65 iu/ml

DFI, Doppler flow imaging.

97% specificity. These results were confirmed in another study by the same group (Davies et al, 1993), but a lower specificity (89%) at the 200 cut off level was found. A combination of criteria is thus more accurate than an individual one in diagnosing ovarian cancer.

Schutter et al (1994) combined pelvic examination, TVS and serum CA-125 in postmenopausal women presenting with a pelvic mass. They found that the individual accuracy of each exploration was quite similar (76, 74 and 77%, respectively). Using logistic regression analysis, they found that pelvic examination was the single most relevant factor, followed by CA-125 (with a cut off level of 35 iu/ml) and ultrasonography (using Finkler's score with a cut off level of 7). When all three examination methods were negative, no case of cancer was found. The important finding of this study is that a number of patients (53 of 228 in the series) can be preoperatively classified as certainly benign. However, combining the examinations improves specificity if all test results are positive, but the sensitivity is low. If only one test is positive, the sensitivity is high, but the specificity is low, leading to unnecessary referral to a gynecological oncologist and aggressive surgery. Guidelines for the gynecologist are provided in *Table 21.2*.

Canis et al (1994) presented data allowing the comparison of the diagnostic value of ultrasonography, CA-125 and laparoscopic diagnosis (*Table 21.3*), clearly showing that laparoscopic diagnosis is both more sensitive and more specific than noninvasive investigations.

Table 21.3 *Comparison of the sonographic, CA-125 and laparoscopic findings with the pathological report*

Pathology	n	Ultrasonography (% not purely anechogenic)	CA-125 (% ≥ 35 iu/ml)	Laparoscopy (% suspicious)
Functional	122	22.9	7.1	1.8
Organic, benign	561	29.1*	17.6†	3.8
Borderline	11	54.6	37.5	100
Suspicious or malignant	7	100	50	100

* *Including 111 mature teratomas, 91% of them showing a sonographic appearance that is not purely cystic.*

† *Including 82 endometriomas. The positivity rate of CA-125 was 32.9% in this group.*

Reprinted with permission from The American College of Obstetricians and Gynecologists and adapted from Canis M (1994) Laparoscopic diagnosis of adnexal cystic masses: a 12-year experience with long-term follow up. Obstet Gynecol 83: 707.

IS ANY SURGERY NECESSARY?

Functional cysts do not require surgery because they usually disappear within 6 weeks to 3 months. Unnecessary surgery for functional cysts may induce adhesions and increase the risk of recurrent functional cysts in some patients. As a consequence, only persistent or obviously organic masses (large cyst, dermoid cyst, endometriosis, suspected cancer) should be proposed for surgery. If an incidental cyst is found during diagnostic laparoscopy for pelvic pain or infertility, the diagnosis of functional cyst is usually easy (fine cyst wall, citrine or hemorrhagic fluid, retinoid vascularity of the inner surface); however, cytological examination of the cyst content and biopsy of the wall are required to document the diagnosis. Any suspicious sign or suggestion of an organic mass at cytological or histological examination requires early reoperation.

Small (3 cm or less in diameter) clear cell cysts with low CA-125 in menopausal patients are almost certainly benign. Laparotomy and even laparoscopic surgery should be considered as overtreatment in such cases, as they involve a morbidity obviously in excess of the benefit. The choice is between conservative management and aspiration under ultrasound guidance. Conservative management requires repeat examination after 3 and 12 months to affirm that the volume of the cyst is unchanged. Aspiration requires one interventional ultrasonography and one follow up ultrasound examination after 3 months to rule out early recurrence. The decision depends on the likely compliance of the patient in attending for follow up ultrasound examination, the patient's preference, and the accessibility of the cyst to ultrasound guided aspiration.

IS SCREENING OF OVARIAN CANCER USEFUL?

The feasibility of screening using noninvasive techniques such as TVS and CA-125 determinations has been investigated. Screening programs have not demonstrated suf-

ficient accuracy to provide a reliable and cost effective means of detecting early ovarian cancer in the general population, in which the false positive rate is unacceptably high considering the sensitivity and specificity of currently available tests. A randomized screening study would require at least 100 000 subjects over 45 years of age for 6 years to demonstrate a 50% reduction in mortality. It is, however, likely that in a high risk group of patients selected on the grounds of family history of ovarian and/or breast and/or colon cancer, the prevalence of cancer is high enough to warrant screening programs and to lower the false positive rate.

IS THE LAPAROSCOPIC APPROACH ACCEPTABLE?

The standard opinion is that laparoscopic surgery is not suitable for ovarian cancer. Regardless of the level of caution exercised, it is possible that an early malignant tumor may be submitted to laparoscopic surgery. Spillage must therefore be avoided in all cases. The use of an endoscopic bag to retrieve cysts through the abdominal wall is mandatory. Frozen sections are required to rule out invasive tumors in cases of macroscopically suspicious ovarian cysts. If these rules are respected, the fear that the laparoscopic operation will impair the outcome of the patient with cancer must be considered to have been overemphasized in the literature (Berek, 1995).

Recent data concerning the use of laparoscopic surgery in the staging and surgical therapy of ovarian cancer are available (Querleu and Leblanc, 1994). Although this technique is still under investigation, it must be stressed that laparoscopic surgery is acceptable in the hands of those gynecological oncologists committed to laparoscopy, provided that they can ensure surgical therapy and staging procedures similar to those obtained by laparotomy.

In conclusion, *Figures 21.14–21.16* summarize the data presented in this chapter and provide guidelines for the general gynecologist confronted by the adnexal mass.

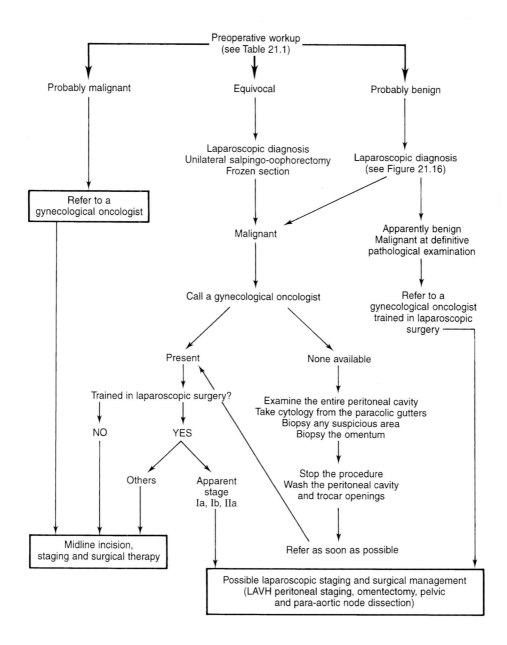

***Figure 21.14**: Avoiding laparoscopic mismanagement of ovarian cancer. LAVH, laparoscopically assisted vaginal hysterectomy.*

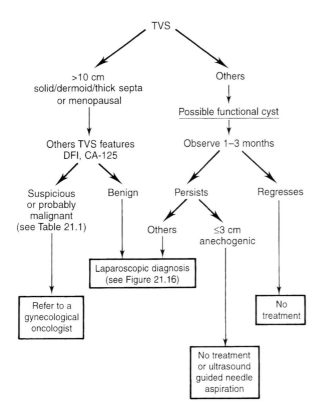

Figure 21.15: Management of the clinically benign adnexal mass. TVS, transvaginal sonography; DFI, Doppler flow imaging.

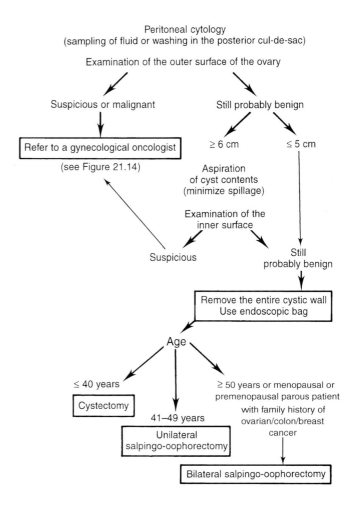

Figure 21.16: Management of the probably benign (at preoperative workup) adnexal mass.

REFERENCES

Audra P, Dargent D, Akiki S et al (1991) Ponction échoguidée des kystes de l'ovaire. Possibilités et limites. *Rev Fr Gynecol Obstet* **86**: 672–675.

Benacerraf BR, Finkler NJ, Wojciechowski C & Knapp RC (1991) Sonographic accuracy in the diagnosis of ovarian masses. *J Reprod Med* **35**: 491–495.

Berek J (1995) Ovarian cancer spread: is laparoscopy to blame? *Lancet* **346**: 200.

Blanc B, Boubli L, D'Ercole C & Nicoloso E (1994) Laparoscopic management of malignant ovarian cysts: a 78-case national survey. Part I: preoperative and laparoscopic evaluation. *Eur J Obstet Gynecol Reprod Biol* **56**: 177–180.

Botta G & Zarcone R (1995) Transvaginal ultrasound examination of ovarian masses in premenopausal women. *Eur J Obstet Gynecol Reprod Biol* **62**: 37–41.

Bromley B, Goodman H & Benacerraf BR (1994) Comparison between sonographic morphology and Doppler waveform for the diagnosis of ovarian malignancy. *Obstet Gynecol* **83**: 434–437.

Campbell S, Bhan V, Royston P et al (1989) Transabdominal ultrasound screening for early ovarian cancer. *BMJ* **299**: 1363–1367.

Canis M, Mage G, Pouly JL et al (1994) Laparoscopic diagnosis of adnexal cystic masses: a 12-year experience with long-term follow-up. *Obstet Gynecol* **83**: 707–712.

Cohen CJ & Jennings TS (1994) Screening for ovarian cancer: the role of noninvasive techniques. *Am J Obstet Gynecol* **170**: 1088–1094.

Curtin JP (1994) Management of the adnexal mass. *Gynecol Oncol* **55**: S42–S46.

Davies AP, Jacobs I, Woolas R et al (1993) The adnexal mass: benign or malignant? Evaluation of a risk of malignancy index. *Br J Obstet Gynaecol* **100**: 927–931.

Depriest PD, Shenson D, Fried A et al (1993a) A morphology index based on sonographic findings in ovarian cancer. *Gynecol Oncol* **51**: 7–11.

Depriest PD, Van Nagell JR, Gallion HH et al (1993b) Ovarian cancer screening in asymptomatic postmenopausal women. *Gynecol Oncol* **51**: 205–209.

Finkler NJ, Benacerraf B, Lavin PT et al (1988) Comparison of serum CA 125, clinical impression, and ultrasound in the preoperative evaluation of ovarian masses. *Obstet Gynecol* **72**: 659.

Fleischer AC, Rodgers WH, Kepple DW et al (1993) Color Doppler sonography of ovarian masses: a multiparameter analysis. *J Ultrasound Med* **12**: 41.

Granberg S, Wilkland M & Jansson I (1989) Macroscopic characterization of ovarian tumors and the relation to the histologic diagnosis: criteria to be used for ultrasound evaluation. *Gynecol Oncol* **35**: 139–144.

Hata K, Hata T, Manabe A et al (1992) A critical evaluation of transvaginal Doppler studies, transvaginal sonography, magnetic resonance imaging, and CA-125 in detection of ovarian cancer. *Obstet Gynecol* **80**: 922–926.

Hulka JF, Parker WH, Surrey M et al (1992) Management of ovarian masses: AAGL 1990 survey. *J Reprod Med* **37**: 599.

Jacobs I, Oram D, Fairbanks J et al (1990) A risk of malignancy index incorporating CA-125, ultrasound and menopausal status for the accurate preoperative diagnosis of ovarian cancer. *Br J Obstet Gynaecol* **97**: 922–929.

Kroon E & Andolf E (1995) Diagnosis and follow-up of simple ovarian cysts detected by ultrasound in postmenopausal women. *Obstet Gynecol* **85**: 211–214.

Kurjak A, Predanic M, Kupesic-Urek S & Jucik S (1993) Transvaginal color and pulsed Doppler assessment of adnexal tumor vascularity. *Gynecol Oncol* **50**: 3–9.

Lerner JP, Timor-Tritsch LE, Federman A & Abramovitch G (1994) Transvaginal ultrasonographic characterization of ovarian masses with an improved, weighted scoring system. *Am J Obstet Gynecol* **170**: 81–85.

Luxman D, Bergman A, Sagi J & Davis MP (1991) The postmenopausal adnexal mass: correlation between ultrasonic and pathologic findings. *Obstet Gynecol* **77**: 726–727.

Maggino T, Gadducci A, D'Addario V et al (1994) Prospective multicenter study on CA-125 in postmenopausal pelvic masses. *Gynecol Oncol* **54**: 117–123.

Maiman M, Seltzer V & Boyce J (1991) Laparoscopic excision of ovarian neoplasms subsequently found to be malignant. *Obstet Gynecol* **77**: 563–565.

Malkasian GD, Knapp RC, Lavin PT et al (1988) Preoperative evaluation of CA-125 levels in pre-menopause and post-menopause patients with pelvic masses: discrimination of benign from malignant disease. *Am J Obstet Gynecol* **159**: 314–346.

Moran O, Menczer J, Ben-Baruch G et al (1993) Cytologic examination of ovarian cyst fluid for the distinction between benign and malignant tumors. *Obstet Gynecol* **82**: 444.

Nezhat F, Nezhat C, Welander CE & Benigno B (1992) Four ovarian cancers diagnosed during laparoscopic management of 1011 women with adnexal masses. *Am J Obstet Gynecol* **167**: 790–796.

Querleu D & Leblanc E (1994) Laparoscopic infrarenal node dissection for restaging of carcinomas of the ovary or fallopian tube. *Cancer* **73**: 1467–1471.

Querleu D, Capron C, Chevallier L & Bruhat MA (1993) Complications of gynecologic laparoscopic surgery. A French multicenter collaborative study. *N Engl J Med* **328**: 1355.

Sassone AM, Timor-Tritsch IE, Artner A et al (1991) Transvaginal sonographic characterization of ovarian disease: evaluation of a new scoring system to predict ovarian malignancy. *Obstet Gynecol* **78**: 70–76.

Schincaglia P, Brondelli L, Cicognani A et al (1994) A feasibility study of ovarian cancer screening: does fine-needle aspiration improve ultrasound specificity? *Tumori* **80**: 181.

Schneider VL, Schneider A, Reed KL & Hatch KD (1993) Comparison of Doppler with two-dimensional sonography and CA-125 for prediction of malignancy of pelvic masses. *Obstet Gynecol* **81**: 983–988.

Schutter EMJ, Kenemans P, Sohn C et al (1994) Diagnostic value of pelvic examination, ultrasound, and serum CA-125 in postmenopausal women with a pelvic mass. *Cancer* **74**: 1398–1406.

Steinkampf MP, Hammond KR & Blackwell RE (1990) Hormonal treatment of functional ovarian cysts: a randomized, prospective study. *Fertil Steril* **54**: 775–777.

Trimbos JB & Hacker NH (1993) The case against aspirating ovarian cysts. *Cancer* **72**: 828–831.

Valentin L, Sladkevicius P & Marsal K (1994) Limited contribution of Doppler velocimetry to the differential diagnosis of extrauterine pelvic tumors. *Obstet Gynecol* **83**: 425–433.

Westhoff C & Randall FC (1991) Ovarian cancer screening: potential effect on mortality. *Am J Obstet Gynecol* **165**: 502–505.

Wolf SI, Gosnik BB & Feldsman MR (1991) Prevalence of simple adnexal cysts in postmenopausal women. *Radiology* **180**: 65.

22 *Diagnosis of adhesive disease*
CL Kowalczyk, DA Johns and MP Diamond

■ INTRODUCTION

It is well known that pelvic adhesions play a major role in female infertility; adhesions may interfere with ovum pick-up by the Fallopian tube, may create a spatial interference between the ovary and tube, cause fixation of one or both organs in the pelvis, or the tube/ovary may be encapsulated by the adhesions (Bronson and Wallach, 1977; Caspi et al, 1979; Gomel, 1983). Adhesions may also be associated with other conditions such as acute and chronic pelvic pain and small bowel obstruction. Predisposing factors for the development of pelvic adhesions include pelvic inflammatory disease or other pelvic infections, appendicitis, endometriosis, previous ectopic or reproductive surgery and hemorrhage; the most common factor is previous surgery (Diamond and DeCherney, 1987). Unfortunately, the diagnosis of adhesions is usually presumptive until the time of surgery, although newer approaches may provide improvements in our ability to diagnose adhesions preoperatively, as will be described. This inability to diagnose adhesions preoperatively has also grossly limited appreciation by clinicians of how often adhesions develop postoperatively. In this chapter, we will review these issues, as well as grading or characterizing adhesions, which is important to provide a consistent means of communication regarding them. Additionally, we will discuss the process by which adhesions are thought to develop, because an appreciation of this process is likely to be essential to future identification and implementation of new evaluation techniques and treatments.

■ PATHOGENESIS

NORMAL PERITONEAL HEALING

As described by Masterson (1979), the first or inflammatory phase of wound healing involves blood being released from small vessels in the area of injury, followed by vaso-constriction. Vasodilation then occurs, with the release of leukocytes and platelets, histamines, prostaglandins and chemotactic agents. In the second or fibroblastic phase, collagen is deposited by fibroblasts, and there is an increased local concentration of plasminogen activator, which converts the proenzyme plasminogen to plasmin. Plasmin in turn then catalyzes the fibrinolysis of fibrin. The collagen fibrils crosslink, increasing the tensile strength of the repair. In the third or remodeling phase, there is reconstruction of previously laid collagen. This stage can vary in length of time and its quality depends on the availability of blood supply and oxygenation.

A similar process is thought to occur intraperitoneally, but some differences may exist. Raferty (1973a, 1973b, 1979) has described these effects using light microscopy and electron microscopy techniques. The defects in the peritoneum were noted to heal by metaplasia of the underlying connective tissue cells, forming a complete single layer of mesothelial cells within 5 days, in contrast to circumferentially from the edges, as occurs on skin. Specifically, injury to the peritoneum caused an increase in the permeability of blood vessels, resulting in the out-pouring of proteinaceous material and a serosanguineous fluid exudate. At 48 hours after injury, there was no fibrinolytic activity noted and only inflammatory cells were on the wound surface. This formed a fibrinous material that connected to adjacent intraperitoneal structures and became infiltrated by monocytes, histiocytes, polymorphonuclear neutrophils and plasma cells. Mesothelial cells and fibrinolytic activity was observed by day 3, reaching a maximum by day 8. Fibrinolytic activity in normal peritoneum was determined by the amount of plasminogen activator activity; plasminogen activator served to clear the fibrinous deposits. There was then a spontaneous dissolution of the fibrin mass via the fibrinolytic activity of plasminogen activator within a few days, and peritoneal healing was complete.

ADHESION FORMATION

Any alterations in the healing process, such as ischemia, devascularization, persistent bleeding or tissue abrasion, or an inhibition of any portion of the normal coagulation pathway may predispose to the development of adhesions. These injuries cause alterations in the normal healing process. Therefore, crushing injuries, peritoneal stripping, ligating or persistently bloody or oozing surfaces may lead to adhesion formation (Jackson, 1958; Ellis, 1963; Gervin et al, 1973; Buckman et al, 1976a, 1976b).

When this process does not progress smoothly, abnormal peritoneal healing occurs, with resultant adhesions. Mechanistically, fibrinolytic activity is suppressed, the proteinaceous mass is not absorbed and the fibrin persists intraperitoneally. There is then an infiltration and organization of the coagulum by fibroblasts, followed by vascular and cellular ingrowth and collagen deposition. The result is permanent fibrous adhesion formation.

Importantly, there is a difference in adhesion reformation and de novo formation (new adhesions that have formed in areas where they were previously absent); prevention/treatment of the former is more difficult, suggesting a slightly different mechanism of formation or impairment of the normal healing process.

■ SYMPTOMS

Patients will present with a variety of physical complaints that may be associated with pelvic adhesions. The most common complaint is that of chronic pelvic pain, usually described as sharp, intermittent or constant, or as having a pulling sensation in the pelvic area, specifically with activity. Similarly, symptoms may be described during or following intercourse in women with adhesions involving the reproductive tract (or the vaginal cuff in women who have had a hysterectomy). These complaints are usually described as being present throughout the menstrual cycle, although some women with endometriosis or dysmenorrhea may describe luteal phase exacerbation. There may also be complaints of pain with defecation when adhesions involve the bowel, especially the sigmoid colon. Involvement of the intestines, especially the small bowel, may cause complaints of abdominal pain, distension, nausea and/or vomiting, and be associated with partial or complete bowel obstruction. While some patients with severe or extensive adhesions have complaints of pelvic pain, others with only minimal adhesive disease will complain of similar severe symptoms. Conversely, other patients with varying degrees of adhesions from mild to severe will have no complaints of pelvic or abdominal discomfort of any kind. On physical examination, there may be tenderness to movement of the uterus, adnexa and/or other pelvic structures involved in adhesions. There may also be an impression of a nonmobile mass or a decrease in mobility of the uterus of other structures appreciated on pelvic examination. Unless associated with bowel obstruction, adhesions do not usually present as acute abdomens with signs such as guarding, rebound or rigidity.

The difficulty in the diagnosis of adhesions stems from the inconsistency of symptoms and physical findings in patients, the coexistence of other pathology, as well as the difficulty in establishing the diagnosis with current noninvasive methods. A history of previous infection, appendicitis or endometriosis or previous pelvic/abdominal surgery are predisposing factors to adhesion formation. This is secondary to disruption of the normal healing process via tissue trauma, ischemia and/or a decrease in normal fibrinolysis. The differential diagnosis of adhesions for pelvic pain requires an investigation of other pelvic structures that may elicit the pain. A thorough gynecological examination, potentially including transvaginal ultrasonography, may help identify reproductive tract abnormalities that may cause or be associated with the pain, such as ovarian cysts, hydrosalpinx, ectopic pregnancies, etc. A gastrointestinal workup to rule out irritable bowel syndrome, Crohn's disease, appendicitis, diverticulitis or carcinoma should be performed and the patient should be referred to a gastroenterologist if appropriate symptoms so warrant. A genitourinary evaluation may also be in order to detect urinary infections, stones or obstruction. A musculoskeletal examination and history of recent strenuous physical activity to warrant such pain should also be investigated. Finally, many psychosomatic complaints manifest as pelvic pain and may require further psychological evaluation.

■CLINICAL INVESTIGATIONS

NONINVASIVE METHODS

In gynecology, preoperative diagnosis of adhesions may be inferred by certain radiological tests but requires confirmation by surgical intervention. Hysterosalpingography is most commonly used to evaluate the normalcy of the uterine cavity and to document tubal patency. The most common indications for such testing are during routine workup for recurrent abortion and for infertility. A normal hysterosalpingogram (*Figure 22.1a*) shows a normal intrauterine contour and bilateral tubal filling with contrast medium, with diffuse spillage into the peritoneal cavity. On the delayed film there is uniform disbursement of contrast medium into the pelvis (*Figure 22.1b*). In contrast, one suspects adhesions during hysterosalpingography when there is localization of contrast medium after tubal spill into the peritoneal cavity either during the examination (*Figure 22.2a*) or on the delayed film (*Figure 22.2b*). While one report has suggested that peritubal adhesions can be suspected on hysterosalpingography in 75% of laparoscopically documented cases, this has not been our clinical experience. The most common finding in this situation is loculated spill, but peritubal adhesions may also appear as tubal convolutions in a fixed position in the pelvis (Karasick and Goldfarb, 1989). Other factors may contribute to this finding – such as normal bowel positioning. This technique, therefore, has neither the advantage of direct visualization nor the opportunity to treat the adhesions once identified.

Another noninvasive test that may suggest the presence of adhesions in the pelvis is sonohysterography or

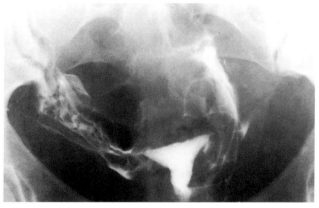

22.1a

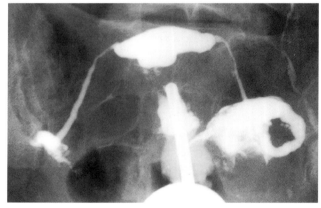

22.2a

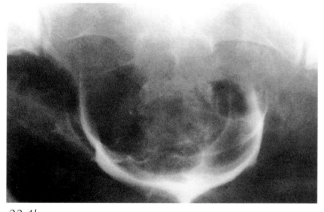

22.1b

Figure 22.1: *(a) Hysterosalpingogram showing a normal uterine cavity with tubal fill and diffuse spillage after instillation of contrast. (b) On the delayed film there is uniform distribution of contrast in the peritoneal cavity.*

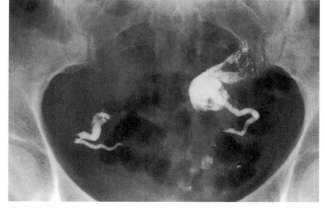

22.2b

Figure 22.2: *(a) Hysterosalpingogram showing a normal uterine cavity and tubal fill but loculation of the perfusion medium at a localized area around the left tube, suggesting peritubal adhesions. (b) Delayed film.*

hydrogynecography. A sonohysterogram utilizes the instrumental techniques of hysterosalpingography (i.e. cannula or tubing placed into the cervical os for dye injection), but the internal contour of the uterus and patency of the Fallopian tubes are documented by ultrasonography using a saline (or other) solution as the medium. In this situation as well, a uniform desplacement of fluid into the pelvis is normally observed, while loculation of fluid in the pelvis is suggestive of adhesions. In patients with infertility and pelvic pain, Maroulis et al (1992) were able to identify 84% of laparoscopically documented cases of pelvic adhesions.

The possibility of this fluid localization being caused by normal bowel positioning and the inability to remove the adhesions serve as potential pitfalls to this technique as well.

The diagnosis of adhesions is difficult to determine for other subspecialties as well. The use of ultrasonography versus computed tomography (CT) for the diagnosis of an ovarian mass and detection of adhesions was evaluated in gynecological oncology. Ozasa et al (1986) compared prospectively 25 cases of clinically suspected ovarian masses for the presence of pathology. While the ultrasound was able to identify adhesions to the uterus only in selected cases, CT was useful in identifying adhesions to the uterus as well as other adjoining structures. Marin et al noted benefit in the diagnosis of abdominal adhesions by the use of prelaparoscopic echography. After a pneumoperitoneum was established, echography was implemented intraoperatively to detect the presence of intra-abdominal adhesions by noting the distribution of gas and pneumoperitoneal chambers. This method was successfully applied in 39 patients and in 38% of the cases an alternate trocar insertion site was chosen, subsequently avoiding abdominal adhesions (Marin et al, 1987). Recently, transabdominal ultrasonography has been employed by Uberoi et al to detect the presence of adhesions and perhaps bowel attached to the anterior abdominal wall. Adhesions cause a reduction in bowel motility within the intraperitoneal cavity relative to the anterior abdominal wall, referred to as the visceral slide (Uberoi et al, 1995). Although it was previously reported that this technique had a 100% detection rate (Kodama et al, 1992), this study, incorporating the evaluation of visceral slide during spontaneous respirations

(SRSL) and exaggerated respiration (ESL), observed bowel movement of only 1–2 cm, and noted a much less positive correlation. They determined that although ultrasound can detect adhesions postoperatively, the sensitivity is poor and there are considerably higher false negatives and false positives noted at the outcome (with SRSL, sensitivity 21%, specificity 94%, accuracy 76%; ESL, sensitivity 20%, specificity 76%, accuracy 63%) (Uberoi et al, 1995). While many of these possible diagnostic interventions seem promising, they are not consistently accurate and thus their routine use has not been implemented.

Perhaps the most diagnostic radiological test is the KUB (kidneys, ureters, bladder) performed in the patient with bowel obstruction. (KUB is the colloquial term for a plain anteroposterior radiograph of the abdomen.) In such subjects, multiple air–fluid levels are often identified, which confirm the diagnosis suggested on physical examination by such findings as distension, tympany and high pitched bowel sounds. However, patients with obstruction represent only a very small proportion of the population who suffer morbidity due to scarring.

SURGICAL CONFIRMATION

Thus, to definitively document the presence of pelvic adhesions, surgical intervention is usually required. At laparoscopy, direct visualization with manipulation of the pelvic and abdominal organs using an atraumatic probe will identify cohesive (*Figure 22.3*), dense (*Figure 22.4*) or filmy (*Figure 22.5*). adhesions. An incision is made in the umbilical area and a Veress needle is introduced. To verify placement into the abdominal cavity and to possibly detect periumbilical adhesions, the aspiration test or hanging drop test can be applied. In the aspiration test, a syringe is filled with saline and is attached to the Veress needle. Once the Veress needle is introduced into the abdominal cavity, the syringe is aspirated. If there is no reaspiration, either the peritoneal cavity has not been entered or the Veress needle is obstructed by an organ or adhesions (Semm, 1987). Similarly, the hanging drop test is incorporated once the Veress needle is in place; a drop of saline is placed on the end of the open Veress needle. The abdominal wall is then lifted and if the saline remains in the top of the Veress needle there

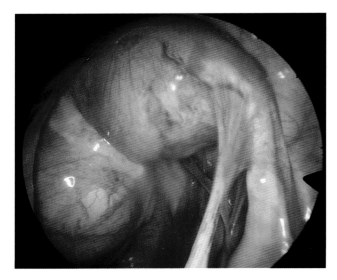

Figure 22.5: Laparoscopic view of filmy adhesions at the isthmic segment of the Fallopian tube.

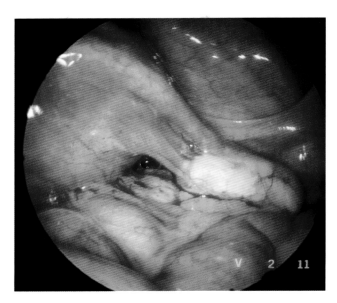

Figure 22.3: Laparoscopic view of cohesive adhesions after ovarian cystectomy.

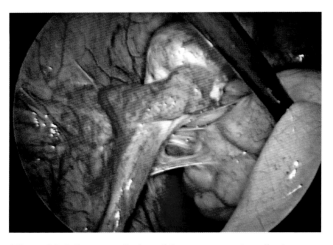

Figure 22.4: Laparoscopic view of dense postoperative adhesions from the rectosigmoid and ovary to the pelvic side wall.

may be adhesions or organs against the needle tip, or the abdominal cavity has not been entered (Fear, 1968). Another variation of the aspiration test uses a 16 Fr spinal needle attached to a syringe. After carbon dioxide has been introduced into the abdomen with the Veress needle, the spinal needle is sequentially inserted in the peritoneal cavity in a semicircular fashion about the umbilicus and air is aspirated into the syringe by retraction. A positive aspiration of CO_2 gas indicates free space in the cavity, whereas the inability to aspirate CO_2

gas may be suggestive of adhesions or other form of obstruction and subsequent trocar placement should be avoided in that area. In such a situation, other sites that have been described are the left upper quadrant adjacent to approximately the ninth intercostal space, the posterior cul-de-sac or through the uterine fundus. (Discussion of these techniques is beyond the limits of this chapter.) The minilaparotomy (open laparoscopy) has the theoretical advantage of direct visualization in diagnosis of adhesions; however, to our knowledge, it has never been documented that the possibility of complications secondary to Veress and/or trocar insertion is avoided. The adhesions can be more directly manipulated and more difficult areas (in the cul-de-sac and behind densely adhered adnexa) can be more extensively evaluated by direct visualization; neither may be possible by laparoscopy. Laparoscopy and minilaparotomy have the advantage, in addition to diagnosis of adhesions, of providing the opportunity for some therapeutic benefit through adhesiolysis. Recently, microlaparoscopy or 'office laparoscopy' has been introduced as a less invasive method of entering the abdomen than laparoscopy. Often performed under intravenous sedation using 1–2 mm instruments, this procedure may provide a lower cost method of evaluating the pelvis, with less resultant patient morbidity. Future evaluations will be necessary to determine its risk of complications and cost effectiveness and to identify its appropriateness compared with other forms of laparoscopy.

■ CLASSIFICATION

In describing adhesions, it is important to be consistent in definitions among surgeons; the following classification system for postoperative adhesion development has been suggested as a method of providing uniform criteria for the assessment of the efficacy of surgical techniques, equipment, instruments and or adjuvants, as the efficacy of any of these variables may be altered by whether an adhesion was lysed at that site, as well as where operative procedures were performed (LaMorke and Diamond, 1993).

Type 1:   de novo adhesion formation – development of adhe sions at site that did not have adhesions initially.

Type 1a: no operative procedure at site of adhesion formation.

Type 1b: operative procedure performed at site of adhesion formation.

Type 2:   redevelopment of adhesions at sites at which adhesiolysis was performed.

Type 2a: no operative procedure at site of adhesion formation (other than adhesiolysis).

Type 2b: operative procedure performed at site of adhesion reformation (in addition to adhesiolysis).

Equally important, in order to communicate universally regarding the site, type and extent of adhesions noted at the time of surgery, Diamond et al established a comprehensive grading system (*Figure 22.6*) (Adhesion Scoring Group, 1994). When compared with the American Fertility Society (AFS) adhesion classification system, this comprehensive system allowed for concordance by a greater number of surgeons, each of whom reviewed the same surgical videos (*Figure 22.7*), thus establishing the degree of interindividual variation. Corson et al (1995) evaluated the intraindividual variation for the same videotapes reviewed at different times and observed a strong correlation. Interestingly, the surgeon who performed the surgical procedures scored the second-look videos as having the lowest adhesion scores,

	Adhesions	<1/3 enclosure	1/3–2/3 enclosure	>2/3 enclosure
Ovary	R Filmy	1	2	4
	Dense	4	8	16
	L Filmy	1	2	4
	Dense	4	8	16
Tube	R Filmy	1	2	4
	Dense	4*	8*	16
	L Filmy	1	2	4
	Dense	4*	8*	16

R, right; l, left
* If the fimbriated end of the Fallopian tube is completely enclosed, change the point assignment to 16

(a)

Location	Severity	Extent
Anterior abdominal wall (1–4):		
1 Left side to ____	____	____
2 Right side to ____	____	____
3 Incision line to ____	____	____
4 Above incision to ____	____	____
Anterior cul-de-sac (5–8):		
5 Over Uterus to ____	____	____
6 Over bladder to ____	____	____
7 Left side to ____	____	____
8 Right side to ____	____	____
*9 Posterior uterus to ____	____	____
*10 Posterior cul-de-sac to ____	____	____
*11 Pelvic sidewall Left-Left to ____	____	____
*12 Pelvic sidewall-Right to ____	____	____
*13 Posterior broad ligament-Left to ____	____	____
*14 Posterior broad ligament -Right to ____	____	____
*15 Round ligament to tube-Left to ____	____	____
*16 Round ligament to tube-Right to ____	____	____
*17 Ovary-Left to ____	____	____
*18 Ovary-Right to ____	____	____
*19 Tube-Left to ____	____	____
*20 Tube-Right to ____	____	____
21 Small bowel to ____	____	____
22 Large bowel to ____	____	____
*23 Omentum to ____	____	____

Severity

0 = no adhesions present

1 = filmy, avascular

2 = some vascularity and/or dense

3a = cohesive, falls apart upon touch

3b = cohesive, visible dissectable planes & can be separated with minimal dissection

3c = cohesive, no visible dissectable planes & requires extensive dissection for separation

Extent

0 = no adhesions present

1 = mild (covering ≤ 25% total area/length)

2 = moderate (covering 26–50% total area/length)

3 = severe (covering ≥ 51% of total area/length)

* Modified MCASM locations

(b)

Figure 22.6: (a) The American Fertility Society adhesion scoring method (AFSASM) and (b) the more comprehensive adhesion scoring method (MCASM). The asterisks in (b) indicate the 13 or 23 sites that correspond to the area of the pelvis likely to be involved with tubal and ovarian adhesions. From Adhesion Scoring Group (1994) Improvement of interobserver reproducibility of adhesion scoring systems. Fertil Steril 62: 984–998. Reproduced with permission of the publisher, the American Society for Reproductive Medicine (formerly The American Fertility Society).

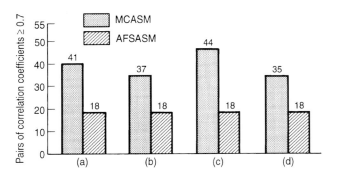

Figure 22.7: Number of pairs (n = 55) of gynecological surgeons with correlation coefficients of adhesion scores ≥ 0.7 utilizing the AFS adhesion scoring system and for each of the four ways of scoring using the more comprehensive adhesion scoring method: (a) addition of the severity plus extent of all 23 sites; (b) multiplication of the severity times extent at all 23 sites; (c) addition of the severity plus extent at 13 sites; and (d) multiplication of the severity times extent at 13 sites. From Adhesion Scoring Group (1994) Improvement of interobserver reproducibility of adhesion scoring systems. Fertil Steril 62: 984–988. Reproduced with permission of the publisher, the American Society for Reproductive Medicine (formerly The American Fertility Society).

suggesting that subconsciously surgeons may wish (and believe) they have achieved better success than would other reviewers.

■ CONCLUSION

In this chapter, normal wound healing as well as the pathophysiological process of adhesion development have been reviewed. A number of insults to the peritoneal surfaces, including a variety of abdominal and pelvic infections, endometriosis and abdominal/pelvic surgery, may cause adhesions; an adequate patient history is important to discern these predisposing factors in her diagnosis. Adhesions may in turn cause a number of clinical manifestations, such as pelvic pain, infertility and bowel obstruction, that warrant investigation. Physical examination, although suggestive of adhesive disease by symptoms, a decrease in uterine mobility or tenderness/fullness in certain areas of the pelvis, requires further workup to evaluate other possible etiologies for the pain. The use of hysterosalpingography and sonohysterography may suggest the presence of adhesions but the

diagnostic tool most appropriate in the evaluation and possible treatment of adhesions is through surgical intervention. The diagnosis and subsequent therapy of adhesions remains a clinical dilemma in many cases; further research and development of newer approaches to the diagnosis of adhesions are required to provide more specific identification and treatment of this process.

REFERENCES

Adhesion Scoring Group (1994) Improvement of interobserver reproducibility of adhesion scoring systems. *Fertil Steril* **62**: 984–988.

Bronson RA & Wallach EE (1977) Lysis of periadnexal adhesions for correction of infertility. *Fertil Steril* **28**: 613.

Buckman RF Jr, Buckman PD, Hufnagel HV & Gervin AS (1976a) A physiologic basis for the adhesion-free healing of deperitonealized surfaces. *J Surg Res* **21**: 67–76.

Buckman RF, Woods M, Sargent L & Gervin AS (1976b) A unifying pathogenetic mechanism in the etiology of intraperitoneal adhesions. *J Surg Res* **20**: 1–5.

Caspi E, Halpern Y & Bukovsky I (1979) The importance of peritoneal adhesions in tubal reconstructive surgery for infertility. *Fertil Steril* **31**: 296.

Corson SL, Batzer FR, Gocial B, Kelly M, Gutmann JN & Maislin G (1995) Intra-observer and inter-observer variability in scoring laparoscopic diagnosis of pelvic adhesions. *Hum Reprod* **10**: 161–164.

Diamond MP & DeCherney AH (1987) Pathogenesis of adhesion formation/reformation: application to reproductive pelvic surgery. *Microsurgery* **8**: 103–108.

Ellis H (1963) The aetiology of post-operative abdominal adhesion: an experimental study. *Br J Surg* **50**: 10–16.

Fear RE (1968) Laparoscopy: a valuable aid in gynecologic diagnosis. *Obstet Gynecol* **31**: 297–309.

Gervin AS, Puckett CL & Silver D (1973) Serosal hypofibrinolysis: a cause of postoperative adhesions. *Am J Surg* **125**: 80–88.

Gomel V (1983) Salpingoovariolysis by laparoscopy in infertility. *Fertil Steril* **40**: 607.

Jackson BB (1958) Observations on intraperitoneal adhesions: an experimental study. *Surgery* **44**: 507–514.

Karasick S & Goldfarb AE (1989) Peritubal adhesions in infertile women: diagnosis with hysterosalpingogram. *AJR* **152**: 777.

Kodama I, Loiacono LA, Sigel B et al (1992) Ultrasonic detection of viscera slide as an indicator of abdominal wall adhesions. *J Clin Ultrasound* **20**: 375–380.

LaMorte AI & Diamond MP (1993) Adhesion formation – laparoscopic surgery. In Diamond MP, Zerega GS, Linsky CB & Reid RL (eds) *Gynecologic Surgery and Adhesion Prevention*, pp 51–58. New York: Wiley Liss.

Marin G, Bergamo S, Miola E, Caldironi MW & Dagnini G (1987) Prelaparoscopic echography used to detect abdominal adhesions. *Endoscopy* **19**: 147–149.

Maroulis GB, Parsons AK & Yeko TR (1992) Hydrogynecography: a new technique enables vaginal sonography to visualize pelvic adhesions and other pelvic structures. *Fertil Steril* **58**: 1073–1075.

Masterson BJ (1979) Wound healing in gynecologic surgery. In Masterson BJ (ed.) *Manual of Gynecologic Surgery*. New York: Springer.

Ozasa H, Noda Y, Mori T, Togashi K & Nakano Y (1986) Diagnostic capability of ultrasound versus CT for clinically suspected ovarian mass with emphasis on detection of adhesions. *Gynecol Oncol* **25**: 311–318.

Raferty AT (1973a) Regeneration of parietal and visceral peritoneum: a light microscopal study. *Br J Surg* **60**: 293–299.

Raferty AT (1973b) Regeneration of parietal and visceral peritoneum: an electron microscopal study. *J Anat* **115**: 375–392.

Raferty AT (1979) Regeneration of peritoneum: a fibrinolytic study. *J Anat* **129**: 659–664.

Semm K (1987) *Operative Manual for Endoscopic Abdominal Surgery.* [Translated and edited by Friedrich ER.] Chicago: Year Book Medical.

Uberoi R, D'Costa H, Brown C & Dubbins P (1995) Visceral slide for intraperitoneal adhesions? A prospective study in 48 patients with surgical correlation. *J Clin Ultrasound* **23**: 363–366.

23 *Pelvic floor relaxation*
SL Stanton

■ INTRODUCTION

Pregnancy and delivery are believed to be the major causes of prolapse. Stretching of the pudendal nerve and its perineal branches during late pregnancy and delivery lead to denervation of the levator ani (pubovisceral muscle) and urethral and anal sphincters, and the passage of the fetus through the birth canal adds mechanical trauma to these muscles.

Prolapse may be classified anatomically according to the pelvic compartment in which it is situated and to the degree of severity. The anterior compartment contains the bladder and urethra (cystocele or cystourethrocele). The middle compartment contains the uterus, or vault if a hysterectomy has been performed, and enterocele (small bowel). The posterior compartment contains the rectum (rectocele). It may be academic to attempt to distinguish between vault descent and an enterocele as symptomatology and signs are very similar and only expert imaging and exposure at surgery will determine the correct diagnosis.

Hitherto, prolapse has been graded on a I–III scale. Grade I is equivalent to some descent within the vagina, grade II is descent of prolapse to the introitus and grade III is descent of the prolapse beyond. This may be qualified according to whether the patient is lying or standing and whether at rest or straining. This classification is diffuse and it was difficult to compare data on treatment of prolapse between different clinicians. To overcome this, the International Continence Society Standardization Committee produced a report on standardization of terminology of prolapse and pelvic floor dysfunction (1995) to permit a more accurate description and evaluation of prolapse. It is suggested that the present evaluation with three grades and without any fixed bony markers is replaced by a new classification that uses the hymen as a fixed reference point and the ischial spines as identifiable landmarks. Measurements

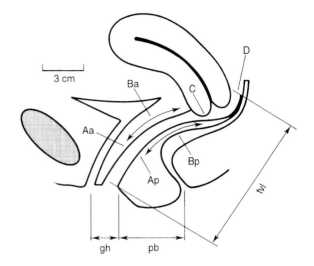

*Figure 23.1: Sagittal section of a female pelvis to demonstrate points for recording prolapse measurements (gh, genital hiatus; pb, perineal body; tvl, total vaginal length). Point **Aa** is in the midline of the anterior vaginal wall 3 cm proximal to the external urethral meatus. Point **Ba** is the most distal position of the upper portion of the anterior vaginal wall from the vaginal vault or anterior vaginal fornix to point Aa. **C** is the most distal (most dependent) edge of the cervix or leading edge of the vault. **D** is the uppermost point of the posterior fornix. **Bp** is the most distal (most dependent) position of the upper portion of the posterior vaginal wall from the vaginal vault or posterior vaginal fornix to point Ap. **Ap** is a point located on the midline of the posterior vaginal wall 3 cm proximal to the hymen. From Bump RC et al (1996) The standardisation of terminology of female pelvic organ prolapse and pelvic floor dysfunction. Am J Obstet Gynecol. Reproduced by kind permission of the International Continence Society Committee on Standardization of Terminology.*

are made between the hymen and two points on the anterior wall, the most distal (dependent) edge of the cervix or vaginal vault, the posterior fornix and two points on the posterior wall (*Figure 23.1*). These are normalized to the level of the hymen by noting the distance between the spines and the plane of the hymen. Measurements are taken at rest and on Valsalva, lying or standing: these variables should be specified. Measurements may be recorded on a 3 × 3 grid (*Figure 23.2*) or line diagram (*Figure 23.3*). Validation of this system has

Point Aa anterior wall	Point Ba anterior wall	Point C cervix or cuff
Genital hiatus	Perineal body	Total vaginal length
Point Ap posterior wall	Point Bp posterior wall	Point D posterior fornix

Figure 23.2: A grid for recording the quantitative description of pelvic organ prolapse. From Bump RC et al (1996) The standardisation of terminology of female pelvic organ prolapse and pelvic floor dysfunction. Am J Obstet Gynecol. Reproduced by kind permission of the International Continence Society Committee on Standardization of Terminology.

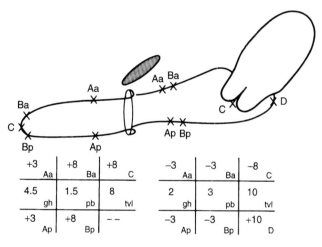

+3 Aa	+8 Ba	+8 C		−3 Aa	−3 Ba	−8 C
4.5 gh	1.5 pb	8 tvl		2 gh	3 pb	10 tvl
+3 Ap	+8 Bp	−−		−3 Ap	−3 Bp	+10 D

Figure 23.3: To show diagrammatic and grid forms of the uterine cervix (right) and complete vaginal vault eversion (left). From Bump RC et al (1996) The standardisation of terminology of female pelvic organ prolapse and pelvic floor dysfunction. Am J Obstet Gynecol. Reproduced by kind permission of the International Continence Society Committee on Standardization of Terminology.

shown accurate site specific measurements with good intraobserver and interobserver reproducibility and a short learning curve; it was acceptable to patients and the extra time to complete this classification did not exceed 3.5 minutes. There was poor to moderate agreement between two examiners in the early stages, but this decreased subsequently (Athanasiou et al, 1995). Schüssler and Peschers (1995) found an interexaminer variability of 25%; however, their numbers were smaller. In both studies the total vaginal length showed the greatest variability.

■ SYMPTOMS

Symptoms may be classified according to each prolapse as general, sexual and specific. Severity of symptoms is not proportional to the size of prolapse and the reason for this is not clearly understood. The general symptoms include 'something coming down', progressively increasing backache or a lower abdominoperineal dragging sensation increased by standing and walking and relieved by lying down. These are due to the anatomical presence of the prolapse and traction on nerve fibers within the peritoneal covering or ligament involved in the prolapse.

The sexual symptoms relate to altered anatomy. Dyspareunia may be due to the prolapse creating a barrier to penetration, or being reduced by the penis or remaining alongside it. Both patient and partner may lose libido when aware of the prolapse and have anxieties about the harmful effects that intercourse might have.

The specific symptoms are as follows.

ANTERIOR COMPARTMENT

Anterior compartment prolapse is mostly cystourethrocele with a cystocele alone occurring less frequently. A urethrocele on its own is extremely rare but may follow unsuccessful prolapse surgery. The most common symptom is stress incontinence due to descent of the bladder neck and failure of the sphincter mechanism to remain competent. There may be difficulty in initiating voiding and incomplete bladder emptying may occur with a large cystocele. Digitation of the vagina may be employed to empty the bladder. Voiding difficulty occurs if the bladder neck is fixed as the bladder descends, leading to kinking of the proximal urethra. If there is a residual urine, infection may occur, revealed by dysuria, frequency and urgency. Whether urgency and frequency in the absence of urinary tract infection can be due to prolapse is contentious. Stanton and Cardozo (1979) found no significant difference in frequency or urge incontinence after correction of a cystourethrocele by either an anterior repair or colposuspension.

MIDDLE COMPARTMENT

The main symptoms of middle compartmental prolapse are the presence of a lump or 'something coming down', which is the uterus or vault if a hysterectomy has been performed. Rarely, where the vault is thin and intra-abdominal pressure raised, the vault may rupture, leading to acute protrusion of the small bowel through the introitus. The patient may become shocked and this is a surgical emergency because of the risk of small bowel strangulation.

POSTERIOR COMPARTMENT

The symptoms are related to the lower intestinal tract, and may be functional or anatomical. Functional symptoms are due to incomplete bowel evacuation as feces become trapped in the anterior and occasionally posterior outpouching of the rectum. This leads to a feeling of incomplete bowel emptying and some patients may digitate (either rectally or vaginally) or splint the perineum in an effort to overcome this. Constipation is a frequent complaint. If the anal sphincter has undergone denervation or a traumatic injury following childbirth, incontinence of flatus or feces may result. The anatomical symptoms are due to awareness of the rectocele and include the feeling of a lump coming down or discomfort on sitting.

■ CLINICAL INVESTIGATIONS

While important advances in imaging techniques have occurred since the mid-1980s, some radiological procedures have continued to be explored and used; however, real time ultrasound and sector scanning with linear array and three-dimensional probes now produce images of much greater clarity and detail than previously. The greatest accuracy has been achieved with magnetic resonance imaging (MRI), which is not invasive and is nonionizing. It is more accurate than ultrasonography but is a static investigation and therefore depicts anatomy rather than function.

RADIOLOGY

VIDEOCYSTOURETHROGRAPHY

This investigation, which images the anterior compartment, was developed by Enhorning and colleagues in 1964; its widespread use now as a comprehensive urodynamic investigation is largely due to the efforts of Bates

and colleagues (1970) who used it to diagnose stress and urge incontinence. It will demonstrate associated movement of the anterior vaginal wall and quantify it. Urethral sphincteric function can be tested both in the ability to milk back and to remain competent where there is an increase in intra-abdominal or intravesical pressure. The bladder is filled with contrast medium (Urografin 150) at a fast fill rate of 100 ml/min (a neuropathic bladder will be filled more slowly, between 5 and 10 ml/min); a pressure measuring line is placed in the bladder and a further pressure measuring line in the rectum and electronic subtraction allows display of the detrusor pressure (*Figure 23.4*). The patient is then radiologically screened in the erect oblique position. She is asked to cough and any loss of contrast and movement of the urethrovesical junction and bladder base are noted (*Figure 23.5*). She is next asked to void and the flow rate and maximum voiding pressure are recorded. About 25% of women have some difficulty in voiding erect and can complete the voiding phase seated without radiological screening.

Owing to projection it is difficult to measure accurately change in excursion of the bladder neck and bladder base. Abnormalities such as detrusor instability and voiding difficulty are detected by the simultaneous pressure flow recordings. Other disadvantages include the number of staff required, the invasiveness and the dose of irradiation (approximately 2.7 mGy to the ovaries).

DEFECATING PROCTOGRAPHY

There is increasing interest by gynecologists in functional aspects of the lower intestinal tract, particularly when rectocele occurs. A number of methods exist for imaging the posterior compartment: defecating or evacuating proctography to image rectal evacuation will also demonstrate pelvic floor descent and rectocele. Barium contrast medium is injected into the anal canal and either cut films at a rate 1–2 per second or video radiology is used to record the images.

The position of the anorectal junction is related to the pubococcygeal line from the superior aspect of the pubic symphysis to the tip of the coccyx during rest, squeeze and strain without defecation, or to when the anal canal just starts to open. Anterior and posterior rectoceles can be identified and measured in relation to a projected line

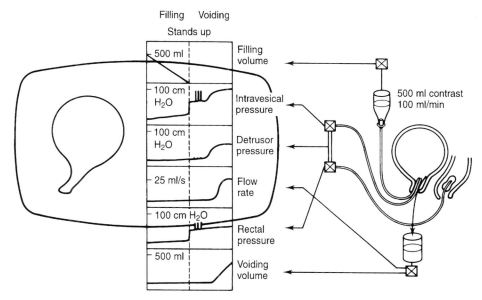

Figure 23.4: *Scheme for videocysto-urethrography. Simultaneous recording of bladder and rectal pressure changes during supine cystometry, combined with a display of bladder filling volume, is shown on the left side of the record. On voiding, the bladder and rectal pressures with the voiding rate and volume are recorded on the right of the trace. The intravesical pressure, detrusor pressure and voiding rate are added to the radiographic image of the bladder (extreme left of the diagram) and recorded with sound commentary.*

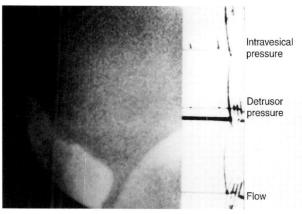

Figure 23.5: *Videocystourethrogram to show stress incontinence due to urethral sphincter incompetence with a cough pressure rise without any detrusor contraction on the detrusor pressure trace. There is a similar rise in the intravesical pressure.*

on the rectum and residual barium in the rectocele may be noted after evacuation. There is a wide variation in measurements from asymptomatic controls and lack of agreement about standardization: the method for measuring some parameters and the validity of many measurements must be questioned (Bartram and Mayhew, 1992). Disadvantages of these techniques are their semi-quantitative nature and the radiation dose, which precludes prolonged and repeated testing.

COLPOCYSTODEFECOGRAPHY (COLPOCYSTOGRAPHY, DYNAMIC CYSTOPROCTOGRAPHY, FOUR-CONTRAST DEFECOGRAPHY)

Simultaneous fluoroscopy of bladder, vagina, rectum and anal canal was first described by Bethoux and Bory in

1962. It involved outlining the bladder, vagina and rectum with barium. The patient was screened in the erect lateral position and measurements were made of the change in position of bladder, vagina and rectum on straining. No pressure measurements were made. The procedure was later modified to include screening during defecation and then Kelvin and colleagues (1994) opacified the small bowel by getting the patient to drink 500 ml of barium. The bladder was filled with 200 ml of contrast medium (Hypaque, 25–50%), the vagina coated with a barium gel and the rectum was filled with a thick barium paste. Fluoroscopy was then performed with the patient sitting on the commode at rest, with the voluntary contraction of the pelvic floor muscle and then during evacuation of bladder and bowel contents (*Figure 23.6*). Finally a postevacuation film was taken at maximum strain. The authors claim to be able to simultaneously image the bladder, vault, vagina, small bowel and rectum while the patient contracts her pelvic floor muscle or evacuates bladder or bowel. Altringer et al (1995) found positive clinical diagnosis was not confirmed by this technique in 75% of patients: 63% had cystocele, 46% had enterocele and 73% had rectocele, which were not detected on clinical examinations. The difficulty with this technique lies in the interpretation of the results: it is hard to believe that an experienced gynecologist would miss between 46 and 73% of prolapse, and, vice versa, find prolapse in 27–75% of patients that

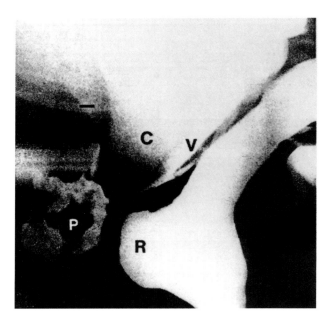

23.6a

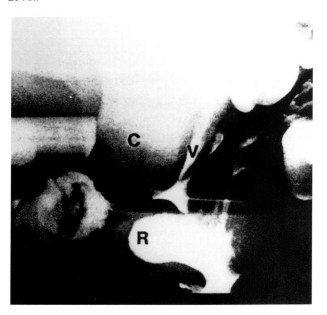

23.6b

Figure 23.6: *Cystocele, rectocele and a sigmoidocele demonstrated by dynamic cystoproctography.* (a) *Lateral radiograph taken during rectal evacuation showing cystocele (C) extending below the inferior margin of the pubic symphysis (horizontal line); a low rectocele (R) is noted. A gauze plug (P) is used to limit barium loss from the vagina (V).* (b) *Lateral radiograph taken after rectal evacuation showing that the cystocele has enlarged because of repeated straining and barium is retained within the rectocele. The rectovaginal space is widened but does not yet contain herniated bowel. Reproduced with permission from Kelvin et al (1994).*

is not confirmed by an imaging study. How many of these fluoroscopic prolapses were symptomatic or required treatment is uncertain. The very artificiality

and complexity of the technique must make interpretation difficult. It would be ideal to have a test–retest or other validation data to determine 'normal values'. No pressure recordings are made either in the bladder or bowel so no urodynamic data or anorectal physiological data is available.

BEAD CHAIN CYSTOURETHROGRAPHY

Bead chain cystourethrography is an established method for determining bladder neck and bladder base position and excursion. A radiopaque material (Hypaque or Urografin) and a slim metallic bead chain are introduced into the bladder and lateral erect radiographs are taken at rest and at maximum Valsalva. The disadvantages include omission of pressure flow measurements so that there is minimal urodynamic data, irradiation (1.6 mGy to the ovaries) and difficulty of obtaining accurate measurements because of projection. Gordon et al (1989) compared it with perineal ultrasound and found good correlation between ultrasound and chain urethrocystograms without significant difference in favor of either. Ultrasound was more accurate irrespective of body mass and was readily available in every gynecological department. Grischke and colleagues (1991) compared chain urethrocystography and simultaneous urethral and bladder pressure measurements and electromyography of the pelvic floor and abdominal wall. They found that chain urethrocystography had a high sensitivity (91%) but low specificity. Both methods supplied different but complementary data.

ULTRASONOGRAPHY

Although the bladder has been imaged by ultrasound for over 30 years, it is only in the last decade that serious attempts have been made to study the pelvic floor and associated pelvic organs. Ultrasound is well recognized for evaluation of pelvic floor muscle function. This includes movement of the bladder neck and base, and the relationship of the bladder base to the posterior vaginal wall. Movement of the bladder neck has been studied using the abdominal route but this is inadequate when the patient is obese or has pronounced prolapse behind the symphysis. The rectal route has been used and allows the extent and type of prolapse to be identified and measured by recording images before and after straining (Richmond et al, 1986). Vaginal ultrasonography (vaginosonography) using high frequency endoprobes (5–7 MHz) is a simple technique for imaging the lower urinary tract. The probe is smaller than the rectal probe but is unsuitable for some patients. Its main disadvantage is that it can interfere with descent of the prolapse on straining. Perineal ultrasonography uses linear array ultrasound (3.5–5 MHz) placed on the perineal region; definition of the bladder neck is improved by using a urethral catheter. Gordon and colleagues (1989) compared perineal ultrasound scanning to lateral chain urethrocystography in the determination of bladder neck descent. Good correlation was obtained between ultrasound and chain urethrocystogram results, with no significant differences in favor of either as a means of localizing the bladder neck. Ultrasound scanning was preferred as it avoided irradiation, was accurate, portable and readily available in most gynecological departments. Creighton and colleagues (1992) developed this further by using perineal ultrasound to quantify vaginal prolapse. They added simultaneous abdominal pressure measurement using a rectal catheter. The patient was sat upright in the lithotomy position, a Foley catheter was introduced to identify the bladder neck and the bladder was filled with 200 ml of saline. Ultrasound measurements were made using the inferior border of the symphysis as a fixed marker, at rest during Valsalva and during coughing. The outline and displacement of the bladder neck and bladder could be clearly seen and measured. Dynamic video screening showed forward rotational movement of the posterior wall and, in some patients, the rectocele appeared to compress the lower urethra when the intra-abdominal pressure was raised. This shows the interrelationships of pelvic floor movement and may explain the appearance of sphincter incompetence in previously continent patients after a successful rectocele repair.

In a more complicated study, Sanders et al (1993) used endovaginal, transrectal and perineal ultrasound to study patients with incontinence and anterior vaginal wall prolapse. Transrectal views were the most sensitive in visualizing the relationship of the urethra to the pubic symphysis and perineal views were the best when there was significant prolapse; endovaginal views were limited if there was urethral, vaginal or rectal prolapse.

To overcome the disadvantages of perineal, endovaginal and transrectal scanning, Koelbl and colleagues (1991) developed the technique of introital sonography, which is intermediate between perineal scanning and vaginosonography. It is carried out simultaneously with urodynamic studies. A standard front viewing vaginal scanner is applied to a small area in the introital region just behind the urethral orifice to scan the bladder, urethrovesical junction and urethra. The small transducer contact area does not interfere with urethral catheterization or voiding and the technique preserves all the advantages of perineal scanning.

MAGNETIC RESONANCE IMAGING

The greatest role of MRI in relation to the pelvic floor is the accurate visualization of different tissues and identification of anatomical completeness. Because it is noninvasive and nonionizing and has a multiplanar imaging capability, it is superior to both computed tomography (CT) and ultrasonography. Muscle can be separated from other tissues and its bulk and integrity clearly visualized and measured. It is not, however, possible to offer high quality moving images. It cannot directly measure function. Most images are made with the patient supine and therefore gravitational effects cannot be used to the best advantage. Some vertical fields, however, exist. Because of the magnetic field it is difficult to measure intra-abdominal pressures accurately.

Either transverse, coronal or sagittal sections can be made and a variety of different imaging conditions used to give different information about tissues. Klutke and colleagues (1990) were the first to use MRI to demonstrate the supportive role of the levator ani extending from the arcuate line of the obturator and fascia to below the urethra, vagina and rectum, uniting with it fibers from the opposite side. Medial extensions from the levator are inserted into the bladder neck and urethra, which support these structures and which seem elongated and even incomplete in women with stress incontinence (*Figure 23.7*). In contrast to this, Kirschner-Hermanns and colleagues (1993) examined 24 stress incontinent patients and six healthy volunteers. They showed that the urethra was not connected to the

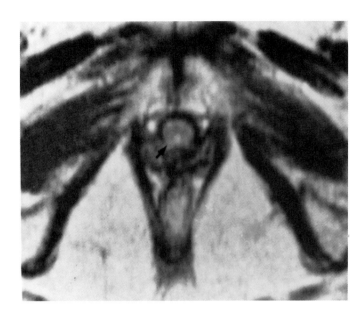

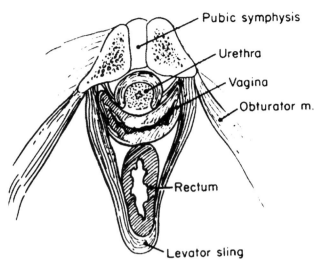

Figure 23.7: Axial magnetic resonance image at the level of the proximal urethra in a patient who had numerous unsuccessful operations for stress incontinence. The arrow shows a deficient area in the smooth muscle capsule surrounding the urethra. Reproduced with

permission from Klutke C, Golomb J, Barbaric Z & Raz S (1990) The anatomy of stress incontinence: magnetic resonance imaging of the female bladder neck and urethra. J Urol 143: 563–566.

levator ani nor fixed to deep perineal muscles. A clearly defined sphincter area was shown and the three layers of the urethra were delineated. Clear distinction of these structures were seen using intravenous GdDTPA (gadolinium diethylene triaminepentaacetic acid) as a contrast agent. Urethral smooth muscle took this up more avidly than the skeletal muscle so the plain MRI of the pelvic floor gave only poor delineation of these details; however, damage from perineal tears were clearly evident. They were able to show that patients with stress incontinence had replacement of muscle by fatty and connective tissue and it is likely that this would also apply to women with prolapse.

Further anatomical details of the levator ani have been presented by Strohbehn et al (1995), who used anatomical cross-sections from female cadavers correlated with multiplanar T_1- and T_2-weighted MRI images from the cadavers and from living patients. They showed the origin and continuity of pubococcygeus and its relationship with the other pelvic floor muscles, endopelvic fascia and external anal sphincter. An intraluminal coil was used in patients but significant distortion of the levator ani muscle was seen as a result of the supine position and interpretation was difficult.

Yang and colleagues (1991) studied 16 controls and 26 patients with stress incontinence and prolapse and took images during mild–maximum pelvic strain and during maximum perineal (levator) contraction. They demonstrated cystoceles, uterine and vault prolapse and rectoceles in patients with otherwise negative clinical findings. Fifteen patients had multicompartmental prolapse. The coefficient between test and retest in the three compartments varied between 0.94 and 0.99 at maximum strain. Straining in the supine position is not, however, the usual way to generate prolapse and may produce quite different results to that in the normal erect position. In addition, no information was given about their treatment results. No comment was made on the integrity of structures. They suggested that the role for dynamic MRI might be in patients with suspected enterocele or when multicompartmental prolapse was present, when there was allergy to contrast media or as a research tool to investigate the biomechanics of pelvic prolapse.

A different approach was taken by Christensen et al (1994) who imaged the change and displacement of the bladder during voluntary pelvic floor contractions in a group of volunteers taught to perform pelvic exercises, in order to identify specific muscle groups that were recruited during voluntary pelvic floor contraction. This enabled them to localize those muscles that failed to be recruited. This may have important implications in the causation of incontinence and prolapse as well as the responsiveness to physiotherapy.

Angulation of the vaginal canal has been the subject of anatomical dissection and radiological studies. MRI can demonstrate the topography of the vaginal canal and Ozasa and colleagues (1992) used sagittal T_1- and T_2-weighted MRI images on 14 patients with prolapse and 19 without. They showed that, in controls, the vagina assumed an angulated or curved shape, with its upper portion bent backward to ride over the levator plate. In patients with prolapse the backward angulation was often absent leading to a straight vagina, confirming the role of the levator in supporting the vagina and producing its angulation.

To determine the changes produced by a sacrocolpopexy to correct middle compartment (vault) prolapse, Monga and colleagues (1994) used a combination of multiplanar fast spoiled gradient echo sequences in the sagittal plane during a Valsalva maneuver and correlated these with preoperative and postoperative urodynamic studies. A sacrocolpopexy was performed and MRI sequences were repeated again. They were able to demonstrate and quantify the changes produced by the sacrocolpopexy in all three compartments. They demonstrated that vault, anterior and posterior compartmental prolapses were improved with upward movement of the anterior and posterior parts of the vagina (*Figure 23.8*).

There are now endocoils that can be inserted into the vagina or rectum and will give superior imaging, especially for the bladder neck and urethra. The biggest criticism of MRI is that it images anatomy rather than function. It is hoped that this can be overcome by using erect MRI, which is being evaluated in some centers. A technique needs to be designed to allow simultaneous intracavity pressure measurement with MRI to enhance its functional application.

SCINTIGRAPHIC DEFECOGRAPHY

Because of these disadvantages, the technique of scintigraphic defecography was developed to provide quantita-

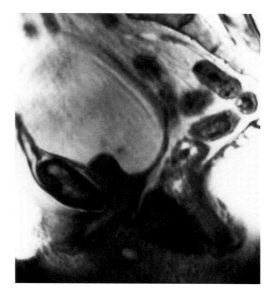

23.8a

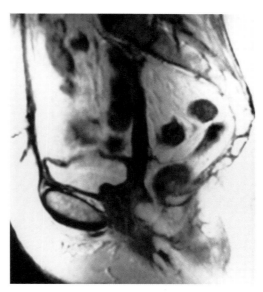

23.8b

Figure 23.8: *Magnetic resonance imaging on a 1.5 T GE Signa Advantage. Resting state images obtained using fast spin echo proton density T_2-weighted and T_1-weighted images in the sagittal plane. Dynamic fast scan images performed with a multiplanar fast spoiled gradient echo during a 15 s Valsalva maneuver. (a) A patient straining down with vault prolapse. (b) A postsacrocolpopexy study with the vault replaced within the pelvic cavity and supported by a Teflon mesh attached to the anterior longitudinal ligament of the first sacral vertebra.*

tive information on the rate and percentage of evacuation and on anatomical abnormalities (Hutchinson et al, 1993). The patient is given 200 ml of a ^{99m}Tc labeled stool, seated on a commode and then static and dynamic images at rest and during evacuation are taken by gamma camera. A line to represent the pelvic floor is drawn between the pubis and coccygeal markers and descent is measured as movement of rectal region of interest (ROI) perpendicular to this plane; it is considered significant if greater than 2 cm. A rectocele is identified by extending a vertical line upwards from the anterior border of the anal canal. Scintigraphic activity anterior to this line was lying within a rectocele and is significant if greater than 2 cm in the anteroposterior plane. The technique differentiates between patients with normal and slow emptying of rectal contents and the rate and extent of emptying from a rectocele (*Figure 23.9*). There are no particular problems associated with the test but it is still embarrassing for the patient and care must be taken to ensure that she is screened in pri-

vacy. A mean of 84 MBq of radioactivity is administered to each subject. Assuming 30% of radionuclide retention, the radiation dose of this technique is considerably less than 1 mSv.

■ CONCLUSION

There is renewed interest in pelvic floor prolapse. Clinical methods of staging are going to become more scientific and will require reliable and practical investigations as support. These should be neither overinvasive nor so artificial that their interpretation becomes suspect.

REFERENCES

Altringer W, Saclarides T, Dominguez J, Brubaker L & Smith S (1995) Four-contrast defecography: pelvic 'floor-oscopy'. *Dis Colon Rectum* **38**: 695–699.

Athanasiou S, Gleeson C, Anders K & Cardozo L (1995) Validation of the ICS proposed pelvic organ prolapse descriptive systems. *Neurourol Urodyn* **14**: 414–415.

Bartram C & Mayhew P (1992) Evacuation proctography and anal endosonography. In Henry H & Swash M (eds) *Coloproctology and the Pelvic Floor*, 2nd edn, pp 146–172. London: Butterworth–Heinemann.

Bates CP, Whiteside CG & Turner-Warwick RT (1970) Synchronous cine/pressure/flow cystourethrography with special reference to stress and urge incontinence. *Br J Urol* **43**: 714–717.

Bethoux A & Bory S (1962) Les mécanismes statiques visceraux pelviens chez la femme a la lumière de l'exploration fonctionnelle du dispositif en position debout. *Ann Chir* **16**: 887–916.

Christensen L, Dewhurst J, Lewis M, Yeh J & Constantinou C (1994) Dynamic 3-D MRI imaging of the pelvic floor. *Neurourol Urodyn* **13**: 354–356.

Creighton S, Pearce M & Stanton SL (1992) Perineal-videoultrasonography in the assessment of vaginal prolapse: early observations. *Br J Obstet Gynaecol* **99**: 310–313.

Enhorning G, Miller E & Hinman F (1964) Urethral closure studied with cineroentgenography and simultaneous bladder–urethra pressure recording. *Surg Gynecol Obstet* **118**: 507–516.

Gordon D, Pearce M, Norton P & Stanton SL (1989) Comparison of ultrasound and lateral chain urethrocystography in the determination of bladder neck descent. *Am J Obstet Gynecol* **160**: 182–185.

Grischke E, Anton H, Stolz W, Fournier D & Bastert G (1991) Urodynamic assessment and lateral urethrocystography. *Acta Obstet Gynecol Scand* **70**: 225–229.

Hutchinson R, Mostafa A, Grant E et al (1993) Scintigraphic defecography: quantitative and dynamic assessment of ano-rectal function. *Dis Colon Rectum* **36**: 1132–1138.

Kelvin F, Maglinte D, Bence J, Brubaker L & Smith C (1994) Dynamic cystoproctography: a technique for assessing disorders of the pelvic floor in women. *AJR* **163**: 368–370.

Kirschner-Hermanns R, Wein B, Niehaus F, Schafer W & Jakse G (1993) Contribution of magnetic resonance imaging of the pelvic floor to the understanding of urinary incontinence. *Br J Urol* **72**: 715–718.

Klutke C, Golomb J, Barbaric Z & Raz S (1990) The anatomy of stress incontinence: magnetic resonance imaging of the female bladder neck and urethra. *J Urol* **143**: 563–566.

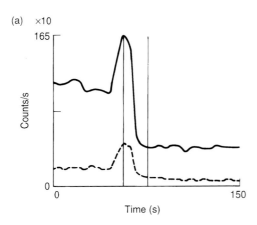

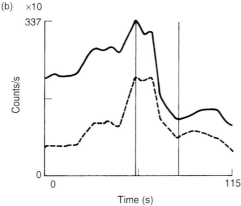

Figure 23.9: (a) *Scintigraphic defecography showing normal rectal emptying (top trace) at a normal rate (3.4%/s). Lower trace shows filling of rectocele that empties almost completely (8% of initial and 20% of final rectal contents).* (b) *Normal rate of rectal emptying (2.3%/s) and evacuation from rectum (top trace) in patient with a large rectocele (lower trace) that retains 28% of initial and 69% of rectal contents at the end of the study. Reproduced by kind permission of D Kumar, St George's Hospital, London.*

Koelbl H, Hanzal E, Bernasachek G (1991) Sonographic urethrocystography – methods and application in patients with genuine stress incontinence. *Int Urogynecol* **2**: 25–31.

Monga A, Heron C & Stanton SL (1994) How does sacrocolpopexy affect bladder function and pelvic floor anatomy? A combined urodynamic and MRI approach. *Neurourol Urodyn* **13**: 378–380.

Ozasa H, Mori T & Togashi K (1992) Study of uterine prolapse by magnetic resonance imaging. Topographical changes involving the levator ani muscle. *Gynecol Obstet Invest* **34**: 43–48.

Richmond D, Suthurst J & Brown MC (1986) Screening of the bladder base and urethra using linear array transrectal ultrasound scanning. *J Clin Ultrasound* **14**: 647-651.

Sanders R, Genadry R, Yang A & Mostwin J (1993) Transabdominal, transvaginal, translabial and transrectal sonographic techniques in the evaluation of stress incontinence. *Neurourol Urodyn* **12**: 304–305.

Schüssler B & Peschers U (1995) Standardisation of terminology of female genital prolapse according to the new ICS criteria: inter-examiner reproducibility. *Neurourol Urodyn* **14**: 437–438.

Stanton SL & Cardozo L (1979) A comparison of vaginal and suprapubic surgery and the correction of incontinence due to urethral sphincter incompetence. *Br J Urol* **51**: 497–499.

Strohbehn K, Ellis J, Strohbehn J & DeLancey J (1995) MRI of the levator ani muscle with anatomic correlation. *Proceedings of the American Urogynecologic Society: 16th Annual Scientific Meeting* October, Seattle.

Yang A, Mostwin J, Rosenshein N & Zerhouni E (1991) Pelvic floor in women: dynamic evaluation with fast MR imaging and cinematic display. *Radiology* **179**: 25–33.

24 Congenital and acquired Müllerian disorders
K Reese, S Reddy and J Rock

■ INTRODUCTION

Uterovaginal anomalies are relatively common congenital disorders, with a reported prevalence of 1–5% (Sorenson, 1988), the timely diagnosis of which is important yet frequently difficult. Associated anomalies are often found in these patients, with up to 40% having associated renal anomalies (Kenney et al, 1984). It has been noted that between 48 and 70% of patients with known urinary tract anomalies have concomitant uterovaginal anomalies (Fortune, 1927; Collins, 1932; Doroshow and Abehouse, 1961). The clinical signs and symptoms that bring these patients to medical attention relate primarily to their uterovaginal anomalies but may also be due to their associated renal anomalies. These presentations include external genital abnormalities, amenorrhea, pelvic mass and/or pain due to outlet obstruction, and, in women of childbearing age, more commonly infertility and obstetric difficulties.

This chapter discusses in detail the common presenting symptoms of genital tract anomalies, followed by a summary of the various imaging and endoscopic techniques available to delineate anomalous anatomy and formulate management plans. It includes a brief description of the problems caused by exposure of the Müllerian system to diethylstilbestrol, and offers a useful classification system that allows the user to describe uterovaginal anomalies based on embryological considerations.

■ CONGENITAL MÜLLERIAN ANOMALIES

THE DIFFERENT ANOMALIES AND THEIR SYMPTOMS

DYSGENESIS OF THE MÜLLERIAN DUCTS

The first type of anomaly results from dysplasia of the Müllerian ducts. This is often described as vaginal agenesis, congenital absence of the vagina or the Mayer–

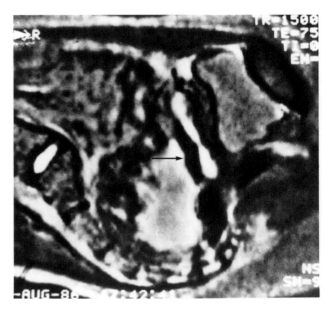

Figure 24.1: *Magnetic resonance T_1-weighted image showing atretic segment of distal cervix (arrow). No vagina is noted.*

Rokitansky–Küster–Hauser syndrome (MRKHS). Patients with MRKHS usually have normal external genitalia and a normal lower vagina but are lacking the middle and upper vagina. Instead of a normal uterus, two rudimentary primordia are present. These uterine primordia may or may not have a functioning endometrium. The Fallopian tubes are typically hypoplastic, but the ovaries and ovarian function are normal (Rock, 1986).

Patients with MRKHS are generally asymptomatic until they reach puberty and have not achieved menses (primary amenorrhea). Two other considerations in the differential diagnosis are imperforate hymen, which should present as a bulging hymen on physical examination, and androgen insensitivity syndrome, which includes absence of the female upper genital tract, blood testosterone elevated to the male range and a 46,XY karyotype. Patients with functioning endometrium in the uterine primordia may complain of cyclic pelvic pain (Rock, 1986) (*Figure 24.1*).

There is a high incidence of associated renal and, to a lesser extent, skeletal anomalies in patients with MRKHS. Patients with disorders of vertical fusion have a lower incidence of renal malformation.

DISORDERS OF VERTICAL FUSION

This developmental defect in embryogenesis involves imcomplete fusion between the downgrowing Müllerian ducts and the upgrowing portion of the urogenital sinus, which would become the vagina. The varied anomalies include transverse vaginal septum, either obstructed or nonobstructed, and may involve cervical dysgenesis or congenital absence of the cervix. (Imperforate hymen is not derived from the Müllerian tissue and will not be discussed in this chapter.)

The incidence of transverse vaginal septum ranges from 1/2000 to 1/7200, and is probably less common than MRKHS, which involves the congenital absence of both vagina and a fully formed uterus (Rock, 1992). Transverse vaginal septum is caused by incomplete vertical fusion, which may occur at any level of the vagina and may vary in thickness. Reported thickness ranges from a thin membrane to a thick atretic segment greater than half the length of the vagina. Rock et al (1982) have reported incidences of location of transverse vaginal septum as 46% in the upper vagina, 35% in the middle vagina and 19% in the lower vagina. Similar incidences were described by Lodi (1951). In general, the thicker vaginal septa are those located closer to the cervix (Rock, 1992). Transverse vaginal septum is associated with fewer urological or other concomitant anomalies than MRKHS. In the older female, diagnosis of an incomplete transverse vaginal septum is generally detected at first pelvic examination. Imaging is not usually indicated for this condition. These patients may have dyspareunia: surgery is only indicated to ease discomfort of coitus, or possibly to relieve potential dystocia in labor.

Uncommonly, in neonates and in young infants, obstructed transverse vaginal septum may lead to serious and life threatening conditions such as hydrocolpos and hydrometrocolpos, caused by the excessive intrauterine stimulation of the infant's cervical mucous glands by maternal estrogen, becoming cystic abdominal masses with resultant urinary and bowel obstruction.

In the adult female with a complete transverse vaginal septum or cervical dysgenesis, the presenting complaint is often that of cyclic abdominal pain and amenorrhea. (If a sinus tract is present, the patient may complain of spotting or a strong discharge odor; if a urethrovaginal tract is present, hematuria may be noted.) This is frequently manifested at puberty because, with the onset of menses, blood will accumulate and result in secondary distension of the vagina and/or uterus. It is important not to delay diagnosis, limiting the possibility of the development of endometriosis with retrograde menstruation due to the obstructed vaginal or cervical canal.

DISORDERS OF LATERAL FUSION

Total failure of lateral fusion may result in a complete duplication of the uterus, cervix and vagina. A partial lack of lateral fusion provides a spectrum of anomalies ranging from a single vagina with a single or double cervix (*Figure 24.2*) to a partial or complete duplication of the uterine fundus (*Figure 24.3*). When lateral fusion occurs but the midline point of fusion is not completely resorbed, a longitudinal septum is present. This septum may involve only part of the uterine fundus or may be complete and extend through the cervix and possibly involve the vagina. Furthermore, these varied disorders of lateral fusion may be obstructed or nonobstructed (Rock, 1992). Correct preoperative assessment of the

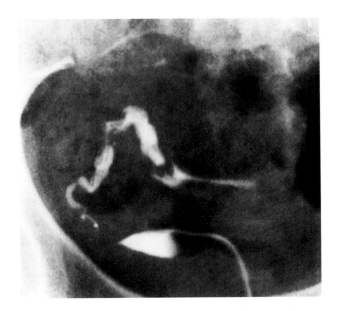

Figure 24.2: Hysterosalpingogram (in a patient with two cervices discovered on routine pelvic examination) shows one uterine horn.

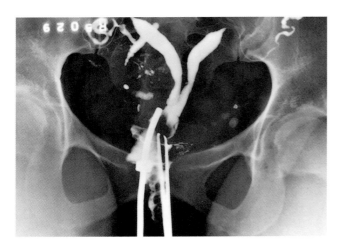

Figure 24.3: Hysterosalpingogram showing a uterus didelphys.

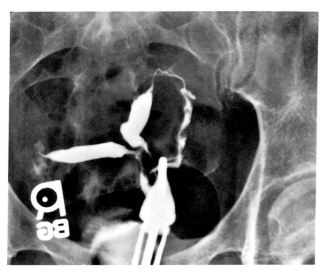

Figure 24.4: Hysterosalpingogram showing a uterus didelphys.

specific anatomical abnormality is imperative; for example, the septate uterus that has been shown to be a cause of recurrent miscarriage is best managed by hysteroscopic incision of the septum, whereas laparotomy and metroplasty is not commonly required for uterus didelphys or a bicornuate uterus.

The symptoms of a lateral fusion defect with unilateral obstruction of the uterine horn or with complete ipsilateral renal genesis will vary, depending on the uterovaginal relationships and the extent of the obstruction (Rock and Jones, 1980). Patients will have cyclic menses from the patent side and complaints ranging from persistent mucopurulent vaginal discharge to spotting to cyclic pelvic pain, and on examination are likely to exhibit findings consistent with a pelvic mass and endometriosis. Treatment will vary depending on the clinical setting

and ranges from excision of the obstructing longitudinal vaginal septum to excision of the obstructed uterine horn (Rock and Jones, 1980).

CLINICAL INVESTIGATIONS

The proper identification of the specific class and subtype of uterine and/or vaginal anomaly is necessary so that one can distinguish those anomalies that carry a high risk of fetal wastage and/or obstetric consequences, and therefore require surgical correction, from their less threatening counterparts. It is also imperative to separate those that can most appropriately be treated by a hysteroscopic approach from those best served by a transabdominal procedure. Advances in cross-sectional imaging modalities have become an aid to preoperative diagnosis. Traditionally the mainstays of diagnosis have included hysterosalpingography (HSG), laparoscopy and occasionally laparotomy, and more recently hysteroscopy.

HYSTEROSALPINOGRAPHY

HSG is best suited to identifying abnormalities of the internal configuration of the uterus; it cannot determine the external contour of the uterus and is therefore quite limited in classifying a particular type or subtype of Müllerian anomaly (*Figure 24.4*). HSG can only image cavities that are patent and communicating and so will miss obstructed, atretic or noncommunicating segments. Reuter et al (1992) reported only 55% success in distinguishing between a septate (*Figure 24.5*) and a bicornuate uterus (*Figure 24.6*). The other negative aspects of the use of HSG include the necessity of exposing the patient to contrast medium and ionizing radiation, in addition to its inability to define extraluminal anatomy. Although cross-sectional imaging techniques may help define external uterine anatomy, surgery (either laparoscopy or laparotomy) is usually needed to define pelvic anatomy completely.

GENITOGRAPHY

This is a more recent radiological technique and is best accomplished by placing the inflated balloon of a Foley catheter in the perineum, with the catheter tip in the vaginal orifice, to infuse contrast into the perineal orifices. It helps to define the anatomy of urogenital sinus-

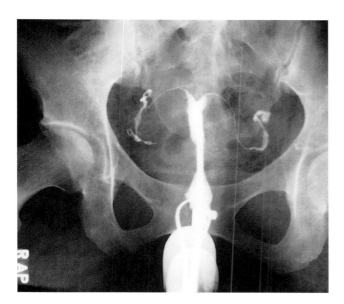

Figure 24.5: Hysterosalpingogram showing a septate uterus.

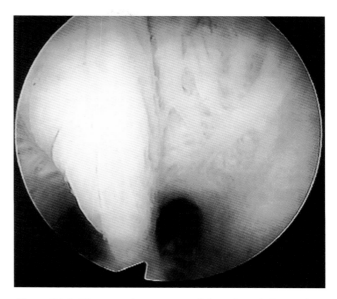

Figure 24.7: Hysteroscopic appearance of the endocervical extension of a complete septum in a septate uterus.

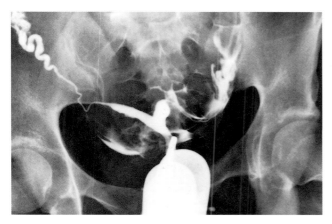

Figure 24.6: Hysterosalpingogram showing a bicornuate uterus.

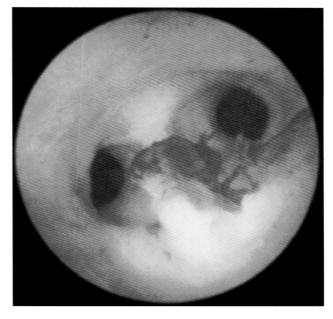

Figure 24.8: Hysteroscopic appearance of a uterine cavity with a partial septum in a septate uterus.

type anomalies and to identify any abnormal structures or communications. Genitography suffers from similar limitations and criticism as HSG (Shatzkes et al, 1991).

ENDOSCOPY/LAPAROTOMY

Once radiological studies have identified patients with Müllerian anomalies, further investigation is often needed to define accurately the patient's true anomaly. This can be accomplished by hysteroscopy and laparoscopy or explorative laparotomy. Operative hysteroscopy is a useful tool in the treatment of uterine septa, which are usually discovered by HSG or diagnostic hysteroscopy. Hysteroscopic diagnosis can also be performed as an adjunct to HSG to determine the exact

intrauterine architecture (*Figures 24.7–24.9*) and to exclude other intrauterine pathology that may simulate anomalies at HSG. Once an intrauterine defect is found, the external contour of the uterus must be examined to differentiate a septate uterus from a bicornuate uterus; as mentioned above, this can be done by laparoscopy (*Figures 24.10* and *24.11*) or occasionally laparotomy. Laparoscopy is most widely used for this purpose and is the initial procedure in these patients.

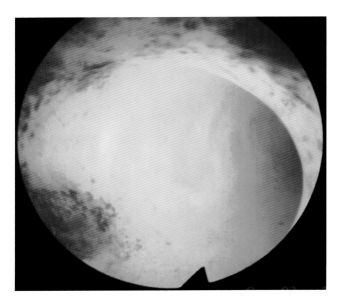

Figure 24.9: *Cornual area of a left unicornuate uterus at hysteroscopy.*

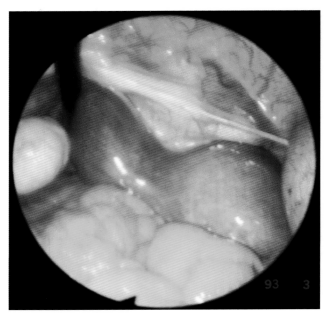

Figure 24.11: *Laparoscopic view of a bicornuate uterus; note the two separate uterine horns of which the right one is somewhat more developed than the left one, probably due to previous pregnancies.*

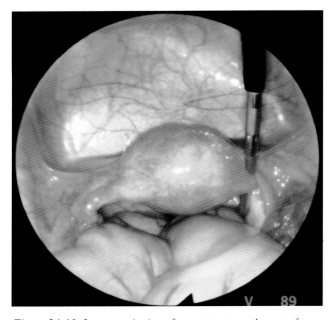

Figure 24.10: *Laparoscopic view of a septate uterus; the outer fundal area has a completely normal configuration.*

Laparotomy is the most invasive method for differentiation of the type of uterine anomaly and as far as possible should be avoided for diagnostic purposes alone. If the anomaly is nonobstructing, as in bicornuate uterus, no further surgical procedure is needed for diagnosis. Patients with visible endometriosis can be treated at the time of laparoscopy. In cases of noncommunicating anomalies laparotomy is usually required, either to create a patent reproductive tract or to remove rudimentary primordia that may rupture in pregnancy or, if they con-

tain functioning endometrium, become painful hematometra. In cases of cervical agenesis in which a functioning outflow tract cannot be maintained, a hysterectomy is indicated to prevent the sequelae of repeat obstruction (Rock et al, 1984). Women with an obstructed cervical canal but otherwise normal anatomy may benefit from a reconstructive procedure (Rock et al, 1995). Both laparoscopy and laparotomy are invasive, costly and carry the added risk of surgery and anesthesia, which has encouraged the search for less invasive methods of investigating the outer configuration of the uterus in cases of anomaly.

Newer modalities have included transabdominal, transvaginal and/or transperineal ultrasonography, hydrosonography, computed tomography (CT) and magnetic resonance imaging (MRI).

ULTRASONOGRAPHY

This technique does not employ ionizing radiation and is noninvasive. Unlike HSG and genitography, it is able to delineate reliably structures both within and external to the reproductive tract. Ultrasonography is particularly useful in delineating dilated, fluid filled structures that are typically found in patients with obstructed uterovaginal anomalies (*Figures 24.12* and *24.13*). It can also document the

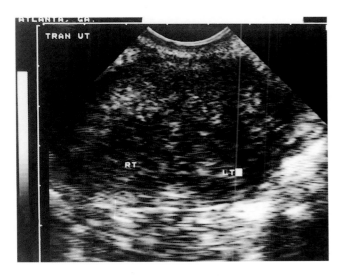

Figure 24.12: Sonographic image showing two uterine cavities.

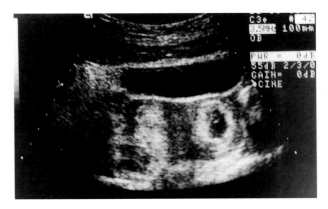

Figure 24.13: Sonographic image showing two uterine cavities, with a gestational sac in one cavity.

presence or absence of kidneys or malpositioning, such as a pelvic kidney. The sensitivity of ultrasound for identifying uterovaginal anomalies ranges from 42 to 87% (Dodson, 1991). This sensitivity is influenced by the examiner's knowledge of all possible uterovaginal anomalies, timing of the menstrual cycle (Reuter et al (1989) believe that the luteal phase ultrasound is a reliable predictor of bicornuate uterus), and the length of time from menarche for the development of hematocolpos and/or hematometra. The sensitivity of transvaginal ultrasonography as compared with endoscopy in evaluating uterovaginal anomalies has not yet been reported (Sabbagha et al, 1994). Transperineal ultrasonography has demonstrated reliability in delineating the length of obstructing segments in a transverse vaginal septum (Scanlan et al, 1990; Meyer et al, 1995). It has been used alone and in combination with transabdominal ultrasonography to delineate the level and extent of vaginal obstruction and the length of the vaginal septum, allowing appropriate planning and operative excision and reconstruction (Graham and Nelson, 1986; Scanlan et al, 1990; Meyer et al, 1995). In some cases, after ultrasound diagnosis of a high thick transverse septum, acute decompression of the hematocolpos via ultrasound guidance may be in order to prepare the patient properly for definitive surgery. The patient is then placed on endometrial suppression and begins vaginal dilation to enlarge the lower vaginal vault in order to facilitate the repair of the septum (Hurst and Rock, 1992). The goal of dilation is to maximize the amount of vaginal mucosa for anastomosis after septum resection.

HYDROSONOGRAPHY OR HYSTEROSALPINGOGRAPHY

This is the combination of sonography of the uterus with artificial distension of the uterine cavity. Studies have found it to be reliable for determining internal uterine architecture as well as myometrial configuration, such as in the case of septate versus bicornuate uterus, but not reliable for determining tubal patency (Van Roessel et al, 1987; Bonilla-Musoles et al, 1992). The addition of a 'water enema' with transabdominal ultrasonography apparently creates a 'sandwich effect', with fluid in both the bladder and rectosigmoid colon, resulting in a more complete definition of interposing structures (Rubin et al, 1978). This could be useful in evaluating the possibility of an obstructed hemivagina. Ultrasound has been found to be useful in the documentation of hematocolpos and/or the absence of a normal uterus in patients with Müllerian dysplasia. Hahn-Pedersen et al (1984) have demonstrated the use of a metal probe in the urethra and rectum to define hydrocolpos. Ultrasonography may demonstrate uterine primordia and the presence of normal ovaries, but it may be less useful in documenting the presence of functional endometrial tissue (Swayne et al, 1986; Rosenblatt et al, 1991; Strubbe et al, 1993). Kaminski et al (1994) presented a case in which transabdominal ultrasound imaging preoperatively suggested a hematocolpos, but at the time of surgery the patient had vaginal and cervical agenesis with a hematometra of the right uterine primordia and a pelvic endometrioma. Transperineal sonography documented the absence of a hematocolpos but could not identify the presence of the right

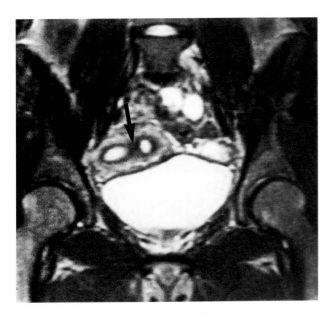

Figure 24.14: Magnetic resonance image shows two separate endometrial cavities separated by a small amount of myometrium (arrow).

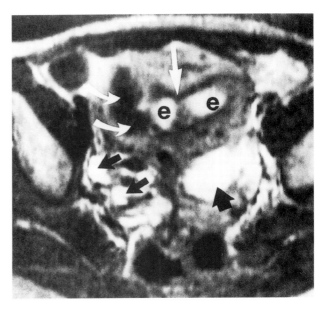

Figure 24.15: Axial magnetic resonance image of a patient with a septate uterus (septum indicated by straight white arrow) between two endometrial cavities (e); also note two intramural fibroids (curved white arrows) and extensive endometriosis in the cul-de-sac (black arrows).

hematometra. MRI would have more precisely identified findings that were confirmed at surgery.

COMPUTED TOMOGRAPHY

CT depends on tissue differences in X-ray attenuation: the attenuation coefficients of calcium, fat, water and air are quite different, so they are clearly separated. Unfortunately, soft tissues usually have only subtle density differences, therefore intravenous contrast is often necessary to improve the separation of normal and abnormal anatomy by differences in vascularity or vascular permeability (McCarthy, 1992). CT can image a number of minor and major renal anomalies adequately; it has insufficient contrast resolution to demonstrate tissue structure within the uterus. CT requires the use of intravenous contrast, with its risk of toxicity – as well as that of ionizing radiation. The limitation of CT to the axial plane alone is a disadvantage in the precise imaging of uterovaginal anomalies (Shatzkes et al, 1991).

MAGNETIC RESONANCE IMAGING

MRI relies on four tissue parameters: hydrogen content (in fat or water), T_1 and T_2 (tissue magnetic relaxation times) and blood flow (McCarthy, 1992). MRI uses no ionizing radiation, has the capability for multiplanar imaging, produces excellent soft tissue differentiation without the use of

contrast agents and is sufficiently sensitive for the diagnosis of thrombotic disease (Kay and Spritzer, 1995). It has been shown to be ideally suited for imaging uterovaginal anomalies because of its ability to differentiate the zonal anatomy of the uterus, cervix and vagina (Mintz et al, 1987; Fedele et al, 1989; Carrington et al, 1990; Doyle, 1992; Pellerito et al, 1992; Wagner and Woodward, 1994).

Two studies by Togashi et al (1987) and Hricak et al (1988) confirmed the accuracy of MRI for precisely imaging the presence or absence of a vagina, especially when utilizing T_2-weighted images optimized in a transverse plane and 5 mm thick sections (*Figure 24.1*). Additionally, MRI should be able to delineate uterine or vaginal septa, noncommunicating horns, hematocolpos, hematometra and cervical and vaginal anomalies (*Figures 24.14* and *24.15*) (Doyle, 1992). MRI has the ability to delineate accurately concomitant anomalies of the renal system. It is also useful in imaging even the most retroverted uteri, which have posed a challenge to ultrasonography. Markham et al (1987) showed that MRI can be used to distinguish between a high transverse vaginal septum and cervical agenesis. It can delineate myometrial tissue between two endometrial cavities. Despite its limitations, which include availability and expense, MRI has become routine in the preoperative evaluation of patients with Müllerian anomalies.

■ ACQUIRED MÜLLERIAN ANOMALIES

THE DES EXPOSED MÜLLERIAN SYSTEM

Diethylstilbestrol (DES) is a synthetic, nonsteroidal estrogen that is structurally similar to estradiol. It was prescribed to approximately 2–3 million women between the 1940s and 1971 because it was believed to be beneficial for treating a range of pregnancy complications, such as stillbirth, postmaturity, toxemia, premature labor and threatened or habitual abortion (Smith, 1948; Smith and Smith, 1949). By 1953, a controlled clinical trial failed to show DES to be beneficial as either a therapeutic or prophylactic agent in pregnancy (Ferguson, 1953). That same year, another paper reassessed an earlier study of DES in treating complications of pregnancy and found that DES exposure in pregnancy actually increased the frequency of stillbirth, premature delivery and spontaneous abortion (Brackbold and Berendes, 1978). Finally in 1971, the Food and Drug Administration (FDA) banned the use of DES in pregnancy following the published report of eight women who developed clear cell adenocarcinoma of the vagina after in utero exposure to DES (Federal Register, 1971). Since then, evidence has accumulated that in utero exposure to DES is also associated with specific anatomical abnormalities of the female genital tract and an increased incidence of infertility and adverse pregnancy outcome.

After the second month of gestation, the uterine stroma differentiates into two distinct compartments: one will become the endometrial stroma, the other the myometrium. It has been proposed that DES may affect the stroma primarily, but then secondarily induce abnormal epithelial changes, in light of evidence that the stroma in the female genital tract has specific inductive effects on the overlying epithelium (Cunha and Fujii, 1981). In the lower genital tract, adenosis, ectropion and squamous metaplasia are more commonly observed due to in utero exposure to DES. DES exposure between the 9th and 20th weeks of the pregnancy may prevent the segregation of the various mesenchymal layers of the uterus, thus causing the clinical conditions of stromal hyperplasia (ridges), hypoplasia (constriction) and an abnormally contoured uterine cavity.

CLINICAL INVESTIGATIONS

HSG has been the standard imaging modality for the assessment of the cervical canal, uterine cavity and tubal patency in infertile, DES exposed women. HSG studies have documented the following upper genital tract anomalies (listed in order of decreasing incidence): T-shaped uterus with a small cavity; T-shaped uterus; T-shaped uterus with a small cavity and constriction rings (Kaufman et al, 1980). HSG has typically shown normal Fallopian tube architecture, but a small surgical series reportedly found a higher percentage of short, distorted Fallopian tubes with pinpoint ostia. This would support the observation that DES exposed women have a higher frequency of ectopic pregnancies than non-DES exposed women (Stillman and Herschlag, 1987). Viscome et al (1980) utilized ultrasonography to document uterine hypoplasia in DES exposed women but were unable to image changes, such as constriction bands or T-shaped cavity, or Fallopian tube configuration. Specific studies reviewing the utility of hydrosonography are not currently available.

Hysteroscopy enables the exact determination of the intrauterine architecture. In typical cases a circular constriction just before the fundal area can be observed (*Figure 24.16*). The cornual areas extend laterally behind this structure and the tubal orifices will only be

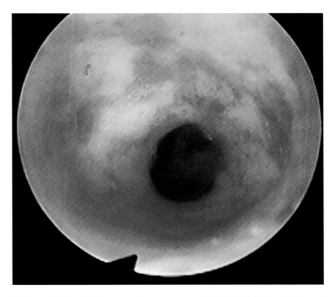

Figure 24.16: Hysteroscopic appearance of a diethylstilbestrol related uterine anomaly; a circular constriction can be observed just before the fundal area.

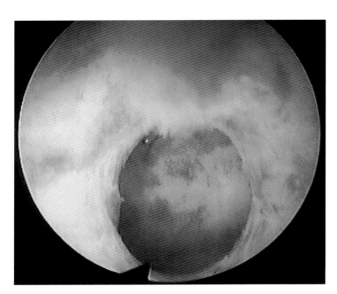

Figure 24.17: The fundal area of the uterine cavity of Figure 24.16. The hysteroscope is just passing through the constricted area; the cornual regions extend laterally and the fundal area shows an arcuate configuration.

visible as the hysteroscope tip passes through the constricted area. The fundal area may have an arcuate (*Figure 24.17*) or even subseptate configuration.

One prospective study of DES exposed women imaged by MRI found that they had a significantly shortened cervix when compared with normal controls. MRI has been used in nonpregnant women to predict cervical incompetence (Hricak et al, 1988). Edelman (1986) has observed that women in whom DES induced changes in vaginal epithelium are seen are 5.1 times more likely to exhibit upper genital tract changes than are unaffected DES exposed women. Similarly, if one notes DES induced cervical changes, then one is 4.5 times more likely to see uterine changes than in unaffected DES exposed women. Menstrual irregularities and oligomenorrhea are also increased in DES exposed women. Additionally, 51% of DES exposed women with an abnormal HSG were found to have a normal pregnancy outcome, as compared with 75% of DES exposed women with a normal HSG.

▪ INTERPRETATION OF FINDINGS

Müllerian anomalies pose diagnostic and therapeutic challenges. To achieve the best outcome the full extent of the anomaly, thus the patient's anatomy, must be known. Once a congenital Müllerian anomaly is defined, careful attention must be paid to the urinary tract because coexisting defects are common. Intravenous urography will show the ipsilateral renal agenesis that is seen on the ipsilateral aspect of the obstructing septum. An intravenous pyelogram will also identify other renal anomalies (pelvic kidney, absence of the ureter, etc.) found in patients with Müllerian anomalies. HSG still remains the gold standard for intrauterine anatomy. Its use is limited to patients with communicating Müllerian anomalies (Maneschi et al, 1991). Sonography has become an accepted modality for delineating the precise nature of the abnormal anatomical relationships in cases of uterus didelphys, obstructed hemivagina and ipsilateral renal agenesis (Chaim et al, 1992). Transabdominal and transvaginal ultrasonography combined with a concurrent water enema may also enhance imaging in cases of possible obstructed hemivagina (Rubin et al, 1978). Ultrasound has been utilized intraoperatively to guide drainage of the longitudinal septum (Sherer et al, 1994). The advances in cross-sectional imaging have added a new weapon to the armamentarium for the diagnosis of Müllerian anomalies. CT can demonstrate uterine and renal anomalies but cannot determine if the cystic contents are hemorrhagic; it does involve exposure to ionizing radiation. MRI can more precisely identify the various soft tissue structures of the uterus and the cervix, and can characterize the hemorrhagic lesions from cystic masses. MRI is also able to depict the renal system accurately. Despite the fact that ultrasonography is less expensive and is appropriate for the initial evaluation of patients, MRI can be most valuable in the presurgical assessment of complicated cases of unilaterally obstructed uterovaginal duplications without a hematocolpos involving cervical agenesis or a uterine horn (Hamlin et al, 1986).

▪ CLASSIFICATION

The current system of classification developed by The American Fertility Society (1988) (now known as the American Society for Reproductive Medicine) is based on the embryological development of the genital tract

The AFS Classification of Müllerian Anomalies

Patient's Name _____ Date _____ Chart# _____

Age _____ G _____ P _____ Sp Ab _____ VTP _____ Ectopic _____ Infertile Yes _____ No _____

Other Significant History (i.e. surgery, infection, etc.) _____

_____

HSG _____ Sonography _____ Photography _____ Laparoscopy _____ Laparotomy _____

EXAMPLES

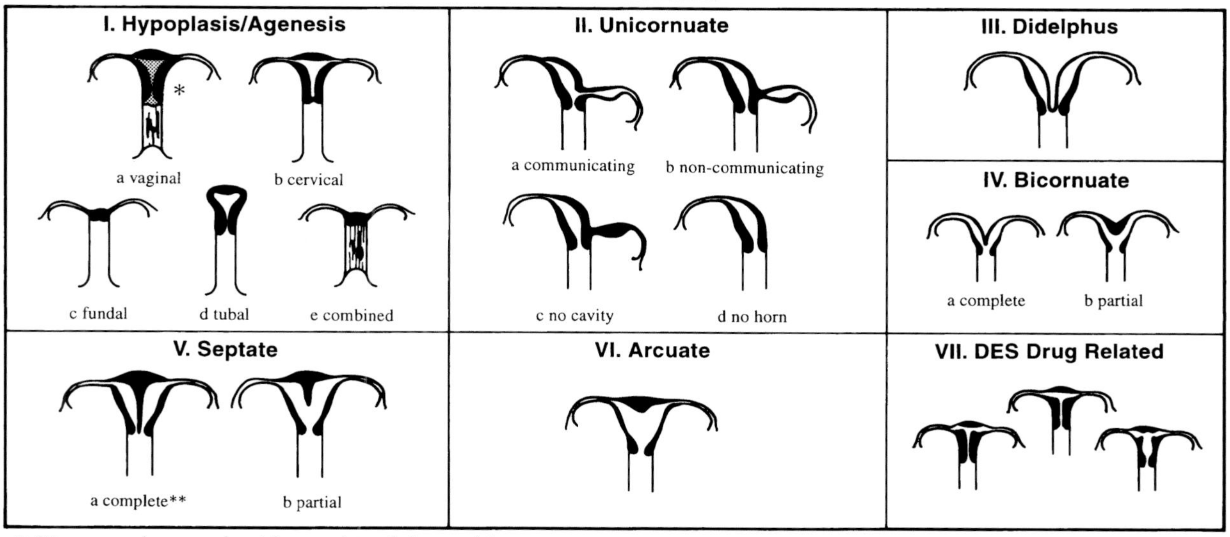

I. Hypoplasis/Agenesis
a vaginal   b cervical
c fundal   d tubal   e combined

II. Unicornuate
a communicating   b non-communicating
c no cavity   d no horn

III. Didelphus

IV. Bicornuate
a complete   b partial

V. Septate
a complete**   b partial

VI. Arcuate

VII. DES Drug Related

* Uterus may be normal or take a variety of abnormal forms.
** May have two distinct cervices

Type of Anomaly
Class I   _____   Class V   _____
Class II   _____   Class VI   _____
Class III   _____   Class VII _____
Class IV   _____

Treatment (Surgical Procedures): _____
_____
_____

Prognosis for Conception & Subsequent Viable Infant*

_____ Excellent   (> 75%)

_____ Good   (50 – 75%)

_____ Fair   (25 – 50%)

_____ Poor   (< 25%)
* Based upon physician's judgement.

Recommended Followup Treatment _____
_____
_____

Additional Findings: _____
_____
_____
Vagina: _____
Cervix: _____
Tubes: Right _____ Left _____
Kidneys: Right _____ Left _____

DRAWING

L   R

*Figure 24.18: The American Fertility Society classification of Müllerian anomalies. From The American Fertility Society (1988) The American Fertility Society classifications of adnexal adhesions, distal tubal occlusion, tubal occlusion secondary to tubal ligation, tubal pregnancies, Müllerian anomalies and intrauterine adhesions. Fertil Steril **49**: 944–955. Reproduced with permission of the publisher, the American Society for Reproductive Medicine (formerly The American Fertility Society).*

(*Figure 24.18*; see also Chapter 29). It allows clinicians to describe anomalies in a uniform and consistent manner. This will assure accurate interpretation of the diagnosis for patients and between colleagues.

REFERENCES

American Fertility Society (1988) The American Fertility Society classifications of adnexal adhesions, distal tubal occlusion, tubal occlusion seondary to tubal ligation, tubal pregnancies, Müllerian anomalies and intrauterine adhesions. *Fertil Steril* **49**: 944–955.

Bonilla-Musoles F, Simon C, Serra V, Sampaio M & Pellicer A (1992) An assessment of hysterosalpingography (HSSG) as a diagnostic tool for uterine cavity defects and tubal patency. *J Clin Ultrasound* **20**: 175–181.

Brackbold Y & Berendes HW (1978) Dangers of diethystilbestrol: review of a 1953 paper. *Lancet* **ii**: 520–525.

Carrington BM, Hricak H, Nuruddin RN, Secaf, Laros RK & Hill EC (1990) Müllerian duct anomalies: MR imaging evaluation. *Radiology* **176**: 715–720.

Chaim W, Kornmehl P, Koppernick G & Meizner I (1992) Uterus didelphys with unilateral imperforate vagina and ipsilateral renal agenesis: the challenge of noninvasive diagnosis. *J Clin Ultrasound* **19**: 583–587.

Collins DC (1932) Congenital unilateral renal agenesis. *Ann Surg* **95**: 715.

Cunha GR & Fujii H (1981) Stromal parenchymal interactions in normal and abnormal development of the genital tract. In Herbst AL & Bern HA (eds) *Developmental Effects of DES in Pregnancy*, pp 179–193. New York: Thieme-Stratton.

Dodson MG (1991) *Transvaginal Ultrasound*, Ch 5. New York: Churchill Livingstone.

Doroshow LW & Abehouse BS (1961) Congenital unilateral solitary kidney: report of 37 cases and a review of the literature. *Urol Survey* **11**: 219–224.

Doyle MB (1992) Magnetic resonance imaging in Müllerian fusion defects. *J Reprod Med* **37**: 33–38.

Edelman DA (1986) *Diethylstilbestrol – New Perspectives*, pp 77–78. Hingham, MA: Kluwer.

Fedele L, Dorta M, Brioschi D, Massari C & Candiani GB (1989) Magnetic resonance evaluation of double uteri. *Obstet Gynecol* **74**: 844–847.

Federal Register (1971) 36: 217.11/10/71. Washington DC.

Ferguson JH (1953) Effect of stilbestrol on pregnancy compared to the effect of a placebo. *Am J Obstet Gynecol* **65**: 592–595.

Fortune CH (1927) The pathological and clinical significance of congenital one-sided kidney defect, with presentation of three new cases of agenesis and one of aplasia. *Ann Intern Med* **1**: 377–380.

Graham D & Nelson MW (1986) Combined perineal–abdominal sonography in the evaluation of vaginal atresia. *J Clin Ultrasound* **14**: 735–738.

Hahn-Pedersen J, Kviat N & Nielson OH (1984) Hydrometrocolpos: current views on pathogenesis and management. *J Urol* **132**: 537–540.

Hamlin DJ, Pettersson H & Moazam F (1986) Magnetic resonance imaging of bicornuate uterus with unilateral hematometrosalpinx and ipsilateral renal agenesis. *Urol Radiol* **8**: 52–55.

Hricak H, Chang YCF & Thurnher S (1988) Vagina: evaluation with MR imaging. *Radiology* **169**: 1351–1353.

Hurst BS & Rock J (1992) Preoperative dilation to facilitate repair of the high transverse septum. *Fertil Steril* **57**: 1351–1353.

Kaminski PF, Meilstrup JW, Ekbladh LE, Shackelford DP & Thieme GA (1994) An unusual presentation of Rokitansky–Mayer–Küster–Hauser syndrome. *J Ultrasound Med* **13**: 911–915.

Kaufman RH, Binder AE & Gerthoffer GL (1980) Upper genital tract changes and pregnancy outcome in offspring exposed in utero to diethylstilbestrol. *Am J Obstet Gynecol* **137**: 299–308.

Kay HH & Spritzer CH (1995) Magnetic resonance imaging in gynecology. In Sciarra JJ (ed.) *Gynecology and Obstetrics*, 2nd edn, Vol 1, Ch 93, pp 1–19.

Kenney PJ, Spirit BA & Leesòn MD (1984) Genitourinary anomalies: radiologic anatomic correlations. *Radiographics* **4**: 233–236.

Lodi A (1951) Contributo clinico statistico sulle malformazion della vagina osservate nella clinica obstetrica e ginecologic di Milano dal 1906 al 1950. *Ann Ostet Ginecol Med Perinat* **73**: 1246–1248.

Maneschi M, Maneschi F & Incandela S (1991) The double uterus associated with an obstructed hemivagina: clinical management. *Adolesc Pediatr Gynecol* **4**: 206–210.

Markham SM, Parmley TH, Murphy AA, Huggins GR & Rock JA (1987) Cervical agenesis diagnosed by magnetic resonance imaging. *Fertil Steril* **48**: 143–145.

McCarthy S (1992) New imaging techniques in gynecology. In Thompson JP & Rock JA (eds) *TE Linde's Operative Gynecology*, 7th edn, pp 279–296.

Meyer WR, McCoy MC & Fritz MA (1995) Combined abdominal–perineal sonography to assist in diagnosis of transverse vaginal septum. *Obstet Gynecol* **85**: 882–884.

Mintz MC, Thickman DI, Gussman D & Kressel HY (1987) MR evaluation of uterine anomalies. *Am J Radiol* **148**: 287–290.

Pellerito JS, McCarthy SM, Doyle MB & Glickman MG (1992) Diagnosis of uterine anomalies: relative accuracy of MR imaging, endovaginal sonography, and hysterosalpingography. *Radiology* **183**: 795–800.

Reuter KL, Daly DC & Cohen SM (1989) Septate versus bicornuate uteri: errors in imaging diagnosis. *Radiology* **172**: 749–752.

Reuter KL, Young SB & Colby J (1992) Transperineal sonography in the assessment of urethral diverticulum. *J Clin Ultrasound* **20**: 221–223.

Rock JA (1986) Anomalous development of the vagina. *Semin Reprod Endocrinol* **4**: 13–31.

Rock JA (1992) Surgery for anomalies of the Müllerian ducts. In Thompson JD & Rock JA (eds) *TE Linde's Operative Gynecology*, 7th edn, pp 603–645. Philadelphia: JB Lippincott.

Rock JA & Jones HW Jr (1980) The double uterus associated with an obstructed hemivagina and ipsilateral agenesis. *Am J Obstet Gynecol* **138**: 339–342.

Rock JA, Zacur HA, Dlugi AM et al (1982) Pregnancy success following surgical correction of imperforate hymen and complete transverse vaginal septum. *Obstet Gynecol* **59**: 448–451.

Rock JA, Schlaff WD, Zacur HA & Jones HW Jr (1984) The clinical management of congenital absence of the uterine cervix. *Int J Gynecol Obstet* **22**: 231–235.

Rock JA, Carpenter SEC, Wheeless R & Jones HW Jr (1995) The clinical management of maldevelopment of the uterine cervix. *J Pelvic Surg* **1**: 129–133.

Rosenblatt M, Rosenblatt R, Coupy SM & Kleinhaus S (1991) Uterovaginal hypoplasia. *Pediatr Radiol* **21**: 536–537.

Rubin AC, Kurtz AB & Goldberg BB (1978) Water enema: a new ultrasound technique in defining pelvic anatomy. *J Clin Ultrasound* **6**: 28–33.

Sabbagha RE, Cohen LS & Crocker L (1994) Sonography of the uterus: vaginal approach. In Sabbagha RE (ed.) *Diagnostic Ultrasound Applied to Obstetrics and Gynecology*, 3rd edn, pp 627–653. Philadelphia: JB Lippincott.

Scanlan KA, Pozniak MA, Fagerholm M & Shapiro S (1990) Value of transperineal sonography in the assessment of vaginal atresia. *Am J Radiol* **154**: 545–548.

Shatzkes DR, Haller JO & Vecek FT (1991) Imaging of utervaginal anomalies in the pediatric patient. *Urol Radiol* **13**: 58–66.

Sherer DM, Rib DM, Nowell RM, Perillo AM & Phipps WR (1994) Sonographic-guided drainage of unilateral hematometrocolpos due to uterine didelphys and obstructed hemivagina associated with ipsilateral renal agenesis. *J Clin Ultrasound* **22**: 454–456.

Smith OW (1948) DES in the prevention and treatment of complications of pregnancy. *Am J Obstet Gynecol* **56**: 821–824.

Smith OW & Smith G (1949) The influence of DES on the progress and outcome of pregnancy based on a comparison of treated with untreated primigravidas. *Am J Obstet Gynecol* **58**: 994–997.

Sorensen SS (1988) Estimated prevalence of Müllerian anomalies. *Acta Obstet Gynecol Scand* **6**: 441–445.

Stillman RJ & Hershlag A (1987) Pathology of infertility and adverse pregnancy outcome after in utero exposure to diethylstilbestrol. In Gondos B & Riddick DH (eds) *Pathology of Infertility*, pp 41–55. New York: Thieme Medical.

Strubbe EH, Willemsen WNP, Lemmens JAM, Thijn CJP & Rolland R (1993) Mayer–Rokitansky–Küster–Hauser syndrome: distinction between two forms based on excretory urographic, sonographic, and laparoscopic findings. *Am J Radiol* **160**: 331–334.

Swayne LC, Rubenstein JB & Mitchell B (1986) The Mayer–Rokitansky–Küster–Hauser syndrome: sonographic aid to diagnosis. *J Ultrasound Med* **5**: 287–289.

Togashi K, Nishimura K, Itoh K et al (1987) Vaginal agenesis: classification by MR imaging. *Radiology* **162**: 675–677.

Van Roessel J, Wamsteker K & Exalto N (1987) Sonographic investigation of the uterus during artificial uterine cavity distention. *J Clin Ultrasound* **15**: 439–450.

Viscome GN, Gonzales R & Taylor KJW (1980) Ultrasound detection of uterine anomalies after DES exposure. *Radiology* **136**: 733–735.

Wagner BJ & Woodward PJ (1994) Magnetic resonance evaluation of congenital uterine anomalies. *Semin US CT MRI* **15**: 4–17.

25 Tubal infertility
I Brosens

■ INTRODUCTION

The outcome of tubal infertility has changed dramatically since the mid-1980s. Microsurgery in the 1970s and operative laparoscopy in the 1980s constituted major advances, and, more recently, the development of in vitro fertilization and embryo transfer (IVF-ET) has created the possibility of pregnancy for women in whom reconstructive surgery was contraindicated or associated with a low chance of pregnancy. Today reconstructive surgery should be offered to women with a good chance of pregnancy, while IVF-ET is the method of choice when the outcome of surgery is poor. The classical exploration of the pelvis by hysterosalpingography and laparoscopy has been the basis on which, for many years, the selection for reconstructive surgery was made. In recent years the direct exploration of the tubal mucosa by salpingoscopy and falloposcopy has provided a more accurate evaluation of the Fallopian tube and improved the selection of patients between reconstructive surgery and IVF-ET.

■ PATHOLOGY OF TUBAL INFERTILITY

Tubal infertility can be caused by different factors, particularly pelvic inflammatory disease, endometriosis and pelvic surgery (*Table 25.1*) and result from obstructive and nonobstructive lesions in the proximal and/or distal part of the Fallopian tube.

PROXIMAL (INTRAMURAL AND ISTHMIC) TUBAL ABNORMALITIES

There are a number of conditions affecting the intramural or isthmic segment that can cause obstructive and nonobstructive lesions. Proximal tubal blocks represent

Table 25.1 *Causes of tubal infertility*

- Pelvic inflammatory disease
- Endometriosis
- Pelvic surgery
- Previous ectopic pregnancy
- Puerperal sepsis
- Septic abortion
- Peritonitis, suppurative appendicitis
- Pelvic tuberculosis
- Adenomatoid tumor

approximately 20% of pathological tubal occlusions (Donnez, 1984). The most common of these are obliterative fibrosis, chronic tubal inflammation, salpingitis isthmica nodosa, endometriosis, tubocornual polyps, tuberculosis, the remnant of chronic tubal pregnancy and tubal sterilization.

Obliterative fibrosis is the most common cause of proximal occlusion and is thought to represent a nonspecific reaction to inflammation or injury of the interstitial or isthmic segments of the tube (Fortier and Haney, 1985). Scanning electron microscopy shows a completely closed lumen due to the replacement of the epithelium by fibrous connective tissue, while the tubal mucosa of the isthmic segment adjacent to the block may be normal or there may be formation of fibrous polyps (*Figure 25.1a*).

Chronic tubal inflammation can be seen in up to 40% of obstructed isthmic segments. The inflammation may involve all three layers, causing the epithelium to become atrophic, the submucosal layers dense and the myosalpinx thickened. The inflammatory lesions are confined to the proximal tube in mild infection but in severe infections there may also be distal involvement, producing agglutination of the ampullary folds and fimbriae and hydrosalpinx formation.

Salpingitis isthmica nodosa. The incidence varies according to populations from 0.5% in Caucasians to 11% in black Jamaicans. It is most frequently found in

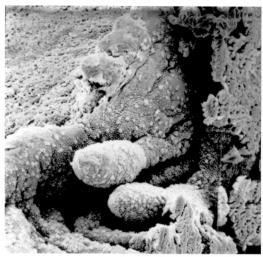

25.1a

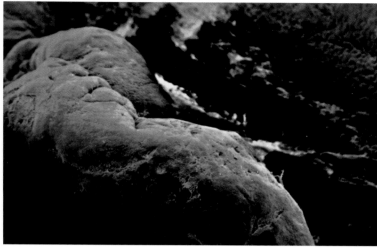

25.1b

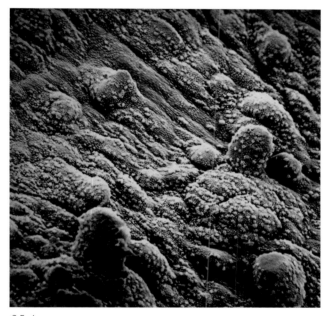

25.1c

Figure 25.1: *Scanning electron microscopy of tubal polyps.*
(a) Tubocornual block: polyps proximal to the block are covered by tubal ciliated cells (×200). (b) Tubocornual polyp showing an endometrial surface epithelium with absence of ciliated cells (×125). (c) Tubal sterilization: the mucosa of the isthmic segment is flattened and multiple small fibrous polyps are seen on the surface (×200).

which have a honeycomb appearance in cross-section. Histological examination reveals glandular formation lined with epithelium similar to that of normal tubal mucosa and surrounded by hyperplastic and hypertrophied smooth muscle fibers.

Endometriosis of the patent Fallopian tube is uncommon. Islands of endometrium are found in between 5.5% (Donnez, 1984) and 19% (Fortier and Haney, 1985) of proximal tubal obstruction.

Tubocornual polyps usually occur in the intramural position but rarely result in tubal occlusion and their association with infertility is debatable (*Figure 25.1b*).

Midtubal obstruction is commonly seen after tubal sterilization or resection of a tubal pregnancy and is rarely found in the unoperated patient after resorption of an ectopic pregnancy or as a segmental defect. Small polyps can be seen after sterilization in the proximal segment adjacent to a block (Vasquez et al, 1980) (*Figure 25.1c*).

DISTAL (AMPULLARY AND FIMBRIAL) TUBAL ABNORMALITIES

Lesions of the distal tube usually include peritubal adhesions and obstructive lesions, which can occur unilaterally but most frequently bilaterally. Obstructive lesions of the ampullary segment, the infundibulum and the fimbriae can be caused by serosal and mucosal adhesions. More exceptionally, obstruction of the distal end is caused by compression of the infundibulum (e.g. ovarian endometrioma) or congenital absence of the fimbriae.

women who have previously had an ectopic pregnancy. It is thought to be the sequel of nonspecific infection, gonorrhea or tuberculosis, but not all patients show evidence of an inflammatory reaction in the Fallopian tube and causes such as a congenital or developmental defect or an acquired form of diverticulosis caused by chronic spasm have been suggested.

The wall of the isthmus is thickened with one or more, white-brown nodules up to 2 cm in diameter,

Histopathologically, the *hydrosalpinx* is distinguished into thick walled and thin walled. In the thick walled hydrosalpinx the wall has a thickness of 10–15 mm and the folds are agglutinated, giving the mucosa a 'honeycomb' appearance due to the numerous pseudoglandular spaces, or thickened with extreme fibrosis and resulting in a rigid tube (*Figure 25.2a,b*). In the thin walled hydrosalpinx the mucosal surface is flattened and the folds are often far apart or show mucosal adhesions, giving the ampullary lumen a web-like appearance in severe cases. The surface shows deciliation and areas of desquamation (*Figure 25.2c,d*).

Genital tuberculosis affects primarily the tubal mucosa of the ampullary segment and causes constrictions of the proximal segment, resulting in a characteristic appearance at hysterosalpingography. The mucosa is affected but caseating granulomas may extend into the myosalpinx, resulting in stenosis and calcification of the tubal wall. The healing of tuberculosis results in a totally

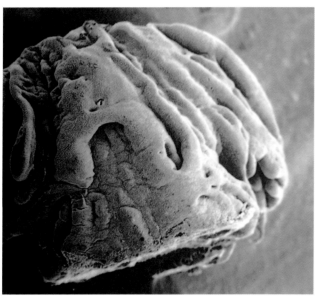

25.2a

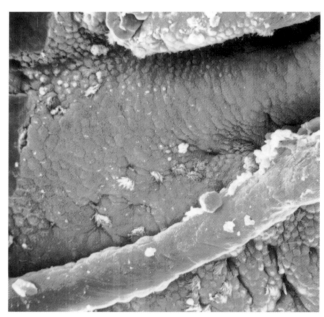

25.2c

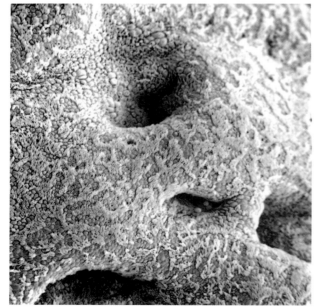

25.2b

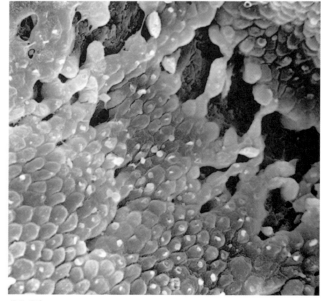

25.2d

Figure 25.2: *Scanning electron microscopy of hydrosalpinx. Thick walled hydrosalpinx: the mucosa of the thick walled hydrosalpinx shows thick adhesions (a) (×26) and has a pseudoglandular,* adenomatous appearance (b) (×250). Thin walled hydrosalpinx: the flattened and deciliated surface (c) (×550) and areas of desquamation (d) (×200) are seen.

obliterated tubal lumen or scarring of the endosalpinx with marked decreased fertility. Indeed, term pregnancies after medical or conservative surgical treatment are extremely uncommon and, if pregnancy occurs, there is a high risk of tubal implantation.

Nonobstructive abnormalities of the distal segment include the tortuous tube and congenital abnormalities. The *tortuous tube* represents segmental dilatations, which may give the appearance of a hydrosalpinx when contrast medium or dye is injected. The abdominal ostium is, however, patent, but the fimbria ovarica is frequently elongated, sometimes being more than 4 cm in length. The abnormality was studied by Moore-White (1960) who obtained histological evidence of aplasia of the myosalpinx. Convoluted tubes are compatible with fertility. *Accessory tubes* are small, nonpatent cylindrical structures attached to the ampulla of a normal sized tube. At their distal end there is a small fimbria-like structure lined with ciliated epithelium. Ectopic pregnancies have been described as occurring in these structures (Beyth and Kopolovic, 1982) and therefore whenever these structures are encountered, particularly in infertile women, they should be removed. *Accessory ostia* are always located in the antimesenteric border of the ampullary segment of the Fallopian tube but their incidence is not known. It is very doubtful that this anomaly plays a role of any significance in infertility.

■ CLINICAL INVESTIGATIONS

The techniques that are currently employed for the investigation and diagnosis of tubal infertility include hysterosalpingography and laparoscopy. Both techniques are used to investigate tubal patency, but in addition yield data on the tubal morphology and tubo-ovarian relationship. Recently, hysteroscopy, salpingoscopy and falloposcopy have been added as tools for the clinical investigation of tubal infertility.

It is the usual practice to perform hysterosalpingography first, before proceeding to laparoscopy, unless the former procedure is contraindicated; however, in patients with a high risk factor for tubal disease, e.g. history of pelvic inflammatory disease or an elevated level of chlamydial antibodies, the use of endoscopy early in the investigation may be preferred.

PROXIMAL TUBAL BLOCK

Proximal tubal block is detected by hysterosalpingography when contrast medium fails to enter the Fallopian tube unilaterally or bilaterally. The absence of tubal filling is frequently not, however, pathological and can be due to myometrial spasm, particularly where there is only unilateral filling of the tubes. A uterine spasm is less likely when the intramural segment is partially or totally outlined. In the presence of a cornual block it is important to assess the intramural segment (*Figure 25.3*).

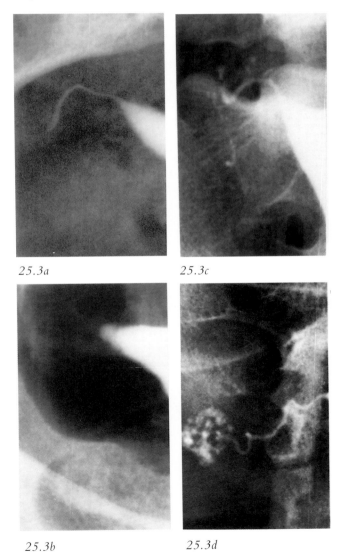

25.3a   25.3c

25.3b   25.3d

Figure 25.3: Appearances of proximal tubal block on hysterosalpingogram: (a) with filling of intramural segment; (b) without filling of intramural segment; (c) with intramural spicules; (d) with nodular spicules. Courtesy of Professor J Donnez.

The problem of whether or not there is true unilateral or bilateral obstruction can be resolved at subsequent laparoscopy when a higher intrauterine pressure can be given under general anesthesia, or, in the case of unilateral block, the patent tube can be occluded by a probe or the uterine spasm can be relieved by an intravenous bolus injection of glucagon. Hysteroscopy, and more specifically selective salpingography and falloposcopy, are new techniques that may provide decisive information about the presence and extent of the obstruction and distal tubal lesions. For a discussion of these techniques the reader is referred to Chapters 5, 11 and 12. In the presence of a true persisting block, laparoscopy and transabdominal salpingoscopy are the appropriate techniques for the exclusion of bipolar lesions (*Figures 25.4* and *25.5*).

DISTAL LESIONS

Sequelae of pelvic inflammatory disease are seen most commonly at the terminal end of the ampullary segment and are distinguished into peritubal adhesions, phimosis (partial occlusion) and hydrosalpinx (complete occlusion). Such lesions are usually bilateral but may be unilateral and of a different degree.

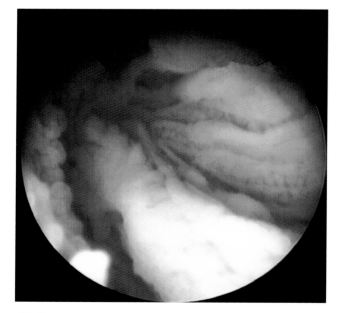

25.4a

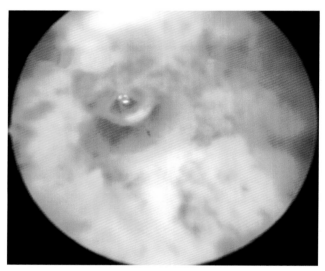

25.4c

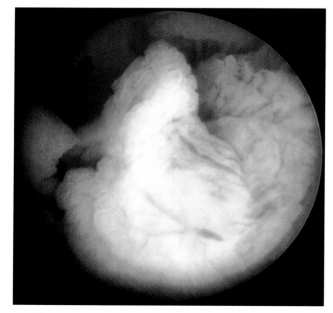

25.4b

25.4d

Figure 25.4: *Endoscopic exploration of bilateral tubocornual block. On the left side: (a) hysteroscopy shows small polyps in the cornu; (b) at salpingoscopy the ampullary mucosa appears normal.*

On the right side: (c) persistence of air bubble in the cornu; (d) at salpingoscopy ampullary mucosal folds are normal.

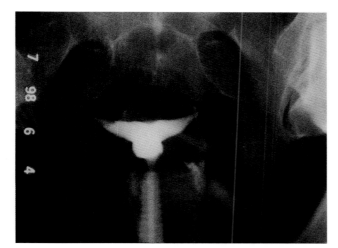

25.5a

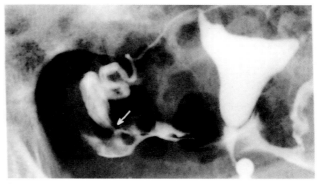

25.6a

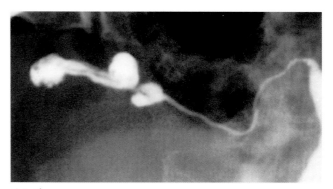

25.6b

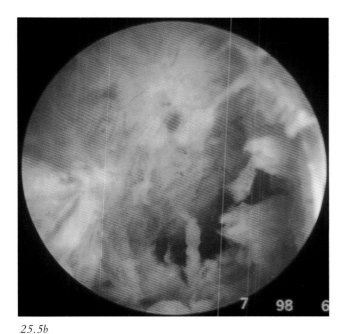

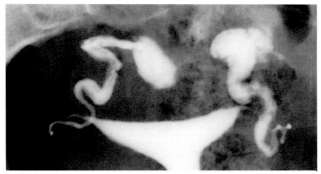

25.6c

25.5b

Figure 25.5: *(a) Bilateral tubocornual block at hysterosalping-ography, with (b) complete destruction of the ampullary folds at salpingoscopy.*

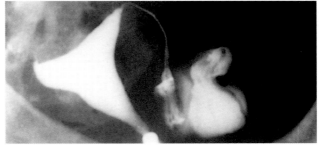

25.6d

Figure 25.6: *Distal tube lesions at hysterosalpingography.*
(a) Filiform peritoneal spilling (arrow) suggests phimosis.
(b) Hydrosalpinx: the regular outline of the ampullary mucosa by the contrast medium suggests preservation of mucosal folds. (c) Bilateral hydrosalpinx with irregular and rigid outline of the ampullary mucosa suggesting thick walled hydrosalpinx. (d) Sactosalpinx. Courtesy of Professor J Donnez.

The patency of the distal tubal end is evaluated on hysterosalpingography by the presence of spillage of the contrast medium (*Figure 25.6*). In cases of complete obstruction there is no spillage of contrast medium and a varying degree of ampullary dilatation on hyster-osalpingography. The diameter can be defined when the tube is distended maximally by the contrast medium. Lesions of the mucosal folds in the ampullary segment may be suspected on the well performed hysterosalpingogram, but the presence and extent of mucosal adhesions are underdiagnosed by this technique (Henry-Suchet et al, 1985; Puttemans et al, 1987).

At laparoscopy the patency of the distal tubal segment is demonstrated by inspection of the fimbriae and the dye test. The degree of distension of the ampulla in the prefimbrial region and the peritoneal spilling are assessed (*Figure 25.7*). Often the obstruction is incomplete or there are peritubal adhesions causing the dye to become loculated, in which case there may be no dilatation of the ampulla. In hydrosalpinx there is complete occlusion of the terminal portion of the Fallopian tube and a variable degree of distension. The thickness and rigidity of the tubal wall are assessed to distinguish between the thin walled and the thick walled hydrosalpinx.

TUBAL MUCOSAL ADHESIONS

Salpingoscopy allows the direct and accurate evaluation of the presence and extent of mucosal adhesions or fibrosis in the ampullary segment (*Figure 25.8*). Adhesions of the ampullary folds occur in 57% of the postinflammatory hydrosalpinges, in 22% of postinflammatory pelvic adhesions and rarely in endometriosis (Brosens, 1996). Serosal adhesions therefore occur more frequently than mucosal adhesions in pelvic inflammatory disease (PID), and in addition there is a poor correlation in severity between them (Vasquez et al, 1995a; Heylen et al, 1996). Laparoscopy therefore tends to overestimate the presence and extent of mucosal adhesions. External inspection of the fimbriae is also discordant with salpingoscopy in PID in approximately one third of cases (Henry-Suchet et al, 1985; Shapiro et al, 1988). Marana et al (1995) have shown that the pregnancy outcome correlates better with the assessment of the tubal mucosal adhesions than with the American Fertility Society classification of pelvic adhesions.

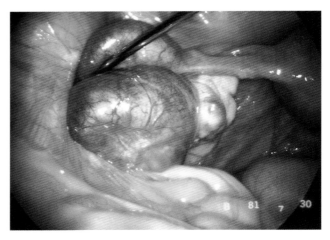

Figure 25.7: Thin walled hydrosalpinx distended by methylene blue. The diameter of the hydrosalpinx can be measured.

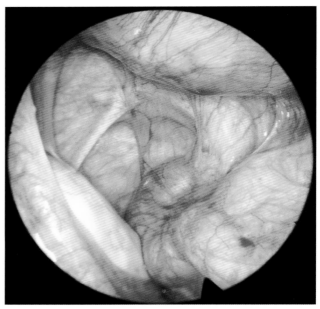

25.8a

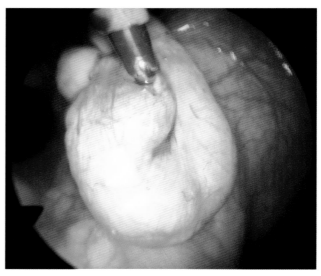

25.8b

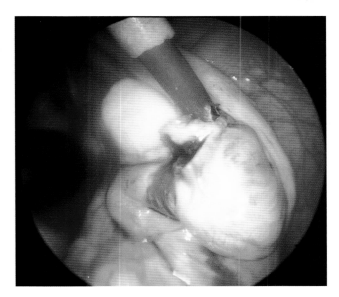

25.8c

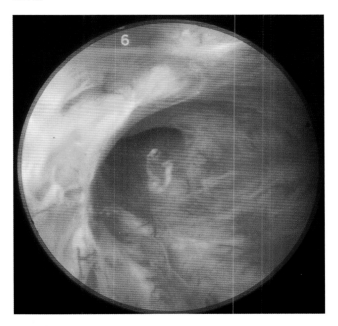

25.8d

Figure 25.8: *Salpingoscopy of the hydrosalpinx: (a) pelvic adhesions with fixation of right hydrosalpinx in the pouch of Douglas; (b) the right hydrosalpinx is mobilized after adhesiolysis; (c) a small incision is made at the terminal end and spilling of methylene blue confirms patency; (d) salpingoscopy shows complete fibrosis of the mucosa, confirming the presence of a thick walled hydrosalpinx.*

SALPINGITIS ISTHMICA NODOSA

In salpingitis isthmica nodosa the radiographic picture usually shows passage of contrast medium or obstruction of the proximal segment with some evidence of branch-

ing channels radiating from the main lumen into the mesosalpinx (*Figure 25.9*). At laparoscopy the isthmic segment appears thickened (*Figure 25.10*) and injection of dye may also lead to serosal staining of the thickened segment. In contrast, lymphatic or vascular intravasation of dye also leads to serosal staining, which is more generalized and involves the uterine fundus (*Figure 25.11*). At salpingoscopy the ampullary mucosa has been found to be normal in 80% of cases (Gürgan et al, 1994).

TUBAL ENDOMETRIOSIS

The radiographic picture of endometriosis is not specific and can result in single obstruction to the passage of the contrast medium or an image similar to that of salpingitis isthmica nodosa, although the punctate pattern may be more pronounced and larger.

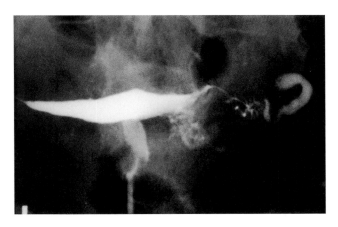

Figure 25.9: *Salpingitis isthmica nodosa: focal lesion in the isthmic segment and abnormal ampullary segment.*

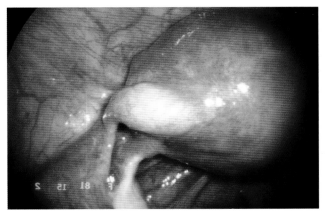

Figure 25.10: *Proximal tubal block. Nodular thickening at the site of the block suggests salpingitis isthmica nodosa.*

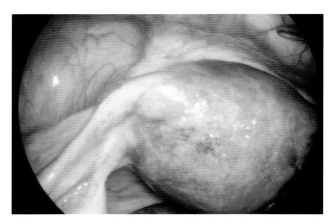

Figure 25.11: Proximal tubal block with intravasation of the myometrial vessels at methylene blue test.

GENITAL TUBERCULOSIS

Genital tuberculosis is usually associated with typical radiological images (*Figure 25.12a,b*):

- most frequently that of a golf-club or tobacco-pouch appearance; usually only the isthmus and proximal ampulla are seen and the isthmic segment has a rigid, irregular appearance;

- beaded appearance: the tube shows alternating segments of stenosis and dilatation;

- the Maltese cross appearance: the tube is rigid and irregular and terminates in the form of a Maltese cross, often surrounded by a halo.

At laparoscopy the fimbriae may appear normal and severe mucosal adhesions may be found at salpingoscopy (*Figure 25.12c*) (Marconi et al, 1992).

UNEXPLAINED INFERTILITY

Unexplained infertility is a diagnosis based on the exclusion of significant pathology after full exploration; however, significant tubal pathology can remain undiagnosed in certain circumstances. Pelvic adhesions, particularly ovarian and fimbrial adhesions, remain undiagnosed by hysterosalpingography. Filmy ovarian and fimbrial adhesions can be missed at laparoscopy when the inspection is made without hydroflotation of the pelvic organs (Nezhat et al, 1995). In 5% of patients with unexplained infertility tubal mucosal adhesions are found at salpingoscopy (Heylen et al, 1995).

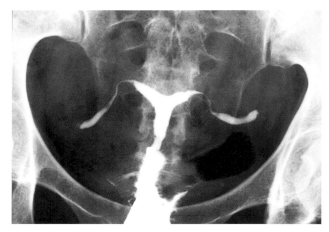

25.12a

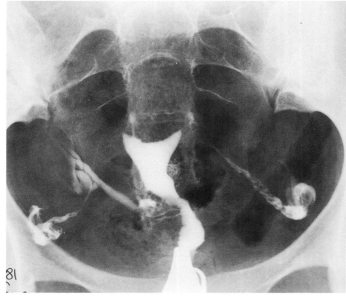

25.12b

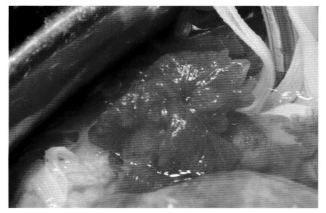

25.12c

Figure 25.12: Tubal tuberculosis: (a) bilateral partial filling and rigid appearance of the ampullary segment; (b) irregular outline of isthmic segment and distended ampullary segment with distal block; (c) the fimbriae are preserved but swollen and agglutinated at the level of the infundibulum.

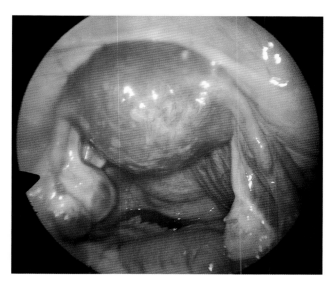

Figure 25.13: Tubal sterilization performed by bilateral ampullectomy eliminates repair.

TUBAL STERILIZATION

For reversal of tubal sterilization the site of tubal sterilization and the remaining length of the Fallopian tube are evaluated by hysterosalpingography and laparoscopy. Silicone rubber bands and spring clips are usually applied on the isthmic segment and result in a loss of 0.5–2 cm of tubal segment. Surgical ligatures and electrosurgery may eliminate a larger segment and before reanastomosis is attempted the site of the sterilization and the length of the remaining tube are assessed (*Figure 25.13*).

OTHER TUBAL ABNORMALITIES

Other tubal abnormalities found at hysterosalpingography and laparoscopy include the tubocornual polyps (*Figure 25.14*), the tortuous tube, accessory ostium, accessory tubes, fimbrial and peritubal cysts and the extrapelvic location of a solitary tube.

■ CLASSIFICATION AND PREGNANCY OUTCOME

PELVIC INFLAMMATORY DISEASE

PROXIMAL TUBAL LESIONS

Proximal tubal lesions can be classified as occlusive and nonocclusive lesions. The proximal blocks with wall abnor-

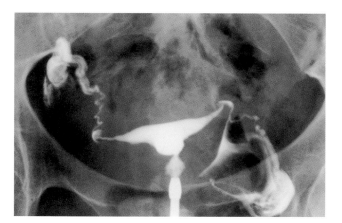

Figure 25.14: Bilateral tubocornual polyps giving an umbrella-like appearance of the tubocornual junction on the hysterosalpingogram and normal patency of both Fallopian tubes.

malities and/or associated distal tubal lesions have a poor pregnancy outcome after reconstructive surgery (*Table 25.2*).

DISTAL TUBAL LESIONS

Distal tubal lesions are classified as nonocclusive and occlusive lesions. Classically four different types of distal occlusion are distinguished:

■ patent tubes with conglutination or phimosis of the fimbrial folds;

■ complete distal occlusion, but the diameter of the ampulla remains normal (less than 15 mm);

■ complete distal occlusion with the ampulla dilated to a diameter of 15–25 mm;

■ complete distal occlusion with the ampulla distended to a diameter of more than 25 mm.

Reconstructive surgery of distal tubal lesions is classified as *salpingolysis* for resection of adhesions reducing the mobility of patent tubes, *fimbrioplasty* for resection of adhesions covering the fimbriae and *salpingoneostomy* for restoring patency of the complete occlusion of the distal tubal segment.

MUCOSAL ADHESIONS

Recent retrospective and prospective studies evaluating the tubal mucosa have shown that the pregnancy outcome is largely determined by the quality of the tubal mucosa (Boer-Meisel et al, 1986; De Bruyne et al, 1989; Dubuisson et al, 1994; Heylen et al, 1995; Vasquez et al, 1995b). Salpingoscopy has led to the recognition of the

Table 25.2 *Pregnancy outcome after anastomosis according to the radiographic picture of the proximal tubal block*

Radiographic picture of proximal tubal block	n	Permeability (%)	Intrauterine pregnancy (%)
No intramural filling	6	83	33
Intramural filling with tapering contrast	38	97	50
Block with branching spicules	7	57	14
Block with nodular spicules	3	33	0

Courtesy of Profesor J Donnez

following five different mucosal fold patterns or stages.

  I   Normal mucosal folds.

  II The major and minor folds are preserved but are wider apart than normal and there is a variable degree of flattening (*Figure 25.15*).

  III The major and minor folds are preserved but there are focal lesions of agglutination or adhesions (more than 50% of the folds are unaffected) (*Figure 25.16*).

  IV Extensive adhesions between more than 50% of the folds (*Figure 25.17*).

  V The pattern of folds is completely lost by fibrosis of the folds and wall (*Figure 25.18*).

Approximately 40% of patients with hydrosalpinx are without ampullary adhesions and in this group salpingo-neostomy results in a 60% intrauterine pregnancy rate

and a 5% tubal pregnancy rate (De Bruyne et al, 1989; Marana et al, 1995).

Focal mucosal adhesions are associated with a decreased intrauterine pregnancy rate and an increased tubal pregnancy rate, giving a ratio of approximately 2:1.

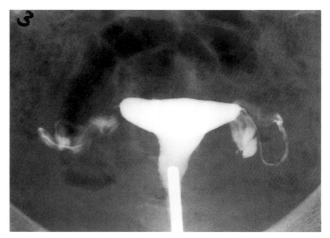

25.16a

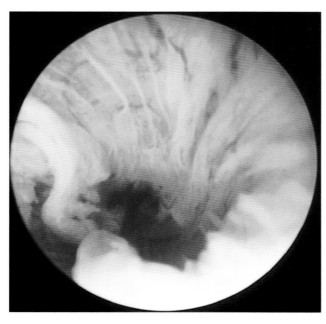

Figure 25.15: *Thin walled hydrosalpinx: salpingoscopy shows distension and flattening of the folds but absence of adhesions and inflammation (hydrosalpinx simplex; stage II of the salpingoscopy classification).*

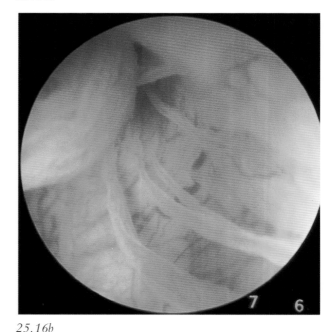

25.16b

Figure 25.16: *(a)–(c) Thin walled hydrosalpinx*

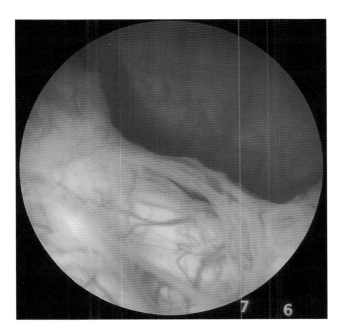

25.16c

Figure 25.16: *(cont.) Thin walled hydrosalpinx. (a) The hysterosalpingogram shows normal outline of tubal mucosa. At salpingoscopy (b) the mucosal folds are preserved but (c) focal adhesions are detected (stage III of the salpingoscopy classification).*

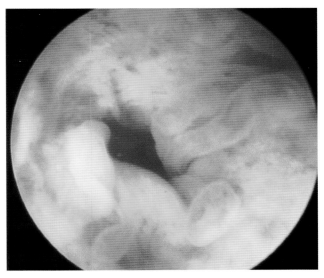

Figure 25.18: *Hydrosalpinx: complete loss and fibrosis of the mucosal folds at salpingoscopy (thick walled hydrosalpinx with adenomatous appearance of mucosa; stage V of the salpingoscopy classification).*

the presence of inflammatory changes (*Figure 25.19*) are absolute contraindications for reconstructive surgery.

TUBAL STERILIZATION

The prognosis of tubal reanastomosis is largely dependent on the length of the remaining tubal segment. A minimum length of 4 cm of tube seems to be necessary

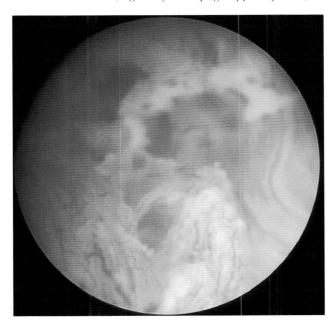

Figure 25.17: *Hydrosalpinx: multiple adhesions between folds at salpingoscopy (hydrosalpinx follicularis; stage IV of the salpingoscopy classification).*

In the presence of extensive adhesions, if the occasional pregnancy occurs, it is likely to be ectopic. When mucosal adhesions are identified in the ampullary segment the preferred treatment is IVF-ET. Extensive mucosal adhesions and fibrosis of the tubal wall or

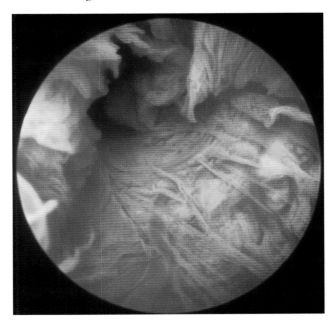

Figure 25.19: *Salpingoscopy shows a hydrosalpinx with distended folds and inflammatory changes of the mucosa.*

for reasonable expectation of pregnancy (Rouzi et al, 1995). No correlation is found between the success of microsurgical reversal and poststerilization isthmic abnormalities such as polyps or distension (Vasquez et al, 1980).

REFERENCES

Beyth Y & Kopolovic J (1982) Accessory tubes: a possible contributory factor in fertility. *Fertil Steril* **38**: 382–383.

Boer-Meisel ME, Te Velde ER, Habbema JDF & Kardaum JWPF (1986) Predicting the pregnancy outcome in patients treated for hydrosalpinx: a prospective study. *Fertil Steril* **45**: 23–29.

Brosens I (1996) The value of salpingoscopy in tubal infertility. *Reprod Med Rev* **5**: 1–11.

De Bruyne F, Puttemans P, Boeckx W & Brosens I (1989) The clinical value of salpingoscopy in tubal infertility. *Fertil Steril* **53**: 339–340.

Donnez J (1984) *La trompe de Fallope: histophysiologie normale et pathologique.* Thesis, Catholic University of Leuven.

Dubuisson JB, Chapron C, Morice P, Aubriot FX, Foulot H & Bouquet de Jolinière J (1994) Laparoscopic salpingostomy: fertility results according to the tubal mucosal appearance. *Hum Reprod* **9**: 334–339.

Fortier KJ & Haney AF (1985) The pathologic spectrum of uterotubal junction obstruction. *Obstet Gynecol* **65**: 93–98.

Gürgan T, Urman B, Yarali H, Aksu T & Kisnisci HA (1994) Salpingoscopic findings in women with occlusive and nonocclusive salpingitis isthmica nodosa. *Fertil Steril* **61**: 461–463.

Henry-Suchet J, Loffredo V, Tesquier L & Pez JP (1985) Endoscopy of the tube (tuboscopy): its prognostic value for tuboplasties. *Acta Eur Fertil* **16**: 139–145.

Heylen SM, Brosens IA & Puttemans P (1995) Clinical value and cumulative pregnancy rates following salpingoscopy during laparoscopy in infertility. *Hum Reprod* **10**: 2913–2916.

Heylen SM, Deyaert V, Deprest J, Puttemans PJ & Brosens IA (1996) Endoscopic evaluation shows no correlation between peritubal and intratubal adhesions in postinflammatory tubal infertility. *Fertil Steril* (in press).

Marana R, Rizzi M, Muzii L, Catalano GF, Caruana P & Mancuso S (1995) Correlation between the American Fertility Society classifications of adnexal adhesions and distal tubal occlusion, salpingoscopy and reproductive outcome in tubal surgery. *Fertil Steril* **64**: 924–929.

Marconi G, Auge L, Sojo E, Young E & Quintana R (1992) Salpingoscopy: systematic use in diagnostic laparoscopy. *Fertil Steril* **57**: 742–746.

Moore-White M (1960) Evaluation of tubal plastic operations. *Int J Fertil* **5**: 237–250.

Nezhat CR, Luciano AA, Nezhat FR, Siegler AM, Metzger DA & Nezhat CH (1995) *Operative Gynecologic Laparoscopy. Principles and Techniques,* p 104. New York: McGraw-Hill.

Puttemans P, Brosens I, Delattin P, Vasquez G & Boeckx W (1987) Salpingoscopy versus hysterosalpingography in hydrosalpinges. *Hum Reprod* **2**: 535–540.

Rouzi AA, Mackinnon M & McComb PF (1995) Predictors of success of reversal of sterilization. *Fertil Steril* **64**: 29–35.

Shapiro BS, Diamond MP & DeCherney AH (1988) Salpingoscopy: an adjunctive technique for evaluation of the fallopian tube. *Fertil Steril* **49**: 1076–1079.

Vasquez G, Winston RML, Boeckx W & Brosens I (1980) Tubal lesions subsequent to sterilization and their relation to fertility after attempts at reversal. *Am J Obstet Gynecol* **138**: 86–92.

Vasquez G, Boeckx W & Brosens I (1995a) No correlation between peritubal and mucosal adhesions in hydrosalpinges. *Fertil Steril* **64**: 1032–1033.

Vasquez G, Boeckx W & Brosens I (1995b) Prospective study of tubal lesions and fertility in hydrosalpinges. *Hum Reprod* **10**: 1075–1078.

26 Diagnosis of ectopic pregnancy
MA Allon, MC Treadwell, DA Johns and MP Diamond

■ INTRODUCTION

The incidence of ectopic pregnancy more than tripled between 1965 and 1985 (Centers for Disease Control, 1984, 1986; Stock, 1988). In 1987 there were 16.8 ectopic pregnancies per 1000 pregnancies (Nederlof et al, 1990). This increased incidence can be explained by the greater prevalence of sexually transmitted diseases, higher rates of tubal ligation and more frequent reconstructive tubal surgery for infertility. The increase in incidence, however, has not paralleled an increase in mortality rate. Looking at past statistics, we note that the fatality rate has decreased from 3.5 to 0.4 deaths per 1000 between the years 1970 and 1985 (Lawn et al, 1988). The decline in fatality rate follows an improvement in diagnostic capabilities made possible with the sensitive quantitative serum beta human chorionic gonadotropin (β-hCG), and the advent of transvaginal ultrasonography. Different treatment options can be implemented in the management of tubal pregnancy and are beyond the scope of this chapter; however, it should be recognized that conservative treatment of ectopic pregnancy has been possible for patients desiring future fertility, and medical therapy as well as expectant management have also been successfully utilized.

Accurate diagnosis of ectopic pregnancy is not without difficulties for the clinician who often encounters a variety of presentations of pregnancy; making the appropriate diagnosis and implementing the proper treatment therefore calls for familiarity with the contributory risk factors.

Knowledge of risk factors that may contribute to the establishment of an ectopic pregnancy are important in order to heighten sensitivity to patients who are at risk for their occurrence. There are several known risk factors, some of which we have been familiar with for several years and others that have surfaced with the increased use of assisted reproductive technology and reconstructive tubal surgery. Women at risk of having an ectopic pregnancy include those with a prior history of salpingitis, prior history of ectopic pregnancy, and infertility due to tubal factor and prior tuboplasty. Previous intrauterine device use and conception after ovulation induction with gonadotropins or in vitro fertilization (IVF) also increase the risk of ectopic pregnancy (Molly et al, 1990). The incidence of ectopic pregnancy after IVF is reported to be between 4 and 5%. Heterotopic pregnancy (combined intrauterine and tubal pregnancy) is seen in 1 in 70 patients after gamete intrafallopian transfer and 1 in 128 after IVF (Molly et al, 1992). The use of clomiphene citrate does not increase the risk of ectopic pregnancy (Grab et al, 1992). Increased risk of ectopic pregnancy is also seen in women with a prior history of tubal sterilization and in women found to have salpingitis isthmica nodosa (Saracoglu et al, 1992). Michalas et al (1992) have found that any pelvic surgery will increase the risk of ectopic pregnancy. Appendectomy increases the risk by a factor of 1.8, ovarian cystectomy by 2.9, and tuboplasty by 6.0. Finally, induced abortion increases the risk of ectopic pregnancy, and the risk is further increased with the increase in number of induced abortions; the reason for this phenomenon remains unclear.

■ SYMPTOMS

The three most common symptoms of ectopic pregnancy are abdominal pain, absence of menses and irregular vaginal bleeding. Pelvic or abdominal pain can be intermittent, varying in intensity, and may be dull, sharp or colicky, as well as either localized or diffuse. Abdominal tenderness is seen in 50% of patients, but rebound tenderness and guarding is less frequent. Findings at bimanual examination are normal in 10% and an enlarged adnexa is seen in one third of patients.

Table 26.1 *Symptoms of women with ectopic pregnancies from the infertility and residents' clinics*

	Infertility clinic (n=38)		Residents' clinic (n=22)	
	No.	%	No.	%
Asymptomatic	5	13.2	0	0.0
Abdominal pain	19	50.0	21	95.5*
Spotting/bleeding > 3 days	5	13.2	11	50.0†
Dizziness	0	0.0	4	18.2‡
Shoulder pain	0	0.0	3	13.6‡

* P<0.001.

† P<0.01.

‡ P<0.05.

Reprinted with permission from Diamond MP, Wider-Estin M, Jones EE & DeCherney AH (1994) Failure of standard criteria to diagnose non-emergency ectopic pregnancies in a noninfertility patient population. J Am Assoc Gynecol Laparosc **1**: 131–134.

Shoulder pain is infrequent and may accompany other peritoneal irritation. Menstrual history is not always consistent, with 15% of patients reporting amenorrhea of more than 12 weeks duration and the same percentage reporting amenorrhea of less than 4 weeks. Abnormal bleeding, however, is seen in 50–80% as corpus luteum support falters and decidua is shed.

It is not uncommon to find patients with significant hypotension without tachycardia; this is seen in 10–90% of patients (Cartright et al, 1984; Snyder, 1990). In these cases, rupture of the tubal serosa with significant hemoperitoneum must be suspected. The altered heart rate response is secondary to the release of vasoactive substances that irritate the peritoneal surfaces and trigger a parasympathetic response, decreasing the pulse rate inappropriately.

▪ CLINICAL INVESTIGATIONS

BIOCHEMICAL MARKERS

Establishing the diagnosis of ectopic pregnancy is often a challenge to the clinician because it can be mistaken for a normal intrauterine pregnancy, a hemorrhagic corpus luteum or a threatened abortion. The most useful test is serum quantitative β-hCG, found to be positive in well over 95% of patients (assay sensitive to second international standard 5 miu/ml). This test, however, will often follow different patterns that can be explained by at least three different clinical presentations, described as follows:

1. The conceptus and corpus luteum may be completely normal but the Fallopian tube is somehow blocked or damaged. The trophoblast may proliferate normally, and secretion of β-hCG and progesterone are similar to normal pregnancy initially (Shepherd et al, 1990). The patient has no symptoms at first but with trophoblast invasion, hematoma occurs and there is a drop in β-hCG and progesterone. Ectopic pregnancy in the distal ampulla can accommodate a large gestation and therefore β-hCG and progesterone may be similar to a normal pregnancy (Stabile and Grudzinkas, 1990).

2. The tube and corpus luteum may be normal but the conceptus is abnormal; for example, a blighted ovum. Here, β-hCG and progesterone are both low early in gestation.

3. The conceptus and tube are normal but corpus luteum function is not. (Norman et al, 1988; Sauer et al, 1988a; Pulkkinen and Jaakkola, 1989). An abnormal corpus luteum will result in reduced levels of hCG, estradiol and progesterone in the early to midluteal phase onward (Hutchinson-Williams et al, 1989).

Interestingly, the utility of the criteria in diagnosing ectopic pregnancy may vary with the patient population being studied. In the evaluation of infertility patients and resident clinic patients at the same medical center, evaluated by the same algorithm, we identified the same most common symptoms; however, abdominal pain, vaginal spotting and/or bleeding for over 3 days, shoulder pain, and dizziness were all more common in the resident clinic patients (Diamond et al, 1994) (*Table 26.1*).

Furthermore, despite case management by the same faculty members, ruptured ectopic pregnancies occurred three times as often among the resident clinic patients. These same patients were also more likely to have surgi-

Table 26.2 *Characteristics of ectopic pregnancies in women from the infertility and residents' clinics*

	Infertility clinic		Residents' clinic	
	No.	%	No.	%
Number ruptured	4	10.5	7	31.8
Treatment by laparoscopy	31	81.6	9	40.9*
Salpingostomy performed	25	65.8	14	63.3
Postoperative hematocrit ≤ 25%	1	2.6	4	18.2
Patients receiving transfusions	2	5.3	4	18.2
Postoperative complications	1	2.6	5	22.7†

* $P < 0.01$.

† $P < 0.05$.

Reprinted with permission from Diamond MP, Wider-Estin M, Jones EE & DeCherney AH (1994) Failure of standard criteria to diagnose non-emergency ectopic pregnancies in a noninfertility patient population. J Am Assoc Gynecol Laparosc 1: 131–134.

cal therapy by laparotomy, and to have more postoperative complications, including the need for a blood transfusion (Diamond et al, 1994)(*Table 26.2*). Thus the patient population may greatly influence the success of early diagnosis of ectopic pregnancy.

With an ectopic pregnancy, while β-hCG levels are less than 25 miu/ml in only 1% of patients, the levels are usually lower compared with those of an intrauterine pregnancy of the same gestational age. Higher β-hCG levels will often correlate with tubal rupture, ectopic size and volume of hemoperitoneum (Cartright et al, 1987; DiMarchi et al, 1989). For further improvement in diagnostic accuracy, some investigators have utilized serum progesterone levels. Progesterone is often abnormally low with ectopic and nonviable pregnancy (Matthews et al, 1986; Yeko et al, 1987; Buck et al, 1988; Sauer et al, 1988a; DiMarchi et al, 1989; Stoval et al, 1989). Stovall and coworkers (1989) reviewed 582 patients with suspected ectopic pregnancy. They found that 81% of 67 patients with ectopic gestation had a progesterone level below 15 ng/ml and 11% of 387 patients with intrauterine pregnancies had levels below 15 ng/ml; however levels of progesterone are not as reliable as serum β-hCG, but may increase the suspicion of ectopic pregnancy and help in the decision to perform a diagnostic laparoscopy.

Other serum chemistries have been evaluated in patients with ectopic pregnancies. Depressed level of placental proteins 12 and 14 may distinguish an ectopic pregnancy from an intrauterine pregnancy. Pregnancy associated plasma protein (PAPP-A), a glycoprotein of placental origin, rises over nonpregnant levels by day 30 of normal gestation (Coddington et al, 1989; Stabile and Grudzinkas, 1990), although levels are usually decreased with ectopic or nonviable intrauterine pregnancy and are nonspecific in discriminating normal from abnormal gestation. CA-125 is 15–50 times higher with tubal rupture and hemoperitoneum (Sauer et al, 1989a; Brumsted et al, 1990) compared with levels found with a normal intrauterine pregnancy. Finally, Sauer and coworkers (1988b) reported on a rapid enzyme immunoassay for urinary pregnanediol-3-glucuronide, which correlated well with serum progesterone and was below the expected levels in 60 patients with ectopic pregnancy. This may be useful when used in conjunction with urinary chorionic gonadotrophin. The use of these tests is currently limited because they lack the specificity and availability of serum β-hCG, which is currently the test of choice.

CULDOCENTESIS

Another diagnostic method is the use of culdocentesis, which is defined as positive when there is aspiration of 0.5 ml (Cartright et al, 1984) of nonclotting blood from the posterior cul-de-sac.

A negative test, however, is the aspiration of at least 0.5 ml of serous fluid, which may be seen in 10% of patients with ectopic pregnancy. The test is inconclusive with failure to aspirate fluid or if the fluid aspirated is blood tinged, which occurs when the needle is improperly positioned in the posterior cul-de-sac. Positive culdocentesis has been seen in 70–90% of patients with ectopic pregnancy (Cartright et al, 1984). Culdocentesis is relatively contraindicated in the case of a retroverted

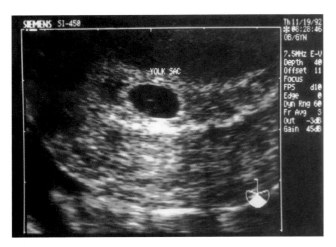

Figure 26.1: Yolk sac of an early intrauterine gestation.

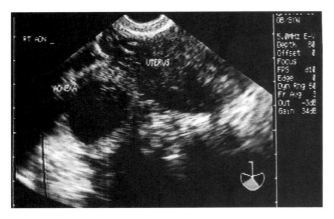

Figure 26.2: Adnexal mass representing a tubal ectopic gestation.

uterus or if a mass is palpated in the cul-de-sac. Currently the technique of culdocentesis is often confined to cases with an indeterminate diagnosis and after an ultrasound has been performed in a hemodynamically stable patient.

TRANSVAGINAL ULTRASONOGRAPHY

The primary role of ultrasound in the evaluation of ectopic pregnancy remains the identification of an intrauterine pregnancy (*Figure 26.1*). The improved resolution of transvaginal sonography (TVS) allows earlier localization of a pregnancy, with demonstration of an intrauterine pregnancy possible as early as 35 days gestation (Fossum et al, 1988). Utilization of TVS allows for the use of lower discriminatory β-hCG levels, 1800 miu/ml (Fleischer et al, 1996), for the identification of a gestational sac in the uterus, as opposed to the 6500 miu/ml level traditionally used for transabdominal scan-

ning (Kadar et al, 1981). In a patient where no intrauterine pregnancy is visualized, the task becomes identification of signs of an ectopic gestation. After implantation, the endometrium will appear prominent. As the decidua sloughs, a pseudocyst may develop; this can precede the onset of vaginal bleeding and must be differentiated from an early intrauterine pregnancy. The pseudocyst tends to be centrally located and may appear irregular. This contrasts with the eccentric location of the early intrauterine gestational sac and does not possess the 'double sac' sign. The association of a pseudocyst with an intrauterine pregnancy is relatively uncommon, occurring in only 4 of 68 women in one series (Nyberg et al, 1983). The identification of a gestational sac outside the uterus provides a definitive diagnosis of ectopic pregnancy. The presence of a tubal ring measuring 1–3 mm with a 2–4 mm concentric, echogenic rim of tissue surrounding a hypoechoic center was described in 23 of 34 patients with unruptured ectopic pregnancy (*Figure 26.2*) (Fossum et al, 1988; Fleischer et al, 1990). A cystic or complex mass may be visualized by ultrasound in 60–90% of patients, and free fluid in the pelvis is seen in 25–35% (Romero et al, 1988; Schwab, 1988). Actual identification of an embryo is much less common and may only occur in less than 15% of ectopics. The use of Doppler flow to improve ectopic identification has been described (*Figure 26.3*). Color flow may be useful for isolating fetal cardiac motion (*Figure 26.4*). Up to 40% of ectopic gestations will have a characteristic trophoblastic flow with slow ascent and slow descent. (Taylor et al, 1986). Color Doppler patterns suggestive of ectopic pregnancy may be detected in the adnexa, yielding sensitivity and specificity of 88 and 97%.

For the diagnosis of a suspected ectopic eccyesis in the hemodynamically stable patient, serial quantitative β-hCG levels should be obtained and TVS is performed when the β-hCG level is greater than 750 miu/ml (second international). An evaluation of an abnormal pregnancy or an ectopic pregnancy is considered when the β-hCG levels are not found to double every 48 hours (Timonen and Nieminen, 1967). Serial β-hCG should be utilized concurrently with ultrasound findings. It must, however, be recognized that in women with an intrauterine pregnancy a normal doubling time for hCG was observed in 77 of 87 (88.5%) (Wiser-Estin et al,

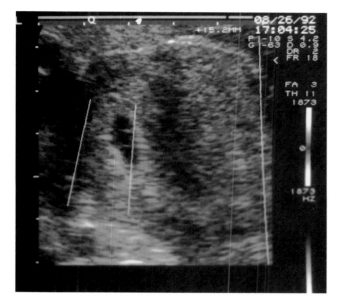

Figure 26.3: *Trophoblastic flow demonstrated by color Doppler identifying an ectopic pregnancy.*

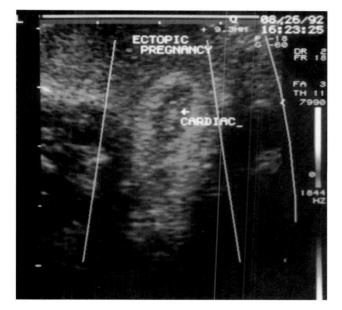

Figure 26.4: *Fetal heart motion identified by color Doppler in an ectopic pregnancy.*

1993). Thus 11.5% of women with a normal intrauterine pregnancy had an abnormal doubling time (*Figure 26.5*). In contrast, 35 of 46 (76.1%) of women with an ectopic pregnancy had a falling or abnormally slow β-hCG pattern. It is important to realize that the remainder of women with an ectopic pregnancy (23.9%), however, had titers that rose appropriately with a normal doubling time (*Figure 26.6*). In distinguishing normal intrauterine pregnancies from ectopic pregnancies a

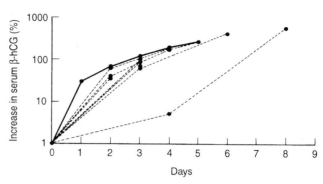

Figure 26.5: *Patients with a normal intrauterine pregnancy but abnormal rates of rise of β-hCG.* •···• *Individual subjects;* •—• *minimum increase in β-hCG. Reproduced with permission from Estin MW, DeCherney AH & Diamond MP (1993) Perils in the differentiation of a viable intrauterine pregnancy from an ectopic eccyesis.* Gynaecol Endosc **2:** 223.

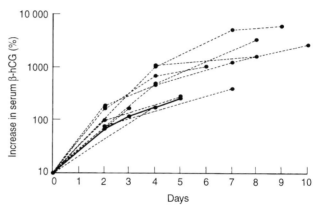

Figure 26.6: *Patients with an ectopic pregnancy with a normal rate of rise of β-hCG.* •···•, *Individual subjects;* •—• *minimum increase in β-hCG. Reproduced with permission from Estin MW, DeCherney AH & Diamond MP (1993) Perils in the differentiation of a viable intrauterine pregnancy from an ectopic eccyesis.* Gynaecol Endosc **2:** 223.

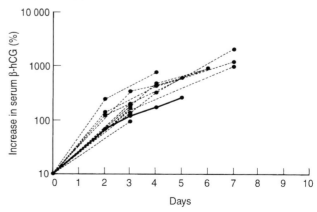

Figure 26.7: *Patients with nonviable intrauterine pregnancies with a normal rate of rise of β-hCG.* •···•, *Individual subjects;* •—• *minimum increase in β-hCG. Reproduced with permission from Estin MW, DeCherney AH & Diamond MP (1993) Perils in the differentiation of a viable intrauterine pregnancy from an ectopic eccyesis.* Gynaecol Endosc **2:** 223.

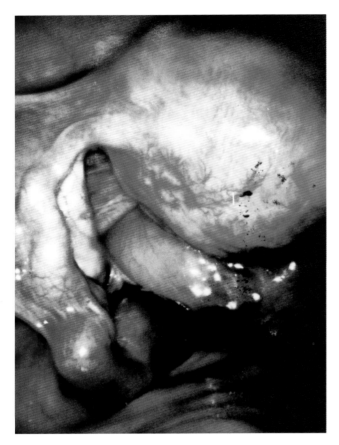

26.8a

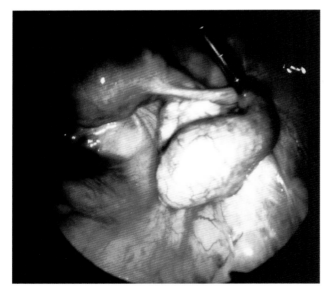

26.8b

Figure 26.8: *Ectopic pregnancies in the ampullary segment of (a) the left Fallopian tube and (b) the right Fallopian tube.*

third situation must also be considered: that of a nonviable intrauterine pregnancy, which can have a normal or an abnormally rising β-hCG level (*Figure 26.7*). Finally,

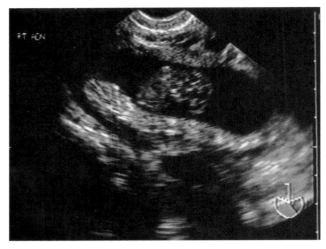

26.9a

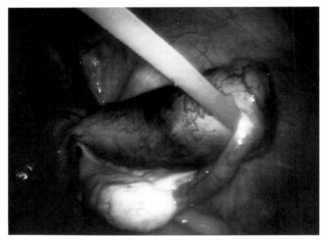

26.9b

Figure 26.9: *(a) Ultrasonographic and (b) laparoscopic views of the same ectopic pregnancy.*

for patients in whom there is a high suspicion of an ectopic pregnancy based on a subnormal rise in β-hCG and in whom a fetal sac is not visualized, a laparoscopy can be performed for diagnostic and/or therapeutic purposes.

LAPAROSCOPY

By far the most common location of an ectopic pregnancy is the ampullary segment of the tube. The appearance of the ectopic pregnancy is that of tubal distension with a purple hue (*Figure 26.8*). The laparoscopic finding should be consistent with the ultrasound scan, as was the case in the patient presented in *Figure 26.9*. Less commonly, the eccyesis may be in the isthmic portion of the tube (*Figure 26.10*), or the interstitial

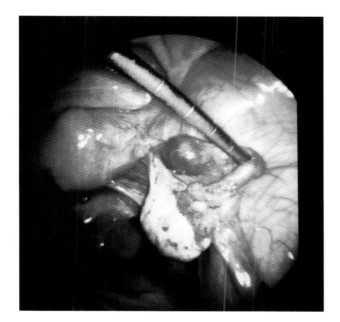

26.10a

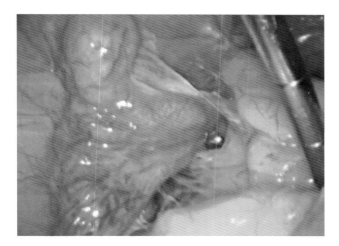

26.10b

Figure 26.10: *Isthmic ectopic pregnancies: (a) unruptured and (b) ruptured.*

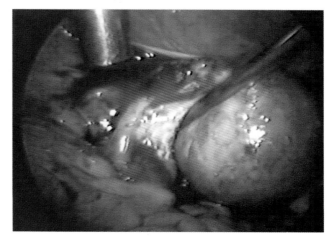

Figure 26.11: *Enlarged interstitial ectopic pregnancy.*

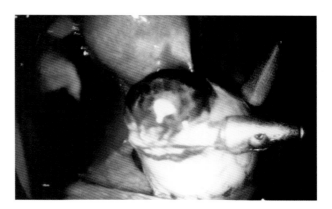

Figure 26.12: *Right ovarian ectopic pregnancy.*

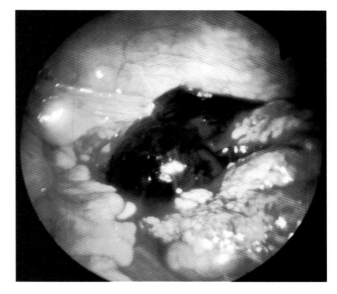

Figure 26.13: *Abdominal ectopic pregnancy with omental implantation.*

portion (*Figure 26.11*). Among the rare locations are an ovarian ectopic (*Figure 26.12*), and an abdominal ectopic with implantation on the omentum (*Figure 26.13*). The latter can also be diagnosed ultrasonographically, as was the case in the patient shown in *Figure 26.14*.

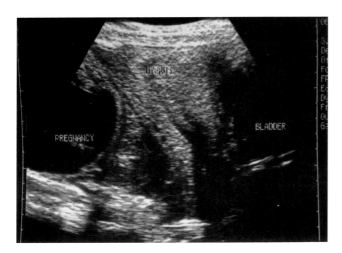

Figure 26.14:Abdominal ectopic pregnancy.

▪ INTERPRETATION AND CLINICAL MANAGEMENT

ROLES OF EXPECTANT MANAGEMENT AND MEDICAL THERAPY IN PATIENTS IN WHOM DEFINITIVE DIAGNOSIS IS DIFFICULT

The earlier diagnosis of ectopic pregnancy has led to an increase in the number of ectopic pregnancies that would otherwise go undetected. The data from medically treated ectopic pregnancies that were followed by hysterosalpingography confirm that tubal patency continued to be maintained. Expectant management relies upon the assumption that patients with a spontaneously resolving ectopic pregnancy terminate their gestation through expulsion of the gestational product from the fimbrial end. Reported frequencies of tubal abortions range from a high of 73% (Marchetti and Kuder, 1946) in the old literature, to the low of 1% (Sherman et al, 1982) found in more recent literature. Sauer and associates (1989b) reported on 36 women who had a laparoscopically documented ectopic pregnancy after 30–56 days of gestation. They enrolled ten patients (27.8%) in a study of nonsurgical treatment. Inclusion criteria were:

- ▪ tubal gestation <3 cm in diameter
- ▪ tubal serosa intact
- ▪ no active bleeding
- ▪ declining β-hCG.

All of the ectopic pregnancies in that study resolved without medical treatment or surgical intervention.

They also noted that the levels of progesterone, estradiol, 17-hydroxyprogesterone and β-hCG were significantly lower in these patients compared with patients with ongoing ectopic pregnancy and viable intrauterine pregnancy, but some overlap between these values did exist. In another study, Ylostalo et al (1992) noted that 57 of 83 (69%) patients with an ectopic pregnancy of under 4 cm in diameter and declining β-hCG levels did not require further surgery. Twenty of their patients required surgery because of clinical symptoms or rising β-hCG levels, while one patient had tubal rupture. Makinen and coworkers (1990) noted a spontaneous resolution in 27 of 33 (82%) women with an ectopic pregnancy and with a β-hCG of <2500 miu/ml and declining. Finally, a study by Mashiach and Oelsner (1982) reported on 13 ectopic pregnancies that were diagnosed by laparoscopy without the initiation of treatment. Three of the 13 (23%) patients required a laparotomy as a result of pain or tubal rupture; the other 10 (77%) had an uneventful follow up with spontaneous resolution of symptoms.

No universal approach currently exists regarding the criteria for expectant management of ectopic pregnancy. Expectant management may be undertaken for a selected group of patients who are asymptomatic, hemodynamically stable with a small diameter (<3.5 cm) ectopic pregnancy, and declining serum β-hCG. Caution should be exercised because tubal rupture can still occur with low and falling serum β-hCG (Tulandi et al, 1991), and these patients should also be closely monitored.

An alternative to expectant management is medical treatment of ectopic pregnancy, which has most commonly been performed using methotrexate. Theoretical advantages of medical treatment include decreased tissue trauma and peritoneal adhesion formation, particularly in patients in whom a definitive diagnosis is difficult. Methotrexate, also known as amethopterin, a 4-amino-*n*-10-methylpteroyl-glutamic acid, is a potent folate antagonist. It acts by inhibiting dihydrofolate reductase and thus preventing the incorporation of thymidylate into DNA during cell division.

Toxicity is seen when serum levels reach a concentration of 2×10^{-8} M and a time threshold of the first 42 hours (Bleyer, 1978). Potential side effects are bone marrow depression, stomatitis, gastrointestinal ulceration and hemorrhage, diarrhea, liver dysfunction, renal toxicity, alopecia, inflammation pneumonitis and anaphylaxis. No major reactions have been reported at the concentration of 1 mg/kg methotrexate used for ectopic pregnancy. Stovall et al (1991) have treated 100 patients with methotrexate given intramuscularly (1 mg/kg body weight) alternating with intramuscular citrovorum factor (0.1 mg/kg) on a daily basis, up to four doses. A more recent approach (Stovall et al, 1993) has advocated administration of a single dose of intramuscular methotrexate (50 mg/m²) without citrovorum rescue. This method was used in 120 women with an intact ectopic pregnancy of < 3.5 cm in the greatest diameter and no side effects were noted with the exception of nausea and vomiting seen in one patient. The treatment was successful in 113 (94.2%) women. Only four (3.3%) patients required a second dose of methotrexate, while seven (5.8%) patients required surgical intervention. No evidence of tubal rupture was noted and tubal patency was identified in 51 of 62 (82.3%) patients. Importantly, following methotrexate therapy, abdominal pain was experienced by 71 (59.2%) patients, four of whom required hospitalization. Utilizing single dose methotrexate, β-hCG levels may rise for at least 3 days after treatment but will begin to decline by day 7 (Stovall et al, 1993). Patients in whom the serum β-hCG level did not decline by 15% between days 4 and 7 would then receive a second dose of methotrexate (50 mg/m² i.m.) on day 7 after the initial treatment. If the serum β-hCG is declining by day 7, the patients would then be followed by weekly titers until their β-hCG levels declined to negativity. Ultrasound follow up after methotrexate treatment was performed by Brown and coworkers (1991), who found that the mass of ectopic pregnancy may remain after the β-hCG titers were negligible and that an increase in mass size would not predict tubal rupture.

Persistent ectopic pregnancy diagnosis

Persistent ectopic pregnancy is seen when there is a continued growth of trophoblastic tissue after conservative treatment (*Figure 26.15*). This may result in elevated β-hCG, recurrence of symptoms, a pelvic mass and possibly delayed hemorrhage. The only reliable method of

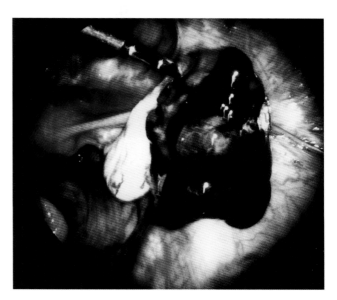

Figure 26.15: Persistent trophoblastic tissue in the right fimbria 2 weeks after salpingostomy.

detecting a persistent ectopic pregnancy is by monitoring the levels of serial β-hCG postoperatively. Currently one will follow β-hCG weekly after linear salpingostomies until the titers are negative: as long as they are declining and the patient is asymptomatic, observation is often sufficient. Serum levels of β-hCG were shown by Kamrava and associates (1983) to be undetectable 24 days after linear salpingostomy. Vermesh and coworkers (1988) demonstrated that, by postoperative day 12, the diagnosis of persistent ectopic pregnancy could be suspected if serum β-hCG levels did not fall below 10% of their initial value. Finally, the time between the initial treatment with salpingostomy and the second operative procedure was found to be between 18 and 60 days with viable trophoblastic tissue seen in the pathology specimen (Kelly et al, 1979; Bell et al, 1987). Ultrasonography can sometimes be used to evaluate patients with persistent ectopic pregnancies (*Figure 26.16*).

The incidence of persistent ectopic pregnancy after laparoscopic conservative treatment is reported to be between zero and 10% (Decherney and Kase, 1979; Kelly et al, 1979; Pouly et al, 1986; Bell et al, 1987; Brumsted et al, 1988). The incidence of persistent ectopic pregnancy after conservative surgery at laparotomy was, however, reported to be between 3 and 5% (Brumsted et al, 1988; Vermesh et al, 1988, 1989; Seifer et

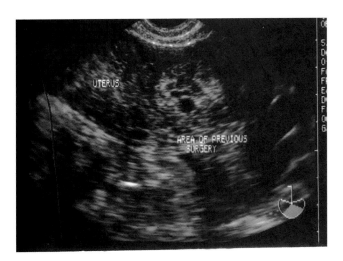

Figure 26.16: *Ultrasonographic appearance of the uterine cornua with a persistent ectopic pregnancy initially treated by a salpingostomy for an interstitial ectopic pregnancy.*

al, 1990). Although the incidence of persistent ectopic pregnancy after conservative laparoscopic treatment may be reported to be higher than that after laparotomy, others may argue that there is no significant difference. Pouly and colleagues (1986) have reported that 15 of 321 (4.8%) patients treated for an ectopic pregnancy with conservative laparoscopic surgery had subsequent persistent disease. The discrepancy in the reported incidence of persistent ectopic pregnancy can be explained by several factors.

The time of ectopic removal might impact on persistent trophoblastic tissue. Seifer and colleagues (1990) have found that early conservative surgical treatment when an ectopic pregnancy measures less than 2 cm and patients have less than 42 days of amenorrhea will result in an increased risk for persistent ectopic pregnancy. This was hypothesized to be due to incomplete evacuation of ectopic pregnancy secondary to poor cleavage planes at the implantation site. To prevent persistent disease, the suggestion of biweekly β-hCG estimations when the ectopic pregnancy is less than 2 cm or there is less than 6 weeks of amenorrhea may be implemented. The evidence of trophoblastic tissue in pathology specimens of surgically treated persistent ectopic pregnancies may suggest incomplete evacuation of the pregnancy. Stock (1991) reviewed eight cases of persistent ectopic pregnancy and found that four of five tubes examined histologically had implantation sites with associated

chorionic villi medial to the cornual border of the previous surgical incision site; therefore, if uncontrolled bleeding is noted, irrigation or exploration of the tube medial to the apparent site of implantation is recommended.

■ CONCLUSION

Ectopic pregnancy has been the second leading cause of maternal mortality in the United States. In recent years, different diagnostic and therapeutic modalities have greatly diminished the morbidity and mortality rate. The earlier diagnosis of ectopic pregnancy, with more sophisticated TVS, more sensitive quantitative β-hCG, advanced laparoscopic techniques and medical therapy, have all contributed to the conservative treatment of this condition.

REFERENCES

Bell OR, Awadalla SG & Mattox JH (1987) Persistent ectopic syndrome: a case report and literature review. *Obstet Gynecol* **69**: 521–523.

Bleyer WA (1978) The clinical pharmacology of methotrexate. *Cancer* **41**: 36.

Brown DL, Felker RE, Stovall G et al (1991) Serial endovaginal sonography of ectopic pregnancies treated with methotrexate. *Obstet Gynecol* **7**: 406–409.

Brumsted J, Kessler C, Gison C et al (1988) A comparison of laparoscopy and laparotomy for the treatment of ectopic pregnancy. *Obstet Gynecol* **71**: 889–892.

Brumsted JR, Nakajima ST, Badger G et al (1990) Serum concentration of CA-125 during the first trimester of normal and abnormal pregnancies. *J Reprod Med* **35**: 499.

Buck RH, Joubert SM & Norman RJ (1988) Serum progesterone in the diagnosis of ectopic pregnancy: a valuable diagnostic test? *Fertil Steril* **50**: 752–755.

Cartright PS, Tuttle D & Vaughn B (1984) Culdocentesis and ectopic pregnancy. *J Reprod Med* **29**: 88.

Cartright PS, Moore RA, Dao AH et al (1987) Serum β-hCG levels relate poorly to the size of a tubal pregnancy. *Fertil Steril* **48**: 679–680.

Centers for Disease Control (1984) Current trends: ectopic pregnancies: United States, 1979–1980. *MMWR* **33**: 201.

Centers for Disease Control (1986) Ectopic pregnancy: United States, 1981–1983. *MMWR* **35**: 289.

Coddington CC, Sinosich MJ, Boston EG et al (1989) Pregnancy-associated protein-A does not improve predictability of pregnancy success or failure over human chorionic gonadotropin levels in early and normal and abnormal pregnancy. *Fertil Steril* **52**: 854–857.

Decherney AH & Kase N (1979) The conservative surgical management of unruptured ectopic pregnancy. *Obstet Gynecol* **54**: 451–455.

DiMarchi JM, Kosasa TS & Hale RW (1989) What is the significance of the human chorionic gonadotropin value in ectopic pregnancy? *Obstet Gynecol* **74**: 851–853.

Diamond MP, Wiser-Estin M, Jones EB & DeCherney AH (1994) Failure of standard criteria to diagnose nonemergency ectopic pregnancies in a noninfertility patient population *J Am Assoc Gynecol Laparosc* **1**: 131–134.

Fleischer AC, Pennell RG, McKee MS et al (1990) Ectopic pregnancy: features at transvaginal sonography. *Radiology* **174**: 375.

Fleischer AC, Manning FA, Jeanty P & Romero R (1996) *Sonography in Obstetrics and Gynecology*. Stanford, CT: Appleton and Lange.

Fossum GT, Davanajan R & Kletzy OA (1988) Early detection of pregnancy with transvaginal ultrasound. *Fertil Steril* **49**: 788.

Grab D, Wolf A & Kunze Sterzik K (1992) Die Ovarielle l. H, stimulation mit Clomifen stellt Kienen Risikofaktor fur eine Extrauterinegraviditat dar. *Zentalbl Gynakol* **114**: 289–291.

Hutchinson-Williams, K, Lunenfeld B, Diamond MP et al (1989) Human chorionic gonadotropin, estradiol, and progesterone profiles in conception and nonconception cycles in an in vitro fertilization program. *Fertil Steril* **52**: 441.

Kadar N, Devore G & Romero R (1981) Discriminating hCG zone: its use in the sonographic evaluation of ectopic pregnancy. *Obstet Gynecol* **58**: 156–161.

Kamrava MM, Taymor ML, Berger MJ et al (1983) Disappearance of human chorionic gonadotropin following removal of ectopic pregnancy. *Obstet Gynecol* **62**: 486–488.

Kelly RW, Martin SA & Strickler RC (1979) Delayed hemorrhage in conservative surgery for ectopic pregnancy. *Am J Obstet Gynecol* **133**: 225.

Lawn HAW, Trash HK, Softballs AF et al (1988) Ectopic pregnancy surveillance: United States, 1970–1985. *MMWR* **37**: 9.

Makinen JI, Kivijarvi AK & Ifjala KM (1990) Success of non-surgical management of ectopic pregnancy. *Lancet* **335**: 1099 (letter).

Marchetti AA & Kuder KA (1946) A clinical evaluation of ectopic pregnancy. *Am J Obstet Gynecol* **52**: 544–553.

Mashiach S & Oelsner G (1982) Nonoperative management of ectopic pregnancy: a preliminary report. *J Reprod Med* **27**: 127.

Mathews CP, Coulsen CB & Wild RA (1986) Serum progesterone levels as an aid in the diagnosis of ectopic pregnancy. *Obstet Gynecol* **68**: 390.

Michalas S, Minaretzis D, Tsionou C, Maos G, Kioses E & Aravantinos D (1992) Pelvic surgery, reproductive factors and risk of ectopic pregnancy: a case controlled study. *Int J Gynecol Obstet* **38**: 101–105.

Molly D, Deambosis W, Keeping D et al (1990) Multiple-sighted (heterotopic) pregnancy after in vitro fertilization and gamete intrafallopian transfer. *Fertil Steril* **53**: 1068.

Nederlof KP, Lawn HAW, Softballs AF, Trash HK & Finches EL (1990) Ectopic pregnancy surveillance, United States, 1970–1987. *MMWR* **39**: 9.

Norman RJ, Buck RH, Kemp MA et al (1988) Impaired corpus luteum function in ectopic pregnancy cannot be explained by altered human chorionic gonadotropin. *J Clin Endocrinol Metab* **66**: 1166.

Nyberg DA, Laing FC, Filly RA et al (1983) Ultrasonographic differentiation of the gestational sac of early intrauterine pregnancy from the pseudogestational sac of ectopic pregnancy. *Radiology* **146**: 755.

Pouly JL, Mahnes H, Mage G et al (1986) Conservative laparoscopic treatment of 321 ectopic pregnancies. *Fertil Steril* **46**: 1093–1097.

Pulkkinen MO & Jaakkola UM (1989) Low serum progesterone levels and tubal dysfunction: a possible cause of ectopic pregnancy. *Am J Obstet Gynecol* **161**: 934.

Romero R, Kadar N, Castro D et al (1988) The value of adnexal sonographic findings in the diagnosis of ectopic pregnancy. *Am J Obstet Gynecol* **158**: 52–53.

Saracoglu FO, Mungan T & Tanzer F (1992) Salpingitis isthmica nodosa in infertility and ectopic pregnancy. *Gynecol Obstet Invest* **34**: 202–205.

Sauer MV, Gorrill MJ, Rodi IA et al (1988a) Corpus luteum activity in tubal pregnancy. *Obstet Gynecol* **71**: 667–670.

Sauer MV, Vermesh M, Anderson RE et al (1988b) Rapid measurement of urinary pregnanediol glucouronide to diagnose ectopic pregnancy. *Am J Obstet Gynecol* **159**: 1531–1535.

Sauer MV, Vasilev SA, Campeau J et al (1989a) Serum cancer antigen 125 in ectopic pregnancy. *Gynecol Obstet Invest* **27**: 164.

Sauer MV, Anderson RE, Vermesh M et al (1989b) Spontaneously resorbing ectopic pregnancy: preservation of human chorionic gonadotropin bioactivity despite declining steroid hormone levels. *Am J Obstet Gynecol* **161**: 1673–1676.

Schwab RA (1988) Ultrasound versus culdocentesis in the evaluation of early and late ectopic pregnancy. *Ann Emerg Med* **17**: 801–803.

Seifer DB, Gutmann JN, Doyle MB et al (1990) Persistent ectopic pregnancy following laparoscopic linear salpingostomy. *Obstet Gynecol* **76**: 1121–1125.

Shepherd RW, Patton PE, Novy MJ et al (1990) Serial beta-hCG measurements in the early detection of ectopic pregnancy. *Obstet Gynecol* **75**: 417–420.

Sherman D, Langer R, Sadovsky G et al (1982) Improved fertility following ectopic pregnancy. *Fertil Steril* **37**: 497–502.

Snyder HS (1990) Lack of a tachycardic response to hypotension with ruptured ectopic pregnancy. *Am J Emerg Med* **8**: 23–26.

Stabile I & Grudzinkas JG (1990) Ectopic pregnancy: a review of incidence, etiology and diagnostic aspects. *Obstet Gynecol Surv* **45**: 335–347.

Stock RJR (1988) The changing spectrum of ectopic pregnancy. *Obstet Gynecol* **71**: 885–888.

Stock RJ (1991) Persistent tubal pregnancy. *Obstet Gynecol* **77**: 267–270.

Stovall TG & Ling FW (1993) Single dose methotrexate: an expanded clinical trial. *Am J Obstet Gynecol* **168**: 1759–1765.

Stovall TG, Ling FW, Cope BJ et al (1989) Preventing ruptured ectopic pregnancy with a single serum progesterone. *Am J Obstet Gynecol* **160**: 1425–1428.

Stovall TG, Ling FW, Gray LA, Carson SA & Buster JE (1991) Methotrexate treatment of unruptured ectopic pregnancy: a report of 100 cases. *Obstet Gynecol* **77**: 749–753.

Taylor K, Ramos I, Feyock A et al (1986) Ectopic pregnancy: duplex Doppler evaluation. *Radiology* **173**: 93.

Timonen S & Nieminen U (1967) Tubal pregnancy: choice of operative method of treatment. *Acta Obstet Gynecol Scand* **46**: 327.

Tulandi T, Hemmings R & Khalifa F (1991) Rupture of ectopic pregnancy in women with low and declining serum β-hCG levels *Fertil Steril* **56**: 786–787.

Vermesh MV, Silva PD, Sauer MV et al (1988) Persistent tubal ectopic gestation: patterns of circulating β-hCG and progesterone, and management options. *Fertil Steril* **50**: 584–588.

Vermesh MV, Silva PD, Rosea GP et al (1989) Management of unruptured ectopic gestation by linear salpingostomy: a prospective, randomized clinical trial of laparoscopy versus laparotomy. *Obstet Gynecol* **73**: 400–403.

Wiser-Estin M, DeCherney AH & Diamond MP (1993) Perils in the differentiation of a viable intrauterine pregnancy (IUP) from an ectopic eccyesis. *Gynaecol Endosc* **2**: 223–226.

Yeko TR, Gorril MJ, Hughes LH et al (1987) Timely diagnosis of early ectopic pregnancy using a single blood progesterone measurement. *Fertil Steril* **48**: 1048–1050.

Ylostalo P, Cacciatore B, Sjosberg J, Kaariainen M, Tenhunen A & Stenaman U (1992) Expectant management of ectopic pregnancy. *Obstet Gynecol* **80**: 345–348.

27 Intrauterine early pregnancy disorders
A Kurjak, S Kupešić and D Zudenigo

■ INTRODUCTION

Until fairly recently ultrasonography in early pregnancy was only performed for the detection of an ongoing early pregnancy and to confirm fetal heart beat. The introduction of transvaginal sonography (TVS) has enabled detailed studies of early embryonic development. Adding color Doppler facilities to TVS has generated a new diagnostic technique. This new method has enabled investigation of the functional state of an early embryo and placenta and has given new insights into the physiology of an early gestation. In this chapter we shall summarize data on ultrasonic assessment of early pregnancy and give an overview of the uteroplacental and fetal circulation in both the normal and abnormal pregnancy.

■ NORMAL EARLY PREGNANCY

Using TVS (*Figure 27.1*) the gestational or chorionic sac can usually be detected at 4 weeks 1–4 days from the last menstrual period (or 15–18 days after ovulation). The average level of serum beta human chorionic gonadotropin (β-hCG) at this gestational age is 400–500 iu/l; the gestational sac measures 4–5 mm and is visualized within the 'shining' endometrium; the gestational sac itself grows by approximately 1–2 mm each day. Transabdominal sonography (TAS) enabled visualization of the gestational sac about 1 week after the vaginal probe produced its first image of the same patient.

The yolk sac becomes evident at 5 weeks gestation and fills about one third of the cross-section of the gestational sac. Its cross-section in a normal pregnancy is always a circle because of its spherical nature (*Figure 27.2*). TAS will consistently detect the yolk sac from 6 weeks onward.

During the fifth week, the embryo measures between 2 and 5 mm and heart beats are clearly visible.

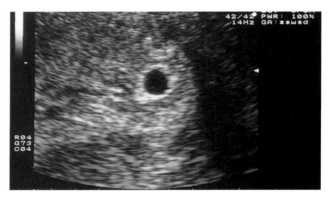

Figure 27.1: *Transvaginal sonogram shows an ovoid structure which represents an early gestational sac at 5 weeks gestation.*

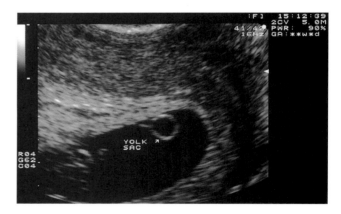

Figure 27.2: *Transvaginal sonogram demonstrating a gestational sac with well-defined, spherical yolk sac.*

Throughout the sixth and seventh weeks (*Figure 27.3*), the fetal pole becomes more evident and from this gestational age onward measurements are available for dating purposes.

During the seventh week a cystic area representing the rhombencephalon can be identified in the brain (*Figure 27.4*). At 6–8 weeks the amniotic membrane can be seen as a thin rounded structure that encircles the embryo.

Using transvaginal color Doppler sonography it is possible to detect and investigate uteroplacental and embryonic blood flow very early in pregnancy (Kurjak

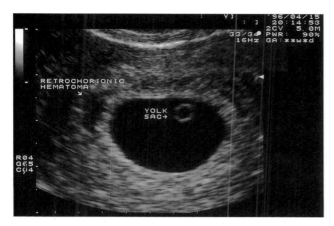

Figure 27.3: *Transvaginal sonogram of a 6 week gestational sac. Note the regular shape and diameter (4 mm) of the yolk sac, and a retrochorionic hematoma on the left side of the gestational sac.*

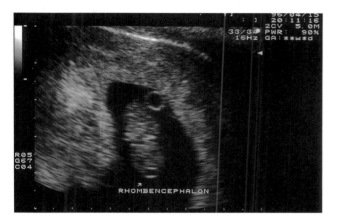

Figure 27.4: *Transvaginal sonogram demonstrates a 7–8 week gestational sac. Note the normal morphology of the embryo and yolk sac. A cystic structure, the rhombencephalon, is shown at the cranial pole of the embryo.*

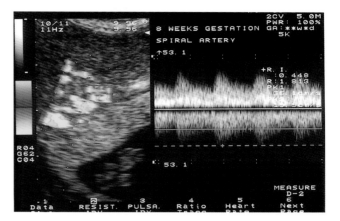

Figure 27.5: *Transvaginal sonogram demonstrates a gestational sac. Note the color coded area representing the spiral arteries (left). The pulse Doppler analysis shows a high velocity and low impedance signal (resistance index (RI) = 0.45) (right).*

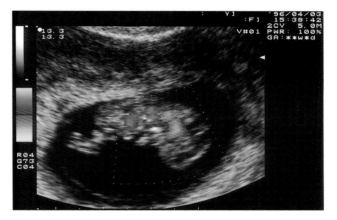

Figure 27.6: *A color image of an embryo at 8 weeks gestation. Vascular signals are obtained from the fetal heart, aorta and cerebral vessels.*

et al, 1993a, 1993b). Spiral artery perfusion can be detected even at 4–5 weeks gestation (*Figure 27.5*). In fetal aorta and umbilical artery it is possible to detect blood flow signals from 6 weeks, and in fetal brain from 7 weeks onwards (*Figure 27.6*). In general, peripheral vascular resistance decreases in all the uteroplacental (uterine, arcuate, radial, spiral and umbilical arteries) (*Figure 27.7*) and fetal vessels (aorta and cerebral arteries) with advanced gestational age; at the same time an increase in blood flow velocity is observed.

■ UTERINE BLEEDING

Roughly 25% of pregnant women have uterine bleeding during the first trimester. It is widely accepted that

more than 50% of these abort spontaneously. Uterine bleeding is only a clinical sign of different pathological conditions: subchorionic hematoma, incomplete abortion, complete abortion, blighted ovum, missed abortion and gestational trophoblastic disease.

SUBCHORIONIC HEMATOMA

A sonolucent crescent-shaped or wedge-shaped structure between the uterine wall and the chorion is subchorionic hematoma (*Figure 27.8*). Physiologically this represents a separation of the chorionic plate from the underlying decidua with a resultant collection of blood between the chorion and decidua. There have been a number of studies on subchorionic hematoma, and

Table 27.1 *Clinical outcome of pregnancies complicated by subchorionic hematoma (SCH)*

Author	n	Pregnancy outcome	Comment
Abu–Yousef et al (1987)	21	7 SpAb 3 PTD 5 severe bleeding, therapeutic abortion	Larger SCH associated with increased risk of poor out come
Baxi and Pearlstone (1991)	5	1 PTD at 24 weeks	Selected group of patients with autoantibodies
Bloch et al (1989)	31	3 SpAb 2 PTD 26 FTD	Size of SCH unrelated to pregnancy outcome
Borlum et al (1989)	86	19 SpAb	Volume of SCH was < 30 ml in 85% patients
Goldstein et al (1983)	10	2 SpAb	Size of SCH unrelated to pregnancy outcome
Jakab et al (1994)	35	8 SpAb	Size of hematoma unrelated to pregnancy outcome
Jouppilla (1985)	33	6 SpAb 3 PTD	Size of SCH unrelated to pregnancy outcome
Mantoni and Pederson (1981)	12	2 SpAb 1 PTD	Larger SCH associated with increased risk of poor out come
Nyberg et al (1987)	46	3 fetal mortality 6 termination of pregnancy 12 PTD	Size of SCH unrelated to pregnancy outcome
Pederson and Mantoni (1990)	23	1 SpAb 2 PTD	Large SCH (> 50 ml) not associated with increased risk of poor outcome
Sauerbrei and Pham (1986)	30	3 SpAb 4 stillbirth 7 PTD	Large SCH (>60 ml) associated with increased risk of poor outcome
Spirit et al (1979)	4	2 PTD 2 FTD	
Stabile et al (1989)	20	0 SpAb	Volume of SCH in all study patients < 16 ml
Ylostalo et al (1984)	16	5 placental abruption	Median duration of pregnancy shorter in patients with SCH

SpAb, spontaneous abortion; PTD, preterm delivery; FTD, full term delivery.

reported results are conflicting. Most of the authors examined the volume of the hematoma. *Table 27.1* summarizes the results of different investigators. Some studies found that the site of the hematoma has a prognostic value for pregnancy outcome (Kurjak et al, 1996). Most hematomas associated with abortion were found in the corpus or fundus of the uterus, not in the supracervical area. Furthermore, it was found that hematomas altered blood flow in spiral arteries by mechanical compression, which was considered as a secondary effect

without influence on pregnancy outcome (Kurjak et al, 1996).

INCOMPLETE ABORTION

Sonographic findings of incomplete abortion vary with the stage of embryonic development at the time of abortion and the amount of the gestational tissue passed. Variable amounts of echogenic debris, choriodecidua and fluid are present within the uterus (*Figure 27.9*).

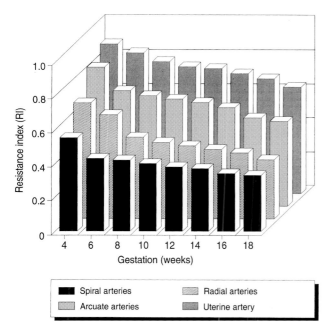

Figure 27.7: Resistance index (RI) values for uteroplacental vessels. A decrease in peripheral vascular impedance with advancing gestational age is shown.

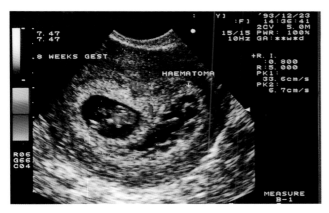

Figure 27.8: Transvaginal sonogram of gestation lasting 8 weeks complicated by retrochorionic hematoma. Spiral artery perfusion and fetal heart action are displayed simultaneously.

This tissue typically appears as echogenic material within the uterine lumen. The choriodecidua is irregular and the gestational sac itself appears 'deflated'. Increased perfusion and low impedance blood flow signals typical of retained products of conception are easily obtainable.

COMPLETE ABORTION

In patients with complete abortion there is a close apposition of relatively thin and regular endometrial inter-

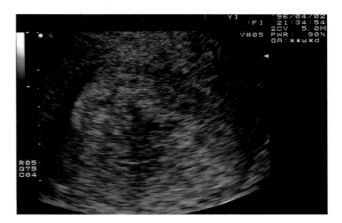

Figure 27.9: Transvaginal sonogram of the uterus in a patient with incomplete abortion. Note the abnormal thickening of the endometrium which represents retained products of conception and blood clots.

face. Although one might argue that ectopic pregnancies may demonstrate this appearance, correlation with β-hCG values may be helpful in confirming a completed miscarriage. In a complete abortion, serial β-hCG values will typically fall precipitously, whereas in ectopic pregnancy this value slowly decreases or reaches a plateau. Color Doppler findings enable confident diagnosis of a complete abortion because there is no increased intracavitary vascularization.

BLIGHTED OVUM AND MISSED ABORTION

A gestational sac of 24 mm or more without a living embryo was considered an anembryonic or empty sac, otherwise termed a blighted ovum (Robinson, 1975). The introduction of TVS has changed these criteria (*Figure 27.10*): with better imaging it is now considered that a 16 mm gestational sac without a fetal pole or any contents should be termed an empty sac.

There are some color Doppler studies on the blighted ovum but results are inconsistent and vary from author to author. It was found that some blighted ova were richly vascularized and that the intensity of color flow corresponded to the trophoblast activity (Kurjak et al, 1991). Abundant color signals possibly indicate which blighted ova will undergo molar changes (*Figure 27.11*).

Missed abortion can be documented by TVS findings of no heart beat in an embryo measuring over 6 mm in

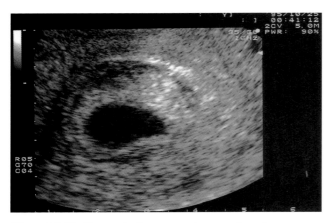

Figure 27.10: *Transvaginal sonogram of an anembryonic pregnancy. An empty gestational sac and a peripheral anechoic structure representing a subchorionic hematoma can be seen.*

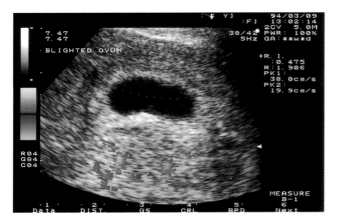

Figure 27.11: *Transvaginal sonogram of a vascularized blighted ovum.*

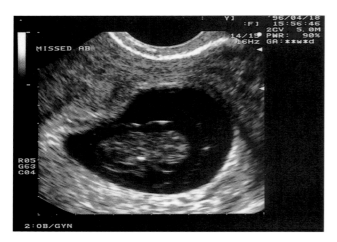

Figure 27.12: *Transvaginal sonogram demonstrating a missed abortion at 8 weeks gestation.*

length (*Figure 27.12*). If the sonographer or sonologist is unsure, the patient should be rescanned 3–4 days later to confirm the observation.

Transvaginal color Doppler can be useful in looking for fetal heart beats in patients suspected of missed abortion. Using this technique, a significantly higher mean uterine pulsatility index (PI) was found in missed abortions compared with normal controls. Intervillous flow was present in 69.6% of the missed abortions of under 12 weeks gestation; this was not found in controls (Jauniaux et al, 1994). In contrast to this initial study, recent Doppler investigations using more sensitive equipment have shown continuous intervillous flow in all normal pregnancies during the first trimester (Kurjak et al, 1995; Kurjak and Kupešić, 1996; Valentin et al, 1996). No difference was found in the Doppler parameters analyzed between the group of patients with missed abortion and those with normal pregnancy (Kurjak and Kupešić, 1996; Valentin et al, 1996). These results shed new light on this very controversial field of early embryonic development, indicating that the establishment of intervillous circulation is a continuous process rather than an abrupt event at the end of the first trimester.

■ GESTATIONAL TROPHOBLASTIC DISEASE

Table 27.2 summarizes the different types of gestational trophoblastic disease.

HYDATIDIFORM MOLE

ULTRASONOGRAPHY

The diagnosis of a complete hydatidiform mole is greatly facilitated by ultrasonography. The entire uterine cavity appears filled with more or less refringent masses and, almost always, there is a total absence of fetal signs. The echoes correspond to the sonic reflections on the surface of the vesicles. This appearance is known as the 'snowstorm' pattern (Gottesfield et al, 1967). The more

Table 27.2 *Histopathological classification of gestational trophoblastic disease*

- Hydatidiform mole
    - Complete
    - Partial
    - With coexistent fetus
- Invasive mole (chorioadenoma destruens)
- Choriocarcinoma

advanced the gestation, the easier and more certain is the diagnosis because the size of the vesicles increases with time. At the beginning of the pregnancy the diagnosis can therefore be missed (Munyer et al, 1981). The application of vaginal ultrasonography permits an earlier diagnosis. Hematomas commonly occur in areas of molar detachment. These accumulations of blood form small echogenic areas that have irregular borders, either inside the mole or, more frequently, along the uterine wall.

When a pregnancy is more than 12 weeks and the fetus is intact, it is not difficult to diagnose a partial mole because the typical 'snowflake' picture is seen in the placental area accompanying the embryo. Nevertheless, this pattern is not typical, as the embryo usually degenerates early and is resorbed (Czernobilsky et al, 1982). The sonographic appearance of the partial hydatidiform mole is thus commonly confused with missed abortion or with a degenerated ovum. The presence of a molar tissue together with an embryo is a sonographic pattern suggestive of a partial mole. There are two other sonographic patterns: (1) the presence of strongly refringent chorial tissue with small cystic areas; and (2) the presence of a large gestational sac with poorly defined inner limits that are surrounded by a strongly refringent ring (Hertzberg et al, 1986).

Sonography can also delineate the theca-lutein cyst that enlarges under the influence of high levels of β-hCG elaborated by the trophoblast. These cysts appear as multiloculated cystic masses that are usually located superior to the uterine fundus or, less commonly, in the cul-de-sac. Theca-lutein cysts appear only with total hydatidiform moles (Munyer et al, 1981), and they may persist in postmolar disease (Woo et al, 1985).

DIFFERENTIAL DIAGNOSIS

At the beginning of the pregnancy it may be impossible to diagnose any type of mole, and only with the use of the vaginal probe may an early diagnosis be established. The mole may remain undetected (Kadar and Romero, 1982; Callen, 1983) or be confused with degenerated ova, which is particularly common with partial moles. The main difference between a partial mole and a blighted ovum lies in the perfect interior delineation of the embryonic sac in the latter. The partial mole usually has a poorly defined sac surrounded by a strongly sonolucent, trophoblastic ring; it shows the remains of an embryo, never seen in a blighted ovum. The image of a missed abortion or a degenerated ovum is similar to that of the partial mole. The picture may be easily confused with postmolar gestational trophoblastic disease or spontaneous abortion because echorefringent and nonhomogeneous chorionic remnants, either located inside the cavity or attached to the uterine wall, are demonstrated. Low or negative β-hCG levels are helpful in differentiating these entities. After curettage, gestational trophoblastic disease, which persists in 20% of patients (Munyer et al, 1981), may exhibit the same appearance. Another consideration is the existence of a mole with a normal twin pregnancy. In this case a normal sac and another with the appearance of a hydatidiform mole are seen. In patients with ectopic pregnancy a dedicually transformed endometrium is visualized. Sometimes, decidua has a similar appearance to a mole because of the presence of a pseudosac and pseudovesicles (Kadar and Romero, 1982). The combined use of quantitative determinations of β-hCG and vaginal sonography may resolve this uncertainty. Color Doppler allows accurate distinction between decidua and trophoblastic tissue, based on the demonstration of the typical trophoblastic blood supply in the latter.

Another diagnostic problem is differentiation between a mole with a live fetus and a hydropic placental degeneration. During an early pregnancy the picture is similar to that of a missed abortion or even a total mole (Hertzberg et al, 1986). In advanced cases, vesicles, cysts, fetal remnants and an abnormal placenta are easily visualized.

Sometimes even a fibromyoma may be confused with a total hydatidiform mole. In addition to the fact that the clinical symptoms are different, when the intensity of the ultrasound is reduced, echoes from the fibromyoma do not disappear, whereas a mole becomes entirely echolucent (Czernobilsky et al, 1982). Furthermore, some partially solid ovarian tumors can simulate the appearance of a hydatidiform mole. Patients with this type of mass can be distinguished from those with molar pregnancies by clinical or laboratory methods because β-hCG is not elevated in nonpregnant conditions. Color Doppler examination seems to further increase the sensitivity of TVS.

Table 27.3 *Mean resistance index values for uteroplacental blood vessels in molar pregnancy*

	Uterine artery	Arcuate artery	Radial artery	Spiral artery	Tumoral vessels
Normal pregnancy	0.82	0.68	0.52	0.48	—
Hydatidiform mole	0.75	0.62	0.47	0.39	—
Invasive mole and choriocarcinoma	0.66	—	—	—	0.30

INVASIVE MOLE AND CHORIOCARCINOMA

ULTRASONOGRAPHY

The sonographic appearance of invasive trophoblastic tissue is that of a focal irregular echogenic region within the uterine myometrium. Irregular hypoechoic areas may surround the more echogenic trophoblastic tissue that corresponds to the areas of myometrial hemorrhage. Due to its proximity to the uterus, myometrial invasion may be precisely delineated with transvaginal scanning.

TRANSVAGINAL COLOR DOPPLER FINDINGS

Transvaginal color Doppler has been reported as a useful diagnostic tool in evaluating gestational trophoblastic disease, which is often associated with increased vascular supply to the placental tissue. Color Doppler may therefore be useful in the diagnosis of myometrial invasion in patients with invasive mole or choriocarcinoma. It seems that the presence of increased blood supply within the myometrial portion can be used to diagnose early invasion, even before it becomes visible on B-mode ultrasonography (*Figure 27.13*).

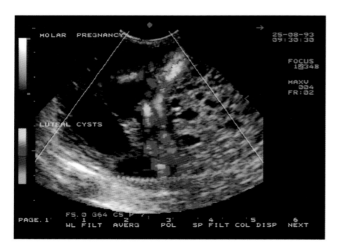

Figure 27.13: Transvaginal sonogram of a molar pregnancy. The 'snowstorm' mass 5 cm in diameter is avascular. Note the prominent area of vascularization on the periphery of the mass, within the myometrium. Bright color signals indicate invasion of the mole. Note the luteal cysts demonstrated on the right ovary.

In invasive mole and choriocarcinoma, trophoblastic invasion into myometrial tissue can be recognized as prominent color coded zones in the myometrium. These zones correspond to dilated spiral arteries and newly formed vessels feeding the tumor. As choriocarcinoma is a malignant tumor, it probably produces its own vessels, contributing to the neovascularization. All of these vessels are characterized by a high velocity and low impedance blood flow pattern.

In patients with gestational trophoblastic disease, impedance to blood flow in uteroplacental vessels is significantly lower than in normal pregnancies (Shimamoto et al, 1987; Taylor et al, 1987; Long et al, 1990; Flam et al, 1991; Kurjak et al, 1994). The highest impedance is obtained in patients with complete mole, while the lowest values occur in choriocarcinoma. *Table 27.3* presents the mean resistance index (RI) values for uteroplacental vessels in patients with different types of disease.

Transvaginal color Doppler is useful in monitoring patients with gestational trophoblastic disease receiving chemotherapy (Aoki et al, 1989; Carter et al, 1993; Hsieh et al, 1994; Zanetta et al, 1996). Results showed negative correlation between β-hCG titer and vascular indices. At the same time, color coded spots representing newly formed vessels disappeared.

Color Doppler can also be helpful in differentiating pathological conditions such as postabortal uterus and other endometrial pathologies from gestational trophoblastic disease (Achiron et al, 1993).

■ CONCLUSIONS

High resolution ultrasonography, and particularly TVS, has changed the approach of both the ultrasonographer and the patient to normal and/or abnormal early embryonic development. Superb visualization has opened up the possibilities of screening for congenital anomalies very early in pregnancy and it is therefore anticipated that new methods for fetal and placental tissue sampling, together with color Doppler investigation, will alter clinical management to a certain extent. Furthermore, color Doppler studies enable confident diagnosis in patients with early pregnancy failure. Increased diagnostic accuracy has been achieved in patients with suspicious ectopic pregnancy and nonspecific adnexal masses on B-mode scan. This modality has become useful in differentiating the types of gestational trophoblastic disease, as well as in following up patients after the chemotherapy. Three-dimensional ultrasonography is another technical improvement that can be potentially useful during the first trimester of pregnancy; however, the clinical role of this and other future developments remains to be defined.

REFERENCES

Abu-Yousef MM, Bleicher JJ & Williamson RA (1987) Subchorionic hemorrhage: sonographic diagnosis and clinical significance. *AJR* **149**: 737–740.

Achiron R, Goldenberg M, Lipitz S & Mashiach S (1993) Transvaginal duplex Doppler ultrasonography in bleeding patients suspected of having residual trophoblastic tissue. *Obstet Gynecol* **81**: 507–511.

Aoki S, Hata H, Hata K et al (1989) Doppler color flow mapping of an invasive mole. *Gynecol Obstet Invest* **27**: 52–54.

Baxi L & Pearlstone M (1991) Subchorionic hematomas and presence of autoantibodies. *Am J Obstet Gynecol* **165**: 1423–1426.

Bloch C, Altchek A & Levy-Ravetch M (1989) Sonography in early pregnancy: the significance of subchorionic hemorrhage. *Mt Sinai J Med* **56**: 290–293.

Borlum KG, Thomsen A, Clausen I & Eriksen G (1989) Long-term prognosis of pregnancies in women with intrauterine hematomas. *Obstet Gynecol* **74**: 231–234.

Callen DW (1983) Ultrasonography in evaluation of gestational trophoblastic disease. In Callen PW (ed.) *Ultrasonography in Obstetrics and Gynecology*, pp 259–270. Philadelphia: WB Saunders.

Carter J, Fowler J, Carlson J et al (1993) Transvaginal color flow Doppler sonography in the assessment of gestational trophoblastic disease. *J Ultrasound Med* **12**: 595–599.

Czernobilsky B, Barasch A & Lancet M (1982) Partial moles: a clinicopathologic study of 25 cases. *Obstet Gynecol* **59**: 75–78.

Flam F, Lindholm H, Bui T-H & Lundstrom-Lindstedt V (1991) Color Doppler studies in trophoblastic tumors: a preliminary report. *Ultrasound Obstet Gynecol* **1**: 349–352.

Goldstein SR, Subramanyam BM, Raghavendra BN, Horii SC & Hilton S (1983) Subchorionic bleeding in threatened abortion: sonographic findings and clinical significance. *AJR* **141**: 975–978.

Gottesfeld KE, Leopold GR, Kohorn EI & Blackwell RJ (1967) Diagnosis of hydatidiform moles by ultrasound. *Obstet Gynecol* **30**: 163–166.

Hertzberg BS, Young RH, Jacobs PA & Kohorn EI (1986) Gestational trophoblastic disease with coexistent normal fetus: evaluation by ultrasound-guided chorionic villus sampling. *J Ultrasound Med* **5**: 467–451.

Hsieh FJ, Wu CC, Chen CA, Chen TM, Hsieh CY & Chen HY (1994) Correlation of uterine hemodynamics with chemotherapy response in gestational trophoblastic tumors. *Obstet Gynecol* **83**: 1021–1025.

Jakab A Jr, Juhasz B & Toth Z (1994) Outcome of the first trimester subchorial hematomas. In Tenth International Congress, International Society, *The Fetus as a Patient*, Brijuni, Croatia, **5**: 54 (abstract).

Jauniaux E, Zaidi J, Jurkovic D, Campbell S & Hustin J (1994) Doppler of the uteroplacental circulation in normal and complicated early pregnancies. *Hum Reprod* **9**: 2432–2437.

Joupilla P (1985) Clinical consequence after ultrasonic diagnosis of intrauterine hematoma in threatened abortion. *J Clin Ultrasound* **13**: 107–110.

Kadar N & Romero R (1982) Gray-scale findings in ectopic pregnancy resembling molar pregnancy and missed abortion. *J Clin Ultrasound* **10**: 403–406.

Kurjak A & Kupesic S (1996) Doppler assessment of the intervillous blood flow in normal and abnormal early pregnancy *Obstet Gynecol* (submitted).

Kurjak A, Zalud I, Salihagic A, Crvenkovic G & Matijevic R (1991) Transvaginal color Doppler in the assessment of abnormal early pregnancy. *J Perinat Med* **19**: 155–165.

Kurjak A, Zudenigo D, Funduk-Kurjak B, Shalan H, Predanic M & Sosic A (1993a) Transvaginal color Doppler in the assessment of the uteroplacental circulation in normal early pregnancy. *J Perinat Med* **21**: 25–34.

Kurjak A, Zudenigo D, Predanic M & Kupesic S (1993b) Recent advances in the Doppler study of early fetomaternal circulation. *J Perinat Med* **21**: 136–140.

Kurjak A, Zalud I, Predanic M & Kupesic S (1994) Transvaginal color and pulsed Doppler study of uterine blood flow in the first and early second trimester of pregnancy: normal vs. abnormal. *J Ultrasound Med* **13**: 43–48.

Kurjak A, Laurini R, Kupesic S, Kos M, Latin V & Bulic K (1995) A combined Doppler and morphopathological study of intervillous circulation. The Fifth World Congress of Ultrasound in Obstetrics and Gynecology, Kyoto, 1995. *Ultrasound Obstet Gynecol* **6 (suppl 2)**: 16 (abstract).

Kurjak A, Schulman H, Zudenigo D, Kupesic S, Kos M & Goldenberg M (1996) Subchorionic hematomas in early pregnancy: clinical outcome and blood flow patterns. *J Matern Fetal Med* **5**: 41–44.

Long MG, Boultbee JE, Begent RH, Hanson ME & Bagshawe KD (1990) Preliminary Doppler studies on the uterine artery and myometrium in trophoblastic tumors requiring chemotherapy. *Br J Obstet Gynaecol* **97**: 686–689.

Mantoni M & Fog-Pedersen J (1981) Intrauterine hematoma. An ultrasound study of threatened abortion. *Br J Obstet Gynaecol* **88**: 47–50.

Munyer TP, Szulman AE, Black MF, Merrill JA & Nelson L (1981) Further observations on the sonographic spectrum of gestational trophoblastic disease. *J Clin Ultrasound* **9**: 349–353.

Nyberg DA, Laurence AM, Benedetti TJ, Cyr DR & Schuman WP (1987) Placental abruption and placental hemorrhage: correlation of sonographic findings with fetal outcome. *Radiology* **164**: 457–460.

Pederson JF & Mantoni N (1990) Large intrauterine hematoma in threatened miscarriage. Frequency and clinical consequences. *Br J Obstet Gynaecol* **97**: 75–78.

Robinson HP (1975) Gestational sac: volumes as determined by sonar in the first trimester of pregnancy. *Br J Obstet Gynaecol* **82**: 100–107.

Sauerbrei EE & Pham DH (1986) Placental abruption and subchorionic hemorrhage in the first half of pregnancy: US appearance and clinical outcome. *Radiology* **160**: 109–111.

Shimamo S, Sakuma S, Ishigaki T & Makino N (1987) Intratumoral blood flow evaluation with color Doppler echography. *Radiology* **165**: 683–687.

Spirit BA, Kagan EH & Rozanski RM (1979) Abruptio placentae: sonographic and pathologic correlation. *AJR* **133**: 877–880.

Stabile I, Campbell S & Grudzinskas JG (1989) Threatened miscarriage and intrauterine hematomas: sonographic and biochemical studies. *J Ultrasound Med* **8**: 289–291.

Taylor KJW, Schwartz PE & Kohorn EI (1987) Gestational trophoblastic neoplasia: diagnosis with Doppler US. *Radiology* **165**: 445–448.

Valentin L, Sladkevicius P, Laurini R, Soderberg H & Marsal K (1996) Uteroplacental and luteal circulation in normal first trimester pregnancies: Doppler ultrasonographic and morphologic study. *Am J Obstet Gynecol* **174**: 768–775.

Woo JS, Wong LC & Ho-Kei MA (1985) Sonographic patterns of pelvic and hepatic lesions in persistent trophoblastic disease. *J Ultrasound Med* **4**: 189–193.

Ylostalo P, Ammala P & Seppala M (1984) Intrauterine hematoma and placental protein 5 in patients with uterine bleeding during pregnancy. *Br J Obstet Gynaecol* **91**: 353–356.

Zanetta G, Lissoni A, Colombo M, Marzola M, Cappellini A & Mangioni C (1996) Detection of abnormal intrauterine vascularization by color Doppler imaging: a possible additional aid for the follow up of patients with gestational trophoblastic tumors. *Ultrasound Obstet Gynecol* **7**: 32–37.

Section Two:
Appearances and
Classification of Pathology

PART 2
CLASSIFICATION OF PATHOLOGY

28 *Clinical use of diagnostic imaging and endoscopic techniques*
I Brosens and K Wamsteker

■ CARDINAL SIGNS AND SYMPTOMS OF GYNECOLOGICAL PELVIC DISEASE

Cardinal signs and symptoms:

1　Pelvic pain
 - premenstrual pain
 - dysmenorrhea: primary and secondary
 - dyspareunia
 - acute pelvic pain
 - chronic pelvic pain

2　Abnormal bleeding
 - amenorrhea: primary and secondary
 - oligo-/polymenorrhea
 - menorrhagia
 - intermenstrual bleeding, breakthrough bleeding
 - metrorrhagia
 - postmenopausal bleeding

3　Pelvic mass

4　Pelvic infection

5　Pelvic relaxation

6　Infertility

In all cases general gynecological procedures should be performed:
 - medical history and drug use
 - inspection of lower genital tract
 - careful bimanual examination
 - cervical cytology.

Optionally:
 - laboratory tests
 - vaginal/cervical cultures
 - endometrial tissue sampling.

The diagnostic imaging pathways provide guidelines for the application of different imaging techniques to exlude or diagnose organic lesions, in patients with specific symptoms, which are of frequent occurrence in gynecological practice.

■ ORGANIC CAUSES AND DIAGNOSTIC IMAGING

1 PELVIC PAIN

1.1 ORGANIC CAUSES

- Infection (acute and chronic): blood laboratory, culture
- Pregnancy related: positive hCG
- Endometriosis
- Nonpregnancy related adnexal pathology
- Nonpregnancy related (intra)uterine pathology
- Other intrapelvic gynecological pathology
- Intestinal pathology
- Urinary tract pathology: urine laboratory, culture

1.2 SPECIFIC SYMPTOMS AND PREFERRED DIAGNOSTIC IMAGING

- Pregnancy related

  Positive hCG   TVS/TAS
  - no intrauterine pregnancy: optionally: laparoscopy
- Dysmenorrhea

  Primary: usually idiopathic

  If ovulation inhibition is unsuccessful rule out intrapelvic pathology:
  - obstructive uterine anomaly: TVS/TAS, hysteroscopy, laparoscopy
  - endometriosis: laparoscopy

  Secondary: generally organic or iatrogenic

  To rule out intrapelvic pathology:
  - cervical obstructive factor: TVS, hysteroscopy
  - intrauterine adhesions: hysteroscopy, HSG
  - intracavitary myoma: TVS/TAS, hysteroscopy
  - adenomyosis: TVS, MRI
  - endometriosis: laparoscopy
- Dyspareunia

  To rule out intrapelvic pathology:
  - endometriosis: laparoscopy
  - chronic pelvic inflammatory disease: laparoscopy
  - mass prolapsed in cul-de-sac: TVS/TAS, laparoscopy
- Acute pelvic pain

  To rule out gynecological pathology:
  - pregnancy related (positive hCG):   TVS/TAS, laparoscopy
  - pelvic inflammatory disease: TVS/TAS, laparoscopy
  - other uterine or adnexal pathology: TVS/TAS, laparoscopy

Abbreviations: CT, computed tomography; hCG, human chorionic gonadotropin; HSG, hysterosalpingography; MRI, magnetic resonance imaging; TAS, transabdominal sonography; TVS, transvaginal sonography.

- Chronic pelvic pain

  To rule out gynecological pathology: TAS and TVS

  In addition:

  – intrauterine abnormality: hysteroscopy

  – other uterine abnormality: laparoscopy, optionally hysteroscopy

  – adnexal abnormality: tumor markers, laparoscopy

                                                          optionally color Doppler flow

  – other gynecological abnormalities: laparoscopy

  – specific abnormalities:

    adenomyosis   optionally: MRI

    pelvic congestion syndrome   optionally: uterine flebography

2 ABNORMAL BLEEDING

2.1 ORGANIC CAUSES

- Pregnancy related: positive hCG
- Benign or malignant organic pelvic lesions: vagina, uterus, tubes, ovary
- Extragenital problems (coagulopathies, endocrinopathology, iatrogenic)

2.2 SPECIFIC SYMPTOMS AND DIAGNOSTIC IMAGING FOR GYNECOLOGICAL PATHOLOGY

- Primary amenorrhea

  If congenital anomaly is suspected: TAS, laparoscopy, hysteroscopy

                                                          HSG

                                                          optionally: MRI

- Secondary amenorrhea

  Exclude pregnancy: hCG, TVS

  If intrauterine adhesions are suspected: hysteroscopy, HSG

- Oligomenorrhea/polymenorrhea

  If organic lesions are suspected: TVS, laparoscopy, hysteroscopy

- Menorrhagia/hypermenorrhea

  To exclude:

    – intrauterine pathology: TVS, hysteroscopy, (HSG)

    – other uterine pathology: TAS, laparoscopy

    – adenomyosis: TVS, MRI

- Metrorrhagia/intermenstrual bleeding

  To exclude:

    – (intra)uterine pathology: TVS/TAS, hysteroscopy/histology

    – adnexal pathology: TVS/TAS, laparoscopy

- Postmenopausal bleeding

  To exclude:

    – (intra)uterine pathology: TVS/TAS, hysteroscopy/histology

                                                          optionally: color Doppler flow

    – adnexal pathology: TVS/TAS, laparoscopy

                                                          optionally: color Doppler flow

3 PELVIC MASS

3.1 ORGANIC CAUSES

- Uterine origin (pregnancy, retrodisplacement, leiomyomas, adenomyosis, malignant uterine tumors, congenital anomaly, hematometra-pyometra)
- Tubal origin (paraovarian cyst, ectopic pregnancy, torsion, chronic inflammatory process, tuberculosis, benign neoplasm, tubal carcinoma)
- Ovarian origin (functional cysts, endometrioma, torsion, ovarian abscess, benign neoplasm, malignant tumor)
- Extragenital pelvic origin (inflammatory, hematocele, ascites, urological lesions, gastrointestinal lesions, retroperitoneal lesions, abdominal wall lesions)

3.2 ORIGIN OF MASS AND DIAGNOSTIC IMAGING PROCEDURES

- Uterine: TVS/TAS, hysteroscopy, laparoscopy, (hysterography)
- Tubal: TVS/TAS, color Doppler flow, laparoscopy
- Ovarian: TVS/TAS, color Doppler flow, laparoscopy
- Extragenital: TAS, abdominal X-ray, barium enema, pyelography, laparoscopy
- For all pelvic masses: optionally: CT, MRI

4 PELVIC RELAXATION

DIAGNOSTIC IMAGING PROCEDURES

- Anterior compartment: videocystourethrography, intravenous pyelography, TVS, perineal ultrasonography, cystoscopy, bead chain cystourethrography
- Posterior compartment: defecating proctography, scintigraphic defecography
- Combined: optionally: MRI, colpocystodefecography

5 PELVIC INFECTION

DIAGNOSTIC IMAGING PROCEDURES: TVS/TAS, laparoscopy

6 FEMALE INFERTILITY

DIAGNOSTIC IMAGING PROCEDURES

- Routine investigation: HSG, TVS, laparoscopy
- On indication:
    - suspected intrauterine pathology: hysteroscopy
    - suspected other uterine or adnexal pathology: TAS, laparoscopy
    - specific tubal investigation: salpingoscopy, selective salpingography

29 *International classification systems*
L Cohen, L Keith and JJ Sciarra

■ INTRODUCTION

Recent advances in the electronic transfer of information and medical technology underscore an urgent need for physicians to compare treatment modalities and outcomes using consistent nomenclature. In the past, efforts at comparison were often hampered by the absence of uniform classifications of treatments and/or specific therapeutic endpoints. This circumstance differed considerably from the uniformity afforded by wide use of an international classification system for diseases (ICD-9). This document has undergone nine revisions and is currently available in print as well as in electronic form.

Within the discipline of obstetrics and gynecology, no international format presently exists for comparison of treatment modalities and/or outcome measures. In addition, the few existing classification systems are not universally accepted. Of greater importance, no formal or informal method exists by which the international community of obstetrics and gynecology can evaluate, refine, promulgate or ratify proposed classification systems.

Within obstetrics and gynecology, classification systems have been proposed in one of the three following ways:

- by international organizations such as the International Federation of Gynecology and Obstetrics (FIGO);
- by national societies;
- by individual practitioners who have had no input, advice or sponsorship from organized medicine.

■ SURVEY RESULTS

After determining the absence of any formal or informal database of existing and/or proposed classification systems, we conducted an informal survey of 22 members of the FIGO leadership. The purpose of this effort was to augment our own review and to solicit experienced counsel. The response to our solicitation was 100%. Information was received from individuals in decision making positions at academic centers on six continents. A list of the survey participants is presented in *Table 29.1*. Our survey determined:

- which classification systems for gynecologial diseases or conditions were used internationally;
- respondents' opinions about the use of such systems.

Based on these replies, the FIGO classification of gynecological cancer appears to enjoy the greatest international recognition and use. In addition, the former American Fertility Society (AFS)* staging system for endometriosis enjoys a similar reputation. In contrast, the AFS classification systems for uterine anomalies and adhesions do not have the same degree of acceptance. In other instances, exemplified by trophoblastic disease, different classification systems compete for acceptance, a situation which leads to considerable confusion.

The survey respondents additionally described numerous classification systems that had been proposed over the years, but as yet had not been widely accepted, including those for stress incontinence, pelvic prolapse, intrauterine adhesions and vaginal fistulas.

Perhaps most importantly, the survey reinforced what had been our initial impression, that is, that although classification systems have been available for years, they have little chance of being accepted at a national or international level without peer review and modification. Similarly, it became clear that without national or international sponsorship a specific classification system is unlikely to undergo periodic review and revision

---

* Name changed to the American Society for Reproductive Medicine in 1994. For the purposes of this chapter, we will use former name of American Fertility Society (AFS).

Table 29.1 *Survey participants and corresponding location*

Participant	Location
Professor S Azulkumaran	Singapore
Profesor Guiseppe Benagiano	Switzerland
Professor George Creatsas	Greece
Professor M Elstein	United Kingdom
Professor Mahmoud Fathalla	Egypt
Dr Juan Y Fuentes Jr	Philippines
Professor Lars Hamberger	Sweden
Professor Ho Kei Ma	United Kingdom
Professor Laszlo Kozacs	Hungary
Professor Walter Kuhn	Germany
Dr Timothy Johnson	United States
Dr George D Malkasian Jr	United States
Professor Con Michael	Australia
Dr John O'Loughlin	Australia
Dr Naren Patel	United Kingdom
Professor Joseph Schenker	Israel
Professor Markku Seppala	Finland
Mr Ralph Settatree	United Kingdom
Professor Shirish Sheth	India
Dr Milton Siew Wah Lum	Malaysia
Professor Vit Unzeitig	Czech Republic

when practice patterns or technologies change. This lack of timely review appears to be the most important factor relating to clinicians' disagreements with a system and thus their decision not to use it.

■ INTERNATIONAL CLASSIFICATION SYSTEMS

The development of the present FIGO staging system for gynecological cancer has been long and complex. Initial attempts at classification of gynecological malignancy were undertaken by the League of Nations Health Organization in 1929 (International Federation of Gynecology and Obstetrics, 1994). The original purpose of these discussions was to coordinate the treatment of cervical cancer in order that uniform radiation protocols could be developed. Under the aegis of varying organizations, 11 reports were published on the treatment of gynecological cancer between the years 1929 and 1955. An equal number have been published since 1958, when FIGO took over reporting responsibility.

A recent revision of this classification took place in 1988 and was published in 1989. At that time, it was recommended that cancers of the vulva, uterus and ovary be surgically staged. Subsequent revisions in 1991 and 1994 respectively addressed staging for gestational trophoblastic disease and a revision of the staging system for cervical cancer. At first glance, the frequency of change may appear disconcerting, but it is important to recognize that these changes have been critical in obtaining the present worldwide acceptance of the FIGO staging system for malignancies. In our opinion, this system should serve as a model of the need for periodic review and modification.

■ NATIONAL CLASSIFICATION SYSTEMS

As the FIGO work progressed, the TNM classification system for malignant disease was developed by the International Union Against Cancer. The philosophy of this staging system is that the biological behavior of a malignancy is best described by the size and location of the primary tumor (T), lymph node status (N), and the presence of metastasis (M). The International Union Against Cancer, along with the American Joint Committee on Cancer, published the *Manual for Staging of Cancer* in 1977. Revised editions of this publication appear in 1983, 1988 and 1992 (American Joint Committee on Cancer Staging, 1992).

■ PROPOSED INDIVIDUAL PRACTITIONER'S CLASSIFICATION SYSTEMS

By way of example, we shall describe the present situation in relation to corrective surgery for pelvic relaxation and obstetric vesicovaginal fistulas. Renewed academic interest in surgery for pelvic prolapse became apparent in the late 1980s and early 1990s. Attempts were made to correlate the fascial and vaginal defects seen in cadaver specimens with findings obtained on magnetic resonance imaging (MRI). Work by Delancey (1992) suggested that fascial defects on the pelvic floor can be separated into three distinct groups, all of which relate to the extent of existing support. Such defects have been documented with MRI (Yang et al, 1991; Ozasa et al, 1992). Despite these interesting observations, national and international organizations such as the Society of Gynecologic Surgeons, the American Urogynecologic Society and the International Continence Society, working individually or collectively, have not seen fit to consider organizing a task force to develop a uniform classification system for defects of the pelvic fascia which might achieve either national or international acceptance (Shull, 1995).

The same problem exists for other conditions such as vesicovaginal fistulas. Although these defects are rare in industrialized countries, they are relatively common in developing countries. Many classification systems have been proposed and are still being proposed (Elkins, 1994). As an example, Waaldijik (1995) suggested another classification system for fistulas. Regardless of the merit of individual classification proposals, our survey suggests that they are likely to languish in the literature unless they are adopted by a sponsoring organization. Two other examples of individual practitioner's classification systems will be given later in this chapter.

■ COOPERATION BETWEEN EXISTING CLASSIFICATION SYSTEMS

The occasional coexistence of two competing systems may lead to crossfertilization and enhanced acceptance. For example, in 1988 the FIGO staging system for vulvar malignancy incorporated the TNM scoring system. Similarly, when the fourth edition of the *Manual for Staging of Cancer* appeared in 1992, it incorporated the TNM categories and created corresponding FIGO stages. At present, the FIGO system is the most widely used international classification system, whereas the TNM system is mainly used in the United States for staging gynecological malignancy in order to comply with the reporting requirements of the National Cancer Institute.

The scope of this chapter does not permit us to review either the complete FIGO or the TNM staging for gynecological malignancy. Regardless, it is important to mention that the change from clinical to surgical staging for malignancy of the vulva, uterus and ovary was instituted because appropriate treatment requires knowledge of the size of the tumor, the depth of invasion, lymph node status and metastatic spread. The combined FIGO–TNM classification for staging of vulvar carcinoma is an example of the utility of this process. Prior to the adoption of surgical staging in 1988, patients were often incorrectly staged owing to an inability to properly assess metastatic spread to the inguinal and femoral lymph nodes. This inadequacy in staging led to problems of undertreatment as well as overtreatment. In contrast, the knowledge of lymph node status in this specific disease entity enables the surgeon to adjust the extent of the vulvectomy as well as the nature of adjuvant therapy, if any. In a similar manner, the surgical staging of uterine and ovarian cancer more accurately describes the metastatic spread of these diseases and allows for more appropriate adjuvant treatment and the use and development of new protocols.

■ CONTROVERSY AND FAILURE OF ACCEPTANCE

In all fairness, it should be noted that although the FIGO classification system for gynecological malignancy is widely used, some of its aspects remain controversial. An example is the debate surrounding the classification of trophoblastic diseases. In the United States, the National Institutes of Health (NIH) classification system for gestational trophoblastic disease, published in 1973, was based on work by Hammond and colleagues, which basically divided this disease into nonmetastatic and metastatic categories. The latter category was further subdivided into good prognosis and poor prognosis groups (Hammond et al, 1973). In 1983, a decade after the NIH system was published, the World Health Organization (WHO) Scientific Group published its own classification system for trophoblastic disease based on the work of Bagshawe and colleagues. This latter publication introduced the scoring of high risk characteristics into the classification system of trophoblastic disease.

In 1988, FIGO attempted to establish its own classification system for trophoblastic disease. This attempt failed to achieve wide acceptance because neither the NIH nor the WHO criteria for risk staging was incorporated into this new version. In response to this failure, FIGO modified its classification system in 1992 to recognize the high risk characteristics established by both Hammond and by Bagshawe (Creasman, 1992). Despite this, however, many centers continue to stage trophoblastic disease using either the NIH or the WHO criteria. It would appear that further effort will be required to establish a uniform and internationally accepted classification system for this disease. Work by Lurain and colleagues (1991) suggests that a system incorporating aspects from both the NIH and the WHO classification systems would perform optimally in predicting high risk trophoblastic disease. At the present time, this issue remains unresolved.

At the same time that FIGO was attempting to establish a classification system for trophoblastic disease, the then AFS published six classification systems for specific gynecological diseases, including adnexal adhesions, distal tubal occlusion, tubal occlusion secondary to tubal ligation, tubal pregnancies, Müllerian anomalies and intrauterine adhesions (American Fertility Society, 1988). The purpose of these systems was to provide clinicians with meaningful instruments for comparing operative protocols and techniques. Unfortunately, unlike their now widely accepted scoring system for endometriosis, none of these newer classification systems appears to have received international acceptance.

Perhaps two other papers relating to infertility surgery are worthy of note in this regard. Valle and Sciarra (1988) used the hysteroscope for treatment of intrauterine adhesions, and developed a classification system in conjunction with this study. They were able to correlate subsequent pregnancy rates with the severity of the disease described; however, this classification system has not yet been adopted by other investigators in this field. In a similar fashion, Marana and colleagues (1995) were able to correlate the severity of adnexal adhesions with decreased subsequent pregnancy rates. Whether the system they developed will be used by others is a matter of speculation. In general it would appear that for any classification system not related to life threatening diseases to gain real acceptance, the sponsorship of an international organization such as FIGO is crucial.

The issues related to classification of urinary incontinence are not unique and reflect problems already cited in this chapter. Blaivas and Olsson (1988) proposed a change in the clinical classification system for urinary stress incontinence, describing four distinct anatomical categories and labeling them as types 0–3. This revision was deemed necessary in order to correlate operative success with the anatomical defects found at preoperative workup. Other workers, including Abrams and colleagues (1990), representing the International Continence Society, emphasized the need for the use of standard terminology in the description of lower urinary tract function. Unfortunately, to date neither the proposed revision in clinical classification nor nomenclature has been widely accepted in either clinical practice or published reports. Perhaps these materials are too new to have gained acceptance on a local or national basis. On the other hand, the fact that these proposals have been made by individuals in the first instance and a small society in the second may impede their further acceptance.

▪ STANDARDIZED IMAGE DISPLAY

Although not strictly the subject of this chapter, the need for standardization is further exemplified by the lack of an internationally accepted orientation system for the display of transvaginal ultrasound images. This issue was initially raised by Bernaschek and Deutinger (1989) and reviewed by Sabbagha and colleagues (1994). Simply stated, confusion arises from the fact that individual authors have used four different orientations in displaying sagittal transvaginal images. These are:

- the cervix superior and the bladder to the right;
- the cervix superior and the bladder to the left;
- the cervix inferior and bladder to the right;
- the cervix inferior and bladder to the left.

As noted by Bernaschek, the most anatomically familiar view for the clinician is with the cervix inferior on the image and the bladder on the right side. This approximates a sagittal section on a transabdominal image. These

four orientations are shown in *Figure 29.1*. In view of the worldwide popularity of ultrasonography, an internationally accepted standard orientation would assist clinicians in their interpretation of the literature.

▪ MODEL CLASSIFICATION SYSTEM

The evolution of the AFS classification system for endometriosis, now utilized internationally, is an excellent model to follow in the evaluation and review of a classification system. This example demonstrates how a classification system can grow from one individual's idea to an internationally utilized classification system. In this case, however, it took several years and many revisions before the classification system for endometriosis was internationally accepted. In its present form, it serves as an irreplaceable system for the comparison of endometriosis worldwide and has been of invaluable assistance to physicians and their patients.

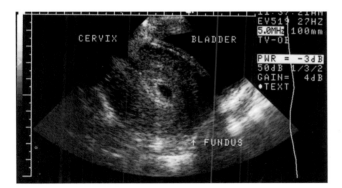

29.1a

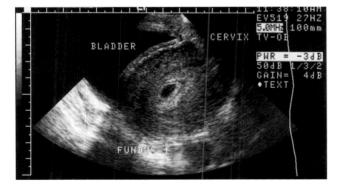

29.1b

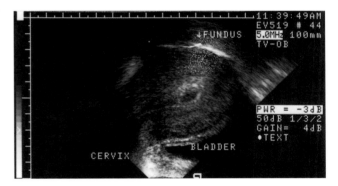

29.1c

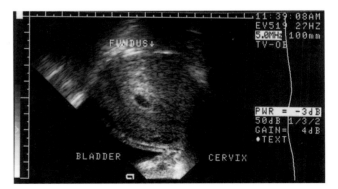

29.1d

Figure 29.1: *This figure displays a 5 week intrauterine pregnancy. The uterus is anteverted. These four transvaginal sagittal images display the four possible orientations available on most machines. They* are: (a) the cervix superior and the bladder to the right; (b) the cervix superior and the bladder to the left; (c) the cervix inferior and the bladder to the right; (d) the cervix inferior and the bladder to the left.

Originally proposed by Acosta and colleagues (1973), this system was deemed unsatisfactory because it understaged the severity of endometriosis in some women. This deficit was addressed by a new classification system proposed by Kistner and colleagues (1977). Despite this revision, many practitioners continued to take issue with either or both systems. In an effort to end this discourse and develop an agreeable classification system, the AFS formed a committee to study the problem and published its first report in 1979. A major revision took place in 1985 (Buttram, 1985). This version is now widely used throughout the world. More importantly, its use has enabled clinicians worldwide to compare their findings and treatment modalities with a uniform staging system.

Buttram's review of the historical evolution of the AFS's classification of endometriosis highlights the need for peer review and modification of classification systems proposed by individuals (Buttram, 1985). It also emphasizes that when a classification system is defined, reviewed and sponsored by a nationally based organization, it is more likely to achieve international acceptance. Despite this encouragement, not all nationally sponsored systems receive international acceptance.

As shown by the references listed in the appendix to this chapter, classification systems receive their initial presentation from diverse sources. These include individually authored articles, chapters in collated textbooks, publications from learned societies, technical bulletins from national societies and, in the rare instance, reports of standing committees of international organizations such as FIGO. Under these circumstances it is not surprising that many excellent suggestions have not received wider recognition.

Those systems currently accepted internationally are shown in *Tables 29.2–29.5* and *Figure 29.2*.

■ CONCLUSION

We believe that sponsorship by a respected organization is critical to the international acceptance of any proposed classification system. The committee system under the forum of national and international organizations appears to be an appropriate means of achieving a mutually satisfactory consensus. The historical evolution of the FIGO gynecological malignancy score clearly demonstrates that continued review and modification of any classification system is important and necessary to ensure its widespread acceptance. In contrast, systems advocated by individual practitioners in specific institutions are less likely to find general acceptance and more likely to be faulted by practitioners at other institutions. In addition to having sponsorship, we believe relevant classification systems should be simple to apply, relevant to clinical practice and subject to periodic review.

We purposely adopted a broad view in the approach to this chapter. Because of this, we included information on a large number of gynecological conditions, some of which have accepted classification systems and others of which do not. We encourage further study and discussion in this area, as we believe that clinicians will benefit from enhanced methods of precise communication.

As we move into the twenty first century, with the heavy emphasis on information systems and outcome based research, it behooves international bodies such as FIGO to take the forefront in evaluating and supporting the development of standardized classification systems. We believe that use of appropriate classification systems at the onset of treatment will allow the medical community of all variations to compare patients, varying treatment modalities and therapeutic outcomes in a more meaningful manner than has been possible in the past.

Table 29.2 *FIGO staging for carcinoma of the cervix uteri*

Stage 0 Carcinoma in situ, intraepithelial carcinoma

Stage I The carcinoma is strictly confined to the cervix (extension to the corpus should be disregarded)

Stage IA Preclinical carcinomas of the cervix, that is, those diagnosed only by microscopy

Stage IA1 Minimal microscopically evident stromal invasion

Stage IA2 Lesions detected microscopically that can be measured. The upper limit of the measurement should not show a depth of invasion of more than 5 mm taken from the base of the epithelium, either surface or glandular, from which it originates, and a second dimension, the horizontal spread, must not exceed 7 mm. Larger lesions should be classified as stage IB

Stage IB Lesions of greater dimensions than stage IA2, whether seen clinically or not. Preformed space involvement should not alter the staging but should be specifically recorded so as to determine whether it should affect treatment decisions in the future

Stage II The carcinoma extends beyond the cervix but has not extended to the pelvic wall. The carcinoma involves the vagina but not as far as the lower third

Stage IIA No obvious parametrial involvement

Stage IIB Obvious parametrial involvement

Stage III The carcinoma has extended to the pelvic wall. On rectal examination, there is no cancer-free space between the tumor and the pelvic wall.

The tumor involves the lower third of the vagina.

All cases with a hydronephrosis or nonfunctioning kidney are included unless they are known to be due to other causes

Stage IIIA No extension to the pelvic wall

Stage IIIB Extension to the pelvic wall and/or hydronephrosis or nonfunctioning kidney

Stage IV The carcinoma has extended beyond the true pelvis or has clinically involved the mucosa of the bladder or rectum. A bullous edema as such does not permit a case to be allotted to stage IV

Stage IVA Spread of the growth to the adjacent organs

Stage IVB Spread to distant organs

Notes about the staging

Stage IA carcinoma should include minimal microscopically evident stromal invasion as well as small cancerous tumors of measurable size. Stage IA should be divided into those lesions with minute foci of invasion visible only microscopically as stage IA1 and macroscopically measurable microcarcinomas as stage IA2, in order to gain further knowledge of the clinical behavior of these lesions. The term 'IB occult' should be omitted.

The diagnosis of both stage IA1 and IA2 cases should be based on microscopic examination of removed tissue, preferably a cone, which must include the entire lesion. The lower limit of stage IA2 should be measurable macroscopically (even if dots need to be placed on the slide prior to measurement), and the upper limit of stage IA2 is given by measurement of the two largest dimensions in any given section. The depth of invasion should not be more than 5 mm taken from the base of the epithelium, either surface or glandular, from which it originates. The second dimension, the horizontal spread, must not exceed 7 mm. Vascular space involvement, either venous or lymphatic, should not alter the staging but should be specifically recorded, as it may affect treatment decisions in the future.

Lesions of greater size should be classified as stage IB.

As a rule, it is impossible to estimate clinically whether a cancer of the cervix has extended to the corpus or not. Extension to the corpus should therefore be disregarded.

A patient with a growth fixed to the pelvic wall by a short and indurated but not nodular parametrium should be allotted to stage IIB. It is impossible, at clinical examination, to decide whether a smooth and indurated parametrium is truly cancerous or only inflammatory. Therefore, the case should be placed in stage III only if the parametrium is nodular on the pelvic wall or if the growth itself extends to the pelvic wall.

The presence of hydronephrosis or nonfunctioning kidney due to stenosis of the ureter by cancer permits a case to be allotted to stage III even if, according to the other findings, the case should be allotted to stage I or stage II.

The presence of bullous edema, as such, should not permit a case to be allotted to stage IV. Ridges and furrows in the bladder wall should be interpreted as signs of submucous involvement of the bladder if they remain fixed to the growth during palpation (i.e. examination from the vagina or the rectum during cystoscopy). A finding of malignant cells in cytologic washings from the urinary bladder requires further examination and a biopsy from the wall of the bladder.

From International Federation of Gynecology and Obstetrics (1988) Annual Report on the Results of Treatment in Gynecological Cancer, *vol. 20. Stockholm: FIGO. Reprinted with kind permission from Elsevier Science Ireland Ltd, Bay 15K, Shannon Industrial Estate, Co. Clare, Ireland.*

Table 29.3 *FIGO staging for carcinoma of the corpus uteri*

Stage IA	G123	Tumor limited to endometrium
Stage IB	G123	Invasion to less than one half the myometrium
Stage IC	G123	Invasion to more than one half the myometrium
Stage IIA	G123	Endocervical glandular involvement only
Stage IIB	G123	Cervical stromal invasion
Stage IIIA	G123	Tumor invades serosa and/or adnexa, and/or positive peritoneal cytology
Stage IIIB	G123	Vaginal metastases
Stage IIIC	G123	Metastases to pelvic and/or para-aortic lymph nodes
Stage IVA	G123	Tumor invasion of bladder and/or bowel mucosa
Stage IVB		Distant metastases including intra-abdominal and/or inguinal lymph nodes

Histopathology – degree of differentiation
Cases of carcinoma of the corpus should be classified (or graded) according to the degree of histological differentiation, as follows:
G1 = 5% or less of a nonsquamous or nonmorular solid growth pattern
G2 = 6–50% of a nonsquamous or nonmorular solid growth pattern
G3 = more than 50% of a nonsquamous or nonmorular solid growth pattern

Notes on pathological grading

1 Notable nuclear atypia, inappropriate for the architectural grade, raises the grade of a grade 1 or grade 2 tumor by 1
2 In serous adenocarcinomas, clear cell adenocarcinomas, and squamous cell carcinomas, nuclear grading takes precedence
3 Adenocarcinomas with squamous differentiation are graded according to the nuclear grade of the glandular component

Rules related to staging

1 Because corpus cancer is now staged surgically, procedures previously used for determination of stages are no longer applicable, such as the findings from fractional D&C to differentiate between stage I and stage II
2 It is appreciated that there may be a small number of patients with corpus cancer who will be treated primarily with radiation therapy. If that is the case, the clinical staging adopted by FIGO in 1971 would still apply, but designation of that staging system would be noted
3 Ideally, width of the myometrium should be measured along with the width of tumor invasion

From International Federation of Gynecology and Obstetrics (1989) Annual report on the results of treatment in gynecological cancer. Int J Gynecol Obstet *28: 189–190. Reprinted with kind permission from Elsevier Science Ireland Ltd, Bay 15K, Shannon Industrial Estate, Co. Clare, Ireland.*

Table 29.4 *FIGO staging for carcinoma of the ovary*

Staging of ovarian carcinoma is based on findings at clinical examination and by surgical exploration. The histological findings are to be considered in the staging, as are the cytologic findings as far as effusions are concerned. It is desirable that a biopsy be taken from suspicious areas outside of the pelvis.

Stage I	Growth limited to the ovaries
Stage IA	Growth limited to one ovary; no ascites present containing malignant cells. No tumor on the external surface; capsule intact
Stage IB	Growth limited to both ovaries; no ascites present containing malignant cells. No tumor on the external surfaces; capsules intact
Stage IC*	Tumor classified as either stage IA or IB but with tumor on the surface of one or both ovaries; or with ruptured capsule(s); or with ascites containing malignant cells present or with positive peritoneal washings
Stage II	Growth involving one or both ovaries, with pelvic extension
Stage IIA	Extension and/or metastases to the uterus and/or tubes
Stage IIB	Extension to other pelvic tissues
Stage IIC*	Tumor either stage IIA or IIB but with tumor on the surface of one or both ovaries; or with capsule(s) ruptured; or with ascites containing malignant cells present or with positive peritoneal washings
Stage III	Tumor involving one or both ovaries with peritoneal implants outside the pelvis and/or positive retroperitoneal or inguinal nodes. Superficial liver metastasis equals stage III. Tumor is limited to the true pelvis but with histologically proven malignant extension to small bowel or omentum
Stage IIIA	Tumor grossly limited to the true pelvis with negative nodes but with histologically confirmed microscopic seeding of abdominal peritoneal surfaces
Stage IIIB	Tumor of one or both ovaries with histologically confirmed implants of abdominal peritoneal surfaces none exceeding 2 cm in diameter; nodes are negative
Stage IIIC	Abdominal implants greater than 2 cm in diameter and/or positive retroperitoneal or inguinal nodes
Stage IV	Growth involving one or both ovaries, with distant metastases. If pleural effusion is present, there must be positive cytological findings to allot a case to stage IV. Parenchymal liver metastasis equals stage IV

* *Notes about the staging*: To evaluate the impact on prognosis of the different criteria for allotting cases to stage IC or IIC, it would be of value to know whether the rupture of the capsule was spontaneous or caused by the surgeon and if the source of malignant cells detected was peritoneal washings or ascites.

From *International Federation of Gynecology and Obstetrics (1989) Annual report on the results of treatment in gynecological cancer.* Int J Gynecol Obstet **28**: 189–190. *Reprinted with kind permission from Elsevier Science Ireland Ltd, Bay 15K, Shannon Industrial Estate, Co. Clare, Ireland.*

Table 29.5 *FIGO staging for carcinoma of the vagina*

Stage 0	Carcinoma in situ, intraepithelial carcinoma
Stage I	The carcinoma is limited to the vaginal wall
Stage II	The carcinoma has involved the subvaginal tissue but has not extended to the pelvic wall
Stage III	The carcinoma has extended to the pelvic wall
Stage IV	The carcinoma has extended beyond the true pelvis or has clinically involved the mucosa of the bladder or rectum. Bullous edema as such does not permit a case to be allotted to stage IV
Stage IVA	Spread of the growth to adjacent organs and/or direct extension beyond the true pelvis
Stage IVB	Spread to distant organs

From *International Federation of Gynecology and Obstetrics (1988) Annual Report on the Results of Treatment in Gynecological Cancer, vol. 20.* Stockholm: FIGO. *Reprinted with kind permission from Elsevier Science Ireland Ltd, Bay 15K, Shannon Industrial Estate, Co. Clare, Ireland.*

AFS Clasification of Endometriosis

Patient's Name _____ Date _____

Stage I   (Minimal) - 1–5
Stage II   (Mild)   - 6–15
Stage III (Moderate) - 16–40
Stage IV (Severe)   - > 40

Laparoscopy _____ Laparotomy _____ Photography _____

Recommended Treatment _____

Total _____

Prognosis _____

PERITONEUM	**ENDOMETRIOSIS**	< 1cm	1–3cm	> 3cm
	Superficial	1	2	4
	Deep	2	4	6
OVARY	R Superficial	1	2	4
	Deep	4	16	20
	L Superficial	1	2	4
	Deep	4	16	20

	POSTERIOR CULDESAC OBLITERATION	Partial	Complete
		4	40

	ADHESIONS	< 1/3 Enclosure	1/3 – 2/3 Enclosure	> 2/3 Enclosure
OVARY	R Filmy	1	2	4
	Dense	4	8	16
	L Filmy	1	2	4
	Dense	4	8	16
TUBE	R Filmy	1	2	4
	Dense	4*	8*	16
	L Filmy	1	2	4
	Dense	4*	8*	16

* If the fimbriated end of the fallopian tube is completely enclosed, change the point assignment to 16.

Additional Endometriosis: _____

_____

_____

_____

Associated Pathology: _____

_____

_____

_____

To Be Used with Normal
Tubes and Ovaries

L   R

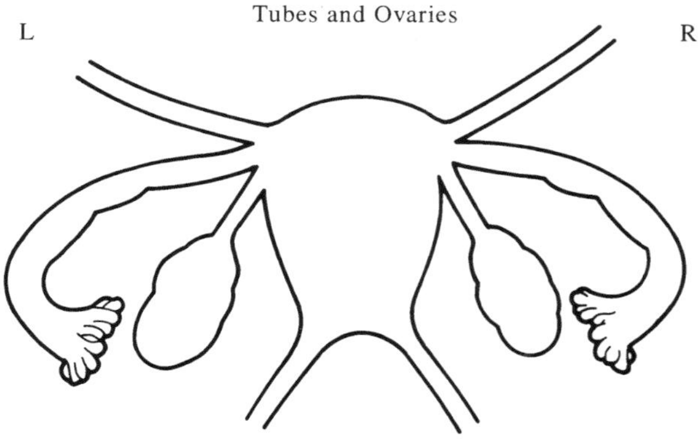

To Be Used with Abnormal
Tubes and/or Ovaries

L   R

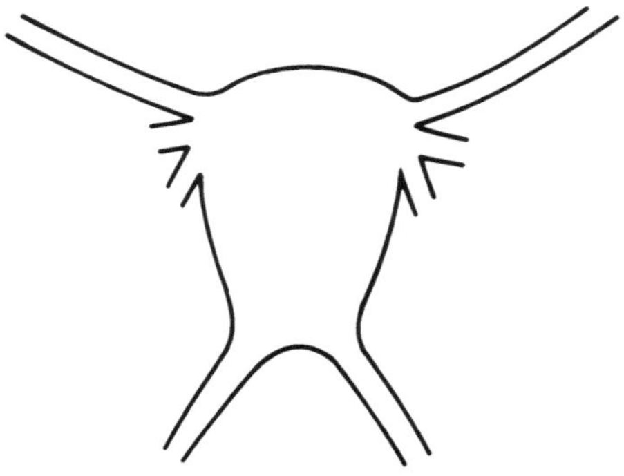

Figure 29.2

EXAMPLES & GUIDELINES

STAGE I (MINIMAL)

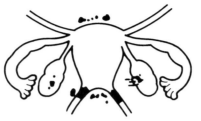

PERITONEUM
Superficial Endo — 1-3cm — 2
R. OVARY
Superficial Endo — <1 cm — 1
Filmy Adhesions — <1/3 — 1
TOTAL POINTS 4

STAGE II (MILD)

PERITONEUM
Deep Endo — >3cm — 6
R. OVARY
Superficial Endo — <1cm — 1
Filmy Adhesions — <1/3 — 1
L. OVARY
Superficial Endo — <1cm — 1
TOTAL POINTS 9

STAGE III (MODERATE)

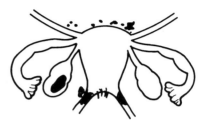

PERITONEUM
Deep Endo — >3cm — 6
CULDESAC
Partial Obliteration — 4
L. OVARY
Deep Endo — 1-3cm — 16
TOTAL POINTS 26

STAGE III (MODERATE)

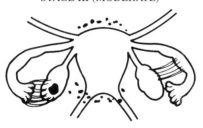

PERITONEUM
Superficial Endo — >3cm — 4
R. TUBE
Filmy Adhesions — <1/3 — 1
R. OVARY
Filmy Adhesions — <1/3 — 1
L. TUBE
Dense Adhesions — <1/3 — 16 *
L. OVARY
Deep Endo — <1cm — 4
Dense Adhesions — <1/3 — 4
TOTAL POINTS 30

STAGE IV (SEVERE)

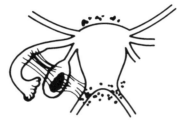

PERITONEUM
Superficial Endo — >3cm — 4
L. OVARY
Deep Endo — 1-3cm — 32 **
Dense Adhesions — <1-3 — 8 **
L. TUBE
Dense Adhesions — <1/3 — 8 **
TOTAL POINTS 52

*Point assignment changed to 16
**Point assignment doubled

STAGE IV (SEVERE)

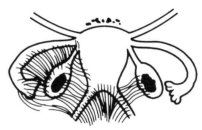

PERITONEUM
Deep Endo — >3cm — 6
CULDESAC
Complete Obliteration — 40
R. OVARY
Deep Endo — 1-3cm — 16
Dense Adhesions — <1/3 — 4
L. TUBE
Dense Adhesions — >2/3 — 16
L. OVARY
Deep Endo — 1-3 — 16
Dense Adhesions — >2/3 — 16
TOTAL POINTS 114

Determination of the stage or degree of endometrial involvement is based on a weighted point sytem. Distribution of points has been arbitrarily determined and may require further revision or refinement as knowledge of the disease increases.

To ensure complete evaluation, inspection of the pelvis in a clockwise or counterclockwise fashion is encouraged. Number, size and location of endometrial implants, plaques, endometriomas and/or adhesions are noted. For example, five separate 0.5cm superficial implants on the peritoneum (2.5 cm total) would be assigned 2 points. (The surface of the uterus should be considered peritoneum.) The severity of the endometriosis or adhesions should be assigned the highest score only for peritoneum, ovary, tube or culdesac. For example, a 4cm superficial and a 2cm deep implant of the peritoneum should be given a score of 6 (not 8). A 4cm deep endometrioma of the ovary associated with more than 3cm of superficial disease should be scored 20 (not 24).

In those patients with only one adnexa, points applied to disease of the remaining tube and ovary should be multiplied by two. **Points assigned may be circled and totaled. Aggregation of points indicates stage of disease (minimal, mild, moderate, or severe).

The presence of endometriosis of the bowel, urinary tract, fallopian tube, vagina, cervix, skin etc., should be documented under "additional endometriosis." Other pathology such as tubal occlusion, leiomyomata, urine anomaly, etc., should be documented under "associated pathology." All pathology should be depicted as specifically as possible on the sketch of pelvic organs and means of observation (laparoscopy or laparotomy) should be noted.

Figure 29.2: The American Fertility Society revised classification of endometriosis. From The American Fertility Society (1985) Revised American Fertility Society Classification of Endometriosis: 1985.

Fertil Steril **43**: 351–352. *Reproduced with permission of the publisher, the American Society for Reproductive Medicine (formerly The American Fertility Society).*

▪ APPENDIX: REFERENCES FOR CLASSIFICATION SYSTEMS OF VARIOUS GYNECOLOGICAL DISEASES

CARCINOMA OF THE CERVIX UTERI

International Federation of Gynecology and Obstetrics (1994) *Annual Report of the Results of Treatment in Gynecological Cancer*, vol. 22. FIGO, Editorial Office Radiumhemmet, S 104 01 Stockholm, Sweden.

American College of Obstetricians and Gynecologists (1991) Clasification and staging of gynecologic malignancies. *ACOG Tech Bull* 155 (May).

CARCINOMA OF THE CORPUS UTERI

International Federation of Gynecology and Obstetrics (1994) *Annual Report on the Results of Treatment in Gynecological Cancer*, vol. 22. FIGO, Editorial Office Radiumhemmet, S 104 01 Stockholm, Sweden.

American College of Obstetricians and Gynecologists (1991) Classification and staging of gynecologic malignancies. *ACOG Tech Bull* 155 (May).

CARCINOMA OF THE OVARY

International Federation of Gynecology and Obstetrics (1994) *Annual Report on the Results of Treatment in Gynecological Cancer*, vol. 22. FIGO, Editorial Office Radiumhemmet, S 104 01 Stockholm, Sweden.

American College of Obstetricians and Gynecologists (1991) Classification and staging of gynecologic malignancies. *ACOG Tech Bull* 155 (May).

CARCINOMA OF THE VULVA

International Federation of Gynecology and Obstetrics (1994) *Annual Report on the Results of Treatment in Gynecological Cancer*, vol. 22. FIGO, Editorial Office Radiumhemmet, S 104 01 Stockholm, Sweden.

American College of Obstetricians and Gynecologists (1991) Classification and staging of gynecologic malignancies. *ACOG Tech Bull* 155 (May).

CARCINOMA OF THE VAGINA

International Federation of Gynecology and Obstetrics (1994) *Annual Report on the Results of Treatment in Gynecological Cancer*, vol. 22. FIGO, Editorial Office Radiumhemmet, S 104 01 Stockholm, Sweden.

American College of Obstetricians and Gynecologists (1991) Classification and staging of gynecologic malignancies. *ACOG Tech Bull* 155 (May).

CARCINOMA OF THE FALLOPIAN TUBE

International Federation of Gynecology and Obstetrics (1994) *Annual Report on the Results of Treatment in Gynecological Cancer*, vol. 22. FIGO, Editorial Office Radiumhemmet, S 104 01 Stockholm, Sweden.

GESTATIONAL TROPHOBLASTIC TUMORS

International Federation of Gynecology and Obstetrics (1994) *Annual Report on the Results of Treatment in Gynecological Cancer*, vol. 22. FIGO, Editorial Office Radiumhemmet, S 104 01 Stockholm, Sweden.

Miller DS & Lurain JR (1988) Classification and staging of gestational trophoblastic tumors. *Obstet Gynecol Clin North Am* **15**: 477–490.

Lurain JR, Casanova LA, Miller DS & Rademaker AW (1991) Prognostic factors in gestational trophoblastic tumors: a proposed new scoring system based on multivariate analysis. *Am J Obstet Gynecol* **164**: 611–616.

World Health Organization Scientific Group (1983) Gestational trophoblastic disease. WHO *Tech Rep Ser* 692.

INTRAUTERINE ADHESIONS

Wamsteker K (1984) Hysteroscopy in Asherman's syndrome. In Siegler AM & Lindemann HJ (eds) *Hysteroscopy: Principles and Practice*, pp 198–203. Philadelphia: JB Lippincott.

Wamsteker K & de Blok S (1993) Diagnostic hysteroscopy: technique and documentation. In Sutton C & Diamond M (eds) *Endoscopic Surgery for Gynaecologists*, pp 263–276. London: WB Saunders.

Valle RF & Sciarra JJ (1988) Intrauterine adhesions: hysteroscopic diagnosis, classification, treatment, and reproductive outcome. *Am J Obstet Gynecol* **158**: 1459–1470.

The American Fertility Society (1988) The American Fertility Society classification of adnexal adhesions, distal tubal occlusion, tubal occlusion secondary to tubal ligation, tubal pregnancies, Müllerian anomalies and intrauterine adhesions. *Fertil Steril* **49**: 944–955.

SUBMUCOUS MYOMAS

Wamsteker K & de Blok S (1993) Diagnostic hysteroscopy: technique and documentation. In Sutton C & Diamond M (eds) *Endoscopic Surgery for Gynaecologists*, pp 263–276. London: WB Saunders.

ENDOMETRIOSIS

Kistner RW, Siegler AM & Behrman SJ (1977) Suggested classification for endometriosis: relationship to infertility. *Fertil Steril* **28**: 1008–1010.

American Fertility Society (1979) Classification of endometriosis. *Fertil Steril* **32**: 663.

Buttram VC Jr (1985) Evolution of the revised American Fertility Society classification of endometriosis. *Fertil Steril* **43**: 347–350.

Acosta AA, Buttram VC Jr, Franklin RR & Besch PK (1973) A proposed classification of pelvic endometriosis. *Obstet Gynecol* **42**: 19–25.

OBSTETRIC FISTULAS

Waaldijk K (1995) Surgical classification of obstetric fistulas. *Int J Gynecol Obstet* **49**: 161–163.

STRESS INCONTINENCE

Blaivas JG & Olsson CA (1988) Stress incontinence: classification and surgical approach. *J Urol* **139**: 727–731.

STANDARDIZATION OF IMAGE DISPLAY

Bernaschek G & Deutinger J (1989) Endosonography in obstetrics and gynecology: the importance of standardized image display. *Obstet Gynecol* **74**: 817–820.

▪ ACKNOWLEDGMENT

The authors would like to acknowledge Ms Crystal L Beecher, Medical Writer and Editor for the Department of Obstetrics and Gynecology at Northwestern University Medical School, for her assistance in locating source materials and for her editorial assistance with this chapter.

REFERENCES

Abrams P, Blaivas JG & Stanton SL (1990) The standardization of terminology of lower urinary tract function. *Br J Obstet Gynaecol* **6: (suppl)** 1–16.

Acosta AA, Buttram VC Jr, Franklin RR & Besch PK (1973) A proposed classification of pelvic endometriosis. *Obstet Gynecol* **42**: 19–25.

American Fertility Society (1979) Classification of endometriosis. *Fertil Steril* **32**: 663.

American Fertility Society (1988) The American Fertility Society classification of adnexal adhesions, distal tubal occlusion, tubal occlusion secondary to tubal ligation, tubal pregnancies, Müllerian anomalies and intrauterine adhesions. *Fertil Steril* **49**: 944–955.

American Joint Committee on Cancer Staging (1992) *Manual for Staging of Cancer*, 4th edn. Philadelphia: JB Lippincott.

Bernaschek G & Deutinger J (1989) Endosonography in obstetrics and gynecology: the importance of standardized image display. *Obstet Gynecol* **74**: 817–820.

Blaivas JG & Olsson CA (1988) Stress incontinence: classification and surgical approach. *J Urol* **139**: 727–731.

Buttram VC Jr (1985) Evolution of the revised American Fertility Society classification of endometriosis. *Fertil Steril* **43**: 347–350.

Creasman WT (1992) Revision in classification by International Federation of Gynecology and Obstetrics. *Am J Obstet Gynecol* **167**: 857–858.

Delancey JOL (1992) Aspects of vaginal vault eversion after hysterectomy. *Am J Obstet Gynecol* **166**: 1717–1728.

Elkins TE (1994) Surgery for the obstetric vesicovaginal fistula: a review of 100 operations in 82 patients. *Am J Obstet Gynecol* **170**: 1108–1118.

Hammond CB, Borchert LG, Tyrey L, Creasman WT & Parker RT (1973) Treatment of metastatic trophoblastic disease: good and poor prognosis. *Am J Obstet Gynecol* **115**: 451–457.

International Federation of Gynecology and Obstetrics (1989) *Annual Report on the Results of Treatment in Gynecological Cancer*, vol. 20. Stockholm: FIGO.

International Federation of Gynecology and Obstetrics (1991) *Annual Report on the Results of Treatment in Gynecological Cancer*, vol. 21. Stockholm: FIGO.

International Federation of Gynecology and Obstetrics (1994) *Annual Report on the Results of Treatment in Gynecological Cancer*, vol. 22. Stockholm: FIGO.

Kistner RW, Siegler AM & Behrman SJ (1977) Suggested classification for endometriosis: relationship to infertility. *Fertil Steril* **28**: 1008–1010.

Lurain JR, Casanova LA, Miller DS & Rademaker AW (1991) Prognostic factors in gestational trophoblastic tumors: a proposed new scoring system based on multivariate analysis. *Am J Obstet Gynecol* **164**: 611–616.

Marana R, Rizzi M, Muzii L, Catalano GF, Caruana P & Mancuso S (1995) Correlation between the American Fertility Society classifications of adnexal adhesions and distal tubal occlusion, salpingoscopy, and reproductive outcome in tubal surgery. *Fertil Steril* **64**: 924–929.

Ozasa H, Mori T & Togashi K (1992) Study of uterine prolapse by magnetic resonance imaging: topographic changes involving the levator ani muscle and vagina. *Gynecol Obstet Invest* **34**: 43–48.

Sabbagha RE, Cohen LC & Crocker L (1994) Sonography of the uterus: vaginal approach. In Sabbagha RE (ed.) *Diagnostic Ultrasound Applied to Obstetrics and Gynecology*, 3rd edn, pp 627–654. Philadelphia: JB Lippincott.

Shull B (1995) Discussion at Central Association of Obstetricians and Gynecologists, Memphis Tennessee, Oct. 1994. *Am J Obstet Gynecol* **172**: 1782.

Valle RF & Sciarra JJ (1988) Intrauterine adhesions: hysteroscopic diagnosis, classification, treatment, and reproductive outcome. *Am J Obstet Gynecol* **158**: 1459–1470.

Waaldijik K (1995) Surgical classification of obstetric fistulas. *Int J Gynecol Obstet* **49**: 161–163.

World Health Organization Scientific Group (1983) Gestational trophoblastic disease. *WHO Tech Rep Ser* 692.

Yang A, Mostwin JL, Rosenschein NB & Zerhouni EA (1991) Pelvic descent in women: dynamic evaluation with fast MRI imaging and cinematic display. *Radiology* **179**: 25–33.

Index

Page numbers in **bold** refer to illustrations, numbers in *italic* refer to tables.